PRINCIPLES AND PRACTICE OF SURGERY

For Churchill Livingstone:

Publisher: Laurence Hunter
Project Editor: Barbara Simmons
Copy Editor: Thérèse Duriez
Indexer: Anne McCarthy
Project Controller: Nancy Arnott
Design Direction: Erik Bigland
Sales Promotion Executive: Marion Pollock

PRINCIPLES AND PRACTICE OF SURGERY

A.P.M.Forrest
Kt MD ChM FRCSE FRCS FRCSG FRSE Hon DSc
(University of Wales; Chinese University of Hong
Kong) Hon LLD (University of Dundee) Hon FRACS
Hon FRCCS (Can) Hon FRCR Professor Emeritus,
University of Edinburgh

D.C. Carter
Kt MD FRCSE FRCSG
Regius Professor of Clinical Surgery, Royal Infirmary
of Edinburgh

I.B. Macleod
BSc MB ChB FRCSE
Honorary Secretary, Royal College of Surgeons,
Edinburgh; Formerly Consultant Surgeon, Royal
Infirmary of Edinburgh

THIRD EDITION

Medical illustrations by Gillian Lee

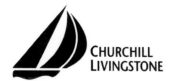
CHURCHILL
LIVINGSTONE

EDINBURGH LONDON TORONTO PHILADELPHIA SYDNEY TOKYO 1995

CHURCHILL LIVINGSTONE
An imprint of Harcourt Brace and Company Limited

© Longman Group Limited 1985
© Harcourt Brace and Company Limited 1998

🖉 is a registered trademark of Harcourt Brace and Company
Limited

First published 1985
Second edition 1991
Third edition 1995
   Reprinted 1995
   Reprinted 1999

ISBN 0 443 04860 6

International Student Edition of third edition 1994
   Reprinted 1995
   Reprinted 1998
   Reprinted 1999

ISBN 0 443 04904 1

British Library Cataloguing in Publication Data
A catalogue record for this book is available from the
British Library.

Library of Congress Cataloging in Publication Data
A catalog record for this book is available from the
Library of Congress.

Medical knowledge is constantly changing. As new
information becomes available, changes in treatment,
procedures, equipment and the use of drugs become
necessary. The author and the publishers have, as
far as it is possible, taken care to ensure that the
information given in this text is accurate and up to
date. However, readers are strongly advised to
confirm that the information, especially with regard
to drug usage, complies with current legislation and
standards of practice.

The
publisher's
policy is to use
**paper manufactured
from sustainable forests**

Printed in China
NPCC/03

−5 OCT 2001

Preface

The continuing success of *Principles and Practice of Surgery* and its companion volume Davidson's classic *Principles and Practice of Medicine* confirms that medical students continue to appreciate textbooks which strike for the middle ground between the synoptic and the encyclopaedic. In compiling the third edition of our book we have striven to delete outdated material and to avoid overburdening the undergraduate with large amounts of non-essential information. We trust that careful editing has maintained a consistent style and a readable account of that which is important in surgery.

The third edition differs in a number of important aspects from its predecessors. For clarity, the book has been divided into sections. Radiographs and clinical photographs have been introduced and the artwork has been revised substantially with the introduction of a large number of new line drawings. Revision boxes have been incorporated, where appropriate, and we hope that the new page design will prove attractive to our readers.

As with earlier editions, a substantial proportion of the book has been written by its editors. We have been fortunate in that most of our contributors to earlier editions have continued to write for us and we are grateful in this regard to Professors G. G. Browning (Head, neck and salivary glands and Mouth, nose, throat and ear), G. D. Chisholm (Urological surgery), J. G. Collee (Infections and antibiotics), E. R. Hitchcock (Neurosurgery), C. V. Ruckley (Peripheral vascular disease), A. A. Spence (Preoperative assessment and preparation, Anaesthesia and the operation and Postoperative care and complications) and D. J. Wheatley (Cardiac surgery), and to Mr J. Dark (The chest and mediastinum), Mr I. M. C. Macintyre (Practical procedures and Medico-legal issues), Dr B. McClelland (Transfusion of blood and blood products) and Mr A. C. H. Watson (Wounds and wound healing and Burns). Dr McClelland contributed the major part of the chapter on the transfusion of blood and blood products for the second edition but was not, unfortunately, appropriately acknowledged. We

were greatly saddened by the recent untimely deaths of Professor E. R. Hitchcock and Professor G. D. Chisholm and wish to acknowledge the very great help and encouragement that they have given to this textbook since its inception.

On this occasion we have introduced new authors or co-authors for a number of key chapters, namely Mr K. C. H. Fearon (Metabolic response to injury, Principles of fluid and electrolyte balance in surgical patients, Principles of surgical oncology), Mr G. Ramsay and Dr R. Jackson (Shock), Dr B. McClelland and Dr R. Green (Transfusion of blood and blood products), Mr I. M. C. Macintyre (Investigation and diagnosis of surgical problems), Dr C. Robertson (Trauma and multiple injury), Mr R. M. R. Taylor (Organ transplantation), Mr U. Chetty (Skin, connective tissues and soft tissues and The breast), Professor J. R. Farndon (Endocrine surgery), Mr O. J. Garden (Nutritional support in surgical patients, Liver and biliary tract, Spleen), and Dr I. Armstrong (Practical procedures).

We are grateful to Laurence Hunter and Barbara Simmons of Churchill Livingstone for continuing to chivy us gently but firmly in the right direction, and to our copy-editor Thérèse Duriez for her immense and patient labours on our behalf. We thank Gillian Lee for the excellence of her artwork and for her ability to make such good sense of the confused directions provided by the editors. Dr Doris Redhead kindly supplied a number of radiographs, Mr Alastair Thompson was a major force in the creation of the Revision Boxes, and Anne McKellar and Carole Tomlinson of the secretarial staff of the University Department of Surgery in Edinburgh University provided invaluable support.

Mr R. M. R. Taylor would like to thank Professor S. Proctor, Consultant Haematologist, Royal Victoria Infirmary, Newcastle upon Tyne, and Mr J. H. Dark for advice and help generously given.

Edinburgh 1995

A.P.M.F.
D.C.C.
I.B.M.

Contributors

Ian Armstrong BSc(Hons) MB ChB FRCA
Consultant Anaesthetist, Royal Infirmary,
Edinburgh

George G. Browning MD ChB FRCSE FRCPSG
Professor and Consultant in Administrative Charge,
Department of Otorhinolaryngology and Head and
Neck Surgery, Royal Infirmary, Glasgow

David C. Carter MD FRCSE FRCSG
Regius Professor of Clinical Surgery, Royal
Infirmary of Edinburgh

Udi Chetty MB ChB FRCS MRCP
Consultant Surgeon, Western General Hospital,
Edinburgh

Geoffrey D. Chisholm ChM PPRCSE FRCS
FCPE FRCPSG Hon FRACS Hon FCS SA
Professor of Surgery, University of Edinburgh,
Western General Hospital; Honorary Consultant
Urological Surgeon; Director, Nuffield Transplant
Unit, Western General Hospital, Edinburgh, UK

J. Gerald Collee CBE MD FRC Path FRCPE
Formerly Professor of Medical Microbiology,
University of Edinburgh, Consultant in
Bacteriology, Lothian Health Board; Consultant
Adviser to the Scottish Home and Health
Department, Edinburgh, UK

John Dark MBBS FRCS
Consultant in Cardiothoracic Surgery, Freeman
Hospital, Newcastle upon Tyne, UK

John R. Farndon BSc MBBS MD FRCS
Professor of Surgery, University of Bristol;
Honorary Consultant Surgeon to Bristol Royal
Infirmary and Honorary Consultant, Southmead
Hospital, Bristol

Kenneth C. H. Fearon MB ChB (Hons) MD
FRCSG
Senior Lecturer and Honorary Consultant, Royal
Infirmary, Edinburgh

A. Patrick M. Forrest Kt MD ChM FRCS
FRCSE FRCSG DSc(Hon) LLD(Hon)
FACS(Hon) FRACS(Hon) FRCS Can(Hon)
FRCR(Hon) FRSE
Professor Emeritus, University of Edinburgh

O. James Garden BSc MB ChB MD FRCSG
FRCSE
Senior Lecturer, University of Edinburgh; Honorary
Consultant Surgeon, University Department of
Surgery, Scottish Liver Transplantation Unit, Royal
Infirmary, Edinburgh

Rachel H. A. Green MB ChB MRCP CTM
MRCPath
Consultant in Transfusion Medicine, West of
Scotland Blood Transfusion Service, Glasgow

Edward R. Hitchcock MB ChM FRCS FRCSE
Late Professor of Neurosurgery, University of
Birmingham

Ruth E. Jackson MB ChB FRCA
Research Registrar, Division of Anaesthesia,
Western Infirmary, Glasgow

D. Brian L. McClelland MB ChB MRCP PhD
FRCP MRCPath
Regional Director, Edinburgh and South East
Scotland Blood Transfusion Service, Royal
Infirmary, Edinburgh

Ian M. C. Macintyre MD FRCSE
Consultant Surgeon, Western General Hospital,
Edinburgh

Ian B. Macleod BSc MB ChB FRCS
Honorary Secretary, Royal College of Surgeons,
Edinburgh; formerly Consultant Surgeon, Royal
Infirmary, Edinburgh

Graham Ramsay MB ChB MD FRCS
Associate Professor of Surgery, Chairman of
Intensive Care, University Hospital, Maastricht,
Netherlands

Colin Robertson MB ChB MRCP FRCS FRCP FFAEM FSA Scot
Consultant in Accident and Emergency Medicine and Surgery, Royal Infirmary; Honorary Senior Lecturer, Faculty of Medicine, University of Edinburgh

C. Vaughan Ruckley MB ChB FRCSE ChM
Consultant Surgeon, Royal Infirmary of Edinburgh; Honorary Professor of Vascular Surgery, University of Edinburgh, UK

Alastair A. Spence MD FRCA FRCPG FRCSE
Professor of Anaesthetics, University of Edinburgh

R. M. Ross Taylor ChM FRCS FRCSE
Consultant Surgeon, Royal Victoria Hospital, Newcastle upon Tyne; Surgical Director, Renal Transplantation, Northern Region, UK

Anthony C. H. Watson MB ChB FRCSE
Consultant Plastic Surgeon, St John's Hospital, Livingston; Honorary Senior Lecturer, University of Edinburgh

David J. Wheatley MD ChM FRCS
British Heart Foundation Professor of Cardiac Surgery; Honorary Consultant Cardiothoracic Surgeon, Royal Infirmary, Glasgow

Contents

Section 1
PRINCIPLES OF SURGICAL CARE

1

The metabolic response to injury

CONTENTS

Following accidental or deliberate injury, a series of changes occur locally and generally which are intended to restore the *status quo*. The local response of inflammation is supported by a generalized response which conserves fluid and provides energy for repair.

The classical view of the metabolic response to injury (as described by the late Scottish physiologist, Sir David Cuthbertson) has an 'ebb' and 'flow' phase. The short 'ebb' phase corresponds to the period of traumatic shock. The 'flow' phase which follows is divided into two parts. The initial *catabolic* phase is characterized by protein and fat mobilization, with an associated increase in urinary nitrogen excretion and weight loss, and usually lasts 3–8 days. It is followed by an *anabolic* phase lasting for some weeks during which protein and fat stores are replenished and weight is regained (the recovery phase).

The changes which follow injury are thought to be due to a complex neuroendocrine and cytokine response designed to conserve fluid, mobilize amino acids from protein for gluconeogenesis and wound repair, mobilize fat for energy production, and upregulate various components of the immune system.

The description that follows concentrates on the catabolic period of the flow phase as this is the period of most concern in the management of patients after operation or serious injury. The problems associated with a prolonged catabolic phase are now seen more frequently as intensive care prolongs the survival of multiply injured and severely septic patients. It is important to stress that for the majority of elective surgical procedures (e.g. cholecystectomy or colectomy), the dominant metabolic changes are those associated with starvation, and that hypercatabolism is only observed following major injury or sepsis, or when complications arise.

FACTORS INITIATING THE METABOLIC RESPONSE TO INJURY

The term 'injury' embraces a wide variety of insults, including trauma, haemorrhage, major sepsis and burns. The precise relationship between factors thought to initiate the response and those thought to mediate it remains uncertain.

Volume depletion

Volume depletion is an important factor initiating some aspects of the metabolic response. Fluid may be lost externally, as in haemorrhage or burns, or it may be sequestered in local oedema at the site of injury or infection. Changes in volume result in changes in plasma osmolality, and these factors lead to an increased sympathetic outflow and increased circulating levels of catecholamines, antidiuretic hormone (ADH, i.e. vasopressin) and aldosterone.

Afferent nerve impulses

Afferent impulses, notably pain, play a significant role. On reaching the hypothalamus they stimulate sympathetic outflow and provoke the release of pituitary hormones. The injury is sometimes anticipated by the patient so that the hypothalamic response is triggered by impulses from higher centres before injury. The importance of afferent nerve impulses is attested experimentally by the observation that the response to a standard limb injury is much reduced by section of the nerves to the limb. Patients undergoing surgery under spinal anaesthesia also show a modified response.

Bacteria and endotoxin

Blood flow to the intestine is particularly sensitive to changes in overall blood volume; a 10% reduction in total blood volume reduces intestinal perfusion by up to 50%. The damage caused by mucosal ischaemia during hypovolaemia is compounded when flow is restored during resuscitation (ischaemia/reperfusion injury) with the result that the gut mucosal barrier may be impaired. This could allow bacterial products (e.g. endotoxin from Gram-negative bacteria) to translocate into the portal circulation, with induction of shock and many of the metabolic changes seen following major injury/sepsis. In major sepsis, bacteria and their products may enter the circulation directly at the site of infection.

Inflammatory response

A variety of endogenous cascade systems are activated both locally and systemically as part of the inflammatory/immune response to tissue injury. This process involves endothelium and activated neutrophils and monocytes. The end-products include prostaglandins, kinins, complement and a variety of cytokines. The cytokines interleukin 1 (IL-1), interleukin 6 (IL-6) and tumour necrosis factor (TNF) are thought to have a major role in inducing aspects of the metabolic response.

FACTORS MEDIATING THE METABOLIC RESPONSE

Many of the metabolic changes observed after major injury (e.g. increased energy expenditure, negative nitrogen balance, hyperglycaemia and insulin resistance) can be reproduced by infusing a 'cocktail' of the counter-regulatory hormones cortisol, glucagon and adrenalin. However, it is now evident that the classical *neuroendocrine response* is complemented by a *cytokine response* (Fig. 1.1), in which inflammatory mediators such as IL-1, IL-6 and TNF contribute to

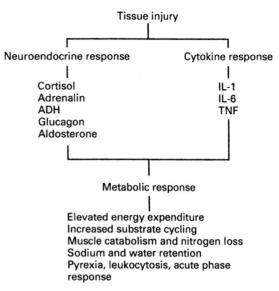

Fig. 1.1   Summary of main events occurring within 48 hours of major injury.

such manifestations as pyrexia and the acute phase response (see below). These two main groups of mediators (i.e. neuro-endocrine hormones and cytokines) do not act in isolation. For example some cytokines can enhance adrenocorticotrophic hormone (ACTH) release from the pituitary, while cortisol can enhance certain end-organ effects of IL-1 and TNF.

FACTORS MODIFYING THE METABOLIC RESPONSE

Many factors modify the magnitude and duration of the metabolic response to injury; the most important are:

- *Severity of injury.* In general the greater the injury, the greater the response. Burns produce a greater response than injuries of comparable size, probably because of the greater heat loss from the burned area.
- *Co-existing disease* such as cancer and renal failure may blunt the metabolic response to injury.
- *Infection* potentiates the metabolic response, and the catabolic phase persists as long as infection remains.
- *Complications* such as deep venous thrombosis, myocardial infarction and pulmonary embolism also potentiate the response.
- *Nutritional status.* Patients in a poor nutritional

state at the time of injury have a modified response. Starvation is common after injury or operation, and its effects interact with those of the metabolic response (see below).

- *Ambient temperature.* Some of the increased metabolic activity after injury is directed towards maintaining body temperature. This is particularly true in patients with thermal burns who lose energy due to evaporation of water from the burned surface. Energy expenditure and the resulting metabolic demands can be reduced if the usual ambient temperature of hospitals in temperate climates (20°C) is raised to 30–32°C.
- *Anaesthesia and drugs.* These may modify the response by affecting the vascular system and hormone production. For example, ether stimulates catecholamine and ADH output, morphine stimulates ADH release, and spinal anaesthesia reduces the initial response by blocking afferent pathways.
- *Other factors.* Meticulous and gentle handling of tissues reduces the severity of operative trauma and thus the postoperative metabolic demand. Prompt and adequate replacement of fluid loss limits liberation of catecholamines, aldosterone and ADH. In some cases, oliguria and sodium retention may be avoided if loss is replaced accurately. Provision of enough calories (energy) and nitrogen minimises the catabolic phase and occasionally prevents weight loss and negative nitrogen balance. However, it is doubtful whether aggressive nutritional support affects wound healing or duration of hospital stay in previously healthy patients undergoing elective surgery. In undernourished patients or those with severe trauma or sepsis, the provision of adequate calories and nitrogen considerably influences recovery. In all patients, prolonged post-traumatic starvation adversely affects convalescence.

CHANGES OCCURRING DURING THE METABOLIC RESPONSE

Pulse and temperature changes

Following injury the pulse rate rises temporarily due to catecholamine release, and there is often a small rise in temperature for 24–48 hours. This reflects a general increase in heat production, accompanied by altered 'setting' of the temperature regulation centre under the influence of IL-1. This pyrexia is not due to infection and does not call for antibiotic therapy.

Metabolic response to injury
- An initial catabolic phase is followed by a more protracted anabolic phase.

- Factors which *initiate* the metabolic response to injury are:
  - fluid loss (volume depletion)
  - afferent nerve (pain) stimuli
  - bacteria and endotoxin
  - the pro-inflammatory cytokine response
  - activated neutrophils and monocytes

- Factors which *modify* the metabolic response to injury are:
  - the severity of injury
  - co-existing disease (e.g. cancer, renal failure)
  - infection
  - nutritional status
  - ambient temperature
  - anaesthesia and drugs
  - miscellaneous factors (e.g. complications, metabolic demand)

Water and salt retention

Oliguria and salt retention is common after injury and normally lasts for 48–72 hours. It is a consequence of ADH and aldosterone release.

Antidiuretic hormone

ADH secretion is increased when:

- Volume receptors in the atria and hypothalamus are stimulated by reduction in blood volume
- Neural stimuli reach the supraoptic nucleus from the injured part
- Increased osmolality stimulates osmoreceptors in the anterior hypothalamus.

ADH acts on the collecting tubules of the kidney, and to a lesser extent on the distal tubule, to promote reabsorption of water. If excess water is administered during this phase, hypotonicity and hyponatraemia result.

Aldosterone

Aldosterone acts on the kidney to conserve sodium and so further reduces urine volume. Aldosterone secretion is increased by the following mechanisms, of which the renin-angiotensin mechanism is much the most important.

1. The juxtaglomerular apparatus of the kidney is

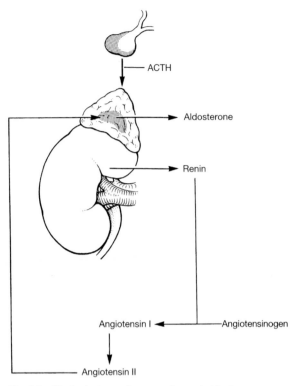

Fig. 1.2 The juxtaglomerular apparatus and aldosterone release.

Aldosterone acts principally on the distal renal tubules to promote reabsorption of sodium and bicarbonate, with a commensurate increase in the excretion of potassium and hydrogen ions. It also affects the exchange of sodium and potassium across all cell membranes, notably those of cardiac and smooth muscle, possibly by modifying the effects of catecholamines on these cells. Large amounts of intracellular potassium are released into the extracellular fluid, and serum levels may rise significantly if renal function is impaired.

In the absence of sweating, the kidneys are the only significant route of excretion of sodium and potassium in healthy individuals. Approximately 50–80 mmol of each ion are excreted in the urine every 24 hours. After injury, urinary sodium losses may fall to 10–20 mmol/24 hours while potassium excretion may rise to 100–200 mmol/24 hours. These changes may persist for 2–3 days, depending on the severity of injury and the amount of fluid and electrolyte replacement, and are taken into account when calculating requirements.

Energy metabolism and substrate cycling

Following severe injury or sepsis, resting energy expenditure may increase by as much as 30%. Contributory factors include the energy needed for increased ion transport, protein synthesis, nerve transmission and 'futile' metabolic cycles (e.g. glucose-lactate cycling, triglyceride turnover and protein turnover). Such increased substrate turnover, although energy dependent, is thought to

sensitive to minor alterations in arteriolar inflow pressure, and secretes renin if inflow pressure falls. Renin acts with angiotensinogen to form angiotensin I, and this is converted to angiotensin II, a substance which stimulates aldosterone production by the adrenal cortex (Fig. 1.2). The macula densa is a specialized area of tubular epithelium immediately adjacent to the juxtaglomerular apparatus which is sensitive to small alterations in the concentration of sodium in urine in the proximal tubule. Any reduction in sodium concentration also activates renin release.

2. A minor role is played by receptors in the right atrium (which are sensitive to changes in circulating blood volume) and by receptors in the carotid artery (which are sensitive to changes in arterial pressure). Any decrease in blood volume and/or drop in arterial pressure results in hypothalamic stimulation and release of corticotropin (ACTH).

3. Aldosterone release may also be triggered by a fall in plasma sodium concentration or a rise in plasma potassium concentration in blood reaching the adrenal cortex. Such changes occur frequently after injury.

Changes occurring during the metabolic response to injury
- Tachycardia and pyrexia lasting for 24–48 hours
- Retention of sodium and water for 2–3 days secondary to aldosterone and ADH secretion
- Increased energy expenditure
- Increased glucose turnover
- Breakdown of skeletal muscle to provide amino acids for gluconeogenesis and hepatic synthesis of other proteins
- Breakdown of adipose tissue as principle energy source after trauma
- Hypercoagulability (with increased risk of thromboembolism) or hypocoagulability

optimize metabolic control. These changes are in direct contrast to starvation where energy expenditure falls and energy/protein reserves are conserved.

Carbohydrate, protein and fat metabolism

Carbohydrate

In the absence of food intake, body carbohydrate stores (liver glycogen) last only 8–12 hours. Nevertheless, following injury there is a period of hyperglycaemia, the duration of which depends on the severity of injury and presence of complications such as infection. Hyperglycaemia results from a combination of breakdown of liver glycogen, increased gluconeogenesis, and insulin resistance. The overall increase in glucose turnover is thought to provide essential fuel for inflammation and repair.

Catecholamines increase glycogenolysis directly and also act indirectly by suppressing insulin release while stimulating that of glucagon. Suppression of insulin release favours release of amino acids from muscle, which are then available for gluconeogenesis. In addition, the effect of insulin on glucose metabolism is inhibited, possibly as a result of raised growth hormone levels. Glucagon is a potent stimulant of hepatic gluconeogenesis but does not significantly affect the efflux of amino acids from skeletal muscle.

Protein

Skeletal muscle is the body's major labile protein reserve. Following major injury, skeletal muscle is broken down to provide amino acids for hepatic gluconeogenesis and to support the synthesis of proteins, including 'acute phase' proteins. This 'acute phase response' involves increased hepatic production of positive acute phase proteins (such as C-reactive protein, fibrinogen and α_2 macroglobulin) and decreased production of negative acute phase proteins (such as albumin and transferrin). It is promoted by cytokines such as IL-1, IL-6 and TNF, and is thought to have a role in fighting bacterial infection and promoting healing.

The normal average daily protein intake is between 80 and 120 g, equivalent to an intake of 12–20 g nitrogen. Of this, approximately 2 g of nitrogen is lost in the faeces and 10–18 g in the urine. After injury, urinary nitrogen losses increase and may reach twice the normal amount after severe trauma or major burns. Nitrogen is lost as urea, so that blood urea concentration rises rapidly if renal function is impaired.

The rise in urinary nitrogen excretion commences soon after injury. After routine elective surgery it may return to normal after 5–8 days, whereas after severe burns or severe sepsis it may persist for many weeks. The patients are usually unable to eat enough protein to match this loss and negative nitrogen balance results. Nitrogen loss can be attenuated by providing energy (calories) and protein by the enteral or parenteral route (Ch. 5).

Negative nitrogen balance is associated with weight loss due to loss of muscle mass. The extent can be calculated as follows:

1 g nitrogen = 6 g muscle protein = 30 g wet muscle mass

A patient with a negative nitrogen balance of 15 g nitrogen a day therefore loses approximately 450 g of muscle mass daily. The provision of carbohydrate calories has a 'protein-sparing effect' by reducing the need for amino acids to act as substrates for hepatic gluconeogenesis.

Fat

Adipose tissue with its large triglyceride store is the principal source of energy following trauma. Catecholamines and glucagon (and to a lesser extent, cortisol and growth hormone) activate adenyl cyclase in fat cells, producing cyclic adenosine monophosphate (cAMP). This in turn activates triglyceride lipase with the breakdown of triglycerides to fatty acids and glycerol. Glycerol provides a substrate for gluconeogenesis, while free fatty acids provide energy for most tissues and for gluconeogenesis. The brain cannot use free fatty acids, but the liver converts free fatty acids to ketone bodies which can support cerebral energy metabolism. A total of 200–500 g of fat may be broken down daily after severe trauma.

The anabolic phase

Following the catabolic phase the patient becomes anabolic with positive nitrogen balance, regain of weight, and restoration of skeletal muscle and fat deposits. The turning point is often obvious clinically in that the patient feels better and his appetite returns, often quite suddenly. Hormones which contribute to anabolism are insulin, growth hormone, androgens and 17-ketosteroids.

Urinary changes during the metabolic response to injury

- Oliguria in response to ADH secretion

- Low urinary sodium excretion due to renal retention of sodium in response to aldosterone secretion

- Increased urinary excretion of potassium. (This should be seen as a 'beneficial' attempt to avoid hyperkalaemia given that tissue injury releases intracellular potassium, as does the mobilization of intracellular water. The renal excretion of potassium also facilitates renal retention of sodium)

- Increased urinary excretion of nitrogen reflects breakdown of muscle protein; each gram of urinary nitrogen is equivalent to 6 g of muscle protein and 30 g of skeletal muscle

---

Changes in blood coagulation

After injury or infection the blood may be hypercoagulable or hypocoagulable. Hypercoagulability appears first and may contribute to the increased incidence of thromboembolism after operation or trauma. It is most marked in the first 12 hours after injury, and increased secretion of ACTH or cortisol may be responsible for increasing the number of platelets and their adhesiveness. Noradrenaline also tends to increase coagulability. Serum fibrinogen levels also rise after injury. In severe sepsis the rise may be prolonged; a rapid fall is associated with a poor prognosis.

Hypocoagulability is associated with increased fibrinolysis and a fall in serum fibrinogen levels. This can lead to generalized bleeding and, though not common, is seen most frequently in severe shock (particularly bacteraemic shock with disseminated intravascular coagulation), after operation on patients with disseminated carcinoma or extensive liver disease, or following cardiopulmonary bypass.

STARVATION AND ITS CONTRIBUTION TO THE METABOLIC RESPONSE

All patients who undergo surgery or suffer severe injury are starved for a period. It is customary to starve patients for 12 hours before operation, and most are unlikely to take *any* food on the day of operation. Patients having operations on the alimentary tract may be unable to take food for some days, and those who develop complications may be unable to eat for days or even weeks. Patients with intra-abdominal disease (e.g. carcinoma of the stomach) may have had an inadequate intake for weeks or months before surgery.

If the surgery is relatively minor and followed by a short period of starvation (e.g. colectomy), the changes in metabolism are similar to those caused by starvation alone. On the other hand, after major trauma there are marked differences.

In acute starvation, intermediate metabolism of protein, fat and carbohydrate is altered to preserve the supply of glucose to the brain by increasing hepatic glycogenolysis and gluconeogenesis. In early starvation, the basal energy requirement of a 70-kg adult is approximately 1800 kcal per 24 hours. The brain uses most of the available glucose, but some is broken down anaerobically in kidney and muscle to provide pyruvate and lactate, which are then recycled to provide glucose by gluconeogenesis. Most of the body tissues use fatty acids and ketones as an energy source.

If starvation is prolonged beyond a few hours, glycogen stores in the liver and muscle become depleted. Muscle protein converted to glucose by gluconeogenesis then maintains the brain's energy supply. This process cannot continue indefinitely, and after 2–3 weeks the brain gradually reduces its glucose consumption and utilizes ketones (produced in the liver from free fatty acids) as an energy source. The amount of muscle protein used falls to about 20 g/day while fat consumption increases. Total energy requirements fall from 1800 kcal to about 1500 kcal/day (Table 1.1). This

Table 1.1 A comparison of energy and nitrogen losses during the different phases of starvation and in the hypermetabolic state*

	Hypermetabolic state	Early starvation	Compensated starvation
Nitrogen loss (gN/day)	24	14	3
Energy expenditure (kcal/day)	2400	1800	1500

*Values are approximate and relate to a 70-kg male.

state of energy and nitrogen conservation is known as compensated starvation.

MANAGEMENT OF THE CATABOLIC STATE

The best way of correcting simple starvation is to feed the patient, preferably by the enteral route, but if need be by the parenteral route (Ch. 5). If major injury or sepsis is the cause of catabolism then prompt resuscitation and adequate surgical treatment are mandatory. Thereafter, if the patient is unable to eat, enteral or parenteral nutritional support should be provided (see Ch. 5). Patients should be mobilized as early as possible as exercise is one of the best stimuli for protein anabolism.

2

Principles of fluid and electrolyte balance in surgical patients

CONTENTS

The majority of surgical patients with fluid and electrolyte problems cannot take in fluid by mouth so that it has to be administered intravenously. The effect of trauma on the secretion of antidiuretic hormone (ADH) and aldosterone necessitates careful control of fluid administration in the early postoperative period. Adequate amounts of water, sodium, potassium and anions (chloride) must be supplied. In a few individuals, particularly those with chronic gastrointestinal tract loss, deficiencies of calcium and magnesium require correction.

Normal water and electrolyte balance

The distribution of body water in a 70-kg male is shown in Figure 2.1. The major extracellular cation is sodium. If intravenous fluids are given as isotonic saline then the contained sodium chloride and water will distribute mainly in the 14 litres of the extracellular space. In contrast, since an isotonic solution of dextrose (5% w/v) does not contain any major ions it will distribute throughout the entire body water (42 litres). Since the dextrose is readily metabolized this is equivalent to giving water alone.

In calculating fluid (and electrolyte) requirements one must know how much the patient has lost so that it can be replaced accurately. A healthy individual loses fluid by three routes: the kidneys, the gastrointestinal tract, and by diffusion from the skin and respiratory passages. In a 70-kg adult approximately 1500–2000 ml of urine is passed in 24 hours, 300 ml of fluid is lost in faeces, and 700–1000 ml is lost as water vapour from the skin and respiratory tract (insensible water loss). The onset of sweating (sensible water loss) greatly increases water loss from the skin. Water is taken in as fluids and in solid foods, and an additional 200–300 ml per 24 hours is provided endogenously by oxidation of carbohydrate and fat (i.e. metabolic water).

In the absence of sweating, almost all the sodium lost is in the urine. Under the influence of aldosterone the kidney can reduce sodium loss to about 10–20 mmol/24 hours. The principal route of potassium excretion is also the kidney, some 60–100 mmol being lost daily in the urine. The kidneys cannot conserve potassium as efficiently as sodium, but in severe potassium deficiency they can reduce losses to 40 mmol per day. The normal daily losses and the requirements to maintain fluid and electrolyte balance are summarized in Table 2.1.

Intravenous administration of normal requirements

When fulfilling normal daily requirements intravenously (Table 2.2), sodium is normally provided as a 0.9% sodium chloride solution, each litre containing 154 mmol sodium and 154 mmol chloride. As 0.9% saline is isotonic with plasma, it is called *normal* or *physiological* saline. For practical

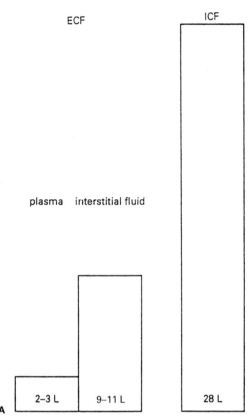

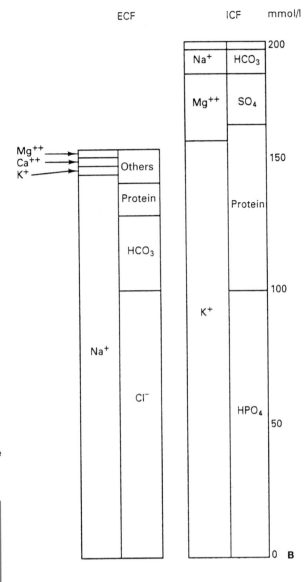

Fig. 2.1 A Distribution of water between the intracellular and extracellular compartments. Values shown are approximate values in a 70 kg man. **B** Distribution of cations and anions in the extracellular and intracellular fluid compartments.

Fluid and electrolyte balance
- The normal daily requirements for water and electrolytes are met by providing:
  1 litre of 0.9% saline (154 mmol Na^+ and 154 mmol of Cl^-), and
  2 litres of 5% dextrose + 60 mmol K^+.

- After injury/surgical trauma the following factors must be considered:
  - potassium replacement is usually unnecessary in the first 2–3 days as hyperkalaemia rather than hypokalaemia is the danger
  - losses of water are increased by:
    hyperventilation (diffusion of water vapour)
    pyrexia (200 ml/1°C/day)
    sweating (also incurs loss of Na^+ 20–70 mmol/l and K^+ 10 mmol/l).
  - secretion of ADH and aldosterone after injury/surgery reduces Na^+ loss to 30 mmol/day while increasing K^+ loss to 120 mmol/day
  - sequestration of fluid at the site of operation/injury may be considerable.

Table 2.1   Normal daily losses and requirements of fluids and electrolytes

	Volume (ml)	Na^+ (mmol)	K^+ (mmol)
Urine	2000	80	60
Insensible loss	700	–	–
Faeces	200	–	–
Minus endogenous water	300	–	–
Requirement	3000	80	60

Table 2.2 Provision of normal 24-hour fluid and electrolyte requirements by intravenous infusion		
Intravenous fluid	Additive	Duration
500 ml 0.9% NaCl	20 mmol KCl	4 hours
500 ml 5% dextrose	–	4 hours
500 ml 5% dextrose	20 mmol KCl	4 hours
500 ml 0.9% NaCl	–	4 hours
500 ml 5% dextrose	20 mmol KCl	4 hours
500 ml 5% dextrose	–	4 hours

purposes, 1 litre of normal saline supplies the daily requirement of sodium. The remaining volume requirement (2 litres) is provided as an isotonic non-electrolyte solution such as 5% dextrose. Potassium can be added to saline or dextrose from ampoules containing 1.5 g potassium chloride (i.e. 20 mmol of potassium and 20 mmol of chloride). Potassium should not be administered faster than 10–20 mmol per hour except in severe potassium deficiency (continuous electrocardiogram (ECG) monitoring is then essential). It must never be given as an intravenous bolus, as cardiac arrest will occur.

Effect of sweating on requirements

Hyperventilation increases insensible water loss, and pyrexia raises water loss from the skin by approximately 200 ml per day for each 1°C rise in temperature. Sweating considerably increases fluid loss by up to a litre an hour. Calculation of the amount of fluid lost by sweating is difficult and repeated weighing of the patient may be necessary. Sweat contains significant amounts of sodium (20–70 mmol/l) and potassium (10 mmol/l), losses which must be taken into account when calculating requirements.

Effect of operation on fluid and electrolyte balance

Following operation, release of ADH conserves water by its action on the distal convoluted and collecting tubules. Urine volume is reduced to 1000–1500 ml for 2–3 days. Attempts to produce a diuresis by giving water in the form of 5% dextrose are unsuccessful and only produce hyponatraemia and possibly water intoxication.

Aldosterone secretion conserves sodium and further contributes to oliguria. In the first 2 days after operation, urinary excretion of sodium falls to approximately 30 mmol/24 hours. Potassium excretion is increased during this period to approximately 120 mmol per day, due partly to the influence of

aldosterone on the kidney and partly because potassium is liberated from damaged body cells and by the mobilization of intracellular water. Further free potassium is provided by the infusion of stored blood, so that serum potassium levels tend to rise in the early postoperative period, particularly if the glomerular filtration rate is reduced. For this reason intravenous potassium should not be given in the first 24–48 hours after operation unless the patient is hypokalaemic or was potassium-deficient pre-operatively.

Sequestration of extracellular fluid (ECF) at the site of operation produces local oedema and temporary loss of fluid from the circulation. Sequestration persists for approximately 48 hours and may involve up to 4 litres of fluid, depending on the severity of the operation or injury. For example, 500 ml may be lost daily after partial gastrectomy. Such sequestration must be taken into account when calculating fluid and electrolyte requirements.

Not all patients require intravenous support following an operation. The majority tolerate 48 hours of fluid deprivation, although at the expense of thirst and a possible increase in the risk of deep venous thrombosis. Patients are more comfortable if fluid losses are replaced but when there is evidence of impaired renal or cardiac function, it is better to err on the side of underhydration rather than risk overhydration, hyponatraemia and/or pulmonary oedema.

Causes of fluid and electrolyte loss from the alimentary tract

The majority of surgical patients requiring intravenous fluid and electrolyte therapy for sustained periods have continuing fluid loss from the gut. This may be due to any of the following circumstances.

Intestinal obstruction. In general, the higher the obstruction in the intestine the greater the fluid loss. This is because fluids secreted by the upper alimentary tract fail to reach the absorptive areas of the distal jejunum and ileum. Thus a patient with a high small bowel obstruction loses fluid more rapidly than one with a low small bowel obstruction. Major fluid loss from vomiting is a late feature of large bowel obstruction.

Adynamic ileus. This condition, in which propulsion in the small intestine ceases, may result from surgical trauma, infection, electrolyte imbalance (particularly potassium, calcium and magnesium deficiency), hypoproteinaemia, retroperitoneal trauma or haemorrhage, hypoxia, head injury or neurosurgical operations, and shock due to different

Table 2.3   Approximate electrolyte concentrations in plasma and various gastrointestinal fluids

	Volume (ml/24 h)	Na^+ (mmol/l)	K^+ (mmol/l)	Cl^- (mmol/l)	HCO_3^- (mmol/l)
Plasma		140	5	100	25
Gastric juice	2500	50	10	80	40
Intestinal fluid (upper)	3000	140	10	100	25
Bile and pancreatic juice	1500	140	5	80	60
Mature ileostomy	500	50	5	20	25
Diarrhoea (inflammatory)		110	40	100	40

causes. Distension of the gut from swallowed air results in increased intestinal secretion and reduced absorptive capacity. Unless the intestinal fluid is removed by nasogastric aspiration, vomiting is persistent.

Intestinal fistula.   Fluid loss from an intestinal fistula may be considerable. As with obstruction, the higher the fistula in the gut, the greater the fluid loss. Fluid loss is not often a major problem with fistulas of the large bowel.

Diarrhoea.   Fluid and electrolyte loss from diarrhoea may be considerable. For example, in cholera some 6–10 litres may be lost each day, resulting in fatal contraction of ECF.

Table 2.3 shows the approximate concentrations of electrolytes in some gastrointestinal fluids and may be used to calculate losses over short periods. There is considerable variation in electrolyte composition, and if gastrointestinal loss continues for more than 2–3 days, all fluid and urine should be collected and sent to the laboratory for accurate determination of electrolyte content.

An example of how short-term requirements may be provided is shown in Table 2.4. In patients requiring replacement for more than 3–4 days, such calculations are likely to be inaccurate. Correction of acid–base imbalance and the provision of parenteral nutrition also have to be considered. Ions other than sodium and potassium may be needed if intestinal fluid loss continues, notably magnesium (up to 1 mmol/kg body weight per 24 hours) and calcium (10–60 ml of 10% calcium gluconate, i.e. 4.5–27 mmol per day).

Patients who have pre-existing fluid and electrolyte deficiency, or who develop deficiencies, should have these corrected by adding the calculated deficit to the normal requirement, usually spreading the replacement over 2–3 days.

Table 2.4   Calculation of short-term fluid and electrolyte requirements of a patient with ileus

Assuming that the patient is in electrolyte balance and is losing 2 litres/24 hours as nasogastric aspirate and 1.5 litres as urine, his 24-hour losses can be calculated as follows:

	Volume (ml)	Na^+ (mmol)	K^+ (mmol)
Urine	1500	80	60
Nasogastric aspirate	2000	240	20
Insensible loss	800	–	–
Minus endogenous water	–300	–	–
Net losses/requirements	4000	320	80

2 litres of normal saline would supply 310 mmol of Na^+ which for practical purposes would supply sodium needs; the remaining 2 litres of fluid would be supplied as 5% dextrose. Thus, in the short-term, provided that urinary losses are normal, replacement of nasogastric losses on a volume-for-volume basis by normal saline gives the required sodium replacement while the volume of urine loss (plus 500 ml) is replaced by dextrose. The required 60–80 mmol of K^+ would be supplied by 4 1.5 g ampoules of potassium choride.

Fluid and electrolyte loss from the gastrointestinal tract

Common causes of fluid and electrolyte loss from the gastrointestinal tract are:
- vomiting
- intestinal obstruction (greater loss from high obstructions)
- adynamic ileus (increased intestinal secretion with reduced absorption)
- intestinal fistula (high fistulas cause the greatest loss)
- diarrhoea (may involve losses of up to 10 l/day)

Appropriate replacement of fluid and electrolytes demands accurate measurement of:
- all overt losses (urine, gastrointestinal and fistula loss, drain fluid)
- due allowance for insensible loss (normally up to 1 litre of water a day by diffusion through skin and airways)
- determination of electrolyte composition of urine and gastrointestinal losses

WATER IMBALANCE

Water depletion

A reduction of 1–2% (350–700 ml) in total body water produces thirst. Clinically obvious dehydration with intense thirst, a dry tongue, and loss of skin elasticity (particularly over the clavicles) signifies a deficiency of at least 1.5–2 litres. Pure water depletion is rare in surgical practice. Water depletion is usually combined with sodium loss, the combination being referred to as 'salt depletion'. The combined loss of sodium and water results in contraction of the ECF volume with circulatory changes (vasoconstriction and tachycardia) as well as the clinical features of dehydration. The most frequent cause of salt depletion is loss of gastrointestinal secretions.

Treatment

Rapid infusion of isotonic saline is indicated.

Water excess

In contrast to pure water depletion, water excess is not uncommon in surgical practice, particularly in elderly postoperative patients who receive too much water in the face of persisting ADH secretion. Renal excretion of sodium continues despite the dilutional hyponatraemia. This contrasts with the hyponatraemia of sodium depletion, in which urinary sodium excretion is minimal and the patient shows the clinical signs of reduction in blood volume. Patients with water excess look comparatively well.

Acute renal failure may produce a similar picture if water administration is continued in the face of oliguria. Chronic starvation can also produce dilutional hyponatraemia, in this case resulting from excess production of water from the metabolism of body fat in the presence of elevated ADH levels. There is also an increase in aldosterone activity, and total body sodium may actually be increased. A similar effect may be produced by chronic liver disease or congestive cardiac failure.

Inappropriate secretion of ADH can occur in a number of conditions, including sepsis, severe pulmonary infection, ectopic secretion by tumours of lung or pancreas, and disease/trauma involving the brain and meninges.

Treatment

If dilutional hyponatraemia due to water excess is recognized, administration of any water by mouth or intravenously (as 5% dextrose) should cease so that the patient can 'dry out'. Electrolyte replacement should continue.

SODIUM IMBALANCE

Sodium is the principal extracellular cation, and changes in its total amount or its concentration affect the volume and tonicity of the ECF. Sodium concentration is the main indicator of ECF tonicity. The concentration of other ions, e.g. Cl^-, HCO_3^-, K^+, is also affected by acid–base changes and renal function, and therefore does not reflect dilutional change in the same way as sodium (which is relatively uninfluenced by these factors).

In most clinical situations which involve sodium excess or deficit there is a combination of volume and tonicity change, either simultaneously or in sequence. It is artificial to consider changes in sodium without at the same time taking into account changes in its solvent, i.e. water. In general terms the significance of an elevated or low serum sodium concentration can best be determined from a study of the patient's history.

Sodium depletion

Causes

Acute sodium loss may be due to:

- Haemorrhage or plasma loss
- Acute gastric dilatation (the patient may lose up to 1 litre of ECF per hour over a period of 3–5 hours)
- Massive diarrhoea, e.g. cholera, staphylococcal or pseudomembranous enterocolitis.

Chronic sodium loss may occur as a result of chronic diarrhoea, protracted ileus, ileostomy or chronic renal disease. As indicated above, true dilutional hyponatraemia can occur with a normal total body sodium but an excess of water. As the fluid lost in these conditions is isotonic, there is contraction of ECF volume, along with features of dehydration (thirst, oliguria and concentrated urine).

Treatment

Mild dilutional hyponatraemia is harmless and does not call for the administration of sodium. In malnourished patients it is corrected by an adequate caloric intake.

In more severe sodium depletion, it is essential that isotonic fluids are used for replacement. If water or hypotonic solutions are administered orally or intravenously, ADH continues to conserve water, the ECF becomes hypotonic and serum sodium concentration falls further. If sodium concentration drops to below 110 mmol/l there is considerable risk of convulsions and water intoxication. Patients with major trauma or sepsis are likely to have persistent excess ADH activity and are particularly liable to this form of hyponatraemia.

Isotonic fluid replacement is continued while the patient 'dries out'. Treatment with hypertonic saline is only considered if the serum sodium has fallen to 110 mmol/l or convulsions have developed. Sodium levels are corrected slowly; too rapid changes may worsen the situation. Excess urinary loss of sodium due to chronic renal disease may require an increased intake of sodium.

Sodium excess

Causes

True sodium excess is usually iatrogenic, and is due to continued excessive administration of sodium in the face of persisting aldosterone activity. This is particularly likely to occur in the postoperative or postinjury period. ECF volume is expanded, increasing the risk of circulatory overload and pulmonary oedema. Hypernatraemia associated with a true excess of sodium is relatively uncommon but may occur in primary (Conn's syndrome) or secondary hyperaldosteronism. It occurs more frequently as a result of abnormal loss of water or hypotonic fluids:

- Pure water loss from skin or lungs. The classic example is a shipwrecked sailor without access to water who may compound the situation by drinking sea water (which is hypertonic). In clinical practice pure water loss may occur in patients supported on a ventilator without adequate humidification.
- Loss of hypotonic fluid. Sweat is hypotonic, and if excess sweating is not compensated for by taking fluid, hypernatraemia results. Gastro-intestinal secretions are sometimes also hypotonic, particularly in babies. Frequently the loss is replaced with drinking water, which can result in hyponatraemia; if only isotonic saline is given, true sodium overload with hypernatraemia can develop.

The consequences of hypernatraemia are extreme thirst and confusion proceeding to coma. The severity of the thirst is such that hypernatraemia is rare in the conscious patient who has access to water.

Treatment

Sodium excess is best treated by giving pure water orally or 5% dextrose intravenously. The temptation to correct abnormal sodium concentrations rapidly should be resisted, as sudden changes in the tonicity of ECF can prove dangerous.

POTASSIUM IMBALANCE

Potassium is the principal intracellular cation. Its *intracellular* concentration is 150 mmol/l. Only 60 mmol of the body potassium content (3500 mmol) is extracellular, its concentration in ECF varying around 4.0 mmol/l. Levels below 2.4 mmol/l and above 6.0 mmol/l are dangerous and may cause cardiac arrest. Increasing the intake or output of potassium produces only slow changes in serum potassium concentrations. Rapid equilibration of intra- and extracellular potassium and efficient renal excretion guard against sudden changes in circulating concentrations. However, alterations in acid–base balance affect these exchanges and may produce rapid changes in extracellular potassium concentration.

Water and salt imbalance in surgical patients
- Pure water depletion is rare; the usual problem is salt and water loss as in diarrhoea.
- Sodium is the key to understanding fluid and electrolyte balance; it is the principal cation in ECF and the major determinant of ECF volume and tonicity.
- Water excess is a particular problem in the elderly following operation, and is a consequence of giving too much water intravenously (as 5% dextrose) in the face of increased ADH secretion.
- Sodium depletion may be associated with convulsions when serum sodium levels fall beneath 110 mmol/l, and is a particular problem in patients with sepsis or major trauma. Sodium levels should be corrected slowly with isotonic saline; hypertonic saline is inadvisable unless sodium levels are extremely low.

Effect of acid–base changes on potassium balance

Derangement in acid–base balance changes potassium balance within and outside the cell. Conversely, changes in potassium balance have secondary effects on acid–base balance.

Acidosis. Excess of hydrogen ions in the ECF causes hydrogen ions to move into the cells in exchange for an equivalent amount of potassium ions, which move out into the ECF. The serum potassium concentration rises and there is increased potassium excretion in the urine. If acidosis continues, a considerable deficit in total body potassium may result.

If the acidosis is corrected rapidly, without at the same time providing potassium ions, serum potassium levels may fall catastrophically as potassium returns to the cells. This dangerous situation can develop within a few hours and applies equally to metabolic and respiratory acidosis.

Alkalosis. In alkalosis the exchange of potassium for hydrogen ions takes place in the opposite direction. Hydrogen ions move out of the cell in exchange for potassium ions, which move in. Further, the kidneys conserve hydrogen ions at the expense of increased urinary loss of potassium. Hypokalaemia follows.

When the deficiency of potassium becomes severe, the kidney again allows the excretion of hydrogen ions so that potassium is conserved. This *paradoxical aciduria* results in worsening alkalosis. Adequate replacement of potassium ions is an essential part of treatment.

Effect of potassium imbalance on acid–base balance

Potassium excess and deficiency have secondary effects on acid–base balance because of the exchange of potassium for sodium and hydrogen ions across the cell membrane. For every three potassium ions withdrawn from the intracellular compartment, two sodium ions and one hydrogen ion enter the cell. In states of potassium deficiency there is thus a developing intracellular acidosis and extracellular alkalosis. Conversely, when there is potassium excess with an increase in movement of potassium into the cell, sodium and hydrogen ions are kept out, leading to an extracellular acidosis.

Potassium depletion

Causes

Acid–base balance abnormalities apart, potassium depletion results from inadequate intake or increased loss.

Inadequate intake. The kidney cannot conserve potassium as efficiently as it does sodium. Even in the absence of potassium intake, urinary loss of potassium continues at approximately 40 mmol per day. This loss is borne primarily by the cells; serum potassium levels are maintained until late in the deficiency state.

A special example of inadequate intake occurs in patients who are in an anabolic state, particularly when receiving intravenous nutrition. The formation of normal cellular components requires potassium, which can be supplied only from the ECF. If potassium intake is not increased (up to 100–200 mmol per day), hypokalaemia may rapidly develop.

Increased loss. This may occur through factors affecting the kidney, e.g. administration of diuretics, excessive secretion of aldosterone (primary and secondary hyperaldosteronism and the response to stress) or other adrenocortical steroids, or chronic loss of gastrointestinal secretions (e.g. from diarrhoea, malfunctioning ileostomy). In these situations, potassium loss greatly exceeds nitrogen loss, indicating that the potassium comes mainly from the ECF. The ratio of potassium to nitrogen in the urine may be as high as 10:1. Hypokalaemia develops

---

Potassium and fluid and electrolyte balance

- Potassium is the principal intracellular cation; 98% of total body potassium is intracellular and serum potassium concentrations are a poor index of total potassium content.

- The body normally contains some 3500 mmol of potassium; as much as one-third of this potassium content may be lost in conditions such as pyloric stenosis.

- The normal serum potassium concentration is 3.6–5.1 mmol/l; levels below 2.4 mmol/l and above 6 mmol/l are associated with the danger of cardiac arrhythmias and arrest.

- ECF acidosis causes H^+ to move into the cells while K^+ moves out; the resultant hyperkalaemia increases potassium loss and reduces total body potassium content.

- ECF alkalosis causes H^+ ions to move out of the cells in exchange for K^+. The resulting hypokalaemia is compounded by the renal conservation of H^+ at the expense of increased urinary potassium losses.

more rapidly than when potassium loss is due to starvation alone.

The principal effect of hypokalaemia is impaired muscle contractility. There is generalized muscle weakness and ileus. The associated extracellular alkalosis may produce features of tetany with signs of neuromuscular irritability, including a positive Chvostek sign. Sensitivity to digitalis is increased, so that it must be used with great care. Electrocardiographic changes include an increased QT interval, depressed ST segment and inverted T waves. If the serum potassium falls below 2 mmol/l, cardiac arrest may occur.

Treatment

Adequate replacement of potassium ions is essential. In severe deficiency states the recommended maximum rate of intravenous administration (10 mmol/hour) may be exceeded. Cardiac monitoring should then be instituted. Adequate provision of chloride ions (as NaCl) is necessary to correct the alkalosis.

Potassium excess

Causes

Potassium is lost from the body mainly through the kidney. Normal daily potassium intake and urinary excretion each approximate to 60–100 mmol. In the presence of normal renal function it is almost impossible to raise serum potassium levels by increasing oral intake. However, excessive or too rapid parenteral administration (>15 mmol/hour) may overwhelm the renal excretory mechanism and lead to hyperkalaemia.

Impaired renal function can lead to a rapid rise in serum potassium concentration even when potassium intake is reduced or prevented. Release of potassium from cell breakdown may compound the problem in the postoperative catabolic phase. The rise in serum potassium which occurs in acute renal failure is approximately 0.1–0.5 mmol/l per day.

The clinical picture of hyperkalaemia is surprisingly similar to that of hypokalaemia. There is muscle weakness, loss of tendon reflexes and development of paralysis. Sensitivity to digitalis is impaired. Electrocardiographic changes include peaked T waves, an increase in the P-R interval and widening of the QRS complex. Cardiac arrhythmias may develop. If the serum potassium exceeds 7.0 mmol/l, ventricular fibrillation may supervene.

Treatment

All administration of potassium is stopped. Hyperkalaemia may be temporarily counteracted by the administration of other cations. In an emergency, intravenous administration of 50–100 ml 10% calcium gluconate, 100 ml 1-molar sodium bicarbonate or 100 ml 5% sodium chloride will improve the clinical features for an hour or two.

A slower but longer-lasting depression of serum potassium levels may be achieved by slow (over 4 hours) intravenous infusion of 250 ml 25% glucose with 20 units soluble insulin, which 'drives' potassium back into the cells. This treatment may be continued for up to 24 hours.

Ion exchange resins may be administered orally or rectally but if the serum potassium approaches 7 mmol/l, haemodialysis is indicated.

ACID–BASE BALANCE

Metabolic acidosis

Metabolic acidosis is common in surgical practice and is usually a consequence of impaired tissue perfusion as in shock. It is potentiated by renal failure. Metabolic acidosis should be suspected by the onset of deep rapid respirations in a volume-depleted patient. The diagnosis is confirmed by measurement of arterial hydrogen ion concentration, blood gases, and standard bicarbonate (Table 2.5).

Treatment

Therapy is directed towards restoring tissue perfusion. Infusion of bicarbonate is only required when the plasma standard bicarbonate level is less than 15 mmol/l (normal value 24–32 mmol/l). The amount of bicarbonate required is calculated on the basis that 2 mmol of bicarbonate will raise the standard bicarbonate level of each litre of cellular fluid by 1 mmol/l, and that the ECF constitutes

Table 2.5 Changes associated with mixed patterns of acid–base upset

	H^+	Pa_{CO_2}	Standard HCO_3
Metabolic acidosis	↑	↓	↓
Respiratory acidosis	↑	↑	normal
Metabolic alkalosis	↓	normal or slightly ↑	↑
Respiratory alkalosis	↓	↓	normal

approximately 20% of body weight. For example, the amount of bicarbonate required to raise the plasma standard bicarbonate level from 10 mmol/l to 27 mmol/l in a 70-kg patient is:

$$(27 - 10) \times 70 \times 20/100 \times 2 = 476 \text{ mmol}$$

In practice only half of this amount is given slowly over 2 hours, and the standard bicarbonate level is rechecked after 4 hours before further administration is considered. As an 8.4% solution of sodium bicarbonate contains 1 mmol of bicarbonate per ml, the volume required can be calculated easily if an 8.4% or 4.2% solution is used. Care must be taken not to overload the patient with sodium and to correct the fall in serum potassium which tends to occur after bicarbonate therapy. As many such patients are potassium depleted, potassium replacement is an important consideration.

Acute renal failure and cardiac arrest produce severe metabolic acidosis and are considered elsewhere in this volume.

Metabolic alkalosis

Transient metabolic alkalosis follows injury and can occur in shock, but the most frequent surgical cause is gastric outlet obstruction. The loss of acid from the stomach is compensated initially by renal conservation of hydrogen ion and an associated increase in potassium output. Thus patients with metabolic alkalosis are always potassium-deficient, and many are severely hypokalaemic. Conversely, patients with potassium depletion from other causes often develop metabolic alkalosis.

The management of gastric outlet obstruction consists of stopping all oral intake, hourly gastric aspiration, correction of dehydration by normal saline, potassium replacement, and surgical relief of the underlying cause.

Respiratory acidosis

Respiratory acidosis is common in surgery as a consequence of oversedation or postoperative chest complications. Management is directed towards relief of the underlying chest condition, supplemented if need be by assisted ventilation. The administration of bicarbonate is not indicated.

Respiratory alkalosis

There are many causes of respiratory alkalosis.

Table 2.6   Causes of respiratory alkalosis encountered in surgical practice
Hyperventilation on a mechanical ventilator or under anaesthesia Pain and apprehension (hysteria) Small areas of pulmonary atelectasis Multiple pulmonary emboli Central nervous system injury Septicaemia (particularly Gram-negative septicaemia)

Those encountered in surgical practice are listed in Table 2.6. The underlying cause should be sought and treated. Sustained respiratory alkalosis has a poor prognosis, usually because of the severity of the underlying condition.

Mixed patterns of acid–base imbalance

Many patients have a mixture of respiratory and metabolic components in their acid–base imbalance. Measurement of arterial blood gas tension, hydrogen ion and standard bicarbonate concentrations helps to reveal the contribution of the metabolic and respiratory components (see Table 2.5).

MONITORING OF PATIENTS WITH FLUID AND ELECTROLYTE PROBLEMS

The parameters shown in Table 2.7 should be estimated daily. Serum protein should also be measured twice a week, and in special circumstances losses of magnesium and calcium should also be measured. Determination of serum and urine osmolalities is useful in patients with severe disorders of hydration.

Table 2.7   Parameters monitored in patients with fluid and electrolyte problems

Parameters measured daily
   Urine volume
   Serum sodium, potassium, bicarbonate and urea concentrations
   Volume of losses from the gastrointestinal tract
   Haemoglobin concentration and haematocrit
Parameters measured daily in patients with complex problems
   Arterial H^+ concentration, Pa_{CO_2} and standard bicarbonate
   Urinary sodium and potassium excretion
   Gastrointestinal sodium and potassium loss
   Body weight

3
Shock

CONTENTS

DEFINITION OF SHOCK

Regardless of the underlying cause, shock is characterized by an acute alteration of the circulation in which inadequate perfusion leads to cellular damage and dysfunction or failure of major organ systems. The clinical features of shock are so variable that they cannot be used to define the shock state. Although the terms 'hypotension' and 'shock' are often taken to be synonymous, cellular perfusion may be inadequate despite a normal blood pressure. Perfusion describes not only blood flow but also implies the supply of substrates (including oxygen) and the removal of waste products. Use of the term 'inadequate' rather than 'reduced' is important since blood flow and substrate supply may be increased in hypercatabolic states (e.g. trauma and sepsis) and yet inadequate for the metabolic demands of the tissues.

All patients with shock can be regarded as having an inadequate (although not necessarily reduced) cardiac output (Fig. 3.1). There are only two causes: pump failure and peripheral circulatory failure, the latter being due to loss of circulating volume (true hypovolaemia) or to vasodilatation (apparent hypo-

Fig. 3.1 Classification of the mechanisms underlying the shock process.

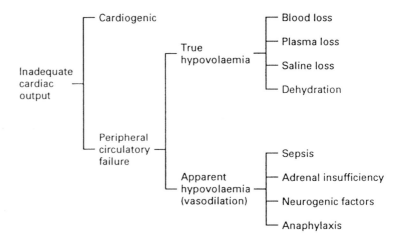

18

volaemia). The major categories of shock within these groupings are cardiogenic, hypovolaemic and septic.

Shock can be thought of as several 'vicious cycles' offset by several compensatory mechanisms (Fig. 3.2). In the absence of early and complete resuscitation, the vicious cycles can become self-perpetuating leading to progressive cellular injury, organ dysfunction and death. Compensatory mechanisms such as vasoconstriction are physiological responses to low-output shock which help to maintain blood flow and perfusion pressure in vital organs. However, it is these very compensatory mechanisms that initiate the changes that ultimately lead to organ damage. Vasoconstriction affects different vascular beds to varying degrees and some organs, notably those in the splanchnic circulation, take the brunt of the hypoxic injury that results from regional hypoperfusion. Tachycardia is another compensatory mechanism which increases cardiac output. However, tachycardia may increase myocardial oxygen demand at a time when arterial pressure is low and myocardial oxygen supply is decreased. It is hardly surprising that patients with coronary artery disease often develop myocardial ischaemia during shock.

Pathophysiology of shock
- *Inadequate* but not necessarily *reduced* tissue perfusion
- Cardiac output inadequate to meet tissue demands because of:
  - pump failure
  - peripheral circulatory failure
- Peripheral circulatory failure may result from:
  - loss of circulating volume (true hypovolaemia) as in burns or bleeding, or
  - vasodilatation (apparent hypovolaemia) as in septic shock.

CAUSES OF SHOCK

Hypovolaemia

Hypovolaemia is an important cause of low-output shock in which low venous return leads to low cardiac output. It may result from any of the following causes:

Haemorrhage is a common cause of hypovolaemia, its effects varying with the duration and severity of

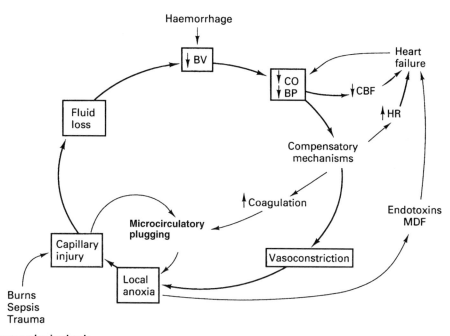

Fig. 3.2 Vicious cycles in shock
BV = blood volume, CO = cardiac output, BP = blood pressure, CBF = coronary blood flow, HR = heart rate, MDF = myocardial depressant factors.

blood loss, the patient's age and myocardial condition, and the speed and adequacy of resuscitation.

Loss of gastrointestinal fluid may result from vomiting and diarrhoea, from fistulae, and from sequestration of fluid in the bowel lumen in intestinal obstruction.

Trauma and infection increase capillary permeability with local sequestration of fluid and oedema. In addition to causing hypovolaemia, trauma and infection may also lead to sepsis.

Burns lead to direct loss of fluid from the burned surface and tissue fluid sequestration.

Renal loss of water and electrolytes (e.g. in sodium-losing chronic nephritis, diabetic ketosis or Addisonian crisis) is an occasional cause of shock.

Surgical factors can contribute to hypovolaemia. For example, mechanical bowel preparation, fasting prior to anaesthesia, and insensible fluid losses during prolonged operations, may all contribute.

Pump failure

Primary impairment of cardiac function may result from myocardial infarction, acute arrhythmias, acute cardiomyopathy, and acute valvular lesions (caused by aortic dissection or trauma). *Secondary* impairment can result from cardiac tamponade producing constriction of the heart, or major pulmonary embolism with obstruction to right ventricular outflow. In all shock states, myocardial performance is affected adversely by reduced coronary arterial perfusion and in some cases by circulating myocardial depressant substances.

Shock due to sepsis

The pathophysiology of septic shock is imperfectly understood. It is most frequently associated with Gram-negative bacillary infection, although Gram-positive organisms and fungi are sometimes responsible. Sepsis may also complicate situations such as major trauma and burns in the absence of infection (i.e. non-bacterial sepsis).

A large number of primary and secondary mediators are implicated in sepsis, and the condition is best thought of as a state of uncontrolled intravascular inflammation. In Gram-negative infection, endotoxin from the bacillary cell wall is thought to be the main trigger for mediator release. In cases of sepsis where Gram-negative infection is not present, endotoxin absorbed from the patient's own gastrointestinal tract may be responsible. Factors such as ischaemic-hypoxic injury may lead to breakdown of the gut mucosal barrier, allowing absorption of endotoxin from Gram-negative gut organisms.

In response to endotoxin, tissue macrophages, neutrophils and endothelial cells all produce mediators which may contribute to the shock state. The list of potential mediators includes complement-derived anaphylotoxins (C5a, C3a), bradykinin, prostaglandins, leukotrienes, thromboxane, histamine, beta-endorphins, tumour necrosis factor (TNF), platelet activating factor (PAF) and interleukins. Most of these mediators are involved in the normal 'beneficial' inflammatory response to infection and injury. It is not understood what tips the balance to produce the 'malignant' uncontrolled intravascular inflammation that characterizes sepsis.

In contrast to our imperfect understanding of some aspects of its pathophysiology, the haemodynamic response to sepsis is well characterized. The primary response is a fall in systemic vascular resistance (SVR) due to loss of vascular tone and vasodilatation, particularly at the level of the precapillary sphincters. Arteriovenous shunting may divert blood from the nutrient capillaries. The decrease in SVR reduces the afterload on the heart and leads to a reflex increase in cardiac output (in the presence of a healthy myocardium). Thus, in early sepsis, blood pressure may be well maintained. In the later stages, the heart may be unable to maintain an adequate output in the face of a falling SVR, so that blood pressure falls. Fluid loss due to increased capillary permeability also contributes to hypotension.

Anaphylaxis

Anaphylactic reactions are produced by IgE

Septic shock
- Most frequently due to Gram-negative organisms but can be due to Gram-positive bacteria or fungi.

- Endotoxin from bacillary cell wall has central importance in septic shock due to Gram-negative infection and may be derived from:
  - organisms at site of infection
  - gut organisms following hypoxic/ischaemic damage to the mucosal barrier.

- Haemodynamic response is fall in *systemic vascular resistance* due to loss of tone and vasodilatation.

- Reflex increase in cardiac output may maintain blood pressure and produce a hyperdynamic circulation (at least in the early stages) so that the patient can appear deceptively well with pink perfused extremities.

antibodies which adhere strongly to tissues and to mast cells in particular. Anaphylactic shock follows the parenteral injection of an antigen (e.g. drugs such as penicillin, foreign sera or insect stings) to which the individual has been previously sensitized. Activation of mast cells releases histamine and serotonin, and with systemic kinin activation this leads to capillary vasodilatation and permeability. In contrast to sepsis, the fall in SVR is so sudden and profound that blood pressure falls markedly. Prompt treatment with adrenaline, hydrocortisone and an antihistamine is required.

Neurogenic factors

True neurogenic shock follows spinal transection or brainstem injury with loss of sympathetic outflow beneath the level of injury and consequent vasodilatation. The rapid increase in size of the vascular bed, including venous capacitance vessels, leads to reduced venous return and reduced cardiac output.

Pain may make an important contribution to shock in patients with trauma, particularly those with fractures. Pain increases the output of catecholamines, with adverse effects on the microcirculation and regional blood flow. Fractures should be immobilized early in patients with multiple injuries.

The most frequently cited example of neurogenic shock is the vasovagal attack or faint, in which intense vagal activity produces marked bradycardia and a fall in cardiac output. The circulation returns rapidly with involuntary assumption of the horizontal position. The transient nature of vasovagal attack removes it from the true spectrum of shock.

Endocrine factors

Although adrenal failure is in itself a potent cause of shock (due to the sudden withdrawal of circulating cortisol and aldosterone), the role of the adrenal cortex in the production of shock by other causes is debatable. Acute adrenal failure may occur in severe meningococcal sepsis (Waterhouse-Friedrichsen syndrome).

PATHOPHYSIOLOGY OF SHOCK

Hypovolaemia is the commonest cause of shock. Its onset may be sudden and obvious, as for example in major haemorrhage, or more gradual and obscure, as for example when fluid replacement is inadequate after surgery. Release of catecholamines as part of the sympathetic response to hypovolaemia has important effects on the macrocirculation (heart and great vessels) and the microcirculation (tissue blood flow at capillary level). Failure to correct the initiating factor means that the sympathetic response persists, leading to reduced tissue perfusion, regional or generalized hypoxia, and consequent metabolic changes.

Effects on the macrocirculation

Diminished venous return activates baroreflexes which increase heart rate and cause peripheral arteriolar constriction. These reflexes are supplemented by rising levels of catecholamines and angiotensin-II. The increase in heart rate improves cardiac output, while increased peripheral (systemic) resistance helps maintain arterial blood pressure. Thus a normal blood pressure may be maintained for some time, especially in young patients, yet regional tissue perfusion may not improve, or may actually worsen, because of the peripheral vasoconstriction.

Peripheral vasoconstriction is most marked in the skin and splanchnic circulation. This tendency to preserve blood flow and perfusion pressure in vital central organs has been described as the 'sympathetic squeeze'. The characteristic clinical picture is of cold pale clammy skin with collapsed veins, the sweating being due to sympathetic sudomotor activity. Splanchnic vasoconstriction is of crucial importance in that the ischaemic gut is a potent source of endotoxin and other mediators, while ischaemia may compromise the metabolic functions of the liver.

Most patients with sepsis present a different clinical picture from those with hypovolaemia. The circulation is usually hyperdynamic in that the cardiac output is higher than normal and the extremities are warm. As already discussed, vasodilatation at precapillary level is responsible for the fall in SVR. Once again, systolic pressure may be relatively well maintained if the myocardium is healthy and can cope with the fall in afterload. A small arteriovenous oxygen difference indicates that oxygen utilization is impaired in sepsis.

Myocardial function is adversely affected in all forms of shock, largely due to low coronary arterial flow and myocardial hypoxia. Local and generalized metabolic acidosis together with alterations in plasma electrolyte concentrations, alter cardiac contractility and may provoke arrhythmias.

In cardiogenic shock, the overall clinical picture is

one of low cardiac output. In left ventricular failure, pulmonary artery wedge pressure rises (see below) and pulmonary oedema may be manifested by tachypnoea, dyspnoea and in some cases, hypoxia. Right ventricular failure leads to raised central venous pressure (CVP).

Effects on the microcirculation

As stated above, the catecholamine-induced vasoconstriction seen early in hypovolaemic shock is not uniform and the brunt of the initial microcirculatory changes is borne by the skin, muscle and gut. The renal response depends on the rapidity of onset of hypovolaemia; the slower the onset, the greater the opportunity for autoregulation and diversion of flow to juxtaglomerular capillaries. The magnitude of the reduction in blood flow through some of these tissues is often *not* reflected in any of the routine haemodynamic measurements. For example, a 10% reduction in blood volume occurring gradually over an hour may produce negligible changes in heart rate and systolic blood pressure, but a profound reduction in splanchnic blood flow and oxygen delivery.

The microcirculatory response to shock can be complicated by underlying pathological changes in the blood vessels (e.g. hypertension and atherosclerosis) or impaired by general anaesthesia, sedatives or other drugs. Maldistribution of tissue perfusion is of fundamental importance, but its pathogenesis is imperfectly understood. Even when flow to an organ or region appears adequate, blood may be traversing 'preferred-route' capillaries rather than nutrient vessels. Furthermore, oxygen extraction and utilization may be impaired at a cellular level in sepsis. Other factors which can impair microcirculatory flow (especially in sepsis) include: increased red cell and platelet adhesiveness, reduced red cell deformability, increased neutrophil adhesiveness with margination (leading in some cases to capillary plugging), endothelial cell swelling, altered capillary permeability, and increased blood viscosity (particularly when hypovolaemia is due to causes other than blood loss, e.g. burns).

In most cases of shock, the coagulation time is shortened and this is of benefit in hypovolaemia due to bleeding. However, in severe sepsis the combination of platelet aggregation, stickiness, sludging and slow flow may lead to intravascular coagulation. Coexisting activation of the fibrinolytic cascade can cause consumptive coagulopathy, the syndrome being known as disseminated intravascular coagulation (DIC). This significantly worsens microcircula-tory flow leading to worsening hypoxia, local metabolic acidosis and cell death. DIC can produce the apparent paradox of a patient with a marked bleeding tendency suffering simultaneously from severe intravascular coagulation.

Neurohumoral response

The central nervous system (CNS) initiates the homeostatic response to acute injury, including fluid loss. Multiple afferent stimuli (arterial and venous pressures and volume, osmolality, pH, hypoxia, pain, anxiety and tissue damage) reach the hypothalamus where they are integrated and relayed to the sympathetic nervous system and adrenal medulla. At the same time, the anterior pituitary initiates the hormonal response which characterizes the metabolic response to injury. Vasopressin (also known as antidiuretic hormone (ADH)) and adrenocorticotrophic hormone (ACTH) are usually regarded as the principle stress hormones. ACTH is released into the bloodstream in response to corticotrophin-releasing factor, vasopressin and adrenalin. ACTH stimulates the production of cortisol which plays a major role in the initial protection from the effects of hypovolaemia.

The initial endocrine response in shock is the release of catecholamines and angiotensin, with later increases in the plasma concentrations of such hormones as cortisol, growth hormone, glucagon, vasopressin and aldosterone. The combined effect is mobilization of energy reserves and conservation of salt and water. While these mechanisms can be regarded as protective in the short term, they lead ultimately to breakdown of cellular integrity.

A number of other substances are released in shock, particularly when it is prolonged or complicated by trauma or sepsis. Histamine and plasma kinins are vasodilators which increase capillary permeability, while serotonin and histamine may contribute to the pulmonary vascular response. Activation of Hageman factor (factor XII) promotes complement activation, and also initiates the generation of kinins from inactive precursors (kininogens) by proteolytic enzymes (kallikreins) released from leucocytes and injured tissues. Potential local mediators of microvascular injury include arachidonic acid metabolites, plasma and phagocyte-derived proteases (particularly elastase), fibrin degradation products, and toxic oxygen radicals released by activated leucocytes. Cytokines (e.g. TNF and interleukins) released from macrophages also mediate many of the metabolic and microcirculatory changes of sepsis and complicated shock.

Cellular dysfunction

To function, cells must extract energy from glucose. This process occurs in the mitochondria and the energy is stored in the form of adenosine triphosphate (ATP) while free hydrogen is released. Energy is readily released from ATP for cellular protein and enzyme synthesis, maintenance of the sodium pump, and cell reproduction. The 'sodium pump' is an ion exchange pump which has crucial importance in functions such as transmission of nerve impulses and glandular secretion. Failure of the pump allows sodium to accumulate within the cell, and when water follows the osmotic gradient, cellular swelling and disruption follow.

Oxygen is necessary to remove most of the hydrogen released during energy generation (Fig. 3.3). In shock, oxygen is lacking at cellular level and other hydrogen receptors soon become saturated. Energy transformation in the Krebs' cycle is then impaired, and lactic acid which cannot be dehydrated to pyruvate accumulates. The cell has to rely on anaerobic glycolysis for energy production, and this gives a poorer yield of ATP than aerobic glycolysis. Consequently, vital cell functions deteriorate: protein and enzyme synthesis fails, sodium leaks into the cell while potassium leaks out, lysosomal membranes break down with intracellular release of proteases, esterases and phosphatases, and the cell dies. If such changes are widespread, organ failure becomes manifest and recovery becomes increasingly unlikely.

Acid–base balance

Accumulation of lactic acid from anaerobic metabolism leads eventually to generalized metabolic acidosis. An elevated blood lactate or low pH reflects inadequate tissue perfusion and as resuscitation proceeds, lactate levels should fall towards normal. Metabolic acidosis is compensated to some degree by buffers and by respiratory and renal mechanisms. However, renal compensation is impaired in shock as a result of reduced renal blood flow, and renal failure in itself greatly increases the tendency to acidosis. Acidosis stimulates chemoreceptors to increase respiratory rate and thereby 'blow off' carbon dioxide. In early shock, anxiety-induced hyperventilation can actually result in respiratory *alkalosis*, and a 'mixed' picture may be present, necessitating careful evaluation of arterial pH, P_{CO_2} and bicarbonate concentrations ('blood gases'). However, it must be stressed that the primary acid–base disturbance in shock is a *metabolic acidosis*

resulting from anaerobic metabolism, perhaps with an element of respiratory compensation through hyperventilation.

Effects on various organs and systems

The 'sympathetic squeeze' reduces the effects of shock on vital organs at the expense of the periphery. However, this sparing is relative and important effects on various organ systems are discernible.

Nervous system

The earliest sign of cerebral hypoxia is restlessness, which may progress to confusion, stupor and coma. Unless hypoxia is prolonged the effects are usually rapidly reversible. Patients recovering from severe sepsis often exhibit encephalopathy, with confusion and poor cognitive function, which may take weeks to reverse.

Kidneys

Increased knowledge and improved management have reduced the incidence and mortality of renal failure in shock, although it remains a serious complication.

A fall in urine output is the most frequent effect of shock on the kidneys. This results initially from reduced renal blood flow, together with the volume-conserving actions of vasopressin and aldosterone. If the shock state continues, the renal tubule cells suffer chemical and structural damage. *Oliguria* is defined as production of less than 400 ml of urine in 24 hours, *anuria* as the production of less than 20 ml in 24 hours. In clinical practice, the minimum acceptable urine output is 0.5 ml/kg body weight per hour; many clinicians use a bedside 'rule of thumb' of 30 ml/hour. As recovery occurs, oliguria gives way to a marked diuresis. In some patients, particularly those with sepsis, acute renal failure with rising blood urea and creatinine occurs in the face of a normal or high urine output, without a preceding oliguric phase (i.e. high output renal failure).

If oliguria is simply the consequence of volume conservation, the urine has a normal to high specific gravity and low sodium concentration; this situation is managed by increasing fluid administration. Extensive tubular damage is denoted by urine with a low specific gravity, increasing sodium concentration, and osmolality close to that of plasma. In practice, if the urine:plasma osmolality ratio exceeds 1.4:1, inadequate perfusion is the cause of the oliguria. A rise in blood urea in the presence of adequate hydration and blood pressure indicates acute renal parenchymal damage.

Other factors which contribute to renal damage in shock include intravascular coagulation, jaundice, hyperkalaemia and nephrotoxic drugs such as aminoglycoside antibiotics. Acute renal failure is usually reversible provided the primary cause of shock is controlled; ultrafiltration or dialysis provide support while recovery is awaited.

Respiratory system

Pulmonary gas exchange can be impaired by a number of factors in shock. For example, in cardiogenic shock it is impaired by left ventricular failure leading to pulmonary oedema, while lung contusion, rib fractures, pneumothorax and haemothorax may all impair exchange after trauma. In addition, shock may give rise to a non-specific but well-defined syndrome of acute respiratory failure known as the adult respiratory distress syndrome (ARDS). Synonyms for ARDS include 'shock lung' and 'noncardiogenic pulmonary oedema'; the latter is a useful description since the clinical and radiological features of ARDS resemble those seen in pulmonary oedema, but measurements of pulmonary artery wedge pressure (see below) exclude a cardiac cause. The diagnosis of ARDS can only be made after pneumonia, pulmonary oedema and pulmonary contusion have been excluded.

The pathophysiology of ARDS is complex and the mediators mentioned earlier may play a role. In the *early phase*, the major factors are pulmonary vasoconstriction (affecting particularly the postalveolar venules) and increased capillary permeability. This results in leakage of protein-rich fluid into the alveolar space. Capillary leakage can be rapidly reversible, but occasionally it persists and there is a *late phase* of proliferation characterized by pulmonary fibrosis.

A ventilation-perfusion (V/Q) mismatch may occur in all forms of shock. Excess secretion or inadequate ventilation can cause plugging of small bronchioles and atelectasis, so that alveoli are perfused but not ventilated. Alternatively, hypovolaemia and reduced perfusion pressure may mean that ventilated alveoli are not perfused. Thus, a combination of pulmonary oedema, V/Q mismatch and later sequelae such as surfactant loss, leads to inadequate pulmonary gas exchange in ARDS. The resulting hypoxia may have profound consequences in patients in whom oxygen delivery to the tissues is already compromised by haemodynamic factors.

Increased capillary permeability secondary to endothelial damage occurs in virtually all organ systems in shock, and ARDS should be viewed as the pulmonary manifestation of multiple organ failure.

Heart

Myocardial performance is adversely affected in shock as a result of reduced coronary arterial perfusion, particularly in patients with coronary artery disease. Hypoxia limits aerobic metabolism in the myocardium, and acidosis depletes myocardial stores of noradrenaline. Contractility and ventricular function may be further impaired by humoral agents acting directly on the myocardium, particularly in sepsis.

Gut

Splanchnic blood flow is markedly reduced in shock and paralytic ileus is common. Gastrointestinal bleeding from stress ulceration (see Ch. 28) was once common during the intensive care of septic patients. Its incidence has decreased steadily as techniques of resuscitation have improved. A more important consequence of ischaemic-hypoxic injury to the gut is breakdown of the barrier to endotoxin.

Liver

The vital metabolic functions of the liver, including its role as the main site of conversion of lactate to pyruvate, may be severely compromised by ischaemia-hypoxia. This results mainly from splanchnic vasoconstriction and portal venous oxygen desaturation; 50% of the liver's oxygen supply and 70% of its blood flow comes from the portal vein. In the early stages of shock, ischaemic-hypoxic injury to the liver is reflected in elevated transaminase levels, while multiple organ failure is often characterized by cholestasis. Kupffer cells are an important part of the reticulo-endothelial system, which as a whole is important for detoxification, phagocytosis and antibody formation. All of these functions may be impaired as organ blood flow is reduced in shock. Since the Kupffer cells sit as a filter between an ischaemic splanchnic bed and the systemic circulation, impairment of their phagocytic and detoxification functions may have particular importance.

Adrenal glands

The adrenal glands play a fundamental role in the

response to injury or infection, and in shock the production of catecholamines and corticosteroids is normally well maintained. Acute pathological changes in the adrenals are rare in shock, although necrosis can occur in the Waterhouse-Friedrichsen syndrome (see above).

CLINICAL SYNDROMES OF SHOCK

Clinical features

The majority of patients with shock have a low cardiac output; the exception is septic shock where the cardiac output is usually high. The classical appearance of a patient with low-output shock is that seen after haemorrhage. The features are partly due to loss of circulating volume and partly to intense sympathetic stimulation. The patient is pale and has a rapid thready pulse and cold clammy extremities. The peripheral veins are collapsed due to reduced filling and sympathetic venoconstriction. The respiratory rate is increased due to chemoreceptor stimulation. The patient becomes restless as a result of cerebral hypoperfusion, and confusion and coma can supervene. Urine output is low.

The effect of haemorrhage on blood pressure depends on the duration and magnitude of blood loss, the patient's age and cardiovascular status, and the speed and adequacy of resuscitation. Initially, the systemic blood pressure is maintained, and may actually increase, particularly in young patients. Up to 25% of circulating volume can be lost without affecting systolic pressure because of the intense vasoconstriction, and to a lesser extent, the shift of fluid from interstitial to intravascular space.

The key to *early diagnosis* is to look for signs of decreased tissue perfusion. For example, in the absence of a head injury an alteration in conscious level is a useful early sign of decreased cerebral perfusion; capillary refill time can be assessed by observing the return of colour after pressure on the nail beds or ear lobes; cool extremities or a widening gap between core and peripheral temperature reflects decreased skin perfusion; and a fall in urine output indicates decreased renal perfusion. In addition, the respiratory rate normally increases before significant tachycardia or hypotension develop. In situations where accurate measurement of blood pressure is possible, an early fall in pulse pressure (difference between systolic and diastolic) reflects the rise in diastolic pressure due to vasoconstriction.

Specific features of cardiogenic shock

Cardiogenic shock shares many of the features associated with haemorrhagic shock. Although there is no primary loss of circulating volume, cardiac output falls and catecholamine-induced vasoconstriction still produces cold clammy extremities. The picture is modified, however, by elevation of cardiac filling pressures leading, in the case of left ventricular failure, to pulmonary oedema.

Specific features of septic shock

The early features of sepsis are subtle and a high index of suspicion is essential as diagnosis is difficult without invasive monitoring. The patient may look remarkably well, largely due to the pink well-perfused extremities. In postoperative patients, early diagnosis often depends on blood gas or lactate measurements. It is all too easy for inexperienced personnel to treat restlessness with sedation rather than appropriate resuscitation.

Changes in core temperature in sepsis are variable. Infected patients may present with pyrexia but peripheral vasodilatation and a cool ambient temperature can lead to excessive heat loss and low core temperature. Thus, the patient may be hypothermic or hyperthermic and it is useful to monitor core–peripheral temperature gradient.

The *early* features of sepsis (Table 3.1) are predominantly due to peripheral vasodilatation and redistribution of blood flow. The low SVR leads to reflex increase in cardiac output so that blood pressure is maintained. The *later* features begin to resemble those of low-output shock as the heart fails to maintain a high output in the face of falling SVR or hypovolaemia secondary to capillary permeability.

Table 3.1	Clinical features of sepsis	
Early	Late
Restlessness and slight confusion	Decreased conscious level
Tachypnoea	Tachypnoea
Tachycardia	Tachycardia
Low SVR*	High SVR
High cardiac output	Low cardiac output
Systolic BP normal or slightly decreased	Systolic BP less than 80 mmHg
Oliguria	Oliguria
Elevated blood lactate	Elevated blood lactate
Warm dry suffused extremities	Cold extremities
SVR = systemic vascular resistance	

The fact that high SVR and low cardiac output are listed as late clinical features of sepsis in Table 3.1 requires explanation. While it is true that cardiac output is often low in patients who present late, it is almost always possible to raise output to above-normal levels by aggressive resuscitation. However, it is now recognized that a low cardiac output in aggressively resuscitated patients is an end-stage feature.

PRINCIPLES OF MANAGEMENT

Restoration of adequate perfusion at cellular level is the essential aim of treatment. Initial attention to ABC (airway, breathing and circulation) must always precede a survey of the patient looking for the underlying cause of shock. In practice, the initial resuscitation of patients with any form of shock is influenced more by the nature of the associated physiological disturbances than by the specific underlying cause. On the other hand, the success of treatment depends largely on detection and elimination of the underlying cause (e.g. arrest of bleeding or drainage of a source of sepsis). The mainstays of early treatment are infusion of fluid and oxygen administration with the aim of improving cardiac output and oxygen transport.

Hypovolaemic shock

Initial assessment

A clinical history is always part of the initial assessment, but may be difficult or impossible to obtain when consciousness is disturbed as a result of head injury, alcohol intake or decreased cerebral perfusion. In trauma, useful information may be obtained from witnesses. Physical examination must be carried out in a logical sequence to avoid serious oversights.

In many instances the combination of overt fluid loss and inadequate or no replacement makes the diagnosis of hypovolaemia straightforward. In some patients the diagnosis is less obvious because of prior resuscitation or a multifactorial aetiology. Hypovolaemia is best assessed by considering the history and clinical examination in conjunction with estimation of apparent or observed losses, measurements of haematocrit, heart rate, pulse volume, arterial and venous pressure, and assessment of tissue perfusion. As stressed above, it is the indices of tissue perfusion which are most useful in the early management of hypovolaemia. One should not be misled into thinking that a patient is well-perfused simply because the blood pressure and heart rate are normal. On the other hand, a lucid patient with rapid capillary refill, warm dry skin, and a good urine output is unlikely to have significant hypovolaemia.

Monitoring and instrumentation

The success of early monitoring depends on the frequent measurement of simple haemodynamic indices and assessment of tissue perfusion, as just outlined. The following guidelines apply to all forms of shock.

Venous access. Good venous access must be obtained early by inserting at least two large-bore peripheral cannulae. Access is normally obtained in the antecubital fossa or via the cephalic vein at the wrist. If vasoconstriction makes it difficult to gain access, a 'cut-down' can be performed in the antecubital fossa or on the long saphenous vein in front of the medial malleolus. In profoundly shocked patients it may be necessary to obtain the initial access by cannulating the femoral vein percutaneously in the groin.

Bladder catheterization. A bladder catheter is inserted transurethrally unless there is a possibility of urethral injury (as in severe pelvic fractures), or when dealing with young children. Under these circumstances, a suprapubic catheter is inserted once the bladder has filled. The urinary catheter is attached to a graduated collecting device (urimeter) so that output can be measured hourly.

Electrocardiogram (ECG) monitoring. ECG monitoring will detect arrhythmias and myocardial ischaemia. It is indicated particularly in primary cardiogenic shock, myocardial dysfunction secondary to ischaemia, direct thoracic injury, and

---

Clinical features of hypovolaemic shock
- Clinical appearances of hypovolaemic shock result primarily from loss of circulating volume (with diminished tissue perfusion and hypoxia) and excessive sympathetic stimulation.
- The patient appears pale, restless and confused.
- Peripheral circulatory changes include a rapid thready pulse with cold clammy extremities, collapsed peripheral veins and prolonged capillary refill time.
- Respiratory rate is increased early as a consequence of chemoreceptor activity.
- Urine output is diminished.

sepsis. Arrhythmias are more likely when there is electrolyte or acid–base disturbance.

Pulse oximetry. A pulse oximeter attached to a finger or ear lobe allows transcutaneous estimation of oxygen saturation of haemoglobin. The screen normally gives a digital read-out of percentage saturation. The accuracy of such peripheral probes depends on good peripheral perfusion. However, in poorly perfused patients, good equipment gives a visual or audible warning of a poor signal, so providing a useful index of both oxygen transport and tissue perfusion.

Central venous catheterization. A catheter can be inserted percutaneously via the internal jugular or subclavian veins so that it lies in the superior vena cava, thus allowing measurement of CVP. In the initial resuscitation of an overtly hypovolaemic patient time must not be wasted inserting a central venous catheter. Furthermore, the bore of the catheter is usually too small for rapid infusion, while inadvertent damage to the apical pleura during insertion may lead to a pneumothorax, a potentially fatal complication in a non-resuscitated patient. However, following the initial administration of fluid and oxygen, measurement of CVP can be useful.

In a shocked patient, a low (<5 mmHg) or even negative CVP indicates the need for more fluid. At the other extreme, a very high CVP (>20 mmHg) indicates cardiac failure and the need for diuretics, vasodilators or inotropic agents. In practice, static measurement of CVP can mislead. For example, a young patient may have an apparently normal CVP (say 10 mmHg) as a result of vasoconstriction. A 'fluid challenge' can resolve doubt. This is performed by measuring CVP before and after the administration of a small fluid bolus. If the CVP does not rise, further fluid can be given safely; a significant rise in CVP suggests myocardial failure or dysfunction and avoids inadvertent over-transfusion.

Core and peripheral temperature measurement. Using one's own hand to assess skin temperature is useful in shocked patients. If thermistors are used to measure core and peripheral temperatures, the core–peripheral gradient provides a useful index of skin perfusion. Core temperature measurement also detects hypothermia, as in trauma patients who have lain in a cold environment, particularly following water immersion.

Fluid administration

The type of fluid lost in shock has little influence on the choice of fluid for initial replacement. 'Colloid'

> **Assessment of the shocked patient**
> - Monitor clinical appearance noting restlessness and confusion (cerebral hypoxia), respiratory rate and state of the peripheral circulation.
> - Monitor pulse rate, systemic blood pressure, hourly urine output and central venous pressure.
> - Gain valuable additional information by monitoring or periodically checking:
>   - blood urea and electrolyte concentrations
>   - haemoglobin concentration, white cell count and haematocrit
>   - arterial blood H^+ ion and gas concentrations
>   - blood lactate levels
>   - pulse oximetry
>   - core and peripheral temperature
>   - pulmonary capillary wedge pressure.
> - Remember to send appropriate samples for bacteriological examination (e.g. blood, urine, sputum, drain fluids) when sepsis is suspected.

---

and/or 'crystalloid' can be used in the first instance regardless of whether shock is due to bleeding, burns or gastrointestinal upset. Red cell concentrates may be needed later, preferably after cross-matching although uncross-matched group O Rhesus negative blood may be needed in extreme situations. Successful initial resuscitation depends more on the rapidity and adequacy of fluid replacement than on the choice of regimen.

'Colloids' are fluids containing solute particles larger than MW 30 000. In clinical practice this means the particles remain within the intravascular space, being retained by the capillary membrane. The duration of vascular expansion achieved depends largely on the molecular weight of the solute particles. Colloid particles may be natural (albumin) or synthetic (gelatins, starch or dextrans).

'Crystalloids' are sodium-containing solutions that have solute particles with a molecular weight of less than 30 000. Following infusion, crystalloid solutions equilibrate rapidly with the interstitial space (in which sodium is the main cation), and so have to be infused in amounts which exceed estimated loss by a factor of 3–4 times. It should be noted that 5% dextrose solution is not a crystalloid but merely water rendered isotonic by adding glucose. Infused 5% dextrose equilibrates not only with the interstitial space but with the much larger intracellular space, making it quite useless for resuscitation but ideal for correction of dehydration.

Infusion of large volumes of fluid can cause dilution of clotting factors (factors V and VII, fibrinogen and platelets) and coagulopathy may need correction by transfusion of fresh frozen plasma and/or platelets. Some synthetic colloids, notably dextrans, can compound coagulopathy. If massive transfusion is needed, hypothermia must be avoided by using blood-warming equipment.

If hypovolaemic shock proves refractory to fluid replacement and oxygen administration, the following factors may be responsible:

- Underestimation of the degree of hypovolaemia
- Failure to arrest haemorrhage
- Presence of cardiac tamponade or tension pneumothorax
- Underlying sepsis
- Secondary cardiovascular effects due to delay in instituting treatment.

Metabolic control

Urea and electrolyte levels are required to establish a baseline and monitor progress. Arterial pH and blood gas measurements are essential to assess hypoxia, hypercapnia and acid–base balance. Blood lactate levels are a good index of cellular hypoxia and hepatic function.

Acid–base balance rarely requires pharmacological correction. *Metabolic acidosis* associated with inadequate perfusion will correct rapidly once cardiac output is improved, indeed its disappearance is a marker of adequate resuscitation. Bicarbonate is occasionally required when pre-existing hyperkalaemia is exacerbated by a decreasing extracellular

pH as a result of metabolic acidosis. Even in this situation, bicarbonate should only be given if the metabolic acidosis is severe (pH <7.2 and base excess >−10), and even then, only in amounts which will partially correct the acidosis. Overzealous administration of bicarbonate can produce a left-shift in the oxyhaemoglobin dissociation curve (Fig. 3.3). Although this may improve oxygen uptake in the lungs, it may also impair its release at the low levels of oxygen tension found in the tissues (although this is offset by local acidosis). *Respiratory acidosis* with an increase in arterial P_{CO_2} usually indicates the need for endotracheal intubation and assisted ventilation. *Metabolic alkalosis* occasionally results from impaired renal handling of bicarbonate or transfusion of large amounts of stored blood (citrate is metabolized to bicarbonate in the body).

Analgesia

Effective analgesia must not be withheld from hypovolaemic patients, particularly when they have been injured. Morphine probably remains the most useful drug despite its potential side-effects. There is no place for subcutaneous or intramuscular injection of any narcotic drug in hypovolaemic shock since impaired blood flow means that absorption is dangerously unreliable and unpredictable. Increments of morphine (e.g. 2 mg) are administered intravenously every 2–5 minutes until pain control is satisfactory. The effect of intravenous injection is short and the dose may have to be repeated every 30–60 minutes. Such careful admin-

Fig. 3.3 Shifts in the oxygen dissociation curve in response to pH changes (NB. pH in a central vessel may not reflect tissue pH).

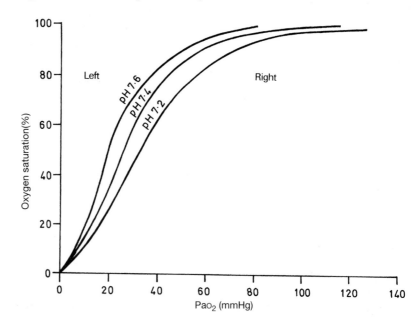

istration of analgesics should not interfere with assessment of conscious level, and reduces anxiety and suffering.

Infiltration of local anaesthetics and regional nerve block deserve consideration in the acute situation. For instance, a femoral nerve block can be performed rapidly and gives good pain control in patients suffering from a fractured femur.

Summary

The mainstays of resuscitation in hypovolaemia are simply the *provision of enough fluid and oxygen.* Adequacy of provision is guided by simple indices of tissue perfusion, supplemented later by basic monitoring and assessment of oxygenation. Pharmacological agents are not generally required for haemodynamic support in uncomplicated hypovolaemic shock (unless monitoring reveals myocardial impairment). The need for pharmacological support generally necessitates more invasive monitoring and transfer of the patient to a high dependency unit or intensive care unit (see below).

Management of sepsis

All of the principles just outlined apply to the management of patients with sepsis. Significant hypovolaemia may be present when sepsis is first diagnosed; this may be true hypovolaemia secondary to capillary permeability or relative hypovolaemia due to vasodilatation. However, sepsis is characterized by a low SVR and the resulting decrease in cardiac afterload together with release of multiple mediators makes secondary myocardial ischaemia common. This, together with dysfunction or failure of other organ systems, generally necessitates intensive care. Prolonged mechanical ventilation, enteral or parenteral nutrition, ultrafiltration or haemodialysis, and inotropic support for the cardiovascular system are all typically required.

In severe sepsis it is not uncommon to find evidence of inadequate tissue perfusion (e.g. high lactate levels) despite high cardiac output and oxygen delivery. This is due to maldistribution of oxygen supply and defective utilization of oxygen at cellular level. Careful optimization of oxygen delivery and consumption is essential.

Infection is a frequent, but not invariable, cause of sepsis. Potential sites of infection must be identified, and the responsible organisms identified. Serial blood samples are sent for culture, as are specimens of urine and sputum. Investigations are initiated to detect intrathoracic and intra-abdominal infection or

abscess, and sources of sepsis (e.g. perforated appendix, empyema of gall bladder, or stones in the common bile duct) are treated by appropriate surgery.

Antibiotic therapy is empirical and broad spectrum until microbiological results become available. Appropriate antibiotic therapy is important to prevent sepsis developing in at-risk patients with infection, but has little or no impact on outcome once the full-blown sepsis syndrome has developed with endotoxaemia and mediator release. A large amount of research is at present being devoted to developing antibodies against endotoxin and other mediators in the hope that immunotherapy can be used in patients with sepsis.

Management of cardiogenic shock

Myocardial infarction is by far the commonest cause of cardiogenic shock. Initial therapy must include intravenous narcotics to control pain, treatment of cardiac arrhythmias, provision of adequate oxygenation and correction of metabolic acidosis. Treatment of metabolic acidosis in this situation may require judicious use of bicarbonate, unlike the situation in uncomplicated hypovolaemic shock where acidosis usually corrects promptly once the circulation has been restored. All patients should have continuous ECG monitoring to detect arrhythmias and extension of myocardial damage. Fluid must be infused cautiously in cardiogenic shock, and a pulmonary artery flotation catheter (PAFC or 'Swan-Ganz' catheter) must be inserted to measure pulmonary artery wedge pressure and avoid overload.

Three additional areas require attention:

Management of cardiac failure. Vasodilators may be of benefit if their use is monitored by a PAFC. Some agents (e.g. nitrates) are predominantly venodilators but also improve coronary artery flow; others (e.g. sodium nitroprusside) are predominantly arterial vasodilators. Use of these agents, often in combination, can help to control preload and afterload. Inotropic agents (e.g. dopamine and dobutamine) may be needed for pump failure, a situation where intra-aortic balloon counter-pulsation may sometimes have a role in maintaining the circulation.

Management of arrhythmia. Bradycardia can result from inferior myocardial infarction or atrioventricular block (heart block). It usually requires no treatment but in cardiogenic shock, temporary cardiac pacing will increase heart rate and cardiac output. Tachyarrhythmias may be atrial or ventricular but the rapid rate makes precise diagnosis difficult. A variety of drugs are available to prevent and treat arrhythmias.

Correction of mechanical factors. Cardiogenic shock may be precipitated by mechanical factors such as tamponade, valve rupture or massive pulmonary embolism. Drainage of tamponade, valve replacement and pulmonary embolectomy may have to be considered.

PRINCIPLES OF INTENSIVE CARE MANAGEMENT

Uncomplicated hypovolaemic shock can often be managed satisfactorily without intensive care facilities, but patients with severe trauma, sepsis, cardiogenic shock or shock complicated by secondary myocardial dysfunction, will all benefit from the monitoring and support available in an intensive care unit (ICU). The success of ICU management depends largely on having adequate levels of experienced medical and nursing staff. The correct nurse staffing ratio is one trained nurse per patient at all times. The majority of ICUs in the UK are administered by anaesthetists, but trainees from other disciplines, including medicine and surgery, can enter specialist training in intensive care.

Intensive care falls into two main categories: management of the primary problem necessitating admission and prevention of secondary damage to other organ systems. For practical purposes, the major emphasis is on provision of cardiovascular, respiratory and renal support, although all organ systems require observation and support.

Advanced cardiovascular support

In a ward or emergency room, blood pressure is usually measured with a sphygmomanometer, while CVP is measured using manometer tubing. In the ICU, haemodynamic measurements are made by connecting intravascular catheters to pressure transducers. A slow infusion of heparinized saline prevents clotting, while a three-way tap allows blood to be withdrawn for sampling.

Arterial lines. These are used for continuous monitoring of arterial blood pressure and for withdrawal of arterial blood for gas analysis. In severely shocked patients, the femoral artery may be catheterized, but the radial artery is normally used. Before inserting any catheter into the radial artery it is essential to check that the ulnar artery is patent and supplying the palmar arch.

Pulmonary artery flotation catheters (PAFC). These may not be needed for young patients with uncomplicated hypovolaemic shock, but they are invaluable in patients who need inotropic support or who have sepsis, myocardial impairment, cardiogenic shock, or trauma (particularly thoracic trauma with the possibility of myocardial contusion). A PAFC is a long catheter with two sampling (monitoring) channels, one of which opens at the tip of the catheter while the other opens 30 cm behind the tip (Fig. 3.4). A third channel is used to inflate a balloon at the catheter tip. This balloon is inflated once the catheter is within the superior vena cava and the flow of blood floats it through the right heart and into the pulmonary artery; the balloon can then be deflated and pulmonary arterial pressure can be monitored. If the balloon is inflated with the catheter in the pulmonary artery, it moves on to become 'wedged' in a pulmonary arteriole so that pulmonary capillary wedge pressure (PCWP) can then be measured. PCWP provides an estimate of left atrial filling pressure, i.e. a 'left-sided CVP'. The PAFC also has a thermistor at its tip which measures core temperature and allows calculation of cardiac output by a thermodilution technique.

Thus insertion of a PAFC permits monitoring of right atrial pressure, pulmonary artery pressure,

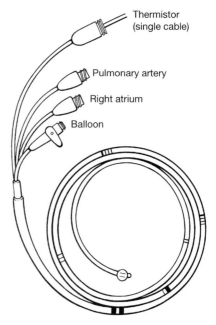

Fig. 3.4 Pulmonary artery flotation catheter (PAFC). Note the two channels for monitoring and sampling, the channel for inflating the distal balloon and the electrical connections for the thermistor.

PCWP, and cardiac output. Pulmonary arterial blood (i.e. mixed venous blood) can be withdrawn for determination of oxygen saturation and content. From these measurements one can calculate systemic vascular resistance, pulmonary vascular resistance, oxygen delivery (DO_2), oxygen consumption (VO_2) and oxygen extraction ratio (OER). Regular measurement of oxygen transport variables allows more comprehensive assessment of the effects of therapy. For example, in a septic patient with a low SVR, a vasoconstrictor such as noradrenaline can raise blood pressure but at the same time diminish tissue oxygenation.

Pharmacological agents. These are only required for cardiovascular support if elimination of surgical causes of shock, restoration of blood volume and red cell mass, and adequate oxygenation fail to restore an adequate cardiac output and oxygen delivery. The drugs used most commonly are inotropic agents (to increase myocardial contractility), with or without vasodilators or vasoconstrictors.

Dopamine. This is a commonly used inotrope because it influences both cardiac output and (in theory) urine output; at higher doses it is also a vasoconstrictor. The response to dopamine is variable and the following should be taken as guidelines only. A dose of 2–5 µg/kg/minute has predominantly 'dopaminergic' effects with improvement in renal and mesenteric blood flow; doses of 5–20 mg/kg/minute produce predominantly inotropic effects; while doses greater than 20 µg/kg/minute have predominantly alpha-adrenergic effects leading to vasoconstriction.

Dobutamine. This acts directly on beta-1-adrenergic receptors and has a more pronounced inotropic action than dopamine and less marked effects on heart rate. Low-dose dopamine is often used in the early stages of resuscitation to maintain renal perfusion, and dobutamine is added if cardiac output has to be augmented. In severe sepsis with a low SVR, high-dose dopamine or noradrenaline may be needed to elevate blood pressure, but vasoconstrictors are only used when the patient is being fully monitored (including use of a PAFC).

Respiratory support

The vast majority of patients admitted to an ICU require assisted ventilation before, or at the time of, admission. An endotracheal tube can be passed through the nose or mouth; the nasal route may be less uncomfortable if ventilation has to be prolonged. All adult endotracheal tubes have an inflatable cuff to allow use of positive pressure and protect the airway from aspiration of oropharyngeal or gastric contents. Although the 'low pressure cuff' limits pressure damage to the trachea, the risk of pressure effects on the larynx mean that surgical tracheostomy is usually performed if intubation is needed for more than 10–14 days.

Positive end-expiratory pressure (PEEP) can be used to improve pulmonary gas exchange by countering the tendency of small airways to collapse at the end of the ventilatory cycle. Continuous positive airway pressure (CPAP) is a recent extension of this concept. Particular difficulties may be encountered in ARDS as the high oxygen concentrations and high gas flow rates needed in patients with stiff lungs may result in dangerously high airway pressures (and barotrauma to the lung).

When 'weaning' a patient from assisted ventilation, the contribution of the ventilator is gradually decreased until the patient is breathing spontaneously. The endotracheal tube is then withdrawn.

Renal support

The incidence of acute renal failure has fallen as resuscitation has become more effective. High output failure is now more common than oliguric failure, an important change since the former has a significantly lower mortality. When acute renal failure does occur, its earliest manifestations are hyperkalaemia and metabolic acidosis. In oliguric failure there is a risk of fluid overload and pulmonary oedema.

Dialysis. This is indicated when the blood urea rises at a rate of 7–10 mmol/day. It avoids severe metabolic acidosis and hyperkalaemia, and the systemic effects of severe uraemia. Excess water, electrolytes and toxins are removed from the blood as it passes over a semipermeable membrane, on the other side of which is an electrolyte solution with a composition similar to that of plasma. In *peritoneal dialysis* the patient's own peritoneum is the dialysing membrane whereas in *haemodialysis* an artificial extra-corporeal membrane is used. Peritoneal dialysis is rarely used in ICU as many patients have intraperitoneal sepsis, have recently undergone gastrointestinal surgery, or have intra-abdominal vascular grafts. In addition, large volumes of fluid in the abdomen can limit diaphragmatic movement and make ventilation difficult. One factor limiting haemodialysis is the frequent occurrence of hypotension in unstable patients.

Ultrafiltration. This can be used sequentially with haemodialysis to overcome the problem of hypotension, and is particularly useful in patients with fluid overload. It has the ability to remove large amounts of plasma without significantly altering osmolality. Anticoagulated blood is pumped through a dialyzer without concurrent use of dialysate and hydrostatic pressure is employed to remove plasma water at rates of 1–3 l/hour.

Without dialysis or ultrafiltration, management of an oliguric patient would be impossible given the need to provide parenteral nutrition, blood and blood products, and drugs, all of which can result in fluid overload.

Dialysis is the most effective way of reducing hyperkalaemia in acute renal failure but a dangerously high potassium level may have to be reduced while dialysis is being established; the following manoeuvres can be used:

1. Sodium bicarbonate will correct metabolic acidosis and encourage potassium transfer into cells
2. Intravenous administration of 50 g glucose with 20 units soluble insulin also favours transfer of potassium into the cells
3. Intravenous calcium gluconate (2–4 g in 500 ml 5% dextrose) should be given if cardiotoxicity due to hyperkalaemia is present or imminent.

Other considerations

Careful cardiovascular and respiratory support is important to prevent secondary damage to other organ systems. Other important aspects of ICU management not covered here include provision of nutritional support and prevention of acquired infection (pneumonia is a particular problem in patients undergoing mechanical ventilation). Psychological care of the patient is vital and includes provision of adequate analgesia (including epidural anaesthesia in some cases), judicious use of sedatives, and most importantly, taking time to talk to the patient and explain procedures and therapies to them, even if the patient appears mentally obtunded.

Organ-system support in shocked patients

Cardiovascular support
- Severely shocked patients frequently require inotropic agents (e.g. dopamine) with or without vasodilators or vasoconstrictors.
- In addition to monitoring basic haemodynamic parameters (pulse, blood pressure), a pulmonary artery flotation catheter is advisable to measure:
  - right atrial pressure, pulmonary artery and capillary wedge pressure
  - core temperature and cardiac output (thermodilution)
  - oxygen saturation in mixed venous blood
- These additional measurements allow calculation of:
  - systemic vascular resistance and pulmonary vascular resistance
  - oxygen delivery and consumption.

Respiratory support
- Endotracheal intubation and positive pressure ventilation is frequently needed.
- Gas exchange is improved if positive end-expiratory pressure (PEEP) is used to counter collapse of small airways at the end of each ventilatory cycle.
- Continuous positive airway pressure (CPAP) may be of additional value.

Renal support
- Hyperkalaemia and metabolic acidosis are early signs of acute renal failure.
- Many patients have high output failure rather than oliguric failure.
- Dialysis is indicated when the blood urea rises at a rate of 7–10 mmol/day.
- Ultrafiltration can be used sequentially with haemodialysis to avoid dialysis-related hypotension and is very useful in patients with fluid overload.

4

Transfusion of blood and blood products

Blood transfusion can be life-saving; there are many areas of medicine and surgery which could not be undertaken without good transfusion support. However, as with any treatment, transfusion of blood and its components carries potential risks which must be outweighed by the patient's need. The magnitude of risk depends on factors such as the prevalence of infectious disease in the donor population, the resources and dedication of the organization collecting, processing and issuing the blood and blood products, and the care with which the clinical team administers these products.

Blood donation

In the UK, whole blood is donated by healthy adult volunteers aged 17–65 years with normal haemoglobin levels. The standard 450 ml donation contains approximately 200 mg of iron, loss which can be withstood readily every 3 months by healthy donors. Blood components (platelets and plasma) can be separated from the donated blood or obtained from the donor as separate products by the use of a cell separator, a process called apheresis. The equipment needed for each procedure makes apheresis expensive so that it is used mainly to collect human leucocyte antigen (HLA)-matched products from specified donors and to obtain plasma containing high levels of specific antibodies (e.g. anti-tetanus immunoglobulin).

Strict donor selection and testing of all donations is essential to exclude blood which may be hazardous to the recipient. All donations are ABO grouped, Rhesus D typed, antibody screened, and tested for hepatitis B antigen and antibody to hepatitis C, human immunodeficiency virus (HIV) I and II and syphilis. Antibody to cytomegalovirus (CMV) is also tested to provide CMV-negative blood for patients such as transplant recipients and premature infants.

BLOOD COMPONENTS

The components which can be prepared from donated blood are shown in Figure 4.1 and their descriptions are as follows.

Whole blood

Donated whole blood is drawn into 60–100 ml of an anticoagulant (citrate)-nutrient (phosphate, dextrose and adenine) solution in which it can be stored for up to 30 days at $4 \pm 2°C$. Despite provision of nutrients, changes in the red cells do occur during storage and the haemostatic properties of the blood decline (Table 4.1). Platelets are non-functional after exposure to 4°C, there are no functional granulo-

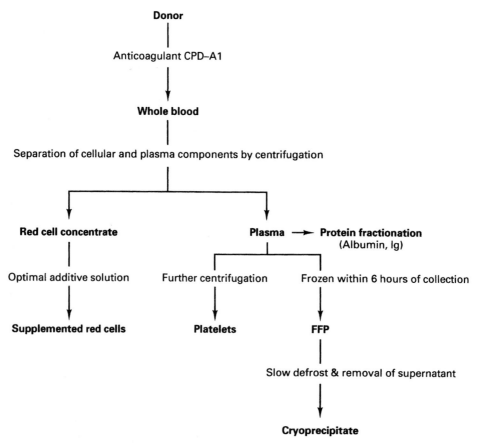

Donor
|
Anticoagulant CPD–A1
|
↓
Whole blood
|
Separation of cellular and plasma components by centrifugation
|

Red cell concentrate   **Plasma** ⟶ **Protein fractionation**
                                                                   (Albumin, Ig)
|
Optimal additive solution   Further centrifugation   Frozen within 6 hours of collection
|
↓   ↓   ↓
Supplemented red cells   **Platelets**   **FFP**
                                                                   |
                                                   Slow defrost & removal of supernatant
                                                                   |
                                                                   ↓
                                                        Cryoprecipitate

Note: Donor whole blood collection bags have satellite packs (2–3) attached and these allow individual products to be processed and collected within a 'sterile' system.

Fig. 4.1   Products which can be obtained from one unit of donated whole blood.

cytes, and concentrations of the labile factors V and VIII decrease quickly in the first week of storage. The blood is not sterilized so that whole blood transfusion can transmit organisms not detected by donor screening.

There are few situations where plasma, proteins and red cells are all needed. Whole blood is an inefficient means of giving haemostatic factors and can cause cardiac failure when used in patients with chronic anaemia. It is indicated when rapid large volume transfusion is needed as in patients who have suffered major trauma. Transfused blood must be ABO and Rh(D) compatible with the recipient.

Red cell concentrate

This concentrate is prepared from a unit of donated blood by removing most of the plasma to leave a haematocrit of 65–75% and final volume of about 300 ml. Packed cells are ideal for use in chronically anaemic patients, and can be given with colloid or crystalloid solutions in acute blood loss. The risk of infection, storage considerations and administration safeguards are those which apply to whole blood.

Supplemented red cells

These are concentrates to which saline, adenine and glucose have been added to give a haematocrit of 55–65% and final volume of 300 ml. The resulting solution has better flow characteristics than concentrated cells but must be used with care in large volume transfusions and renal failure.

Platelet concentrates

Some 50–60 ml of platelets can be produced from a unit of whole blood by centrifugation. The resulting

Table 4.1 Changes in whole blood stored at 2–6°C in CPD-A1

	Storage time (days)			
	0	7	28	35
Red cell viability (%)[1]	> 90	> 90	80	75
Platelet viability (%)[2]	95	0	0	0
Coagulation factors V and VIII (%)[3]	95	30	30	30
Plasma haemoglobin (g/l)	0–0.01	0.1	0.3	0.5
Plasma potassium (mmol/pack)	1.5	5	9	12.5
pH	7.6			7.0

[1] Red cell viability is the proportion of red cells which survive in the circulation 24 hours after transfusion of stored blood.
[2] The loss of functional platelets occurs during the first 48 hours of storage at 4°C.
[3] Other coagulation factors are stable during storage at 4°C.

unit contains more than 55×10^9 platelets and a small amount of red cells and leucocytes, and can be stored on an agitator for 5 days at 20–24°C. An adult is usually given 4–6 of these units, and once pooled, the platelets must be used in 4 hours. Platelet concentrates are not sterile and carry a greater infection risk than whole blood as each transfusion exposes the recipient to the blood of 4–6 donors. Bacterial contamination is also more likely as platelets cannot be refrigerated.

Platelets are infused through a standard blood-giving set over less than 30 minutes. A microaggregate filter should not be used. As the concentrate contains some red cells, it should ideally be ABO and Rh(D) compatible with the recipient. Females of child-bearing age must receive Rh(D) compatible platelets or prophylactic Rh(D) immunoglobulin should be given. Five platelet donations should raise an adult platelet count by $20–40\,000 \times 10^9$/l. Platelet concentrates are indicated in thrombocytopenia, when platelet function is defective, and when there is microvascular bleeding (oozing from mucous membranes, needle puncture sites and wounds) in patients receiving massive blood transfusions.

Fresh frozen plasma (FFP)

Some 200–300 ml of plasma can be removed within 6 hours of donation from a unit of whole blood and stored frozen at –30°C. FFP contains albumin, immunoglobulins and all of the coagulation factors. Like whole blood it carries an infection risk although the risk of cell-borne infection (e.g. CMV infection) is reduced. FFP can be stored at –30°C for a year and is thawed to 37°C before issue.

FFP must be ABO compatible with the recipient and should be given within 4 hours of thawing. The average adult dose is 3–4 units. FFP is used when there are multiple coagulation defects (e.g. disseminated intravascular coagulation (DIC)), for single factor replacement when a heat-treated product is not available, and when there has been an overdose of the anticoagulant warfarin (bleeding and an international normalized ratio (INR) >4.5). It is used occasionally to treat thrombotic thrombocytopenic purpura and pseudocholinesterase deficiency (see Ch. 9), but safer products are available for use as volume expanders or nutritional purposes.

Cryoprecipitate

A single unit of cryoprecipitate can be removed from one unit of FFP after controlled thawing. After resuspension in 10–20 ml plasma, the cryoprecipitate is frozen once more to –30°C. It contains fibrinogen, factor VIII and fibronectin, and can be stored for up to a year.

Cryoprecipitate carries the same basic risk of transmitting infection as FFP, but as an adult dose is normally 10 units, the recipient is exposed to material from 10 donors. ABO compatibility is achieved whenever possible, and the product is infused as soon as possible after thawing. It is used when fibrinogen levels are low, in bleeding associated with uraemia, and in some cases of von Willebrand's disease.

Human albumin

Albumin is prepared by fractionation of large pools of donated plasma. The final product is pasteurized at 60°C for 10 hours and carries no risk of transmitting viral infection. There are no compatibility requirements. A 4.5% and 20% solution are available, each having negligible amounts of potassium and a sodium concentration of 145 mmol/l. 4.5% solutions are used to maintain plasma albumin levels in burns, and are sometimes used in acute blood volume replacement, although crystalloid or non-plasma colloid solution are usually just as effective. 20% solutions can be used when hypoproteinaemia is associated with oedema and is resistant to diuretics (e.g. liver disease, nephrotic syndrome).

20% albumin is hyperoncotic so that there is a risk of acutely expanding the intravascular space and precipitating pulmonary oedema.

Factor VIII and IX concentrates

Purified factor VIII and IX concentrates (containing some factor II and X) are prepared from large pools of plasma. Virus inactivation processes now mean that these products should not transmit HIV I and II or hepatitis B and C, but this may not apply to heat-resistant viruses which have no lipid envelope (e.g. hepatitis A). The concentrates are used to treat factor VIII and IX deficiency. Factor IX concentrates which include other vitamin K-dependent factors may also be used in warfarin overdose. Care must be taken in patients with liver disease as this therapy may be thrombogenic.

Human immunoglobulin

Immunoglobulin (90% IgG) is prepared from fractionation of large pools of plasma from unselected donors or from individuals known to have high levels of specific antibodies. There is no risk of transmitting hepatitis or HIV, and the product can be given intramuscularly or intravenously. The indications are shown in Table 4.2. Intravenous IgG was originally developed as replacement therapy for inherited immunodeficiency states. It is also used to treat immune thrombocytopenia, and other diseases such as the Guillain-Barré syndrome may also benefit from this therapy.

RED CELL SEROLOGY

The red cell membrane is a bilipid layer with which a variety of blood group antigen systems are associated. Over 400 red cell antigens have been described, and although their precise role is uncertain they play a part in the recognition of self from non-self. Of the major antigens, the ABO, Lewis (Le) and P antigens are carbohydrates, the Rhesus (Rh), Duffy (Fy) and Kidd (Jk) antigens are proteins, and the MN system antigens are a combination of glycolipids and carbohydrates.

Table 4.2 Indications and doses for human immunoglobulins

Problem	Patients eligible for IgG	Preparation	Dose
Hepatitis A	Contacts & travellers to endemic areas	Human normal IgG	0.02 ml/kg*
Hepatitis B	Needle-stick or mucosal exposure victims. Should also be immunized	Hepatitis B IgG	1000 iu for adults and 500 iu for children <5 years.
Hepatitis non-A, non-B	Needle-stick or mucosal exposure victims	Human normal IgG or nothing	0.06 ml/kg*
Rubella	Susceptible women exposed in pregnancy (if termination excluded)	Rubella Ig Human normal IgG	10–20 ml 10–20 ml
Varicella zoster	Immunosuppressed contacts Infants exposed to cases Pregnant contacts	Human normal IgG	0.5 ml/kg 0.25 ml/kg 0.2 ml/kg
Rabies Tetanus	Subjects exposed to rabid animals High-risk injuries in non-immune subjects. Treatment of tetanus. Should also be actively immunized	Rabies Ig Tetanus IgG	20 iu/kg 250 iu 500 iu if >24 h delay or heavily contaminated 5000–10 000 iu
Accidental transfusions of Rh(D) positive blood	Women of childbearing age	Anti-D IgG	20–25 µg/ml of transfused blood (if intramuscular route used), 10–15 µg/ml of transfused blood (if intravenous route used)

* In these cases a sensible practice is to give one vial as a standard adult dose.

ABO antigens

Nearly all deaths from transfusion error are due to ABO incompatible transfusion. ABO antigens are present on many cells of the body, and their presence depends on inheritance of allelic genes on chromosome 9 which code for enzymes which change the carbohydrate structures on the cell membrane to the substance known as A or B antigen. In individuals belonging to group O, the gene is silent so that the basic carbohydrate structure is left unchanged. Anti-A and anti-B antibodies are produced only by individuals who lack A or B antigens respectively. These are usually IgM antibodies (naturally occurring) and are present from the age of 3–6 months. IgG anti-A and anti-B (immune) antibodies occur less frequently and follow transfusion or transplacental passage of ABO incompatible red cells, usually in group O individuals. ABO antibodies can react at body temperature and activate complement, and are of major clinical significance as a cause of rapid intravascular haemolysis. For example, transfusion of group A blood to a group B patient results in haemolysis of the transfused red cells because of the anti-A antibodies present in the recipient. Similarly, group O individuals have anti-A and anti-B antibodies in their serum which will react with any donor cells apart from group O cells (see Table 4.3).

Rhesus antigen

This complex blood group system is coded by allelic genes at three closely linked loci on chromosome 1. Rhesus D or no D (termed d), Cc and Ee exist. Rh(D) is by far the most immunogenic of the Rhesus antigens and is the only one currently crossmatched to ensure compatibility in blood transfusion. Individuals who are Rh(D) negative do not normally have anti-Rh(D) is their plasma unless they have been immunized by previous transfusion or pregnancy. More than 70% of Rh(D)-negative patients who are transfused with Rh(D)-positive blood develop anti-Rh(D) antibodies. These are IgG antibodies and do not activate complement, although they do cause extravascular haemolysis. The Fc receptor of the IgG antibody is recognized by the macrophages of the reticulo-endothelial system, and antibody coated cells are removed from the circulation. Rhesus antibodies can cause transfusion reactions and haemolytic disease of the newborn (HDN). It is essential that Rh(D)-negative women of child-bearing age are not transfused with Rh(D)-positive blood.

Other red cell antigens

Kell antigens. These are produced from a precursor substance encoded on the X chromosome. The Kell (K) antigen is present in less than 10% of the population but is very immunogenic, so that the incidence of anti-K antibodies is high in the transfused K-negative population. The antibodies of the K system are IgG antibodies and can cause transfusion reactions and HDN.

Duffy antigens. There are five antigens of which Fy^a and Fy^b are the most important. The antibodies are IgG antibodies and can activate complement causing intravascular haemolysis, resulting in transfusion reactions and HDN.

Kidd antigens. Although weakly immunogenic they produce IgG antibodies which can cross the placental membrane, activate complement, and cause intravascular haemolysis and HDN. Kidd antibodies may be undetectable in pretransfusion compatibility testing, yet sensitized patients can have an anamnestic (anamnesis: the recalling of things past) response at the time of transfusion resulting in a severe delayed haemolytic reaction.

Lewis antigens (Le^a and Le^b). These are present in plasma and are passively absorbed onto the red cell membrane. The antibodies to this system are IgM antibodies and do not cross the placenta to cause HDN. Lewis antibodies are a common cause of incompatibility in ABO matched blood but rarely cause haemolysis as they are not usually reactive at 37°C.

Other blood group antigens. Antigens like those of the MN system give rise to IgM antibodies which are usually only reactive below body temperature and are therefore not clinically significant.

Blood group	Genotype	Frequency (UK) %	Red cell antigen	Serum antibody	Compatible donor blood
A	AA or AO	42	A	Anti-B	A or O
B	BB or BO	8	B	Anti-A	B or O
AB	AB	3	AB	–	AB, A, B or O
O	OO	47	–	Anti-A, B	O only

Table 4.3 The antigens and antibodies of the ABO blood group system

Note: If the patient's blood group is not known, the only blood which may be given is group O. However, never transfuse without compatibility testing unless in extreme emergency.

BLOOD TRANSFUSION

Acute haemolytic transfusion reactions due to ABO incompatibility can be fatal and are most often caused by *errors in identification of the patient at the time of blood sampling or blood administration*. Prior to transfusion the indication must be recorded in the case notes and it is the clinician's responsibility to prescribe the blood and fill out the request form. It is crucial that the patient's identity is established verbally (if this is possible) *and* by checking the patient identification band before blood is taken, and that the sample is labelled fully before leaving the bedside. The blood request form should be clearly and accurately completed, providing the patient's full name, date of birth, and hospital number (each patient must have a unique identification number). This is absolutely essential for emergency admissions who might otherwise be unidentified. In an emergency, the laboratory must be told the quantity of blood needed as soon as possible. In extreme emergency it may be necessary to use Group O Rh(D)-negative blood, although the amount given should not exceed 2 units as the laboratory can normally provide ABO and Rh(D)-compatible blood within 15 minutes of receiving a blood sample.

Compatibility testing

Two major forms of pretransfusion testing are available.

Type and screen involves determining the patient's ABO and Rh(D) type and screening a sample of serum against a panel of red cells of known phenotype for the presence of clinically significant antibodies. The sample is then held for up to 7 days, and if blood is needed it can be provided within 10–15 minutes after rapidly excluding ABO incompatibility. Thus, operations known to require blood transfusion infrequently can be covered without having to keep blood aside for a patient when it is unlikely to be needed.

Crossmatching normally takes about an hour and involves not only typing and screening, but direct testing of the patient's serum for compatibility with red cells taken from the units of blood to be transfused. If the patient has an antibody, its specificity for a particular antigen is determined using a panel of red cells of known phenotype. Once the antibody(ies) has been identified, donor blood is screened and only units negative for the offending antigen(s) can be issued. This process may take

several hours depending on the population incidence of the antigen(s) in question. Cross-matched units are then allocated to the individual patient and held in reserve for 48 hours. If blood is transfused, fresh samples must be provided if additional blood is needed after 48 hours.

Time may not be available in an emergency situation for full cross-matching. Samples can be rapidly ABO and Rh typed and compatible blood released after a rapid test of ABO compatibility while the antibody screen is ongoing. The transfusion form will state that the blood has been released following such a rapid test. If an antibody is discovered subsequently, the ward is notified immediately and full compatibility testing is undertaken.

Blood administration

The transfusion laboratory issues blood with a compatibility report stating the patient's full name, ABO and Rh(D) type, and the unique number of the blood transfusion. The group of each unit is stated with its pack number. Each unit has a compatibility label attached which states the patient's full name, date of birth, hospital number, patient blood group and Rhesus type. The unique donation number and expiry date are also given on each pack.

Before commencing transfusion, the following details must be checked by two individuals, at least one of whom must be a State Registered Nurse (SRN) or medical officer:

- *Full patient identity* on the patient wristband,

Pretransfusion testing
- *Type and screen* determines ABO, Rh(D) status and antibody screen. The sample is then normally held for 7 days thereafter. Compatible blood can be available within 10–15 minutes if needed.

- *Crossmatching* involves typing and screening followed by direct testing of the patient's serum for compatibility with red cells of units to be transfused:
  - normally takes 1 hour but can take several
  - crossmatched units held for 48 hours
  - process has to be repeated if any of the reserved blood is used and further transfusion is deemed necessary.

- *Emergency crossmatching* means rapid ABO and Rh typing with release of 'compatible' blood after checking ABO compatibility and while the antibody screen continues.

compatibility label on the unit of blood and accompanying report form

- ABO and Rh(D) type on the pack, compatibility label and report form
- Donation number on the pack, label and report form
- Expiry date of the pack
- Examination of the pack to ensure that there are no leaks or haemolysis.

If there are any discrepancies, the blood must not be transfused and the laboratory must be informed immediately. If there are no discrepancies, the compatibility form is signed by the person administering the blood and the person checking the documentation. The form is then placed in the casenotes and a copy returned to the blood transfusion laboratory.

Before blood is administered, the pulse rate, blood pressure and temperature should be recorded. Transfusion must be commenced within 30 minutes of removing the blood from the refrigerator and the transfusion of each unit should be completed within 4 hours. The blood is given through a standard administration set containing an in-line filter (170 μm). The set may be primed with 0.9% saline but nothing should be added to the blood. The giving set is flushed with 0.9% saline after each unit has been given. The patient must be observed closely during the first 15 minutes as this is when transfusion reactions are most likely. Pulse rate and temperature are measured every 15 minutes for 1 hour, and hourly thereafter if the patient remains stable. It is advisable to maintain a fluid balance chart in patients having blood transfusions, and pulse rate, temperature and blood pressure should be recorded once transfusion has been completed.

Adverse effects of transfusion

Acute haemolytic transfusion reactions

These potentially lethal reactions are most often due to ABO incompatibility with activation of complement and intravascular haemolysis. Procedural failure such as inadequate identification checks or clerical errors are the major problem; such mistakes are reported in 1/1000–1/2000 transfusions and in reality must be more frequent. The reaction commonly begins very shortly after starting transfusion and even a few millilitres of incompatible blood can be fatal. The patient experiences distress, pain at the infusion site, flushing, abdominal pain and breathlessness. Hypotension ensues with haemoglobinuria, disseminated intravascular coagulation and oliguria leading to acute renal failure.

If an acute haemolytic reaction is suspected *the transfusion must be stopped immediately* and the blood replaced with saline until the situation is fully understood. The next steps in management are outlined in Table 4.4.

Delayed haemolytic transfusion reaction

Patients previously immunized to red cell antigens by transfusions or pregnancy can have antibody levels that are too low to be detected by pretransfusion screening. However, antibody concentrations may rise rapidly in response if the antigen is again transfused and within a few days can attain levels that destroy the transfused cells. The patient presents some 5–10 days later with fever, haemoglobinuria and a falling haemoglobin level. Such delayed reactions occur once every 500 transfusions

Table 4.4 Management of suspected haemolytic transfusion reaction	
Investigation	Therapy

• Double check the labelling of the blood unit with the patient's ID band and with any other identifiers
• Take 30 ml of blood for laboratories
  'Blood Bank' (5 ml anticoagulated)
             (5 ml clotted)
  Biochemistry (10 ml electrolytes)
  Coag Lab (10 ml coagulation screen)
• ECG — evidence of hyperkalaemia
 	
• Arrange repeat coagulation screens
  and biochemistry every 2–4 hours
	• Stop infusion and keep line open with saline but avoid overhydration initially (see 6)
	• Catheterize bladder and monitor urine flow
	• Give frusemide 150 mg i.v.
	• Give saline 100–200 ml
	• Give PPF or saline for replacement
	• If urine flow 2 h after frusemide is < 100 ml/h assume acute renal failure and obtain specialist help
	• If urine flow > 100 ml/h adjust infusion rate to maintain this
	• If hyperkalaemic, start glucose/insulin or resonium A therapy
	• If DIC, give blood product support (platelets and cryoprecipitate) and heparinization may be indicated (5000 units stat i.v. then infuse 1500 unit/h for 6–24 h)
	• If patient needs transfusion use rematched blood. There is no increased risk of a second haemolytic reaction

and the Kidd, Duffy and Rhesus antibodies are commonly implicated. The reaction is seldom fatal but can cause significant morbidity in a patient who is already ill.

Febrile non-haemolytic transfusion reaction

Transfusion-associated fever and rigors are common, especially in patients who have had multiple transfusions or pregnancies. White cell antibodies in the recipient plasma reacting with the donor leucocytes are responsible. The reaction occurs late in the transfusion and is usually mild. Severe reactions may mimic the early stages of acute haemolytic transfusion reaction and it is wise to stop the transfusion until a haemolytic reaction has been excluded. Febrile reactions normally respond to an antipyretic such as paracetamol (500–1000 mg). Recurrent febrile reactions can be unpleasant for the patient and washed red cells or a white cell filter may be needed.

Alloimmunization

Although blood is usually only cross-matched in respect of ABO and Rh(D) antigens, any antigen can give rise to antibodies. This is seldom significant in a surgical patient receiving a single episode of transfusion, but can be catastrophic in a female of childbearing age as such antibodies can cause HDN.

Platelets also have specific antigen systems which can give rise to antibodies and cause the rare condition of post-transfusion purpura. The patient develops severe thrombocytopenia and haemorrhage some 10 days after transfusion. There is a significant risk of intracranial haemorrhage, and high-dose intravenous immunoglobulin or intensive plasma exchange should be considered.

Allergic reactions

Urticaria or itch within minutes of starting transfusion can result from plasma protein reactions. These reactions are occasionally severe and constitute anaphylaxis, particularly in patients with IgA deficiency who have developed antibodies against IgA. Mild reactions respond to an antihistamine alone (e.g. chlopheniramine 10 mg given slowly i.v.) but anaphylactic reactions require urgent therapy. Transfusion is stopped immediately although intravenous fluids are continued. Oxygen is given and adrenaline (0.5–1 mg, i.e. 0.5–1.0 ml of a 1/1000 solution) is administered intravenously, the dose being repeated if necessary. Chlorpheniramine is also prescribed (see above) and a salbutamol nebulizer may be helpful. If the patient does not respond promptly, specialist help is summoned urgently.

Cardiac failure

Fluid overload is common in blood transfusion, particularly in patients with chronic anaemia (who have increased plasma volume) or cardiac dysfunction. It presents as acute left ventricular failure and is treated as such. The problem can be prevented by giving frusemide (20 mg orally or 40 mg i.v.) with alternate units of blood.

Iron overload

This is a risk in patients needing regular transfusion for chronic disease such as thalassaemia or myelodysplasia. Each unit of blood contains 200 mg of iron, and as only 1 mg is excreted daily, a positive balance is easily created. Iron accumulates in the liver, heart, and endocrine organs. Daily chelation therapy (with desferrioxamine) helps to increase excretion.

Graft versus host reaction

This rare complication follows transfusion of viable lymphocytes into an immunocompromised host. It presents 1–4 weeks later with fever, a desquamating rash, abnormal liver function and neutropenia, and has a mortality rate of 80%. It can be prevented by irradiating cellular blood components before transfusion.

Transfusion-associated lung injury

Donor plasma very occasionally contains antibodies which react with the recipient's leucocytes. The patient develops acute breathlessness, fever and chills, the chest X-ray shows nodular infiltration of the hilum and lower lung fields, and assisted ventilation may be needed.

Immune modulation

Blood transfusion may alter the immune system in ways that are not yet clear. Some retrospective studies have shown higher rates of postoperative infection and tumour recurrence in transfused cohorts, although the significance of these reports is still debated. While it is clear that no patient should be transfused unnecessarily, it is equally certain that no one should be allowed to exsanguinate because of these concerns.

Infection and blood transfusion

Although plasma fractions are now treated to inactivate viruses, blood components such as red cells and platelets cannot yet be treated in this way (virus inactivated plasma is now becoming available). However, successive improvements in donor selection and virological screening of donated blood have greatly reduced the risks of transfusion-transmitted infection.

Hepatitis B

All donations in the UK are screened for hepatitis B surface antigen (HBsAg). Occasionally, hepatitis B may be transmitted when the donor is in the early stages of infection and there is not enough antigen to be detected. In future, testing for antibody to the hepatitis B core may reduce this risk.

Hepatitis C

All UK donations are tested for anti-HCV antibody. Roughly 3 in every 10 000 donors test positive and they commonly have a history of drug abuse. The long-term consequences of possessing the antibody are not known but the donor is removed from the blood register.

Human immunodeficiency virus I and II

Infection is detected at a rate of about 0.13/10 000 donors in the UK. Transmission of the virus may still occur in the early phases of the disease when antibody levels are too low to be detected. The estimated risk of transmitting the virus by a blood transfusion in the UK is estimated at 0.1/10 000 units transfused.

Cytomegalovirus

Some 50% of UK donors are positive for antibody to this infection. CMV can cause problems if transmitted to immunocompromised patients and neonates, so that such patients who are CMV negative should receive only CMV-negative blood. A white cell filter can be used if CMV-negative products are not available as the infection is only transmitted by white cells.

Treponemal infection

Donors are screened for this infection. Infectivity of units containing *Treponema pallidum* declines abruptly during storage of blood at 2–6°C.

Bacterial infection

Blood is occasionally contaminated during collection and storage, and is occasionally collected from a bacteraemic donor. Sudden collapse during transfusion is mediated by endotoxin and can be misdiagnosed as an acute haemolytic reaction. Samples should be taken from the patient and the unit of blood for bacteriological culture, and broad-spectrum antibiotics commenced.

Malaria

Donor selection in the UK should prevent potentially infectious units from being donated.

Autologous transfusion

Since immunological and infective complications can result from donated blood, use of the patient's own blood may be considered in certain situations.

Infection and transfusion of blood and blood products

- Risk of infection still exists although it has declined with greater awareness of risks, improved screening, better methods of decontamination, and more judicious use of blood and blood products.

- Risk of viral transmission (hepatitis B, C and HIV) has diminished with routine screening but virus infection may escape detection in the early stages when levels of antigen or antibody are still low. The estimated risk of HIV transmission in the UK is 0.1/10 000 units transfused.

- CMV infection is transmitted by white blood cells. Approximately 50% of UK donors test positive for CMV antibody. CMV-negative blood is used to avoid transmitting infection to transplant recipients and premature infants.

Pre-operative donation

Blood can be withdrawn from otherwise fit patients awaiting elective surgery and stored for up to 35 days. Assuming that the haemoglobin concentration is adequate before withdrawal of each unit, up to 5 units of the patient's own blood can be made available. Sepsis and severe myocardial disease are absolute contraindications to autologous transfusion, and problems may arise if the operation has to be postponed. Autologous units undergo the same testing as allogeneic donations, including the pretransfusion compatibility test, and their use is restricted to the donor.

Isovolaemic haemodilution

Up to 1.5 litres of blood can be withdrawn into anticoagulant before induction of anaesthesia and replaced by saline. The fall in haematocrit reduces the loss of red cells (and haemoglobin) during surgical bleeding while maintaining optimal tissue perfusion. The withdrawn blood can be re-infused during surgery or postoperatively.

Cell salvage

Blood can be collected from the operation site by suction, processed by a cell salvage machine in which it is anticoagulated while the cells are washed, and then returned to the patient. The process is contraindicated in patients with malignancy or sepsis, and is only appropriate when there is substantial blood loss.

Long-term storage

Although the facility is expensive, autologous units from patients with exceptionally rare blood types can be cryopreserved and stored for long periods.

Specific transfusion problems

Rapid transfusion of large volumes of blood

Massive transfusion denotes the transfusion of the equivalent of the circulating blood volume within a 24-hour period (i.e. 10–12 units in an adult). It is needed most often in severe trauma and in bleeding due to gastrointestinal or obstetric disorders. Although massive transfusion restores circulating blood volume and oxygen-carrying capacity, it is frequently complicated by coagulopathy, particularly in patients with an underlying disorder such as liver disease or DIC. The following problems may complicate massive blood transfusion.

Thrombocytopenia. Stored blood contains no functional platelets and consumption and dilution of the patient's own platelets is anticipated in conditions needing massive transfusion. Platelet counts should be kept above $50 \times 10^9/1$ by platelet transfusion. Oozing from venepuncture sites and mucous membranes is a good indication of thrombocytopenia in these circumstances and platelets should not be witheld while a platelet count is awaited.

Coagulation factor deficiency. Stored blood contains little factor V and VIII but has all other factors in amounts adequate for haemostasis. Red cell concentrates and supplemented red cells provide only small amounts of coagulation factors. Dilutional deficiency occurs during blood transfusion, but coagulopathy is more often due to DIC caused by the underlying condition. When tests of the intrinsic and extrinsic coagulation pathways (prothrombin time or INR; and partial thromboplastin time (PTT) respectively) show values greater than 1.5 times control levels and/or a low fibrinogen count (<0.8 g/l), FFP and cryoprecipitate (10–15 ml/kg) should be used as replacement therapy.

Hypocalcaemia. Citrate used as an anticoagulant binds ionized calcium and can lower plasma calcium levels. The liver normally metabolizes citrate rapidly so that this is only a problem in neonates, those with liver disease, and when blood is being infused more rapidly than 100 ml/min. If the electrocardiogram (ECG) shows changes of hypocalcaemia (prolonged QT interval), 5 ml of calcium gluconate should be infused over 5 minutes, the dose being repeated if the ECG remains abnormal.

Hyperkalaemia and hypokalaemia. Red cell degeneration during storage increases the plasma potassium concentration, and rapid transfusion of large volumes of stored blood can cause hyperkalaemia. This may result in cardiotoxicity, particularly in patients with renal failure, hypothermia or extensive muscle damage. After transfusion, red cells normalize their Na/K equilibrium rapidly so that hypokalaemia then becomes the more common problem.

Hypothermia. Rapid transfusion of blood at 4°C lowers core temperature, and in conjunction with other metabolic changes, can cause cardiac arrest. A blood warmer must be used when the transfusion rate exceeds 50 ml/kg/hour in adults and 15 ml/kg/hour in children.

Adult respiratory distress syndrome (ARDS). The risk of developing ARDS is minimized if tissue perfusion is maintained, hypotension is corrected rapidly, and overtransfusion is avoided. Microaggregate filters are indicated when large volumes of stored blood (>7 days) are being transfused or the patient has pre-existing lung disease.

Cardiopulmonary bypass

Platelets and coagulation factors may be activated or lost during extracorporeal circulation during cardiopulmonary bypass at open heart surgery (see Ch. 24), so that FFP and platelet transfusion may be needed to deal with postoperative bleeding. Heparin is used during bypass to prevent clotting in the extracorporeal circuit and is neutralized when surgery is completed. Late onset bleeding (6 hours postoperatively) has been ascribed to heparin leaching out of the tissues and is dealt with by neutralization with protamine. The antifibrinolytic drug, aprotinin, is now used in cardiac surgery to negate the fibrinolytic effect of bypass.

Autoimmune haemolytic anaemia (AIHA)

In this condition, an autoantibody binds to the red cell causing its removal from the circulation. Transfusion is avoided if at all possible in patients with AIHA so as not to stimulate further autoantibody production. Obtaining compatible blood for AIHA patients is difficult as the patient's cells are coated with antibody and during cross-matching, free serum antibody binds to the donor cells giving a false indication of 'incompatibility'. Even more important is the difficulty of identifying potentially significant alloantibodies as these are masked by autoantibody. In such cases the clinician must give a clear indication of the urgency of transfusion as blood may have to be issued before all tests are complete.

In normal transfusion practice, antigen-negative blood is issued if an alloantibody is identified. In the case of AIHA blood, serum of the same major antigen systems as the recipient (i.e. Rhesus and Kell) is issued so that the blood is at least genotype specific. The transfusion slip will indicate that these units are the 'least incompatible' with the patient. Although these units are transfused with special care, serious problems are in fact rare. However, the transfused cells have a reduced half-life.

METHODS OF REDUCING THE NEED FOR BLOOD TRANSFUSION

Non-plasma colloid volume expanders

Solutions of large molecules such as Dextran (see Table 4.5) are an inexpensive colloidal alternative to plasma in first-line management of volume-depleted patients. Anaphylactic reactions are rare and the products carry no risk of viral transmission. Hydroxy-ethyl starch (HES) increases red cell sedimentation rate and can cause difficulty in grouping and compatibility testing, while HES and Dextrans can interact with factor VIII when given in large doses.

In the initial resuscitation of patients with haemorrhagic shock, the adequacy of volume replacement is

---

Massive blood transfusion
- This is defined as the transfusion of the equivalent of the circulating blood volume within a 24-hour period (in practice 10–12 units in an adult).

- Common indications for massive blood transfusion are major trauma, gastrointestinal bleeding and obstetric complications.

- Major problems associated with massive blood transfusion include:
  - underlying coagulopathy
  - thrombocytopenia (stored blood has no platelets)
  - lack of coagulation factors V and VIII
  - hyperkalaemia (although hypokalaemia may develop as transfused red cells normalize their Na/K equilibrium)
  - hypothermia (risk reduced by use of blood warmers).

Table 4.5 Non-plasma colloid volume expanders

Product	Source	Concentration of solution	Average molecular weight	Intravascular persistence	Frequency of acute reactions
Hydroxy-ethyl starch (HES)	Maize starch, chemically modified	6%	450 000 or 265 000	Similar to or longer than Dextran 70	0.1/10 000
Dextran 70	Bacterial product	6%	70 000	50 % of infused volume persists 8 hours	1.5/10 000
Dextran 40	Bacterial product	10%	40 000	Shorter than Dextran 70	0.7/10 000
Urea-bridged gelatin (Haemaccel)	Heat-degraded cattle bone gelatin	3–4%	35 000	50% of infused volume persists 4–5 hours	14/10 000

Data from reviews, Swisher & Petz (1981).

usually of much greater importance than the choice of fluid. A reasonable regimen in adults is 1000 ml of crystalloid (0.9% saline or Ringer lactate solution) followed by 1000 ml of colloid, and then replacement with red cells. In the elderly and those with cardiac impairment, red cell replacement is started earlier to maintain oxygen-carrying capacity without causing fluid overload.

1-desamino-8-D-arginine vasopressin (DDAVP)

This drug releases high molecular weight multimers of factor VIII from endothelial cells when given by slow intravenous infusion (4–5 μg/kg). It can be used as an alternative to blood products in mild to moderate haemophilia A, von Willebrand's disease, and bleeding associated with chronic renal disease. It is usually well tolerated although caution is needed in the elderly with myocardial disease.

Aprotinin

This protease inhibitor exerts an antifibrinolytic effect, inhibiting plasmin, kallikrein and activated protein C. Its use is established in cardiac surgery and it is being assessed in liver transplantation and orthopaedic surgery. Acute allergic effects have been described with repeated dosing, and a prothrombotic tendency may occur.

Fibrin sealant

Such sealants mimic the final stage in the coagulation cascade in which fibrinogen is converted to fibrin in the presence of thrombin, factor XIII, fibronectin and ionized calcium. Freeze-dried steril-ized fibrinogen, fibronectin and factor XIII can be delivered from one barrel of a double-barrelled syringe while thrombin, calcium and aprotinin are delivered from the other. If the two mixtures meet at a surgical bleeding site, the solution clots almost immediately, the clot resolving over a period of days. Fibrin glue has been used in vascular, cardiac and liver surgery and in situations where even small amounts of bleeding can be problematic (e.g. middle ear surgery). The product is *not* for intravenous use.

Future developments

The risk of viral transmission has undoubtedly resulted in the more judicious use of blood and the development of more stringent transfusion policies. Products are being developed continually which can undergo some form of sterilization, and virally inactivated plasma is undergoing clinical trials at present.

Recombinant growth factors are making an increasing impact on blood requirements. For example, recombinant human erythropoietin raises haemoglobin levels in patients with chronic renal failure, while granulocyte/macrophage-colony stimulating factor is undergoing trial as a means of stimulating a granulocyte response in congenital or chemotherapy-induced marrow aplasia.

Although haemoglobin substitutes are being sought actively, no cell free haemoglobin solution is as yet licensed for clinical use. However, there is every expectation that transfusion therapy will be supplanted increasingly by the use of synthetic or biologically engineered substitutes. Until this occurs, administration of human blood products will be required and must be practised responsibly.

5

Nutritional support in surgical patients

CONTENTS

Many patients admitted to hospital or coming to surgery have nutritional disorders. This is particularly true of patients with gastrointestinal disease, underlying malignancy, serious infection, and major injury. Some are admitted with a disease which has caused the nutritional disorder, while others develop nutritional upset during treatment of a disease not normally associated with malnutrition. It is a disturbing fact that the risk of developing a nutritional disorder increases the longer a patient stays in hospital.

Although minor degrees of protein and calorie malnutrition do not appear to affect the outcome of surgery, there is no doubt that major nutritional disorders jeopardize recovery by impairing wound healing, lowering resistance to infection, and prolonging recovery. It is, however, difficult to quantify risk for the individual patient.

Nutritional disorders in surgical practice have two principal components. Firstly, *starvation* can be caused by the effects of the disease, restriction of oral intake, or both. Secondly, there are the *metabolic effects of inflammation*, namely increased catabolism and reduced anabolism. These cause a kwashiorkor-like effect with a low serum albumin concentration, muscle wasting and water retention. While malnutrition may be the result of starvation, in most surgical patients it results from a combination of the two components.

Assessment of nutritional status

Although most patients undergoing surgery, including those with minor degrees of nutritional disorder, can withstand 3–4 days of starvation without obvious detriment, early detection and correction of progressive malnutrition is vital if recovery is not to be jeopardized or delayed.

There are many ways to detect protein-calorie malnutrition, ranging from anthropometry (i.e. body measurements) to the use of isotopic tracers to measure body compartments. Much valuable information can be obtained from simple indices such as:

- Recent unintentional weight loss of 10% or more
- Body weight less than 80% of ideal for height
- Serum albumin less than 30 g/litre
- Total lymphocyte count below 1.2×10^9/litre
- Mid-arm muscle circumference less than 80% of value in comparable population.

It must be stressed that these changes can be difficult to interpret, particularly in the short term, because of confounding factors such as water retention.

Normal nutritional requirements

The recommended daily basal requirements for adults are shown in Table 5.1. Even after quite major surgical procedures, these requirements change little. However, if complications such as ileus or abdominal sepsis develop, catabolism increases and energy requirements rise. Following burns and major injuries, the metabolic requirements increase dramatically from the moment of injury (Table 5.2).

Nutritional requirements are usually estimated from those of normal individuals, taking into account the patient's clinical condition. Energy requirements can be estimated more accurately by

Table 5.1 Recommended daily requirements of water, electrolytes and nutrition

	Per kg body weight	Per 70-kg patient
Water (ml)	35	2450
Non-protein calories	30	2100
Carbohydrate (g)	2.0	140
Fat (g)	3.0	210
Protein (g)	0.7	50
Nitrogen (g)	0.1	7
Sodium (mmol)	1.0	70
Potassium (mmol)	1.0	70
Vitamin B (mg)	0.5	35
Vitamin C (mg)	1.0	70

Table 5.2 Average daily requirements of nitrogen and energy in different metabolic states

Metabolic state	Nitrogen (g/70 kg)	Energy (kcal/70 kg)
Normal	7–9	2000
Starvation	9	1500
Moderate injury	15	2200
Hypercatabolic (e.g. multiple injury, burns)	up to 30	up to 3000

measuring resting energy expenditure by indirect calorimetry (i.e. measuring oxygen consumption and carbon dioxide output). Protein requirements are calculated from urinary nitrogen excretion over a 24-hour period.

Causes of inadequate intake

The ideal way for a surgical patient to take in enough nutrients is for him to eat and drink palatable food. This may not be possible for a number of reasons. The patient may be too weak and anorexic, or have a mechanical problem such as obstruction of the gastrointestinal tract. Patients with increased metabolic demands may have some difficulty in taking sufficient food to meet these demands.

Some patients suffer from what is best described as 'intestinal failure', i.e. a state in which the amount of functioning gut is reduced below a level where it can digest and absorb enough food to nourish the patient. The four principal causes of intestinal failure are:

1. The *short bowel syndrome* which results from massive small bowel resection.
2. *Fistula formation*, in which bowel content is lost externally or short-circuited (internal fistula) before it can be adequately digested and absorbed.

3. *Motility disorders* such as paralytic ileus and chronic intestinal pseudo-obstruction.
4. Extensive *small bowel disease* such as Crohn's disease.

In these difficult cases, specialized nutritional treatment is required if the patient is to remain normally nourished. As a general rule, nutritional treatment is not effective in the presence of active sepsis. The priority in such patients is to eliminate sepsis but attempts must be made to minimize negative nitrogen and calorie balance. The use of exogenous growth hormone, insulin and anabolic steroids has been proposed in this context but has found little application in clinical practice.

Methods of providing nutritional support

Nutrients can be given via the gastrointestinal tract, i.e. enteral nutrition, or intravenously, i.e. parenteral nutrition. Parenteral nutrition is indicated only when enteral feeding is not feasible. Very few patients are not suitable for some form of enteral feeding. Certainly all those who have a normal length of functioning gastrointestinal tract, and most of those who have a reduced amount, can be fed by this route. Furthermore, ingestion of even suboptimal amounts of diet may help to maintain the integrity of the intestinal mucosa, thereby reducing the absorption of endotoxins which may compound the metabolic upset in such patients.

Nutritional status
- Nutrition in surgical patients may be adversely affected by starvation (effects of disease such as oesophageal cancer, restricted intake), effects of inflammation (increased catabolism) and the effects of the operation itself.

- Nutritional status is assessed by weight loss (>10% loss, <80% ideal weight), serum albumin, lymphocyte count and mid-arm muscle circumference.

- Four major surgical causes of intestinal failure are:
  - short bowel syndrome
  - fistula formation
  - motility disorders
  - extensive small bowel disease (e.g. Crohn's disease).

- Nutritional status may be improved by eliminating the source of catabolism (e.g. sepsis) or inadequate intake, by encouraging oral intake in those who can eat, and by considering enteral or parenteral support in those who cannot.

ENTERAL NUTRITION

The first approach is to try to get the patient to take an adequate diet by mouth. If this is prevented by swallowing difficulties, a tube can be passed so that enteral nutrition can be instituted using commercially available liquid feeds. A liquidized normal diet can be used in patients with swallowing difficulties but is unsuitable for tube feeding because it may introduce infection, block the feeding tube, and its nutrient composition is uncertain. In *supplemental feeding* the feed is drunk or infused at regular intervals to complement an otherwise inadequate food intake. *Total enteral nutrition* is indicated in patients who cannot eat or drink normally because of conditions such as those outlined in Table 5.3.

Composition of liquid enteral feeds

The main difference between the available enteral feeds is the way in which the energy and protein content are presented. Liquid whole-protein feeds are cheaper and more palatable than those based on oligopeptides and amino acids (the so-called elemental diets). Oligopeptides and amino acids are said to be better absorbed in patients with shortened or diseased bowel, but there is no evidence for this and the high osmotic load can produce intolerance.

The energy content of most liquid diets is provided in the form of glucose (or other oligosaccharides) or as medium-chain triglycerides such as those found in sunflower seed oil. Other essential nutrients such as electrolytes, minerals, trace metals and vitamins are present in varying amounts. Some feeds do not contain lactose and can be used in patients with lactose intolerance. An ideal nutritionally complete enteral regimen should supply 2000–3000 kcal of energy and 10–15 g of nitrogen a day in 2–3 litres of fluid. The proportion of energy provided by fat should be 30–40%.

Methods of administration of enteral feeds

Nasogastric or nasoenteric tubes

If the patient cannot drink or sip a liquid feed for mechanical reasons, or if he is unconscious or on a ventilator, the preparation can be given by a fine-bore nasogastric or nasoenteric tube. The position of the tube-tip should be checked radiologically, or by injecting air while auscultating over the epigastrium, before nutrients are infused. The tubes are now made of polyurethane or siliconized rubber and are well-tolerated for long periods with none of the risk of oesophageal ulceration or chest complications associated with large nasogastric tubes. Patients who need prolonged enteral feeding can learn to pass a fine-bore tube each evening and feed themselves overnight. When carried out at home this is known as 'ambulatory home enteral nutrition'.

Table 5.3   Conditions which may prevent patients from eating and drinking normally
• Unconsciousness
• Neurological dysphagia
• Inflammatory bowel disease
• Short bowel syndrome
• High intestinal fistula
• Post-traumatic weakness
• Postoperative weakness
• Postirradiation weakness
• Head and neck surgery
• Chemotherapy
• Burns

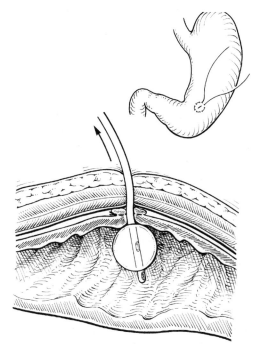

Fig. 5.1   Technique for creating a surgical gastrostomy for feeding purposes. The balloon catheter is inserted obliquely through the stomach wall. The stomach wall is sutured to the parietal peritoneum to avoid the risk of leakage.

Gastrostomy and jejunostomy

If nasogastric feeding is impossible because of disease or obstruction of the upper alimentary tract, nutrients may be given through a tube placed into the gastrointestinal tract below the lesion. Thus a patient with pseudobulbar palsy or an oesophageal fistula can be fed through a gastrostomy (Fig. 5.1), while a patient with a gastric or duodenal fistula can be fed through a jejunostomy.

Specially designed gastrostomy tubes can now be inserted by a combined percutaneous and endoscopic method, and are particularly valuable for prolonged feeding when there is no impairment of gastric emptying. Feeding jejunostomy tubes are more often inserted at the time of laparotomy when the surgeon anticipates that prolonged nutritional support will be needed postoperatively (e.g. patients undergoing oesophagectomy and gastrectomy, or necrosectomy for severe pancreatitis).

Enteral nutrition

- If the patient cannot eat adequate amounts of food, a tube can be used for supplemental or total enteral nutrition.
- Liquid whole-protein feeds are cheaper (and more palatable) than so-called elemental diets. Their energy content is provided in the form of glucose or medium-chain triglycerides, and appropriate amounts of electrolyte, trace metals and minerals, and vitamins are added.
- An ideal daily regimen supplies 2000–3000 kcal of energy and 10–15 g nitrogen in 2–3 litres of fluid.
- If a tube cannot be passed down the oesophagus, gastrostomy and jejunostomy feeding should be considered.
- The main complications of enteral feeding relate to patient tolerance (nausea, vomiting and diarrhoea) and to the insertion site if gastrostomy or jejunostomy is needed.

Complications of enteral nutrition

Just because enteral feeds are administered directly into the gastrointestinal tract, it cannot be assumed that they are free from complications (see Table 5.4). It is advisable to increase the rate of infusion gradually over several days within the limits of the patient's tolerance (e.g. first day 25 ml/h, second day 50 ml/h, third and subsequent days 100 ml/h). Complications can be minimized by careful monitoring and by close co-operation with the dietician.

PARENTERAL NUTRITION

Intravenous feeding is indicated when patients cannot be fed adequately by mouth, nasogastric tube or gastrostomy/jejunostomy, or when they have complete or partial intestinal failure. The problem

Table 5.4 Complications of enteral nutrition

- Gastric retention
- Aspiration
- Nausea and vomiting
- Abdominal cramps and distention
- Diarrhoea
- Gastroenteritis
- Dehydration
- Hyperosmolar coma
- Hyperglycaemia
- Tube displacement
- Leakage around gastrostomy/jejunostomy

may be permanent, as in most cases of the short bowel syndrome, or reversible, as in paralytic ileus or fistula formation. In some cases of short bowel syndrome, the remaining intestine 'adapts' by undergoing mucosal hyperplasia and normal feeding can resume.

Parenteral nutrition can provide the patient's total needs of protein, energy, electrolytes, trace metals and vitamins, i.e. total parenteral nutrition (TPN). The need to restrict volume means that concentrated solutions are used. As such solutions are irritant and thrombogenic, they have to be administered through catheters positioned in large high-flow veins such as the superior vena cava.

Indications for TPN

The chief indications are those already mentioned under 'intestinal failure'. Although pre-operative TPN has been advocated as a means of improving the condition of a patient prior to surgery, there is no good evidence that this affects outcome and there is no consensus regarding the duration of nutritional support. However, it is sensible to commence TPN in any patient with intestinal failure, as soon as the condition is diagnosed. In general, operative removal or eradication of the lesion causing the nutritional disorder is followed by more rapid recovery if nutritional support continues without interruption.

In contrast to pre-operative TPN, there is no doubt that postoperative TPN can be both effective and life-saving when complications develop, especially when these prevent enteral nutrition or are associated with infection. Situations in which TPN is invaluable include prolonged paralytic ileus, gross abdominal sepsis, and in dealing with the greatly increased metabolic demands which follow injury or burning.

TPN should continue until intestinal function has recovered sufficiently to allow nutrition to be maintained by the oral or enteral route. In cases of intestinal fistula, parenteral feeding is continued until the fistula has closed spontaneously or been closed surgically. When enteral nutrition cannot be resumed, the patient can be taught the necessary aseptic techniques to allow 'ambulatory' or 'home TPN'.

Composition of solutions for TPN

Carbohydrate solutions

Many forms of carbohydrate have been used but glucose is now considered to be the best energy source. Concentrations vary from 5–50%; the greater the concentration the more likely it is to be thrombogenic and precipitate diuresis and hyperosmolar problems. In some patients, especially those with infections, insulin has to be given simultaneously to ensure glucose utilization and avoid hyperglycaemia.

Fat solutions

Emulsions used in the United Kingdom are usually prepared from soya bean oil and are available in concentrations of 10% or 20%. They are non-thrombogenic, osmotically inert, and a valuable source of energy, providing 9 kcal/g. Thus, one litre of 20% fat emulsion with its emulsifier provides almost 2000 kcal. Patients with infection find it difficult to metabolize glucose and may need up to 50% of their energy requirement as fat, whereas those without infection may only need a weekly infusion. Fat emulsions are a useful means of reducing the total volume of fluid infused, provide essential fatty acids, and serve as a vehicle for administration of fat-soluble vitamins.

Amino acid solutions

Modern solutions are a mixture of synthetic L-amino acids (rather than protein hydrolysates) and provide between 7 and 17 g nitrogen/litre. There is no ideal formulation; most solutions contain a mixture of essential and non-essential amino acids

and have a composition similar to that of high-grade protein such as egg white.

Mixed TPN solutions

Although TPN can be provided by sequential or simultaneous administration of individual glucose, fat or amino acid solutions, it is now commoner and safer to mix the day's requirements in a 3-litre bag. The bag is made up in the pharmacy under sterile conditions, and its contents are infused over 12–24 hours using a simple infusion pump. To prevent wasteful use of glucogenic amino acids as a source of fuel (energy), non-protein calories must be given in sufficient quantities; the recommended ratio is 150–200 kcal of non-protein energy for every gram of nitrogen.

Fluid and electrolyte needs are also catered for. Many patients on TPN need additional water, sodium and potassium because of excess loss from, say, a high-output fistula. Trace elements and vitamins can also be incorporated and the demands created by infection and excessive loss must be met. An example of the way in which TPN needs are calculated is shown in Table 5.5.

Administration of TPN

Hypertonic solutions have to be infused into a vein with a high flow. Vascular access to the superior

---

Table 5.5 Calculation of composition of solution for total parenteral nutrition

Example: A 70-kg man with a high-output fistula from the duodenum requires intravenous feeding. The daily loss from the fistula is 800 ml of enteric content. He needs a regimen providing approximately:

- 2500 ml of water (normal daily requirement)
- 500 ml of water (partial replacement of fistula loss)
- 70 mmol of Na^+ (approximate normal daily requirement)
- 80 mmol of Na^+ (to replace fistula loss)
- 60 mmol of K^+ (approximate normal daily requirement)
- 40 mmol of K^+ (to replace fistula loss)
- 14 g of nitrogen; and
- 2200 kcal of energy

This can be provided in one 3-litre bag by mixing the following:

- 1 litre of amino acid solution containing 14 g nitrogen, 70 mmol Na^+ and 60 mmol K^+
- 1 litre of 30% glucose solution providing 1200 kcal of energy
- 0.5 litres of 20% lipid emulsion providing 1000 kcal of energy
- 0.5 litres of 0.9% saline containing 75 mmol Na^+ to which is added 40 mmol K^+, trace metals and vitamins

vena cava is normally obtained through the internal or external jugular, subclavian or cephalic vein. Although veins of the lower limb can, and occasionally have to be used, they are best avoided because of the higher risk of thrombosis and infection. The internal jugular vein is approached by direct puncture between the two heads of sternocleidomastoid, while the subclavian vein is punctured above or below the clavicle. The cephalic and external jugular veins are approached by direct cut-down; the former is entered in the deltopectoral groove while the latter is found just behind the sternocleidomastoid muscle. To allow patients greater mobility and to facilitate catheter care, the external portion of the catheter is usually run through a subcutaneous tunnel to emerge through the skin on the anterior chest wall.

Modern cannulae are made of silastic rubber or polyurethrane and are of fine bore. For longer-term feeding a fixed hub (Hickman) catheter is used; this type of catheter has a dacron cuff which secures it in the tunnel without the need for suture fixation. Before use, the position of the catheter-tip is checked radiologically. With good care, a correctly positioned cannula can remain in place for several months or years.

Complications of TPN

Catheter problems

Percutaneous insertion of a catheter may damage adjacent structures and can cause pneumothorax, air embolus and haematoma. Incorrect catheter positioning is excluded by taking a chest X-ray prior to commencing infusion. Sometimes the catheter-tip penetrates the vessel wall resulting in hydrothorax or hydromediastinum, complications which should be suspected if blood cannot be aspirated freely from the cannula. Careless handling of the catheter occasionally results in its fracture with embolization of the tip. The fragment can usually now be recovered by interventional radiological techniques.

Thrombophlebitis

Thrombosis is common when long lines are used, when the catheter tip is not in an area of high flow, and when very hypertonic solutions are infused. The tell-tale signs are redness and tenderness over the cannulated vein, together with swelling of the whole limb and engorgement of collateral veins if the thrombosis is more proximal. Occasionally, a superior mediastinal syndrome develops in patients with superior vena caval thrombosis (see p. 298).

If major vessel occlusion is suspected, the diagnosis is confirmed by venography and anticoagulation is commenced with heparin. If vascular access *has* to be maintained, an attempt can be made to lyse the clot with urokinase. If the clot cannot be dissolved, the cannula must be removed and a new cannula positioned in an unoccluded vein.

Infection

Infection and septicaemia are the most frequent complications of TPN. The usual offending organisms are coagulase -ve staphylococci, *Staphylococcus aureus*, and coliforms, but the incidence of fungal infection is increasing, possibly because many of the patients requiring TPN are also taking broad-spectrum antibiotics. Most catheter infections are the result of poor care of the feeding line. The insertion site must be protected with an occlusive dressing and should be cleaned on alternate days with an antiseptic agent. Drip tubing is changed daily, all connections are protected with a gauze swab soaked in antiseptic solution, and the line must *only* be used for infusion of nutrients and never for taking or giving blood or administering drugs. Great care is taken to avoid contamination when changing 3-litre bags. A Nutrition Support Nurse is invaluable in avoiding catheter sepsis and supervising all aspects of catheter care.

If a patient develops an unexplained pyrexia, the insertion site is inspected for redness and discharge. Blood is taken from a peripheral vein and from the catheter for culture. The catheter is flushed with a heparin-containing solution and feeding is discontinued. If the pyrexia resolves over 24 hours and the cultures are positive, this confirms catheter infection and the line is removed; a new cannula can be inserted after 48 hours to allow TPN to recommence. If there is continuing uncertainty as to the source of infection, intravenous feeding can be recommenced and cultures are taken again if pyrexia recurs. In centres with considerable experience of TPN, attempts are sometimes made to salvage infected lines by flushing them with antibiotic solutions, streptokinase, or absolute alcohol. It must be appreciated that these manoeuvres and the use of systemic antibiotics increase the risk of superinfection with resistant organisms and fungi.

Metabolic complications

An *osmotic diuresis* can result from renal overspill of hyperosmolar solutions. The problem is minimized by slowing the rate of infusion and using fat emulsions routinely in TPN. The urine is tested regularly for glycosuria and if this persists, blood glucose levels should be measured to determine whether the total amount of glucose should be reduced or insulin administered.

Rapid infusion of hypertonic glucose solutions can cause an *acute hyperosmolar syndrome*. This is managed by slowing the infusion and giving insulin. Too rapid cessation of glucose infusion may result in rebound hypoglycaemia. These complications are unusual if 3-litre bags are used and the rate of administration is controlled by an infusion pump.

Hyponatraemia can follow excessive administration of fluid and is avoided by careful monitoring of cumulative fluid balance and periodic measurements of urinary sodium. Potassium supplements are normally contraindicated in the immediate postoperative period (see Ch. 2) and may have to be withheld in catabolic patients. In the 'anabolic phase' following operation or injury, *hypokalaemia* is avoided by potassium supplementation.

Long-term TPN may lead to deficiencies in essential trace substances unless these are provided in adequate quantities. Specific deficiency syndromes are difficult to detect in ill patients. *Zinc deficiency* presents as a skin rash, while *folate deficiency* causes thrombocytopenia as well as anaemia. *Hypophosphataemia* may be a problem in patients receiving glucose only as an energy source; it is avoided by routine use of fat emulsions and provision of phosphate supplements.

Some patients have *sensitivity reactions* to individual components of the nutritional regimen, while others react adversely to overprovision of a particular nutrient. *Abnormal liver function* tests may be related to TPN, but more often signify occult or overt sepsis. Hepatomegaly is a rare result of excessive glucose provision.

Peripheral vein nutrition

Lipid emulsions and isotonic solutions of amino acids are available which are less irritant than conventional TPN solutions and which can be infused into peripheral veins. Such solutions can be used in the short term, but their prolonged use is associated with thrombophlebitis and conventional techniques should be employed if long-term support is needed. Peripheral catheters require the same level of care given to central catheters and the patients must still be monitored for signs of infection or metabolic complications.

Parenteral nutrition
- Parenteral feeding is indicated if the patient cannot be fed orally or enterally. Intestinal failure is the commonest indication.

- The need to restrict volume when using total parenteral nutrition (TPN) means that concentrated solutions are used which may be irritant and thrombogenic. TPN is therefore infused through catheters in high-flow veins (e.g. SVC).

- Glucose is now regarded as the best energy source and concentrations used vary from 5–50%. The higher concentrations are thrombogenic and may precipitate diuresis and hyperosmolar crisis.

- Fat emulsions are used in concentrations of 10–20%. They are a valuable energy source (9 kcal/g), osmotically inert and non-thrombogenic.

- L-amino acids can be used to provide a nitrogen intake of 7–17 g/litre and a mixture of essential and non-essential amino acids is employed.

- The major problems of TPN include complications related to catheter insertion (pneumothorax, air embolus and bleeding), thrombophlebitis, infection and septicaemia, and metabolic complications (e.g. hyperosmolar syndrome, hyponatraemia, hypokalaemia, deficiency syndromes, sensitivity reactions and abnormal liver function).

MONITORING OF NUTRITIONAL SUPPORT

Patients receiving nutritional support are monitored to detect deficiency states, assess adequacy of energy and protein provision, and anticipate complications. Patients receiving enteral feeding require less intense monitoring, but are prone to the same metabolic complications as patients who are fed intravenously.

Pulse rate, blood pressure and temperature are recorded regularly, an accurate fluid balance chart is maintained (remembering not to overlook insensible losses), and the urine is checked daily for glycosuria. Body weight is measured twice weekly. Anthropometry is used to monitor fat stores (triceps skinfold thickness) and lean body mass (mid-arm muscle circumference). Other methods which are not employed routinely include measurement of grip strength (dynamometry) and body compartments by isotopic tracers. Bioelectrical impedance analysis is a bedside technique in which the body's resistance and reactance to an electric current can be used to measure total body water, and hence lean body mass and fat stores.

Serum urea and electrolytes are measured daily, as are blood glucose levels if there is glycosuria. Full blood count, liver function tests, and serum albumin, calcium, magnesium and phosphate are monitored once or twice weekly. Urine is collected over one or two 24-hour periods each week to measure sodium and nitrogen losses. To maintain positive nitrogen balance, nitrogen intake should exceed daily losses by at least 2 g.

6

Investigation and diagnosis of surgical problems

CONTENTS

The diagnostic process in surgical patients is identical to that used in other branches of medicine; a history is taken, the patient is examined, and a differential diagnosis is compiled. Investigations are then planned which will lead to a definitive diagnosis and treatment plan. The length and complexity of the process depends on the nature of the presenting problem. For example, in a patient with a sebaceous cyst it might be confined to a brief history, local examination of the lesion, and if the cyst is to be removed under local anaesthesia, no specific investigations may be indicated. On the other hand, a patient with long-standing abdominal pain will probably require a comprehensive history and examination, and sufficient investigations to justify admission.

Investigation of a surgical patient represents a balance. If medico-legal considerations are uppermost the patient may be over-investigated with unnecessary investigations leading to discomfort, risk and expense. If cost considerations are paramount the patient may be under-investigated. When there is doubt about the need for an investigation, the question should be asked 'how will this investigation influence the patient's management?' If management will not be affected then the investigation is probably unnecessary. Investigations may also be needed to monitor a disease and response to therapy, as for example when endoscopy is used to monitor the response of a gastric ulcer to medical treatment.

EXAMINATION OF THE URINE

Routine analysis

Urinalysis using dipsticks is mandatory on admission and is often indicated when the patient is first seen in the outpatient clinic. Glycosuria may detect diabetes mellitus with its major implications for anaesthesia and surgery. Microscopic examination of the urine may help to define the cause of abdominal pain (e.g. pus cells in pyelonephritis, red cells or abnormal crystals in renal colic) and can monitor the progress of a disease and its response to treatment (e.g. red cell count as a reflection of recovery from renal injury, cast count in monitoring rejection of a kidney transplant).

Specific gravity

Urine specific gravity can be measured on one drop of urine using a portable refractometer. Despite its potential value (e.g. in distinguishing between oliguria caused by acute renal tubular failure and that caused by inadequate renal perfusion due to hypovolaemia), the test is seldom used. However, measurement of urine osmolality by freezing-point depression is used to estimate total solid concentration in patients with complex fluid and electrolyte problems.

24-hour collections

Such collections are occasionally indicated to measure the 24-hour excretion of particular substances, including the following:

- Creatinine to measure creatinine clearance as a test of renal function
- Electrolytes (Na^+, K^+, Cl^-) in the assessment of complex fluid and electrolyte disorders such as those due to intestinal fistula
- Calcium to detect hyperparathyroidism or monitor metastatic bone disease
- 11-hydroxycorticosteroids, 17-oxosteroids and oestrogens in the diagnosis of adrenal hyperactivity
- 3-methoxy-4-hydroxymandelic acid (VMA) in the diagnosis of phaeochromocytoma
- 5-hydroxyindoleacetic acid (5-HIAA) to diagnose and monitor the carcinoid syndrome
- Porphyrins to exclude porphyria as a cause of abdominal pain
- Amylase to estimate amylase clearance relative to creatinine in the diagnosis of acute pancreatitis.

EXAMINATION OF THE BLOOD

Venous blood is sampled for full blood count and urea and electrolyte concentrations in all patients having a procedure under general anaesthesia.

Haemoglobin concentration does not reflect the magnitude of acute haemorrhage, as compensatory haemodilution may not be complete for 48 hours. A patient admitted with acute haemorrhage and a low haemoglobin concentration has probably suffered chronic blood loss as well. As a general rule, patients should not undergo surgery unless the haemoglobin concentration exceeds 10 g/dl. Except in an emergency, anaemia of unknown origin should be investigated before surgery. Patients found to be anaemic because of blood loss will benefit from blood transfusion or a course of iron therapy before operation.

For all but minor operations, blood group should be determined. For more major procedures, each surgical service will have rules about the number of units of cross-matched blood that will be held in readiness on the day of surgery.

In patients treated by intravenous infusion and nasogastric aspiration, urea, sodium, potassium and bicarbonate concentrations should be measured daily. Patients with a history of jaundice should have liver function tests (serum bilirubin, aminotransferases, alkaline phosphatase and albumin) and should be screened for hepatitis B surface antigen (HBsAg). A positive HBsAg test indicates potential infectivity and the need to take precautions against spillage of, and contamination by, the patient's body fluids. Screening of patients suspected of being infected with human immunodeficiency virus (HIV) for HIV-antibodies can only be performed with the patient's consent.

Bioassays employing bacteria (e.g. determination of serum B_{12} and folate) are affected by antibiotics and should be deferred until the course of antibiotic therapy has been completed.

EXAMINATION OF THE STOOL

Examination of the abdomen is incomplete without digital rectal examination (Fig. 6.1), and any faeces on the examining glove should be inspected and tested immediately for the presence of occult blood using Haemoccult test cards.

Inspection of a stool sample is helpful in patients with diarrhoea. Slime (mucus) and blood point to an inflammatory process, clay-coloured stools to obstructive jaundice, and pale bulky or frothy stools to malabsorption. Microscopic examination is also indicated in diarrhoea and may reveal pus cells, trophozoites, cysts of *Entamoeba histolytica*, and worms such as *Giardia lamblia*. Undigested meat fibres point to malabsorption while there may be preponderance of coccal organisms in certain superinfections of the intestine. Bacteriological culture of the stool for enteric pathogens is essential in patients with diarrhoea.

BACTERIOLOGICAL INVESTIGATIONS

Bacteriological investigations are helpful in the following situations:

1. Direct smears and cultures of body fluids, tissues, exudates and excreta may provide evidence of infection. The bacteriological swab is an inefficient sampling device; if it is used it should be well loaded with material and sent to the laboratory without delay. Fragments of necrotic or devitalized tissue and specimens of frank pus in small bottles or capped syringes usually yield more useful information.

2. Determination of the type and antibiotic sensitivity of an infecting organism is necessary for rational antibiotic therapy. Ideally, antibiotics should

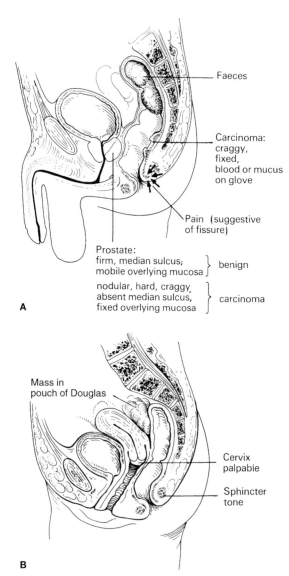

Faeces

Carcinoma:
craggy,
fixed,
blood or mucus
on glove

Pain (suggestive
of fissure)

Prostate:
firm, median sulcus;
mobile overlying mucosa } benign

nodular, hard, craggy,
absent median sulcus,
fixed overlying mucosa } carcinoma

A

Mass in
pouch of Douglas

Cervix
palpable

Sphincter
tone

B

Fig. 6.1 Possible findings on digital examination of the rectum. A Male; **B** female.

not be prescribed until sensitivities are known. When delay could be dangerous, the bacteriologist and clinician can select therapy on a 'best guess' basis, targeting the organism(s) thought most likely to be involved.

3. If a surgical unit develops a 'run' of postoperative infections, the bacteriologist can define precisely the organism responsible, determine its antibiotic sensitivities, and trace its source by examining medical and nursing staff and the ward and theatre environment. The source may prove to be an asymptomatic carrier, a faulty sterilizer or another patient

with sepsis. It is desirable to keep a daily record of the state of all surgical wounds in a designated 'wound book'.

4. Bacteraemia must always be considered as a possible cause of unexplained shock in a surgical patient. Serial blood samples are taken for culture. The ideal time of sampling relative to temperature elevations is still debated, but it is good practice to take one or two samples of blood for culture prior to beginning antibiotic therapy. The organism responsible is often a Gram-negative bacillus originating from the gut, biliary tree or urinary tract.

ENDOSCOPY

Endoscopy is the viewing of the interior of viscera or body cavities by instruments introduced through natural or created orifices. The first endoscopes were rigid, their passage was so uncomfortable that in some sites general anaesthesia was required, and the risk of trauma (e.g. oesophageal perforation during rigid oesophagoscopy) was significant. The development of flexible fibreoptic instruments in which light is transmitted by thousands of fine glass fibres, each coated with an opaque medium, has extended the scope, range and diagnostic accuracy of endoscopy, and now often allows therapeutic intervention. Fibreoptic endoscopes have controllable tips and their flexibility means that they can usually be passed with sedation alone (Fig. 6.2). Most fibreoptic endoscopes have facilities for irrigation and suction, tissue biopsy and photography.

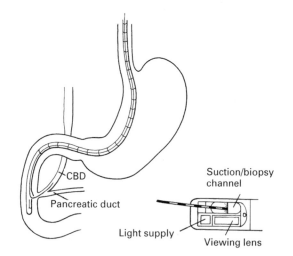

CBD

Pancreatic duct

Suction/biopsy
channel

Light supply

Viewing lens

Fig. 6.2 Endoscopic retrograde cannulation of the pancreatic and biliary ducts (ERCP). CBD=common bile duct.

Upper gastrointestinal tract

Gastroscopes are end-viewing instruments used to examine the oesophagus, stomach and proximal duodenum. The flexible tip means that the instrument can be passed into the stomach and then retroflexed through 180° to inspect the upper lesser curve, cardia and fundus of the stomach.

Gastroduodenoscopes are longer side-viewing instruments which can be negotiated through the pylorus to inspect the duodenum, cannulate the papilla of Vater and inject radio-opaque dye into the biliary tree and pancreatic duct system (i.e. endoscopic retrograde cholangiopancreatography (ERCP); see Fig. 6.3). This technique has been a major advance in the diagnosis and management of patients with biliary and pancreatic disease, especially those with biliary tract obstruction due to gallstones or malignancy. Cytological examination of bile and pancreatic juice may also assist the diagnosis of malignancy.

Choledochoscopes are slimmer endoscopes 3–4 mm in diameter which are used to inspect the interior of the bile ducts during operation and detect residual calculi. The instruments have a wide channel down which a 'stone catcher' can be passed to retrieve stones; the instrument can also be passed postoperatively down drain tracks to achieve the same purpose.

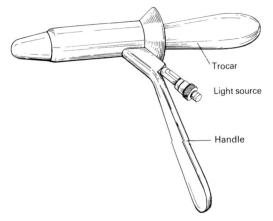

Fig. 6.4 Proctoscope.

Lower gastrointestinal tract

The *proctoscope* is a short instrument (10 cm) which is used to inspect the anal canal and lower rectum (Fig. 6.4). Haemorrhoids can be injected or banded, while carcinomas can be biopsied. Proctoscopy is normally undertaken with the patient lying in the left lateral position with the knees drawn up into the chest. It is always preceded by careful inspection of the perineum and digital rectal examination. The

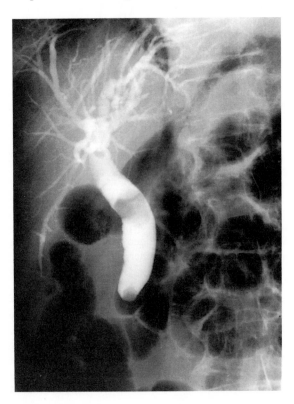

Fig. 6.3 Endoscopic retrograde cholangiopancreatography (ERCP) demonstrating multiple stones within the biliary tree. The endoscope has been withdrawn to enable clear visualization of the lower end of the bile duct which is markedly dilated. These calculi were removed successfully by balloon extraction following sphincterotomy.

instrument is well lubricated with KY jelly and introduced gently so that it passes upwards in the direction of the axis of the anal canal. Painful conditions such as acute anal fissures are associated with marked spasm and proctoscopy is usually impractical without general anaesthesia.

Although flexible *sigmoidoscopes* are now available, sigmoidoscopy is usually still carried out with a rigid steel or plastic instrument. This is 25–30 cm long and used to inspect the rectum and distal sigmoid colon while the bowel is gently distended with air. Sigmoidoscopy is also carried out with the patient in the left lateral position and is preceded by digital rectal examination to relax the sphincters and make sure that faecal loading is not present. If the rectum is full, examination is deferred pending bowel preparation. The lubricated instrument is passed gently through the anal sphincter with its obturator still in place. The obturator is then removed, the eyepiece and insufflator are attached, and the instrument is passed upwards under vision for its full length or until further progress is impossible. Negotiation of the rectosigmoid junction (12–15 cm from the anal verge) can be difficult and may not be possible because of discomfort. The mucosa is carefully inspected as the instrument is slowly withdrawn, noting its colour, consistency and any signs of inflammation. In contrast to normal mucosa, inflamed mucosa bleeds when stroked lightly with the instrument or a mounted swab (contact bleeding). It is important to note the presence of abnormal faeces, mucus, pus and fresh or altered blood, all of which may also signify pathology beyond the reach of the instrument. Whenever faeces are encountered, a sample is tested for occult blood. Special forceps are available to take punch biopsies from the mucosa and lesions such as neoplasms. Small polyps can often be removed completely at rigid sigmoidoscopy, while diathermy can be used to fulgurate small mucosal lesions. Larger polyps can be removed by snare polypectomy using a flexible instrument (see below), but large polyps may require general anaesthesia so that the shorter broader operating sigmoidoscope can be used.

If a biopsy is taken during sigmoidoscopy, the patient must not have any form of enema, including barium examination, for at least five days as distension by the enema can perforate the bowel at the biopsy site and even cause air or barium embolization. Some radiology departments delay barium enemas for a week after any sigmoidoscopy, even when no biopsy has been taken.

The *colonoscope* is a fibreoptic instrument 150 cm in length which is used to inspect the entire length of the large bowel. It is particularly useful in patients with colonic polyps, as these are often multiple and difficult to demonstrate radiologically. Abnormal mucosa is biopsied and polyps are removed for histological examination after encircling their base with a snare through which diathermy is applied. The procedure requires meticulous bowel preparation.

The peritoneal cavity

The peritoneal cavity can be inspected through a *laparoscope*. General anaesthesia is preferred so that the abdominal wall can be relaxed for induction of a

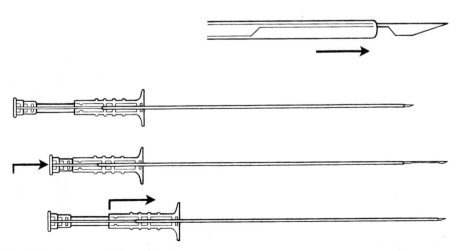

Fig. 6.5 Tru-cut needle for biopsy of solid organs.

pneumoperitoneum. A special needle (Verres' needle) is inserted through the abdominal wall just below the umbilicus, and carbon dioxide is delivered to reach a predetermined pressure (12–15 mmHg). The laparoscope is then inserted through a small subumbilical incision and by appropriate elevation of the head or foot of the table, the various parts of the peritoneal cavity can be inspected. Laparoscopy is particularly useful for:

- Examination of the female pelvic organs and sterilization by tubal diathermy
- Detection of liver metastases (by direct inspection and ultrasonography)
- Biopsy of organs, notably the liver, under direct vision so that a Tru-cut needle can be targeted to areas of obvious pathology (Fig. 6.5)
- Staging of tumours of the digestive tract by detecting peritoneal and lymph node metastases (e.g. pancreatic cancer)
- Investigation of ascites.

Laparoscopy is well-tolerated even by frail patients and causes little discomfort. In patients who have undergone laparotomy, adhesions may limit the view and bowel adhering to the abdominal wall can be perforated during insertion of the instrument. Laparoscopy is used increasingly in the differential diagnosis of abdominal pain and as a means of carrying out such procedures as cholecystectomy, appendicectomy and bowel resection.

The respiratory tree

Laryngoscopes with a curved or flat blade are used to inspect the pharynx and larynx, suck out secretions and other material in unconscious patients, and pass an endotracheal tube.

The *bronchoscope* is used to inspect the trachea and larger bronchi under local or general anaesthesia. Use of a rigid instrument allows large biopsies to be taken and pus or secretions can be aspirated in patients with pulmonary collapse or severe chest infection after surgery. Flexible fibreoptic bronchoscopes are smaller and can be passed through the nose under local anaesthesia; they allow inspection of smaller bronchi and may detect more peripheral lesions although substantial biopsies cannot be taken (Fig. 6.6).

The *mediastinoscope* is a rigid instrument which is inserted through a short transverse incision in the

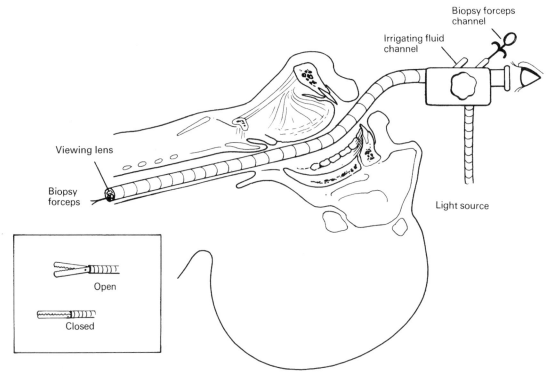

Fig. 6.6 Fibreoptic bronchoscopic biopsy.

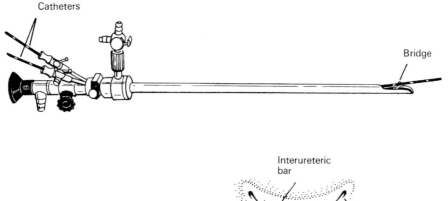

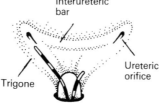

Fig. 6.7   Cystoscope and ureteric catheterization.

suprasternal notch to inspect and biopsy mediastinal tissues. The finding of involved mediastinal nodes contraindicates surgery in patients with bronchogenic carcinoma.

The *thoracoscope* is similar to the laparoscope and is used to inspect the pleural space. Pleural or peripheral lung lesions can be biopsied, and thoracoscopy is used increasingly for therapeutic purposes including resection of the oesophagus or portions of lung.

The urinary system

The interior of the bladder may be inspected by introducing a rigid or flexible fibreoptic *cystoscope* through the urethra (Fig. 6.7). The bladder is distended with distilled water, and forceps or diathermy loops can be passed through the instrument to allow biopsy or fulguration.

The ureteric orifices can be seen and cannulated with fine catheters so that radio-opaque dye can be instilled to visualize the renal pelvis and ureter (retrograde pyelography). Flexible fibreoptic *ureteroscopes* can also be passed up the ureter to inspect small lesions in the upper urinary tract. Alternatively, a *nephroscope* can be passed percutaneously through the renal substance to visualize the renal pelvis and extract calculi.

The urethra can be examined with a *urethroscope* in patients who have sustained urethral trauma or developed urethral strictures or prostatic disease.

DIAGNOSTIC IMAGING

Principles of radiology

X-rays are produced by bombarding a tungsten target with an electron beam (Fig. 6.8). An image can be produced on a fluoroscopic screen which is activated by X-rays to produce light, or a silver precipitate can be made on photographic plate or film coated with an emulsion sensitive to light or X-rays. An X-ray film is normally enclosed in a cassette

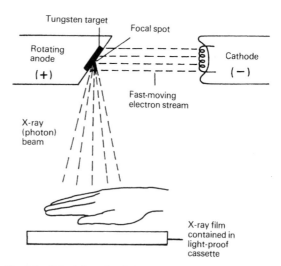

Fig. 6.8   Principles of radiology.

containing a fluorescent screen so that the released light reinforces the action of X-rays on the film.

The intensity of an image depends on the ability of target substances to absorb X-rays. Metals absorb them completely and are absolutely radio-opaque; fat and air are poorly absorbent and therefore almost radiolucent. Passage of X-rays through solid objects also depends on the electromagnetic properties of the X-rays, their quantity and the time of exposure. By varying the kilovoltage of the machine and exposure time, tissues of varying densities can be visualized.

As an X-ray plate gives a two-dimensional reproduction of a three-dimensional target, radiologists frequently take additional films at 90° to the original plane (e.g. when X-raying bones or obtaining anteroposterior and lateral views of the chest). Varying obliquities of projection help to demonstrate tissues at varying depths from the X-ray tube.

Tomograms are made by moving the X-ray tube and film in opposite directions around a fulcrum in the plane of the object under study. The shadow of structures outwith that plane can be intentionally blurred so that only the plane being examined is in focus. Each film represents a 'slice' or section of the body. This technique is the basis of computed axial tomography (CT; see below).

Moving organs or flowing contrast material can be studied by serial radiographs taken on rapid-change cassettes or by continuous viewing on a fluoroscopic or television screen. These techniques are particularly valuable in investigations such as coronary angiography or the study of deglutition.

Dangers of ionizing radiation

Radiological investigations expose patient and staff to potentially harmful radiation, underlining the need to avoid unnecessary investigations. Radiation received by staff is monitored constantly by a small badge containing an X-ray film, and protective lead aprons are worn whenever staff are in an exposed situation. The hands of radiologists are particularly vulnerable and lead gloves are worn when appropriate.

Elective radiological investigation must be avoided during pregnancy and during the first 10 days following menstruation in women of child-bearing age (the '10-day' rule) to avoid irradiation of an unsuspected and recently conceived fetus.

Special radiological techniques

In addition to plain films of the chest and abdomen,

X-ray studies using contrast media are used extensively in diagnosis.

Contrast studies

The differing densities of body tissues and their contained liquids and air normally provide contrast between adjacent structures. These natural contrasts can be augmented by introducing air, barium sulphate, or iodine-containing media into body cavities and hollow viscera, and by oral or parenteral administration of radio-opaque materials which are secreted or excreted in body fluids.

Barium suspensions may be swallowed to outline the oesophagus, stomach or small intestine or introduced by enema to outline the large intestine. In a *barium swallow* the radiologist concentrates on the oesophagus and oesophagogastric junction, in a *barium meal* he concentrates on the oesophagogastric junction, stomach and proximal duodenum, whereas in a *barium meal and follow-through*, barium is followed down the small intestine. In a *small bowel enema*, barium is instilled directly into the small bowel through a tube placed in the duodenum, thus avoiding the need to await gastric emptying.

Relatively small amounts of barium are used in contrast studies and fine mucosal abnormalities are detected more readily if air is insufflated to distend the organ and spread the barium thinly (i.e. 'air contrast' or 'double contrast' studies). A relaxing agent such as the anticholinergic drug, hyoscine butylbromide (Buscopan), is occasionally used to allow distension of the duodenum in hypotonic duodenography. If there is any clinical evidence of obstruction or perforation, barium can compound obstruction or cause dense adhesions if it escapes into the peritoneal cavity. In these circumstances, water-soluble iodine-containing 'Gastrografin' is preferred.

A variety of iodine-containing agents are available for contrast radiology of hollow viscera, ducts, blood vessels and other conduits. Water-soluble compounds excreted by the kidneys are used in excretion urography and can be injected to outline the vascular tree (arteriography or venography), sinus tracts (sinography) and duct systems (e.g. pancreatography). Compounds prepared in an oily base are particularly suitable for lymphangiography as they are trapped by phagocytes and allow serial X-ray of lymph nodes over a period of months. Iodine-containing fluids of varying solubility can also be used to mix with body fluids and outline joints (arthrography), the spinal canal (myelography) or ventricles of the brain (ventriculography).

Iodine compounds which are excreted by the liver

are also available. The fat-soluble compound Telepaque is given orally to outline the gallbladder (oral cholecystography), while the water-soluble compound Biligrafin is injected intravenously to outline the bile ducts (intravenous cholangiography). As both investigations depend on hepatic excretory function, they are of no value in patients with jaundice, and have been largely superseded by the use of ultrasonography in the detection of gallstones and diagnosis of the cause of biliary obstruction (see below). Intravenous cholangiography is limited further by the fact that iodine-containing dyes can produce potentially fatal allergic reactions when injected intravenously, and by the poor quality of the cholangiograms obtained. High-quality cholangiograms can now be obtained by direct injection of contrast into the biliary tree following endoscopic cannulation of the papilla of Vater (ERCP) or through a needle inserted percutaneously into the intrahepatic bile ducts (percutaneous transhepatic cholangiography (PTC).

Computerized tomography (CT scanning)

In CT scanning, a slit beam of X-rays is directed at points on the circumference of a narrow transverse section of the body (Fig. 6.9). These rays fall sequentially on multiple scintillation crystal detectors with photomultipliers, each of which feeds impulses into a computer to build up a picture of the section being examined. The picture can be displayed on a console, printed out, or stored on disc or tape. The dose of radiation to the skin is similar to that received in routine radiology. Minor difference in tissue density can be detected, and resolution is fine (one point on the matrix represents an area 0.75×0.75 mm).

CT scanning has revolutionized the investigation of intracranial, intrathoracic and intra-abdominal disease (Fig. 6.10), and interference caused by respiratory and cardiac movement can be minimized by 'gating' images synchronously with respiration or heart beat. Discrimination is improved by intravenous injection or ingestion of iodine-containing media to enhance contrast.

Ultrasonography

Tissues vary in their capacity to absorb sound. When an ultrasonic wave strikes the interface between two

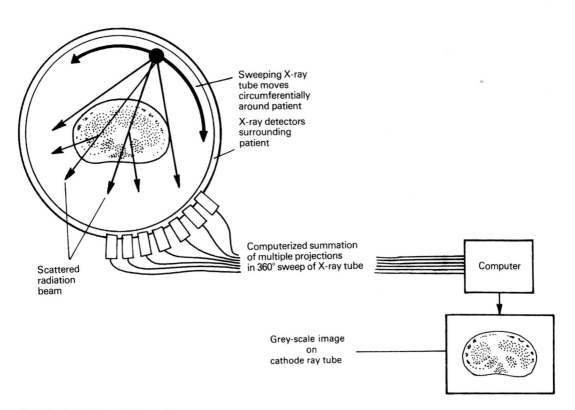

Fig. 6.9 **Principles of CT scanning.**

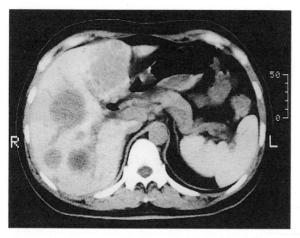

Fig. 6.10 CT scan of abdomen showing multiple hepatic metastases in a patient with colorectal cancer.

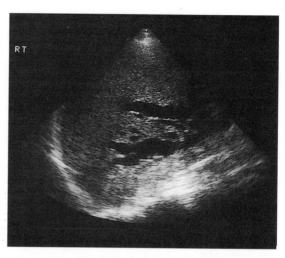

Fig. 6.11 Ultrasound examination showing dilatation of the intrahepatic biliary tree.

media of differing acoustic impedance, some of the energy is reflected as an ultrasonic echo. The echo is recorded by a detector in the line with the source of the ultrasonic beam and can be displayed on an oscilloscope as an unidimensional wave (A scan). If a sweeping beam is used, a two-dimensional black and white picture can be constructed (B scan); modulation of the image according to the amplitude of the reflected wave produces a picture of varying shades of grey (grey-scale ultrasonography) and colour. Multiple generators and detectors in different planes can be used to construct an ultrasonic tomogram and three-dimensional images are also possible. It also can be used for guidance of biopsy needles.

Ultrasonography is non-invasive, carries no radiation risk and has high resolution. It is used commonly in surgical practice to determine whether a mass is solid or cystic, assess the biliary system (Fig. 6.11), detect liver metastases, detect space-occupying intracranial lesions and displacement of the falx cerebri, define intracardiac anatomy, and monitor progress of pseudocysts, deep-seated abscesses or aneurysms.

Ultrasonic flow meters employ the Doppler principle to assess blood flow. Movement of red cells causes a shift in the frequency of the signal reflected from their interface with fluid blood. The meters consist of a transducer (which contains an ultrasonic transmitter and receiver), a receiver, audio-amplifier and loudspeakers. When the transducer is placed over a vessel such as a vein, flow is audible whereas obstruction produces silence. In the normal limb, squeezing the leg distal to the transducer augments venous flow and causes a roar from the loudspeaker. A similar system is used to assess flow in arteries.

Colour flow Doppler ultrasonography displays blood moving towards the transducer in a different colour to that moving away from it, the colour varying according to the velocity of the blood being imaged. The technique has found great application in investigation of cardiovascular disease and in assessing patency of the portal vein and hepatic artery before and after liver transplantation.

Echocardiography is also used to obtain time-based tracing of movements of heart valves and chamber walls and to detect intracardiac lesions.

Magnetic resonance imaging (MRI)

MRI does not involve ionizing radiation and is harmless. It images hydrogen nuclei throughout the body, hydrogen having the most magnetic nucleus of the elements and making up two-thirds of the atoms in all living tissues. An MRI scanner consists of a magnet with a field strength about 20 000 times that of the earth's magnetic field, and which causes the hydrogen nucleus to realign its polarity. The change in alignment causes the nucleus to emit the absorbed energy as radiowaves which can be detected by a short-wave antenna and receiver and converted into images. Slices of tissue of varying thickness can be imaged in multiple planes to produce an image which appears three-dimensional. Details of tissue consistency can be provided by measuring 'relaxation times', i.e. the rate at which the signal from the hydrogen nuclei fades (or relaxes) after stimulation. MRI can scan in any plane and is particularly useful in visualizing the brain. Bone can be suppressed on MRI scanning, allowing clear visualization of structures embedded in bone such as the inner ear, spinal canal and pituitary fossa. MRI has the disadvantages that it is expensive, time-consuming and unsuitable for patients with pacemakers or metallic implants.

Radioactive isotopes and scintiscans

Tracer studies

Isotopes emitting beta- or gamma-rays can be used as trace substances to measure the body pool of their non-radioactive counterparts. For example, body fluid compartments may be measured by injecting small amounts of a radioactive substance, allowing time for equilibration, counting the isotope concentration, and then calculating its volume of distribution using the 'dilution principle'. Assuming that the substance is evenly distributed and not excreted or metabolized, the amount injected (Q) equals the product of (S) and V, where (S) is the concentration of the dissolved substance and V is the volume of distribution. Thus,

$$Q = (S)V$$

and as both Q and (S) are known, the volume is given by:

$$V = Q/(S)$$

The turnover of labelled proteins and other substances can also provide information on metabolism and organ function.

Scintiscans

Gamma-rays penetrate tissues for several centimetres, and can be detected by an external counter. This usually consists of a detector which emits scintillations of light when exposed to gamma-irradiation, and the scintillations are then magnified by photomultiplier circuits and counted or displayed visually. A mobile detector can be used (as in a rectilinear scanner) or multiple detectors can be used in a fixed device (as in the gamma camera). The pattern of emissions can be printed on paper or displayed on an oscilloscope.

Scintiscans are used to visualize organs which selectively concentrate ingested or injected isotopes, and to study blood flow through an organ or region. Isotopes with a short half-life and rapid excretion are used to prevent radiation damage.

Liver scans. The liver can be visualized by injecting substances such as ^{131}I-labelled Rose Bengal which are concentrated by hepatocytes, or by injecting colloidal particles such as ^{99m}Tc-labelled sodium pertechnicate which are removed by the Kupffer cells of the reticulo-endothelial system. In normal liver, these isotopes are distributed normally whereas lesions such as liver metastases appear as areas of diminished uptake. These techniques had a low sensitivity in detecting liver metastases and have now been superseded by ultrasonography and CT scanning. Similarly, simultaneous liver and lung scans are now seldom used to detect subphrenic abscesses.

The compound ^{99m}Tc-labelled HIDA is excreted into the biliary system following intravenous injection and can be used to assess bile flow from the liver in patients before and after repair of bile duct strictures.

Lung scans. In 'perfusion scans', microaggregates of albumin labelled with ^{131}I or ^{99m}Tc are injected intravenously to outline the pulmonary circulation. In ventilation scans, ^{133}Xe (xenon) is inhaled to outline the bronchi and alveoli. An area of diminished uptake on the perfusion scan with a normal ventilation scan indicates pulmonary embolization, whereas postoperative atelectasis diminishes both perfusion and ventilation and produces an abnormality on both scans. A ventilation scan should be performed whenever interpretation of a perfusion scan is in doubt.

Thyroid scans. Radioactive isotopes of iodine are trapped selectively by thyroid acinar cells but uptake determinations have been replaced by measurement of circulating thyroid hormones in the diagnosis of hyper- and hypothyroidism. Scanning with ^{131}I is used to detect localized increase or decrease in uptake in patients with a thyroid nodule, but ^{99m}Tc-sodium pertechnicate is now preferred as it is easier to prepare and gives a lower radiation dose. A nodule is 'hot' if it takes up the isotope to a greater degree than the surrounding gland, 'cool' if the concentration is the same, and 'cold' if it is less. A hot nodule is most likely to be a benign adenoma, whereas a cold nodule is likely to be a cyst, degenerate benign nodule or cancer.

Total body scans after injection of ^{131}I are used to detect metastatic lesions in patients with thyroid cancer.

Brain scans. The higher vascularity of brain tumours results in a relatively high uptake of radiolabelled substances such as ^{131}I-serum albumin, ^{99m}Tc-sodium pertechnicate and ^{113m}In chelate. Haematomas show increased but slow uptake whereas benign cysts have little uptake. CT scans have now largely replaced brain scans.

Skeletal scans. Increased turnover of bone minerals in areas of osteoblastic activity can be demonstrated by intravenous injection of bone-seeking isotopes such as ^{99m}Tc-labelled diphosphonates. Osteoblastic activity surrounding bone metastases can be detected months before radiological change. Areas of increased uptake may also be seen in Paget's disease, arthritis and at fracture sites.

Venous thrombosis. Incorporation of fibrinogen in deep venous thromboses can be detected using ^{125}I-labelled fibrinogen. This technique requires serial scans and has been of more value in clinical trials of prophylactic regimens than in clinical diagnosis.

HISTOLOGICAL AND CYTOLOGICAL DIAGNOSIS

In many situations, a sample of tissue must be obtained for histological or cytological examination before a definitive diagnosis can be made. This is particularly important in differentiating between benign and malignant disease and in the diagnosis of diseases of the liver and kidney.

Cytology

Cytology is the examination of the architecture of cells. Immunocytochemistry can be used to detect the presence of specific products and markers which may help in the diagnosis of malignancy. Two main methods are used to obtain cells for examination.

Exfoliative cytology

Cells shed by the epithelium lining hollow viscera or ducts can be obtained from secretions or excretions. As the cells are suspended individually or in clumps, the recognition of abnormalities depends on cellular as opposed to tissue morphology, and experience and skill is needed in interpretation. Exfoliative cytology is readily applied to diseases of the upper gastrointestinal, respiratory, and genitourinary tracts.

Needle aspiration cytology

A 21-gauge needle is attached to a 10-ml syringe and inserted into the tissue to be sampled. Suction is applied and the needle advanced several times through the tissue so that cellular material is drawn into its shaft. The needle and syringe are then withdrawn and the contents of the needle are squirted onto a slide using a fresh syringe and smeared with another slide before fixation (Fig. 6.12). Apart from obtaining material for cytological examination, needle aspiration can be used to differentiate cysts from solid swellings so that operation can frequently be avoided. Radiological screening or ultrasonic guidance can be used to direct the needle into a deep-seated lesion.

Histopathology

Histopathology is the examination of the architecture of a tissue and its cellular components.

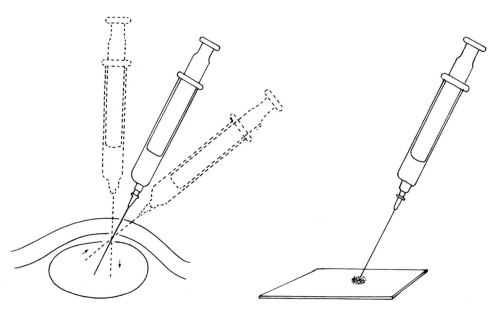

Fig. 6.12   Needle-aspiration cytology.

Immunohistochemistry can be used to detect specific products such as hormones and other polypeptides, and is used predominantly as an aid in the diagnosis of malignancy. A variety of methods are available to obtain a representative sample (biopsy) of tissue.

Needle biopsy

The Tru-cut needle (Fig. 6.5) is used to obtain a core of tissue from organs and tissues such as the liver, kidney and muscle. It is also used to biopsy solid tumours e.g. of the breast. The closed needle is advanced towards the area of interest. The outer sheath is held firm while the inner needle is advanced. The sheath is then slid over the needle into the closed position. The Tru-cut needle is then withdrawn enclosing a core of tissue in the cut-out section behind the needle point. Two hands are required to take a Tru-cut biopsy, although biopsy guns are now available which allow the core to be obtained with one hand while the tissue is held firm with the other.

Specially designed cannulae with cutting edges are used for bone and marrow biopsies.

Drill biopsy

Drill biopsies can be taken by a small sharp cannula attached to a high-speed compressed air drill which rotates at up to 20 000 r.p.m. The technique is cumbersome, noisy and seldom used.

Punch biopsy

Punch biopsy forceps are used to obtain tissue from skin tumours, lesions within the mouth and nose, and tissues accessible to endoscopy. The biopsies obtained using flexible fibreoptic endoscopes are small and multiple samples should always be taken.

Crosby capsule biopsy

The Crosby capsule is used occasionally to obtain samples of small bowel mucosa in patients with malabsorption. The capsule consists of a small metal cylinder attached to a long tube to which suction can be applied. It is swallowed and its position monitored radiologically; when it is in the desired position, suction is applied and a portion of mucosa is drawn into the capsule. A guillotine within the cylinder is used to snip off and retain a biopsy. The capsule can then be withdrawn or the tubing can be cut and the capsule recovered from the faeces.

Modifications of the Crosby capsule now allow biopsy specimens to be sucked up the tube so that multiple samples can be taken.

Open biopsy

Open operation may be needed if a lesion is inaccessible, when closed methods are thought to be dangerous, and when a large piece of tumour is required. The biopsy can be obtained by incision (i.e. cutting into the abnormal tissue to obtain a sample) or excision (i.e. removing all of the abnormal tissue). Immediate histological examination of frozen sections is indicated when a diagnosis is required urgently on samples taken at operation.

SURGICAL EXPLORATION

It may still be necessary on occasions to resort to open operation to establish the presence, extent and nature of disease. This is not an admission of diagnostic failure and when used appropriately, may save numerous expensive, time-consuming and uncomfortable investigations. Furthermore, the findings at operation coupled with immediate histological diagnosis may allow a diagnostic procedure to be converted into a therapeutic one.

POPULATION SCREENING

Screening of normal populations for early evidence of disease has been used to detect malignant disease of the uterine cervix, lung and breast. In Japan, radiological and endoscopic screening has led to the early diagnosis of gastric cancer, and has reduced mortality.

Screening is expensive and its benefits have to be balanced against its costs. The condition sought must be sufficiently common and serious to pose an important health problem, and its natural history must be understood. There must be a recognizable early stage of the disease, and evidence that treatment at that stage will confer more benefit than later treatment. The method of screening must be safe, acceptable to patients, non-invasive whenever possible, and have a high sensitivity (i.e. it should detect more than 90% of established lesions) and specificity (i.e. a low false positive rate). If a high-risk group can be identified, screening can be concentrated on those most likely to benefit from it.

Before launching any large-scale screening

programme, it is essential to demonstrate that early detection will indeed reduce the mortality caused by the disease in question. This usually requires several prospective controlled trials in which the mortality of the disease in the population offered screening is compared to that found in randomly allocated controls.

TESTS OF FUNCTION

Many disease processes produce aberrations in function rather than anatomical changes. Simple biochemical tests of organ function (see Table 6.1) include the use of plasma urea and creatinine levels to reflect renal function, and of serum bilirubin and albumin to reflect liver function. Some abnormalities may reflect altered function in more than one organ or tissue; for example, a raised alkaline phosphatase level can be caused by disease of the liver, bone or intestine.

More complex biochemical investigations are available to study the synthetic, secretory, absorptive and excretory functions of organs. It is important to remember that some organs and tissues have other than biochemical functions. For example, the gut has motor activity, a nerve conducts impulses, and a muscle contracts. Measurement of intraluminal pressure, electrical impulses and the effects of stimuli are all used to study disease processes. Many of these techniques have originated in laboratories devoted to physiological research. Their role in investigation will be discussed elsewhere.

Table 6.1 Normal laboratory values in human blood samples

Biochemistry		
sodium	132–144	mmol/l
potassium	3.3–4.7	mmol/l
CO_2	24–30	mmol/l
urea	2.5–6.6	mmol/l
creatinine	55–150	μmol/l
glucose	3.6–5.8	mmol/l
calcium	2.1–2.6	mmol/l
bilirubin	2–17	μmol/l
alanine aminotransferase (ALT)	10–40	u/l
alkaline phosphatase	40–125	u/l
albumin	36–47	g/l
amylase	50–300	u/l
Haematology		
Haemoglobin	M130–180	g/l
	F115–165	g/l
MCV (fl)	76–100	
MCH (pg)	27–32	
White blood count	4–11	$\times 10^9/l$
Platelet count	150–350	$\times 10^9/l$
Prothrombin time	10.5–14.5	seconds
expressed as International Normalized Ratio (INR) therapeutic ratio	2.0–4.5	
Activated partial thromboplastin time (APTT)	28–40	seconds
therapeutic ratio	1.5–2.5	
Arterial blood gases		
H^+	36–44	nmol/l
bicarbonate	21–27.5	mmol/l
pCO2	4.4–6.1	kPa
pCO2	12–15	kPa

7
Infections and antibiotics

CONTENTS

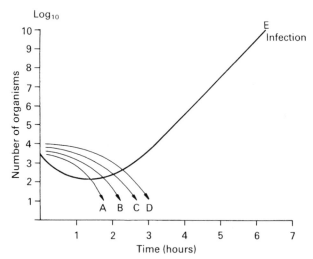

Fig. 7.1   In contamination a number of different species (A, B, C, D, E) may be present in small to moderate numbers. In infection one (or more) species expresses a survival advantage and multiplies to produce a significant challenge (E).

Wound infection

An open wound is invariably contaminated with organisms which may be derived endogenously from the patient's skin or exogenously from an external source such as the soil or air, or the hand of an attendant. The outcome of the microbial challenge depends on many factors, including the circumstances of contamination.

If contamination is minimal, as in an elective surgical incision performed under good conditions on a patient in good general health, the defences of the host cope completely. If contamination is severe, and particularly when other adverse factors operate, the challenge may rapidly result in a fulminating and overwhelming infection unless prompt and adequate action is taken to counter it. Such conditions arise for example with a lacerated wound following a road accident in an elderly person or a perforated lesion of the colon in a debilitated patient.

Contamination usually denotes the passive presence of a relatively small number of various species of bacteria. When one or more contaminants have a survival advantage over the others and replicate in the wound, *infection* is initiated and microbial pathogenicity is expressed (Fig. 7.1). There may be bacterial invasion, toxin production or a combination of these. Less commonly there may be viral or fungal infection.

Thus a wound infection implies the implantation of a potentially infective inoculum under conditions that allow the organisms to evade or overcome host defences; it is a function of the number of organisms in the inoculum, their quality or nature, and the efficacy of local and general host defence mechanisms.

Predisposing factors

Factors that predispose to or promote infection include:

- Contamination with potential pathogens
- Foreign material in the wound
- Virulence-enhancing effect of some materials such as soil, calcium salts and iron salts
- Delay in primary attention
- Pathogenic synergy (see later)
- Devitalized tissue
- Oedema/pressure/constriction
- Impaired blood supply
- Extravasation of tissue fluids and blood
- Host factors lowering resistance, e.g. age, debility, obesity, immunocompromised states, diabetes, alcoholism.

Several of these factors are more likely to be present in accidental wounds, and prompt and adequate surgical treatment should be given before the stage of bacterial contamination has led to bacterial proliferation and passed into that of active infection. Ideally this should be within 1–2 hours of injury and must include thorough cleansing of the wound with removal of all debris (surgical toilet) followed by excision of all devitalized tissue (debridement). If primary surgical care is not given within 6 hours, infection must be presumed.

Factors concerned with healing, and problems of wound management are considered in Chapter 12.

Tissue oxygenation

Primary host defences against wound infection include phagocytosis and intraleucocytic microbicidal systems. Effective phagocytosis, good tissue perfusion and oxygenation are requirements for optimal operation of these defences. All wounded tissue is less aerobic than normal tissue; impaired oxygenation persists for some days until healing is established. If the patient is initially shocked, tissue perfusion is further constrained and a vicious circle may result (Fig. 7.2).

Signs of infection

It is important to detect infection in a wound early. Cardinal local signs include erythema, warmth, oedema, tenderness and possibly serous or seropurulent exudate. The patient's temperature may rise and local tenderness may increase with pain and muscle guarding in the affected part.

Pyogenic organisms provoke a polymorphonuclear leucocytosis. The erythrocyte sedimentation rate (ESR) increases and the level of C-reactive protein rises. If the infection is severe, with early progression to bacteraemia and septicaemia, the

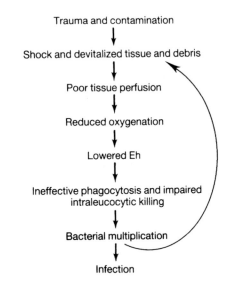

Trauma and contamination

↓

Shock and devitalized tissue and debris

↓

Poor tissue perfusion

↓

Reduced oxygenation

↓

Lowered Eh

↓

Ineffective phagocytosis and impaired intraleucocytic killing

↓

Bacterial multiplication

↓

Infection

Fig. 7.2   The 'vicious circle'. Association of factors that may be involved in the change from contamination to infection in a wound. Eh = oxidation-reduction potential

patient may quickly and insidiously develop bacteriogenic or 'septic' shock (see below) with facial pallor giving way to an ominous, slightly cyanotic flush. As the blood pressure falls and perfusion of vital organs is reduced, the patient's mental state changes from one of anxious malaise to clouded consciousness and then coma. Multiple organ failure and death ensue. The time course of these events may be as short as a few hours.

When an operation involves an unavoidable and significant microbial challenge to the tissues, as in colonic surgery, it is standard practice to protect the patient by giving antimicrobial prophylaxis to cover the period of challenge. It is important that this should be for as short a time as possible. For example, a suitable antibiotic may be given just before operation and continued for 1–2 days postoperatively, but not for longer.

Septic shock

A range of shock syndromes are associated with a considerable spectrum of microbial challenges. These are variously described as *bacteraemic, septicaemic,* or *septic shock.* Other synonyms such as *Gram-negative shock* and *endotoxic shock* reflect the fact that Gram-negative bacteria are often (but not invariably) responsible and that bacterial lipopolysaccharide endotoxin is thought to be a significant mediator or at least significantly involved in a final common pathway.

While Gram-negative sepsis is more commonly associated with septic shock, Gram-positive sepsis may be as well. The possibility of septic shock should be considered whenever cardiovascular instability is evident in a patient with major infection, or in a postoperative or injured patient in whom a major infection may be developing. The condition may present suddenly, but some patients become progressively shocked over a period of time. Clinical awareness and prompt action are essential.

Two phases are recognized although in a fulminating case the patient's condition may deteriorate so rapidly that the dramatic features of the second phase may be all that is noted.

The *hyperdynamic* phase is characterized by tachycardia, hyperventilation, warm dry extremities, but an ominous degree of hypotension. The patient may be anxious and restless, and then confused, lethargic, drowsy and weak.

The patient's colour may progress to a curious facial flush with a slightly mauve cyanotic tinge heralding the transition to the *hypodynamic* phase. Here there is cyanosis, marked hypotension, vasoconstriction, oliguria and mental confusion, followed by multiple organ failure, coma and then death.

The pulmonary component of multiple organ failure is the adult respiratory distress syndrome (ARDS) with acute dyspnoea and hypoxaemia, widespread infiltrates in the lungs with increased permeability and inflammatory changes, and pulmonary oedema. ARDS may be associated with a range of causes. In at least 50% of patients the cause is septicaemia and the mortality rate in this group is very high. ARDS as a complication of septicaemia is sometimes loosely called 'septic lung'. The term denotes acute respiratory failure in a patient with sepsis or septic shock, but the lung is not primarily involved in the bacterial infection and is reacting as one of the components of multiple organ failure.

In septic shock, the organs that fail include the heart, the lungs, the brain, the kidneys and the liver.

Tumour necrosis factor (TNF)

TNF is a macrophage factor (synonym: cachectin) with several known activities. It inhibits lipid uptake by adipose tissue and is involved in the wasting (cachexia) typical of chronic diseases. It is a pyrogen, like bacterial endotoxin, and it induces the synthesis of interleukin 1.

Bacterial endotoxin is a potent inducer of TNF. Thus a cascade of mediators of the components of the septic shock syndrome includes TNF as a key factor.

Hospital infections

Patients who remain in hospital for some time acquire hospital organisms on the skin, in the nose and mouth and in the gut. Such hospital strains of bacteria may have evolved a special facility for colonization and infection. A patient who is unwell and old has both reduced tissue and reduced general resistance, and is more susceptible to colonization and infection. The length of stay of such a patient in an acute hospital must be kept to a minimum.

After any prolonged series of inpatient investigations it is wise to allow patients to return home before surgical treatment so that their normal flora can be restored away from the hospital environment.

Sites of colonization

It is possible to monitor the acquisition of flora and this may be of clinical value, e.g. in the preparation of a patient for intestinal surgery or before treatment with cytotoxic agents. Hospital practice often fails to recognize the significance of a patient's endogenous flora in relation to both potential protective and potential pathogenic effects. For example, long-stay patients, particularly when old, should not be treated in an acute surgical ward, as dispersal of acquired skin flora, e.g. from an infected bedsore, into the ward environment and onto surfaces in toilet areas, poses dangers to other patients.

The 'colonization resistance' of the gut is markedly reduced by some forms of antibiotic therapy, so that the opportunities for exchange of antibiotic resistance between strains and species of gut bacteria are increased.

Hospital microbial challenges

Hand-borne or surface-mediated challenges

The hands of patients and staff are of great importance in conveying microbial challenges. Related hazards and possible control measures are summarized in Table 7.1. Some sophisticated measures, such as special containment facilities, are costly but simple methods of control are not, yet they are often neglected.

Air-borne challenges

Potential microbial challenges from air and effective measures to control them are listed in Table 7.2. Some basic control measures are not unduly expen-

Table 7.1 Hand-borne challenges and contact hazards, and possible control measures

Hazard	Control measures
Hand contact (Direct and mediate contact)	Hand-washing Antiseptics and disinfectants Gloves No-touch techniques
Trolley surfaces, etc. Contaminated instruments Contaminated solutions	Disposable or 'dedicated' instruments Adequate staff adequately trained Adequate facilities
Shared facilities e.g. shared toilets, basins, towels	Separate facilities Special containment facilities

Table 7.3 Ingested challenges, associated problems and possible control measures

Hazard	Control measures
Contaminated hospital food	Strict food hygiene
Contaminated special diet formulations	Good, easily cleaned equipment Safe kitchen practices
Contaminated drug preparations	Bacteriological monitoring Trained staff
R-factor transmission from animals	Control of antibiotics Care in food preparation

sive and if applied conscientiously reduce the advantages of more sophisticated measures, such as unidirectional filtered air-systems, to marginal proportions.

Ingested challenges

Significant microbial challenges may be delivered to the gastrointestinal tract in hospital (Table 7.3). Food hygiene is of paramount importance and hospital catering systems must be of a high standard. The numbers of organisms delivered to our patients in hospital food may be unacceptably high. Resistant organisms may reach the gut of patients as a result of the multiplication of animal strains that contaminate some foods.

Table 7.2 Air-borne hazards, associated problems and possible control measures

Hazard	Control measures
Contamination of ward and theatre air	Ventilation in theatre and ward Adequate interspace in ward
Transmissible respiratory infections	Attention to anaesthetic equipment, respirators, etc.
Wound dressing	Avoidance of contamination by restriction of this procedure in ward
Bedmaking Floor polishing Toilet flushing, etc.	Avoidance of generation of air-borne particles Avoidance of use of aerosols Treatment of fabrics Control of dangerous dispersers
Hot-air blowers	Filtration and laminar-flow systems Special containment facilities

Inoculated challenges

Infection with hepatitis B virus is an important example of the serious potential hazard of skin-penetrating injuries in all clinical staff. This arises from cross-contamination with blood or other body fluids from a patient with a recognized infection or one who may be a known or unknown carrier. Many other pathogenic agents can be transmitted by accidental inoculation of blood or blood products. In surgical staff, punctures of surgical gloves occur in up to 30% of operations, and skin-penetrating injuries with needles and knives are common events demanding constant caution. Currently attention is focused on the viruses of hepatitis B, non-A non-B hepatitis, and the acquired immunodeficiency syndrome (AIDS) as infecting agents. The carrier rate for hepatitis B in the UK is around 0.1%, while in some countries in Africa and Asia it is as high as 5–15%. In high-risk groups in the UK and USA (some immigrants, drug addicts, patients with Down's syndrome, male homosexuals) the carrier rate is 5–10%. Surgeons, obstetricians, dentists, haematologists and their staff, laboratory workers and workers in transfusion services are particularly at risk and should take care to avoid skin-penetrating injuries in circumstances in which contamination with blood or blood products or other body fluids is likely. Active immunization with three injections of hepatitis B vaccine is recommended for all those at risk.

The infective state of a patient or carrier in relation to hepatitis B is demonstrated by the detection of hepatitis B surface antigen (HBsAg), and in particular hepatitis B 'e' antigen (HBeAg) in the serum.

If a non-immunized person has a skin-penetrating injury with likely hepatitis B contamination, emergency (postexposure) passive protection can be given by intramuscular injection of hyperimmune hepatitis B immunoglobulin (HBIgG) within 48 hours.

Hazards associated with intensive care

Special infective hazards may be posed by a variety of procedures performed in an intensive care unit, including the use of ventilators and respirators, nasogastric tubes, suction apparatus, intravenous lines, percutaneous needles, and catheters. It is paradoxical that our most severely compromised patients should be exposed to such inadvertent challenges.

Pathogenic potential of microbes

Exaltation and attenuation

When an organism is serially passaged in vivo, its virulence may be exalted and its capacity to spread from one host to another increased.

The concept of increased pathogenic potential as a result of exaltation in vivo must be linked with the ability of some commensal or opportunist bacteria to acquire and pass on new potentially dangerous genetic information. This may affect an organism's ability to colonize, to infect, to produce toxin or to gain multiple antibiotic resistance. The 'hospital staphylococcus' illustrates some of the alarming possibilities that result when an organism acquires new genetic material in the course of its colonization. Gram-negative bacilli, especially klebsiella organisms, have also demonstrated a potential for dangerous genetic exchange. The extending range of beta-lactamases in such widely different genera as *Haemophilus*, *Neisseria* and *Bacteroides* is a matter for concern. The transmission of organisms from patient to patient must be rigorously avoided. Hand-washing on the ward is critical, as is the wearing of disposable gloves in situations where transfer of flora from one patient to another may occur.

Pathogenic synergy

Two or more organisms may combine forces in a mixed infection and demonstrate enhanced aggression and virulence. Examples include acute ulceromembranous gingivitis (Vincent's infection), Meleney's synergistic gangrene and various fuso-spirochaetal or mixed infections with anaerobic components, all of which may lead to progressive destruction of tissue or a fulminating invasive infection. Mixed infections are common in a wide range of conditions, e.g. cerebral, dental, lung and pelvic abscess and peritonitis. When bacteroides organisms are present in such infections, they interfere with normal phagocytic mechanisms and inhibit intraleucocytic bactericidal systems. This may partly explain the observed synergistic action of co-existing pathogens.

Asepsis

Surgical ritual

In surgical areas, clear and specific instructions must be given on pre-operative skin cleansing of the patient and on adequate disinfection of the operation site (see Ch. 8). The relative advantages of masks, gowns and drapes at operation are debated and the limitations of these precautions should be understood. Only suitable materials should be used.

There should be a clear disinfectant policy and an antibiotic policy to ensure that antimicrobial agents are used sensibly on the wards and in the operating theatres. Strict adherence to the principles of sterilization and disinfection is essential when cleansing and processing surgical instruments and anaesthetic equipment.

Sterilization

This is an absolute term denoting complete removal or inactivation of viable microorganisms (protozoa, fungi, bacteria and viruses). It can only be achieved by strict attention to detail. Instruments or articles can be classified as sterile if they have been subjected to any of the following.

- Wet heat in an autoclave at 121°C for 20 minutes or at a higher temperature for a shorter time (HTST) to provide an equivalent exposure (Fig. 7.3).
- Dry heat in a hot-air oven at 160°C for 1 hour (see Fig. 7.3).
- Gamma-radiation under strictly controlled conditions.
- Special sterilizing chemicals, liquids or gases, such as formaldehyde, glutaraldehyde or ethylene oxide, under strictly controlled conditions.

Some transmissible agents are now known to challenge these conventional assumptions, e.g. those responsible for Creutzfeldt-Jakob disease.

Disinfection

This denotes a significant reduction in the numbers of organisms present, particularly those that might cause infection. With few exceptions, chemical disinfectants are not sterilizing agents. *Antiseptics* are relatively mild disinfectants that can be used on living tissues without causing undue harm.

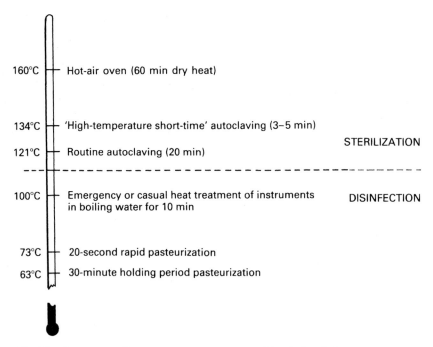

Fig. 7.3 A summary of heat-treatment temperatures (after Collee, J. G. 1981 in *Applied Medical Microbiology*, p. 104. Blackwell, Oxford).

Disinfection and preparation of the skin for surgery. Before a surgical incision is made in intact skin, the transient and resident flora at the operation site can be markedly reduced by thorough cleansing and then largely inactivated by the application of a suitable antibacterial agent. This will inactivate vegetative forms of bacteria only; it cannot be expected to kill bacterial spores. Accessible vegetative bacteria on the skin can be quickly inactivated by applying 70% ethanol, or 70% isopropyl alcohol, in water. Another antiseptic such as chlorhexidine or iodine 1–2% may be incorporated into the application. It is the alcohol at its optimum concentration of 70% in water that achieves a quick kill of vegetative bacteria.

Surgical sepsis

Postoperative wound infection

Bacterial infection of a surgical wound is still a common postoperative complication. The following generalizations reflect current experience in Britain.

Clean wounds in healthy tissue should heal promptly. With adequate facilities, an infection rate of less than 2% should be the aim of a good surgical team. Infections with *Staphylococcus aureus* occur from time to time. A series of such infections in a surgical unit suggests that a member of the team may be a carrier of *Staph. aureus*. Infections with coagulase-negative staphylococci are particularly associated with the implantation of heart valves, orthopaedic prostheses, or other artificial materials.

Abdominal wounds. Per-operative antimicrobial prophylaxis has significantly reduced the incidence of infection in abdominal surgery. Operations on the oesophagus, stomach and proximal small bowel are at risk of infection with oropharyngeal flora such as cocci, bacteroides organisms and coliform bacteria. A 10% infection rate is not uncommon, especially if gastric achlorhydria allows bacterial multiplication in the stomach. This has special relevance to patients receiving cimetidine or other secretory inhibitors.

Colorectal surgery and operations on patients with complicated appendicitis are associated with higher postoperative infection rates, ranging from 5% to 20% or more. Coliform bacteria and bacteroides organisms are common pathogens, often acting synergistically. Mixed infections with faecal streptococci and proteus or pseudomonas organisms pose special problems in clinical management.

The hazard of infection can be reduced by careful choice of antimicrobial prophylactic agents and meticulous preoperative preparation of the patient. Acute emergency cases are at special risk.

Antimicrobial prophylaxis is also important in surgery of the biliary tract, where potentially infective organisms include faecal streptococci, coliform bacteria, pseudomonas organisms and *Clostridium perfringens*. Despite antimicrobial measures, infection rates of 5–10% are still recorded in such patients.

Peritonitis

Chemical ('abacterial') peritonitis arises when irritant substances such as pancreatic juice, gastro-duodenal contents or blood gain access to the peritoneum. Staphylococcal infection sometimes follows surgical intervention.

Various bacteria may be associated with a primary infection. Peritonitis occurring as a complication of continuous ambulatory peritoneal dialysis (CAPD) is a special problem.

Infections most commonly associated with peritonitis secondary to perforation of an abdominal or pelvic viscus are due to aggressive elements of the commensal flora. These infections are mixed: coliform bacteria, bacteroides organisms and Gram-positive cocci are usually prominent. Clostridia are sometimes involved. Pure anaerobic infections without coliform or facultative bacteria may be encountered, especially in pelvic abscesses.

Pelvic inflammatory disease

This is a cause of much morbidity in female patients, who are especially prone to pelvic infection. It is most commonly acquired from the genital tract with inflammation in the region of the uterus, fallopian tubes and ovaries, giving rise to symptoms and signs of local peritoneal irritation. As in other forms of pelvic sepsis, there may be mixed coliform organisms and anaerobes, usually bacteroides and/or anaerobic cocci. Chlamydial infection is common and must not be missed. Pelvic sepsis in male or female patients may follow peritoneal infection arising from a non-genital source, e.g. a perforated appendix.

Burns

Burned areas of skin are highly vulnerable to bacterial colonization with organisms such as *Streptococcus pyogenes* (group A beta-haemolytic streptococcus), various staphylococci and coliform organisms (including pseudomonas), proteus bacteria and faecal streptococci.

Bacteraemia, septicaemia and septic shock

These may occur postoperatively after abdominal or genitourinary operations, following invasive manipulations, or in patients in intensive care after serious injuries or major surgery. Blood culture can be helpful in identifying the pathogens and guiding therapy, but it is necessary to start active antimicrobial treatment on a 'best-guess' emergency basis.

Urinary tract and respiratory tract infections are discussed elsewhere in this volume.

Pressure sores

Ulceration of the skin over pressure areas in immobilized patients results from ischaemia. There is direct pressure on small blood vessels which causes endothelial damage leading to activation of the clotting system. Predisposing factors include vascular disease, anaemia, obesity, incontinence, malnutrition, loss of cutaneous sensation, chronic debilitating disease, and imposed restriction of movement associated with the control of fractures.

Prevention requires careful teamwork and vigilance. A sheepskin or other special mattress (e.g. a water ripple mattress) may be necessary to avoid uneven distribution of the patient's weight. The skin should be kept dry and clean. Treatment of a pressure sore includes cleansing and the application of water-miscible preparations containing dimethicone (a silicone). Dietary supplements of vitamin C and oral zinc may help to promote good healing.

ANAEROBIC INFECTIONS

Tetanus

Clostridium tetani is an anaerobic spore-forming bacillus that occurs in soil and faeces and may contaminate an accidental wound. Survival of anaerobic bacilli in a wound is favoured by hypoxia, the presence of haematoma, soil and foreign bodies, and devitalized tissue. Failure to cleanse and excise the wound, coupled with ill-judged primary closure, provides favourable conditions for clostridial spores to germinate and for the bacteria to multiply and produce toxins.

When infection is established, the tetanus bacillus contributes little to local wound inflammation. However, it produces an exotoxin (tetanospasmin) which increases muscle tone, resulting in exaggerated responses to trivial stimuli and intermittent muscular spasms. These progress to generalized muscular spasms. In 30% of cases the initial injury may be a minor puncture wound so small as to be ignored by the patient.

The incubation period between injury and development of symptoms varies from a few days to 3 months. Most cases declare themselves within 2 weeks. The onset period is that between the first symptom and the onset of generalized muscle spasms. The prognosis is better if the incubation and onset periods are long.

Clinical presentation

The clinical presentation is often insidious. Tingling or ache or stiffness in the wound area is usually the first symptom. Jaw movements become restricted (hence the traditional name 'lockjaw'), facial muscle spasms produce a sardonic grin (risus sardonicus) and the muscles of the neck and back become stiff. Dysphagia, laryngeal spasm and spasm of the chest wall muscles and diaphragm can compromise ventilation and threaten life.

In severe cases, painful muscle spasms become more widespread and increase in frequency and duration. Arching of the back muscles can produce a state known as 'opisthotonos'. Sphincter spasm may cause micturition difficulties.

The patient remains conscious, although consciousness is frequently clouded. Muscle spasms are painful and exhausting and may be triggered by minor stimuli. The temperature is normal or only slightly elevated despite profuse sweating and tachycardia. These features are due to sympathetic overactivity, which may also cause worrying swings in blood pressure.

It is important to appreciate that these are the clinical features of a severe attack. Some cases are milder and do not progress to the full spectrum of generalized muscle spasms.

Diagnosis

Diagnosis is essentially clinical, but is supported by the demonstration of typical slender bacilli with drumstick spores in material from the devitalized wound tissue, and confirmed by the demonstration of tetanus toxin in cultures by toxin-antitoxin neutralization tests in mice.

Prevention

Tetanus is a preventable disease. Its low prevalence in countries with well-developed medical services depends on prompt and adequate attention to

---

Tetanus (1)

- *Clostridium tetani* is an anaerobic spore-forming bacillus found in soil and faeces.

- Tetanus may develop from small contaminated puncture wounds which may be so small that they are ignored by the patient (one-third of cases).

- Survival in wounds is favoured by hypoxia and by haematoma formation, devitalized tissue, and the presence of soil and foreign bodies.

- Failure to cleanse, excise and debride wounds favours multiplication of the organism and liberation of exotoxin.

- Tetanus contributes little to local inflammation but exotoxin increases muscle tone leading to muscle spasms and exaggerated responses to trivial stimuli.

- The incubation period varies from a few days to 3 months (usually less than 2 weeks) and the longer the incubation period and delay to the onset of spasms, the better the prognosis.

---

wounds (Figs 7.4 and 7.5) and programmes of active immunization.

Active immunization of all children in Britain is achieved by the use of a combined vaccine, the so-called triple vaccine (diphtheria, pertussis, tetanus vaccine), which includes adsorbed tetanus toxoid and is given in three doses within the first year of life. The first and second injections are separated by an interval of 6–8 weeks and the third is given about 4–6 months later. Booster injections of adsorbed toxoid should be given at 5 and 15 years and thereafter at 10-year intervals until middle age. In this way they can maintain lifelong immunity.

If possible, the immunization record of all patients with lacerated wounds should be checked. Patients immunized more than 5 years ago are given a booster injection of 0.5 ml of adsorbed toxoid (the need for this is debatable if the period since their last booster is less than 5 years). A full course of active immunization with toxoid is advisable if there is any doubt regarding past immunization, and immediate protection by simultaneous passive immunization is necessary if the patient has not been previously immunized.

Passive immunization with equine immune globulin (anti-tetanus serum; ATS) is associated with the risk of hypersensitivity and should now be abandoned if human immune globulin is available.

Human tetanus immune globulin (HTIG) is available in many countries to give immediate transient protection to non-immune patients. Its use is reserved for those considered to be tetanus-prone

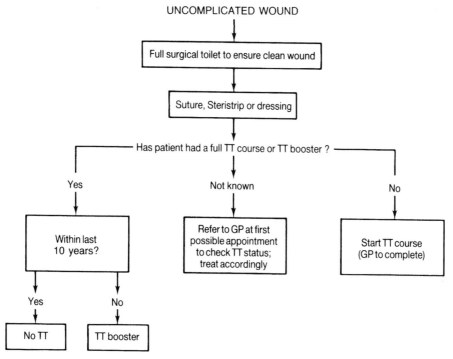

UNCOMPLICATED WOUND

Full surgical toilet to ensure clean wound

Suture, Steristrip or dressing

Has patient had a full TT course or TT booster ?

Yes — Not known — No

Yes: Within last 10 years?

Not known: Refer to GP at first possible appointment to check TT status; treat accordingly

No: Start TT course (GP to complete)

Yes — No

No TT — TT booster

Fig. 7.4 Management of uncomplicated wounds, including tetanus prophylaxis schedule.
TT = tetanus toxoid (adsorbed); GP = General practitioner. (Collee, MacLeod and Little, and Lothian Health Board, 1987)

and then as an adjunct to active immunization and antibiotic treatment (see below). An intramuscular injection of 250–500 i.u. is given at a site distant from that used for the toxoid and from a different syringe.

Tetanus-prone wounds are those complicated by delay in treatment of more than 6 hours; stab and other puncture wounds; animal or human bites; penetrating wounds; and wounds heavily contaminated with agricultural or horticultural materials or soil. They require particular care in their assessment. Following wound toilet they are carefully excised as necessary. Local antisepsis with an iodophor is advised. The wound should not be sutured but drawn together with Steristrips or lightly packed. Delayed primary closure should be considered in 4–5 days.

The assessment of puncture wounds is difficult, and adequate excision and exploration is not always practical. Such wounds should be regarded as potentially contaminated (see Fig. 7.5).

Antibiotic prophylaxis

A dose of long-acting penicillin should be given just before the wound is cleaned and explored. If the patient is allergic to penicillin or a more prolonged course of antibiotic is considered advisable, erythromycin 500 mg twice daily is given for 5 days, the first tablet being administered just before wound toilet. It must be stressed that antibiotic treatment does not replace the need for basic surgical care of the primary wound, but it may be a necessary adjunct.

Tetanus treatment

Treatment of tetanus is intensive and must begin as soon as the diagnosis is made.

Destruction of the infecting organism and neutralization of the toxin. At least 10 000 units of human tetanus immune globulin is given by slow intravenous infusion diluted in saline. The wound is excised, cleaned and left open. Penicillin 1 mega-unit 6-hourly by intramuscular injection or intravenous infusion, and metronidazole 1 g rectally 8-hourly by suppository will kill surviving bacteria and prevent further production of toxin. The first dose of antibiotic and the antitoxin should be given immediately, and before wound excision if possible.

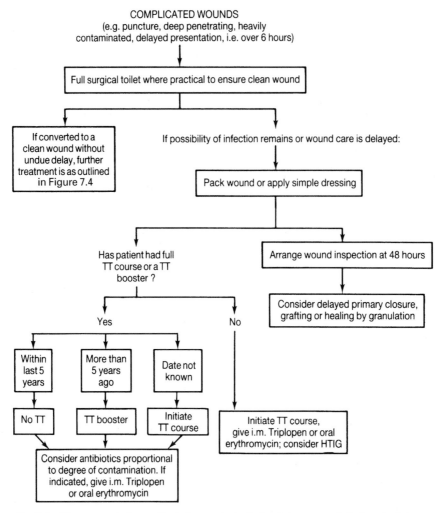

Fig. 7.5 Management of complicated wounds, including tetanus prophylaxis schedule.
TT = tetanus toxoid (adsorbed); HTIG = human tetanus immunoglobulin. (Source as 7.4)

The duration of antibiotic therapy depends on the individual response of the patient and bacteriological guidance. A case can be made for giving a further dose of 5000 units of antitoxin after a few days.

Life support.   The effects of toxin that has been fixed to receptors in the nervous system must be countered if the patient is to survive. He is nursed well-sedated in a quiet, shaded, intensive care room. Muscle spasms are controlled by tubocurarine or other neuromuscular blocking agents which necessitate intubation and assisted ventilation. Tracheostomy may be required to relieve respiratory embarrassment and is best performed early in the disease. Diazepam and chlorpromazine are given to depress excitability and control spasms and to help the patient to cope with a terrifying experience.

The patient is in a hypercatabolic state and nutrition must be maintained. A nasogastric tube facilitates feeding and lessens the risk of aspiration. Regular turning is necessary to avoid pressure sores and to keep the patient's chest clear.

Intense sympathetic activity can be controlled by beta-adrenergic blockers, which also control arrhythmias and labile blood pressure.

Several weeks of such intensive therapy may be required.

Gas gangrene and other clostridial infections

Clostridium perfringens (previously called *Cl. welchii*) is the principal cause of clostridial myonecrosis or

profound systemic upset and quickly threaten the affected limb and life of the patient.

Infection typically takes 2–3 days to become manifest, sometimes as an unexplained deterioration in the patient's general condition. The wound and surrounding tissues must be inspected, after removal of plaster casts if need be. A brown seropurulent discharge with characteristic odour, oedema, crepitus and pain on examination support the diagnosis, which is confirmed microscopically by the presence of Gram-positive rods. Subsequent culture and special tests determine the species involved. *Cl. septicum* and *Cl. novyi* (*Cl. oedematiens*) can be detected directly by immunofluorescence microscopy with special stains.

Blood culture sometimes helps to establish the diagnosis and to guide management.

Prevention

As for tetanus, prompt and adequate primary wound care by excision and debridement is essential. Con-

gas gangrene. Other clostridial species alone or in combination may be associated with gas gangrene, often in concert with facultative organisms. The organisms form spores which reside in soil and faeces, and contaminate skin and clothing. They are strict anaerobes and their growth is favoured by failure to debride contaminated wounds.

The pathogenic clostridia of the gas-gangrene group produce a number of toxins, including phospholipase (lecithinase), collagenase, proteinases, hyaluronidase, lipase and various haemolysins. These toxins and aggressins devitalize cells, destroy the local microcirculation and favour dissemination of infection along tissue planes with active destruction of muscle. When the products of the infection gain entry to the systemic circulation, the patient's initial anxiety gives way to a clouding of consciousness and delirium. There is tachycardia, pallor and jaundice, with subsequent circulatory collapse and death.

The spectrum of infection extends from superficial contamination of an open wound, through invasion of subcutaneous tissue, the production of crepitant cellulitis and localized painful myositis, to the full-blown picture of clostridial myonecrosis and gas gangrene. Localized forms of infection need not be associated with signs of systemic upset, or there may be relatively mild upset with fever and tachycardia. Diffuse myositis and gas gangrene produce

taminated wounds must not be closed by primary suture. Penicillin remains the prophylactic antibiotic of choice, with erythromycin as a good alternative. Polyvalent gas gangrene antitoxin was once available but its efficacy was in doubt and allergic reactions were common. It is no longer used.

Treatment

An established infection is treated radically. The wound is opened widely, fascial compartments are freely incised and dead tissue is meticulously removed. Devitalized muscle must be excised widely until bleeding viable tissue is encountered. In some cases, amputation is inevitable.

Wounds are loosely packed and left open, to be closed only when they appear healthy. Wide tissue defects may require subsequent tissue reconstruction and skin grafting. Amputation stumps are also left open in the first instance.

The patient is shocked and frightened. Intensive supportive therapy to correct and maintain fluid and electrolyte balance is necessary. Hypovolaemia is common and multiple transfusions may be required. Antibiotic therapy is essential. Penicillin is given in very high dosage together with metronidazole to control anaerobes. Additional antibiotics may be needed to control components of mixed infections that may be encountered. Intensive antibiotic therapy should be started before radical surgery, but not at the expense of losing valuable time.

The use of hyperbaric oxygenation in a pressure chamber has reduced mortality but is not a replacement for adequate surgery and the other measures described above. An increased arterial Pa_{O_2} cannot drive oxygen into dead tissues or eradicate established infection in devitalized tissues. However, it has a favourable effect in critical situations, when it may limit the amount of radical surgery required.

A particular mixed form of clostridial infection follows penetrating injury to the colon or rectum, the source of infecting organisms being the bowel. The mixed infection is likely to include clostridia and bacteroides organisms, anaerobic cocci, faecal streptococci, coliform bacteria and pseudomonas organisms. Wide debridement, free drainage, intensive antibiotic therapy and a proximal colostomy are essential measures.

Progressive bacterial gangrene and necrotizing fasciitis

These form a spectrum of advancing bacterial gangrene which may occur after a seemingly trivial injury or an operation, typically in the lower abdomen or perineum.

Progressive bacterial gangrene (bacterial synergistic gangrene, dermal gangrene, Meleney's gangrene) involves only the skin and advances relatively slowly. A variety of organisms have been incriminated, and synergistic action between a microaerophilic streptococcus and associated organisms is considered important. Predisposing factors include general debility, diabetes and hypoxia.

Necrotizing fasciitis (Fournier's gangrene) affects primarily the subcutaneous fat and deep fascia of the perineum or abdomen. The skin dies as a result of thrombosis of its blood supply. It is a rapidly advancing, frequently fatal disease. The rapidity and extent of tissue destruction are very alarming. The initial cellulitis is associated with the appearance of dusky purple patches in its centre which progress to skin necrosis. There may be crepitus. The patient becomes very ill and develops septic shock.

Treatment. It is important to determine the haemoglobin, blood glucose, blood urea and electrolyte concentration. Shock must be corrected with intravenous infusions. Blood, swabs and excised tissue are sent for culture. Diabetes should be considered and, if present, brought under control.

Intravenous antibiotics are started immediately; a combination of large doses of benzylpenicillin, metronidazole and gentamicin or tobramycin is recommended. These are modified in the light of culture reports as they become available.

As soon as the patient's condition allows it, radical excision of the affected area, including skin, subcutaneous tissue and deep fascia, is performed. The patient returns to theatre daily for inspection and further necessary excision until the infection is under control. The resulting defect in the skin and deep fascia, which frequently is very large, requires skin grafting.

Other anaerobic infections

The Gram-negative non-sporing anaerobic pathogens include bacteroides organisms (*Bacteroides fragilis, Porphyromonas (Bacteroides) melaninogenicus* etc.) and fusobacteria such as *Fusobacterium necrophorum*. These often occur in association with anaerobic cocci and other facultative organisms in a wide range of mixed putrefactive infections, including cerebral abscess, periodontal disease, ulceromembranous gingivitis and dental abscess, cancrum oris, Ludwig's angina, aspiration pneumonia, lung abscess, infected bite wounds, synergistic gangrene, Fournier's gangrene (necrotizing fasciitis), peritonitis, pelvic abscess, perianal and ischiorectal abscess, balano-posthitis, vaginitis/vaginosis and decubitus ulcers.

The common anaerobic component of many of these infections must be appreciated if the results of treatment are not to be disappointing. In some cases there is alarming pathogenic synergy which overwhelms the patient if effective treatment is delayed.

ANTIMICROBIAL MANAGEMENT OF WOUND INFECTIONS

It is important to know when a wound is being significantly colonized by a potential pathogen. Regular inspection of wounds is essential, and bacteriological assistance should be sought when necessary. The decision to treat a wound infection should be based on clinical judgment and should not be an automatic response to a positive culture report. In some cases, removal of a suture at an inflamed point (minor stitch abscess) may be all that is needed to allow host defences to operate. Similarly, the isolation of coliform bacteria from a mild superficial infection of an abdominal wound need not call for active antimicrobial therapy if the patient's general condition does not indicate any constitutional upset. On the other hand, a positive blood culture obtained from a patient with signs of impending shock, or the isolation of a significant pathogen (e.g. *Strep. pyogenes*) from a wound with signs of regional lymphadenitis, calls for immediate and positive antimicrobial treatment.

Inconsistent or incompatible findings must be discussed with senior experts. For example, a report on a secondary plate culture obtained after a specimen of pus has been subjected to enrichment culture in cooked meat broth might yield a profuse, almost pure growth of *Clostridium perfringens* derived from spores contaminating skin adjacent to the wound. If the wound is giving no clinical cause for alarm and the patient's general condition is satisfactory, a diagnosis of gas gangrene is most unlikely to be justified. Heroic treatment must not be instituted on the basis of such evidence.

Suggestions for specific antibiotic therapy are given in Table 7.4, and initial ('best-guess') therapy is indicated in Table 7.5. The antibiotic sensitivities of common anaerobic pathogens are outlined in Table 7.6.

Table 7.4   Antibiotics in surgery: suggestions for specific therapy 1994

Organism	First choice	Alternatives
Staphylococcus aureus (coagulase-positive staphylococcus)	Flucloxacillin	Erythromycin, cefuroxime, fusidic acid, clindamycin, Augmentin
Coagulase-negative staphylococci including *Staph. albus*	Vancomycin	?Teicoplanin
Streptococcus pneumoniae (the pneumococcus)	Benzylpenicillin	Erythromycin
Streptococcus pyogenes (group A β-haemolytic streptococcus)	Benzylpenicillin	Erythromycin
Streptococcus faecalis (the enterococcus)	Ampicillin (amoxycillin)	Gentamicin with penicillin or ampicillin; trimethoprim
Bacteroides species	Metronidazole	Augmentin, erythromycin, clindamycin
Escherichia coli 1. Sepsis including bacteraemia 2. Urinary tract infection	Gentamicin* or cefuroxime Cefuroxime or trimethoprim	Cefotaxime, ceftazidime Gentamicin*, cefotaxime, ceftazidime, cotrimoxazole, ampicillin
Haemophilus influenzae	Ampicillin (amoxycillin)	Trimethroprim, erythromycin, Augmentin, chloramphenicol (meningitis)
Klebsiella species	Gentamicin* or cefuroxime	Cefotaxime, ceftazidime, ciprofloxacin, imipenem
Proteus species	Gentamicin*	Cefotaxime, ceftazidime
Pseudomonas aeruginosa	Gentamicin*	Azlocillin, ceftazidime, ciprofloxacin
Clostridia	Benzylpenicillin, metronidazole	Erythromycin, clindamycin
Clostridium difficile	Vancomycin (oral)	Metronidazole

* or other aminoglycoside (tobramycin, amikacin, netilmicin).
? = possible

Table 7.5   Initial ('best-guess') therapy for acute infections

Type of infection	Antibiotic
Chest infection Probable pathogens:	
Streptococcus pneumoniae (pneumococcus)	Benzylpenicillin
Haemophilus influenzae	Ampicillin (amoxycillin), Augmentin
Staph. aureus	Flucloxacillin
Enterobacteria	Gentamicin*, cefuroxime
Urinary tract infection	
1. Relief of acute, but not dangerous infection	Trimethoprim, ampicillin, Augmentin
2. Emergency treatment of potentially severe pyelonephritis	Gentamicin*, cefuroxime, cefotaxime, ceftazidime
Wound infection	
1. Abdominal and pelvic	Gentamicin* with benzylpenicillin and metronidazole, *or* metronidazole with 2nd or 3rd generation cephalosporin
2. If *Staph. aureus* suspected	Flucloxacillin *or* cefuroxime *or* erythromycin
3. Amputations and ? gas gangrene	Benzylpenicillin, metronidazole
Septicaemia and septic (bacteriogenic) shock	Gentamicin* with benzylpenicillin and metronidazole. Consider ceftazidime, chloramphenicol
Severe pseudomonas infections	Gentamicin* plus azlocillin *or* piperacillin. Ciprofloxacin, ceftazidime

Note: these suggestions are for occasions when immediate treatment is necessary. Therapy must be adjusted as bacteriological investigations proceed.
* or other aminoglycoside (tobramycin, amikacin, netilmicin).

Table 7.6   In-vitro activity of antimicrobial drugs against anaerobic bacteria

Antibiotic	Relative activity* against		
	B. fragilis	Anaerobic cocci	Clostridia
Metronidazole	++++	++++	++++
Penicillin	± (often R)	++	++
Amoxycillin plus clavulanic acid (Augmentin)	+++	+++	+++
Erythromycin	+	++	+++
Clindamycin	+++	++++	++
Chloram-phenicol	++++	++++	++++
Tetracycline	+	+	+
Cephradine	+	++	++
Cefuroxime	+	+++	++
Cefotaxime	+	++	+
Cephamycins	+++	++	+++
Imipenem	+++	++++	++++
Gentamicin	R	R	R

* ±, +, ++, +++, ++++ indicate increasing degrees of activity.
R = resistant.
Data from Dr Brian Watt, Medical Microbiology, Edinburgh University Medical School.

ties for the individual patient and for the community.

The choice of therapy should be positively determined. Some organisms associated with certain illnesses are almost invariably sensitive to certain antibiotics. For example, the haemolytic streptococcus (*Strep. pyogenes*) is always sensitive to benzylpenicillin. On the other hand, hospital staphylococci are frequently resistant to penicillin and a range of other drugs. Antibiotic sensitivity tests are necessary to guide the clinician in many cases. It is reasonable to initiate therapy on clinical evidence but the drugs selected must be reviewed once the bacteriological report is available. When an antibiotic has been selected, an adequate dose must be given by the recommended route at the correct time intervals. In hospital practice, there is often a disturbing difference between the practical interpretation of '8-hourly' and 'three times a day'.

When an organism acquires resistance to an antibiotic, it has an advantage over others of the same species in the presence of the relevant antibiotic. If the antibiotic is used extensively or carelessly in a ward, resistant organisms may become predominant.

It is important to restrict the use of an antibiotic where possible and to ensure that body fluids from patients receiving antibiotics are disposed of carefully so that residual antibiotic is not irresponsibly

PRINCIPLES GOVERNING THE CHOICE AND USE OF ANTIBIOTICS

Antibiotics should be used with care. The clinician should attempt to recognize self-limiting infections while taking account of the potential toxicity and cost of any antibiotic. As antibiotic resistance is increasing, antibiotic abuse carries collective penal-

distributed into the ward or adjoining rooms, where it may influence the bacterial flora of patients, staff and the environment.

The staphylococcal menace of the last two decades has been largely controlled, but staphylococci with multiple resistance (MRSA) are a threat. Many other bacteria exploit mechanisms of resistance to gain inroads into the patient they invade.

In general, an effort should be made to use a single effective antibacterial agent in the treatment of a particular infection. If a combination of antibiotics is used, the decision should be based on positive evidence that this is rational. In some cases, for example when a patient is seriously ill and a mixed infection is likely (as in acute peritonitis), it may be necessary to give more than one antibiotic to cover a likely combination of pathogens. This blunderbuss strategy should be reserved for such desperate situations and should be rationalized at the earliest opportunity in the light of the patient's progress and available bacteriological guidance.

Antibiotic policy

A policy for the use of antibiotics is desirable. It must be kept under regular review because of continuing changes in the patterns of bacterial resistance to antibiotics. In conjunction with the hospital bacteriologists, the resistance patterns of all pathogens isolated from sputum, urine, bile, pus and blood should be regularly recorded and periodically reviewed, e.g. at 6-monthly intervals. A policy may then be devised which restricts the use of those antibiotics to which resistance is developing. Knowledge of resistance permits more appropriate use of antibiotics in circumstances where it is necessary to give 'blind' treatment, for example in life-threatening infections where antibiotics must be prescribed before the results of culture and sensitivity tests are known. The following guidelines should be observed when prescribing antibiotics.

- Select an antibiotic to which the known or presumed pathogen is likely to be fully sensitive. The spectrum of an antibiotic should be known accurately. A broad-spectrum antibiotic is avoided if a suitable narrow-spectrum antibiotic is available.
- Restrict the use of antibiotics to which resistance is developing (or has developed).
- Antibiotics that are used systemically should not be used topically.
- Antibiotics should be given in full dose by an appropriate route and at the correct intervals.

- With only a few rare exceptions (e.g. lung abscesses) antibiotics are not used to treat abscesses without also ensuring that effective surgical drainage is achieved.
- The side-effects of antibiotics should be known and monitored.
- Expensive antibiotics are not used if equally effective and cheaper alternatives are suitable.

Prophylactic use of antibiotics

The prophylactic use of antibiotics is established in the following situations.

Chronic bronchitis

Patients with chronic bronchitis subject to intermittent exacerbations may be given prophylactic antibiotics before a planned operation. The matter is fiercely debated and opinions are divided. Amoxycillin or cefuroxime are favoured by some workers. The use of epidural anaesthesia has special advantages for these patients. Prophylactic antibiotics are commenced shortly before operation and discontinued soon afterwards.

Antibiotic policy

- Antibiotics should be avoided in self-limiting infections and due consideration should be given to expense, toxicity, and the need to avoid emergence of resistant strains.

- Choice of therapy is determined positively by knowledge of the nature and sensitivities of the infecting organism(s). Therapy may be initiated on clinical evidence but must be reviewed in the light of culture/sensitivity reports.

- Single agents are preferred to combination therapy, and narrow-spectrum agents are preferred to broad-spectrum agents whenever possible.

- Adequate doses must be given by the recommended route at correct time intervals.

- Antibiotics which are used systemically must not be used topically.

- With few exceptions (e.g. lung abscess), antibiotics should not be used to treat abscesses unless adequate surgical drainage has been achieved.

- Body fluids from patients receiving antibiotics must be disposed of carefully to avoid the emergence of antibiotic-resistant strains in staff, patients and the environment.

Tetanus

Patients with tetanus-prone accidental wounds are given prophylaxis as described on page 75, but the wounds must still be treated by meticulous debridement or, if treatment is delayed, by excision.

Gas gangrene

Patients with ischaemic limbs that require major surgery are at considerable risk of developing gas gangrene. Benzylpenicillin is given 1 hour preoperatively and continued 6-hourly for 3–5 days.

Meningitis

Patients with compound skull fractures and technically compound basal skull fractures involving the paranasal sinuses, the mastoid air cells or the middle ear are at risk of developing meningitis. Ampicillin and flucloxacillin are given for several days. The antibiotic cover for basal fractures is continued until cerebrospinal fluid rhinorrhoea or otorrhoea ceases.

Prevention of endocarditis

Patients with congenital, rheumatic or degenerative valve disease, septal defects, or prosthetic heart valves are at risk of bacterial colonization if bacteraemia occurs. Before any operation that might expose them to such a risk they are given prophylactic antibiotics to cover the following procedures.

For dental treatment under local anaesthesia outside hospital, amoxycillin 3 g orally 1 hour before the procedure, and a second oral dose of 3 g 6–8 hours after treatment, is recommended. If the patient is allergic to penicillin, erythromycin 1.5 g is given orally 1–2 hours before the procedure and 0.5 g orally 6 hours after treatment.

For dental procedures in hospital under general anaesthesia, amoxycillin 1 g by intramuscular injection just before induction of anaesthesia followed by 0.5 g orally 6 hours later is recommended. Penicillin-allergic patients are given erythromycin lactobionate 1 g intravenously before induction and 0.5 g orally every 6 hours in the following 24 hours. Alternatively, vancomycin 1 g given intravenously over 20 minutes (starting 30 minutes before the procedure) provides equivalent cover to a penicillin-allergic patient.

Patients with prosthetic valves should always be referred to hospital for parenteral prophylaxis to cover dental procedures. Amoxycillin 1 g by intra-

muscular injection plus intramuscular gentamicin 1.5 mg/kg body weight (if renal function is normal) is given just before induction, and a further dose of amoxycillin 0.5 g is given orally after 6 hours. Penicillin-allergic patients in this category are given vancomycin 1 g intravenously over 20 minutes, starting 30 minutes before the procedure, plus intravenous gentamicin (as above).

For prophylaxis before urinary, gynaecological or colonic procedures, intravenous gentamicin is given as above, and amoxycillin 1 g intravenously 30 minutes before the procedure and twice thereafter at intervals of 8 hours. Erythromycin 0.5 g can be given instead of amoxycillin to a penicillin-allergic patient. Some surgeons add metronidazole cover for gynaecological or colonic procedures.

Before cardiac surgery, intravenous gentamicin should be given as above, and flucloxacillin 2 g intravenously 30 minutes before operation and 6-hourly thereafter for 48 hours. Some surgeons prefer cefuroxime to the flucloxacillin-gentamicin combination.

Gastrointestinal and genitourinary surgery

Patients undergoing gastrointestinal and genitourinary surgery, whether elective or emergency, are at risk of wound infection, intra-abdominal infection and septicaemia. Many methods have been advocated in the past decade to reduce this risk. A single large dose of antibiotic appropriate for the predicted bacterial flora, and administered intravenously on induction of anaesthesia, is probably the most convenient and effective method. Metronidazole alone or in combination with another antibiotic has a good record of success. In heavily contaminated surgery and in emergency surgery, three additional doses at 8-hourly intervals postoperatively may confer further benefit. Antibiotic lavage of the operative field and the incision is another approach to prophylaxis but this is debated and is not universally practised.

Treatment of compound fractures of limbs

As a compound fracture is almost invariably associated with considerable contamination in an area of severely damaged tissue, it is reasonable to give antibiotic cover at once, and preferably before radical wound toilet and debridement if this does not delay essential surgical attention. Opinions differ on the choice of antibiotics. Staphylococci, coliform organisms and anaerobes are likely infecting organisms, often occurring together and with catastrophic potential. Some surgeons rely on penicillin and metronidazole to control at least two of the likely components. Others would use a second or third generation cephalosporin or clindamycin or erythromycin.

Prosthetic implants

Prophylactic antibiotics are obligatory when any prosthetic material is inserted. Staphylococcal infection is the most serious problem, for example in heart valve replacement, cardiac pacemaker insertion, ventriculovenous shunts, aortic grafts, joint prostheses, mammary prostheses or polypropylene mesh repairs of massive abdominal wall defects. However, other bacteria may also be involved, and broad-spectrum cover is usually given immediately pre-operatively and 8-hourly postoperatively for 24 hours. It is important to have informed bacteriological advice.

Immunosuppressed patients

Patients with suppressed immune mechanisms, either as a result of disease or as a result of therapy (e.g. transplant patients), should receive antibiotic prophylaxis when undergoing surgery. The choice of antibiotic is dictated by individual circumstances. Expert microbiological help should be sought.

Treatment of immunosuppressed patients

Prompt *empirical antibiotic treatment* of suspected bacterial infections in immunosuppressed patients is advisable. A combination of an aminoglycoside with an antipseudomonal penicillin or cephalosporin is often relied upon to cover the range of likely organisms. In these patients, it is also important to be on guard against yeast and fungal and protozoal infections and to be aware of problems posed by viruses such as herpes simplex virus, varicella zoster virus and cytomegalovirus. If antifungal treatment is needed, it should not be delayed.

CONTROL OF HOSPITAL INFECTION

An effective hospital infection control programme depends above all on teamwork, conscientiousness and communication. The possible spread of infection from patient to patient or from patients to hospital personnel (or vice versa) should be constantly considered.

Prompt detection and treatment of infection

Day-to-day monitoring in the wards and related areas is essential to ensure that infections are detected and recorded. A wound infection record should be kept in each unit. Ward surveillance is of particular importance in special areas such as intensive care units, baby units, renal units and areas where neutropenic patients are nursed. There must be assured daily links with the laboratory so that the nature of the infecting organisms is known, early notification of a particularly dangerous pathogen is ensured, and trends in antibiotic resistance are monitored. Close co-operation of the control-of-infection officers and control-of-infection nurses with senior staff in the wards, laboratories and associated administrative offices is essential.

Prevention of transmission of infectious agents

Approaches to the prevention of spread of infection in a hospital range from the provision of suitable isolation and containment facilities for those with special infections or at special risk of infection, to the prompt availability of an expert team to mount an immediate investigation and institute necessary changes when the need arises. Prompt diagnosis and treatment of an infection can contribute substantially to the prevention of transmission. Clear policies on such matters as the recording of infection, the correct use of disinfectants, safe disposal of infected material, sterilization of instruments, management of patients who have infections associated with special risks, proper use of antibiotics, and the use of immunizing agents are important in the protection of hospital staff and their patients against cross-infection.

Section 2
THE OPERATION

8

Pre-operative assessment and preparation

CONTENTS

Pre-operative assessment and preparation are an essential part of any surgical procedure. Elective operations should be carried out under optimal conditions with full physical and psychological preparation of a fully informed patient. Emergency operations, on the other hand, may have to be performed in less than ideal circumstances.

OUTPATIENT VISIT

Assessment and preparation begin at the first outpatient consultation. A good referral letter from the general practitioner provides an invaluable assessment based on a long professional relationship between family doctor and patient. The first responsibility of the consulting surgeon is to determine the most probable diagnosis based on a detailed history, full physical examination and results of investigations. Many investigations can be carried out on an outpatient basis but some require admission to hospital.

The decision to recommend operation is made once the diagnosis is known, risks and potential benefits have been assessed, and the relative merits of other methods of management have been considered. The patient must understand the nature of his illness, the implications of surgery, and the prognosis. If he/she is unwilling or unable to comprehend or discuss the question of surgery, a close relative should be involved in the discussion. Potential postoperative morbidity and the effects of surgery on quality of life must be discussed, as well as risk of mortality. Thus, the likelihood of residual deformity

or disability (e.g. from an amputation or artificial stoma) should be discussed frankly from the outset.

The surgeon should indicate the likely duration of hospital stay, convalescence and time off work or household duties. If possible the date for admission should be agreed or at least estimated. The surgeon writes to the general practitioner after each outpatient visit to keep him informed of progress.

Assessment of fitness for operation

The pre-admission clinic

Ideally all patients should be seen at a pre-admission clinic some days before admission. This ensures that undiagnosed conditions such as hypertension and diabetes mellitus are detected in advance so that appropriate treatment can be instituted. Fitness for anaesthesia and surgery are assessed, and current medication may be maintained, stopped or modified, according to need. The patient can then be admitted on the night before, or on the morning of operation, with all necessary investigations completed.

Fitness for anaesthesia. Any disease which increases the risk of surgery and anaesthesia should come to light during the systematic enquiry and examination. Particular attention is paid to cardiovascular, respiratory and renal disorders. Operation should be avoided whenever possible in patients who have recently had a myocardial infarct; the risk of reinfarction doubles if operation is carried out in the first 4–6 weeks, but falls markedly over the next 6–12 months (Fig. 8.1).

The use of drugs is noted, paying particular attention to steroids, insulin, anticoagulants, bronchodilators, antibiotics, psychotropic agents, and drugs used to treat cardiac failure or hypertension. Women of child-bearing age are asked if they are taking the contraceptive pill. Oestrogen-containing oral contraceptives should be stopped (and alternative arrangements made) for 4 weeks before major elective surgery and all operations on the legs, so as to reduce the risk of thromboembolism. If discontinuation is not possible, e.g. after trauma, prophylaxis with

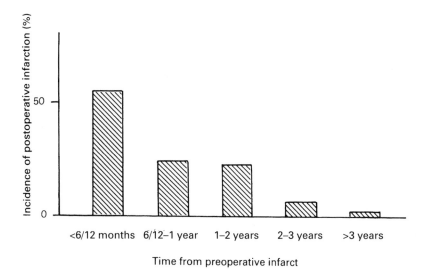

Fig. 8.1   Risk of postoperative myocardial infarction in patients with a pre-operative infarct.

subcutaneous heparin is then considered unless the operation proposed is minor. Elective surgery is avoided in pregnant women because of the risk of miscarriage and exposure to potentially teratogenic drugs.

Allergies and hypersensitivity. Previous adverse or idiosyncratic responses to drugs or other agents must be recorded clearly. Sensitivity to Elastoplast and penicillin is common. Fatal hypersensitivity reactions can be caused by the intravenous injection of iodine-containing imaging agents in sensitized individuals.

Previous operations and anaesthetics. Any complications following a previous operation or anaesthetic should be noted. A history of unexplained jaundice after administration of the volatile anaesthetic, halothane, or prolonged apnoea after the use of the muscle relaxant, suxamethonium chloride, may influence the conduct of anaesthesia. It is recommended that halothane should not be given twice to any patient within a 3-month period unless there is a specific indication for its use. The case notes from previous admissions must be read in their entirety in such cases.

Alcohol and drug abuse. Abuse of alcohol and psychotropic drugs must be recorded as it can affect tolerance to anaesthetic agents, create difficulty in inducing and maintaining anaesthesia, and cause withdrawal symptoms postoperatively.

Smoking. All patients must be encouraged to stop smoking once the decision to operate has been made. The longer the interval between stopping

---

Some factors of importance in preparation for operation

- Following myocardial infarction the risk of reinfarction is maximal over the next 6 weeks. Defer non-urgent operation for 6–12 months if possible.

- Defer elective surgery until hypertension has been controlled.

- Patients with a fixed cardiac output (e.g. aortic stenosis) require particular perioperative care.

- Antibiotic cover is needed in patients with valve disease, septal defects and prosthetic valves to avoid subacute bacterial endocarditis.

- Existing medication must be documented fully, paying particular attention to steroids, insulin, anticoagulants, psychotropic drugs, bronchodilators, antibiotics, and drugs to control cardiac function and hypertension. The long-term risk of stopping medication is often greater than that of continuing.

- Oestrogen-containing contraceptive pills should be stopped for a month prior to elective surgery to reduce the risk of thromboembolic disease.

- In patients with the common cold, elective surgery should be deferred.

- Cigarette smoking should cease for as long as possible before elective surgery.

- Assisted ventilation may be needed if the FEV_1/FVC ratio is less than 50%.

- Sensitivity to drugs (e.g. penicillin, halothane) and other agents (e.g. iodine-containing media, skin preparations) must be recorded.

smoking and surgery, the lower the risk of postoperative chest complications.

Physical examination

General metabolic status

Weight and height are recorded, bearing in mind that the dose of some drugs (e.g. some cytotoxic agents) is determined by body surface area rather than weight. Emaciated malnourished patients withstand surgery poorly and nutritional support may be considered before operation. Nutritional status is assessed by weight loss, serum albumin determination, and measurement of mid-arm muscle circumference as discussed in Chapter 5.

Obese patients present many problems; venepuncture and insertion of venous cannula may be difficult, landmarks are obscured, surgical exposure is tedious, postoperative respiratory problems are common, and the risk of thromboembolism, wound infection and wound dehiscence are increased. Non-urgent operations are best postponed in such cases until substantial weight reduction has been achieved.

The basic requirements regarding haematological and biochemical assessment are outlined in Chapter 6. A coagulation screen is performed if:

- There is a history of a bleeding disorder or undue bleeding at a previous operation
- The patient has received cytotoxic therapy or drugs affecting coagulation
- There is acute or chronic liver disease
- There is purpura or spontaneous bruising.

Respiratory system

The chest is examined clinically and a chest X-ray obtained if there are abnormal signs or symptoms. A chest X-ray is normally obtained routinely in patients over 45 years and in all those undergoing abdominal surgery. This serves as a screening procedure for lung disease and as a baseline if postoperative respiratory problems develop. If there is productive cough, a sputum specimen is sent for bacteriological examination.

Chronic bronchitis and emphysema are associated with intrapulmonary shunting and arterial hypoxaemia, so that arterial Po_2 should be measured. Without special precautions, abdominal or thoracic surgery in such cases can cause life-threatening hypoxaemia. Patients with severe chronic bronchitis may also have carbon dioxide retention. Such individuals form a high-risk group who are likely to

need artificial ventilation postoperatively. As they have a short life expectancy, they should not be considered for anything other than the most urgent operations.

Patients with asthma and bronchospasm may develop postoperative respiratory failure because of the excessive work of breathing. It is important to monitor the degree of airway constriction and, if necessary, lessen the work of breathing by administering bronchodilators such as salbutamol.

The best index of the state of the airways is the ratio of the amount of air that can be expelled in one second (forced expiratory volume (FEV_1)) to the forced vital capacity (FVC), expressed as a percentage (FEV_1/FVC $\times$ 100). A value of less than 50% which cannot be improved by treatment suggests that artificial ventilation is likely to be needed postoperatively. Values above 75% are normal. A crude but useful test is to ask the patient to extinguish a lighted match held 25 cm from the mouth by blowing with the mouth open (not with the lips pursed as when blowing out candles). 'Normal' individuals can achieve enough airflow to extinguish the flame.

Patients producing chronic pus from the bronchial tree (e.g. bronchiectasis) need to be able to cough up secretions and prevent them causing airway blockage and collapse of alveoli. Physiotherapy to encourage coughing and lung drainage is invaluable, and antibiotics are usually prescribed. If pain in the postoperative period is a major impediment to coughing, local anaesthetic nerve blocks may be helpful.

Healthy patients in the acute phase of the common cold should not undergo elective general anaesthesia and surgery. They are likely to receive drugs which will inhibit ciliary action and encourage spread of infection into the distal bronchial tree, with consequent bronchopneumonia.

Cardiovascular system

The cardiovascular system is examined carefully, taking special note of arterial pressure, pulse rate and rhythm, and any signs of right or left heart failure. The fundamental requirement is an adequate flow of oxygenated blood to the vital organs: brain, heart, liver and kidney (see below). Factors which compromise perfusion are reduction in cardiac output (heart muscle disease, reduced coronary flow, or ineffective cardiac rhythm) and reduced flow in diseased major blood vessels.

Patients with cardiac failure are assessed with a view to introducing or modifying treatment so that their cardiovascular system is in optimal condition at the time of surgery. Drugs used to treat cardiac failure, arrhythmias and hypertension should usually be continued throughout the peri-operative period. If hypertension is found for the first time pre-operatively, the blood pressure should be measured 4-hourly over the next 24 hours. If hypertension persists this is an indication to postpone operation until its cause has been established and treatment instituted. In very urgent cases, the advice of a cardiologist is sought with a view to controlling blood pressure rapidly with various combinations of diuretics, beta-blockers, vasodilators and calcium channel blockers. The goal is to achieve a diastolic pressure of 105 mmHg or less. Surgery in untreated hypertensive patients has an increased risk of cerebrovascular accident and myocardial infarction.

Patients with myocardial ischaemia are likely to suffer infarction if anaesthesia increases myocardial oxygen demand, decreases coronary artery blood flow, or both. Drugs or techniques which increase heart rate (and so reduce the filling time for diseased coronary arteries), raise ventricular and diastolic pressure, or alter perfusion gradients must be used with great care. Many anaesthetic drugs have these potentials.

Particular care is needed in patients with a 'fixed' cardiac output such as those with severe aortic stenosis or cardiac tamponade. Even small haemodynamic changes induced by anaesthesia or haemorrhage can lead to sudden cardiac failure, or to myocardial infarction if coronary perfusion is compromised.

Cardiac arrhythmias found pre-operatively should be discussed with a cardiologist. In some cases the problem is not serious (e.g. runs of ventricular extrasystoles can follow sudden withdrawal of nicotine in heavy smokers), while in others it has serious import. Arrhythmias may signal that there is an area of ischaemia or a metabolic or drug problem causing altered movement of potassium across the cell membrane. Atrial fibrillation is common and has a variety of causes, ranging from myocardial ischaemia to thyrotoxicosis. In many cases, the fibrillation cannot be abolished but its effect on ventricular rate may need to be controlled. Patients with heart block may require a temporary pacemaker.

Patients with valve disease, septal defects or prosthetic valves should be given antibiotics before any surgical or dental procedure to prevent subacute bacterial endocarditis. It is important to note that the term 'surgical procedures' includes endoscopy of the gastrointestinal, respiratory and genitourinary tract. Amoxycillin (1 g intramuscularly prior to induction with 500 mg orally 6 hours later) is recom-

mended. Patients at special risk, such as those who have had endocarditis or who have a prosthetic valve, should be given gentamicin (120 mg intramuscularly prior to induction) in addition to amoxycillin. Patients allergic to penicillin can be given vancomycin (1 g intravenously over 60 minutes) with gentamicin.

The concept of available oxygen. The amount of oxygen available to the tissues is the product of cardiac output and total blood oxygen content (the latter being the product of arterial oxygen saturation and oxygen carrying capacity). About 1000 ml oxygen/minute is normally available to the tissues: available oxygen (ml/min) = cardiac output × % saturation of haemoglobin × haemoglobin concentration × 1.34

where: available oxygen is expressed in ml/min
cardiac output in ml/min
haemoglobin in g/dl
1.34 ml is the oxygen carrying capacity of 1g of haemoglobin at 100% saturation.

The resting metabolic demand is usually about 250 ml/minute so that there is an apparently impressive safety margin. However, reduction in all three of the above parameters causes a profound fall in available oxygen, although the reduction in each parameter may not appear significant when taken in isolation. For example, if all three are reduced by one-third, available oxygen falls to only 300 ml/minute.

Hypovolaemia. Loss of intravascular volume from whatever cause (see Ch. 3) leads to a fall in cardiac output. Dilutional anaemia develops and by the time such patients become hypotensive, reduced pulmonary perfusion and a worsening ventilation:perfusion ratio (V/Q ratio) usually produce arterial hypoxaemia. Thus, unless there is life-threatening haemorrhage, an adequate blood volume must be restored before anaesthesia commences.

Hepatic function

All jaundiced patients and those with a history of liver disease, hepatomegaly, splenomegaly, or a high alcohol intake must have tests of liver function, hepatitis B status, and a full coagulation screen.

Urinary system

Postoperative retention can be anticipated in male patients with prostatic hyperplasia. In all elderly males, prostatic size is checked by digital rectal examination, and bladder distension is excluded by abdominal palpation and percussion. Pre-operative investigations are instituted if chronic retention of urine is suspected (i.e. bladder emptying appears incomplete).

Plasma urea and creatinine concentrations are useful but insensitive indicators of renal function. Suspicion of renal disease demands more sensitive tests, e.g. creatinine clearance. A urine sample must always be tested by 'dipstick' before operation for sugar, ketones, bilirubin, urobilinogen and blood. Microscopic examination and culture of urine are indicated if urinary tract infection is suspected or haematuria is discovered.

AIDS and HIV infection

Patients suffering from acquired immunodeficiency syndrome (AIDS) may present for surgery on an emergency basis. There may be varying degrees of organ failure which can influence the conduct of anaesthesia and healing of wounds. The drug azidothymidine (AZT) can have profound effects on both red and white cell formation.

Patients who are HIV (human immunodeficiency virus) positive pose a threat to the operating team and other attendants if blood or tissue fluids such as saliva come into contact with the broken skin of an attendant. Accidental needle puncture of the finger or hand, or damage inflicted by the patient's teeth during examination of the mouth, are potential sources of infection. It is possible for the attending team to take precautions (e.g. wear double gloves, double gowns and goggles) during surgery and procedures such as wound dressing in HIV-positive patients. For this reason there has been debate about whether HIV antibody status should be tested routinely or selectively, and with or without consent in patients coming to surgery. The majority probably favour a selective policy but only after obtaining the patient's informed consent, and when counselling and support can be provided if the test proves positive. Testing without consent is at present regarded as assault in legal terms.

ADMISSION TO HOSPITAL

Many hospitals have admission departments where basic information such as name, address, date of birth, religion, occupation, next of kin, and general practitioner's name and address is recorded in the patient's case notes. If the patient has not already

received a booklet explaining hospital procedure, one is provided.

On arrival at the ward, the house surgeon takes and records a full history and documents the findings of a full physical examination. He or she checks that the results of pre-operative investigations have been received, that the patient understands the nature and implications of the operation that is proposed, and that the consent form has been completed and signed. Some procedures (e.g. operation for breast cancer, or colorectal surgery where a stoma may result) require extensive counselling and this is best undertaken by specially trained personnel (usually a nurse counsellor). Where possible the patient should become fully familiar with appliances that may have to be worn after operation. For example, patients who will need crutches should practise before surgery, while patients who are likely to have a stoma should wear a stoma bag for 24 hours to ensure that its siting is correct when standing, lying down or sitting. Special preparation for certain procedures (e.g. large bowel surgery, see Ch. 28) are instituted.

Arrangements are made to ensure that the immediate relatives are fully informed about the diagnosis, and understand the nature of the operation to be performed and its possible outcome.

THE PRE-OPERATIVE WARD ROUND

On the day before surgery, the surgeon and his team visit the patient with the senior member of nursing staff on duty. The anaesthetist usually visits the patient on the eve of operation, unless pre-operative assessment indicates that an earlier visit is advisable.

Implications for surgical staff

The purpose of the pre-operative visit is to re-examine the patient to ensure that the operation proposed is still appropriate. In the case of unilateral conditions, e.g. breast lumps, hernia and varicose veins, the operation side is marked with an indelible marker. The records are checked to make certain that all essential investigations have been completed and that, if appropriate, blood has been grouped and cross-matched or is available for transfusion. Problems such as diabetes mellitus and impaired coagulation require special attention (see Ch. 11).

The need for intravenous lines, nasogastric tubes and urinary catheters is discussed but where possible these are inserted after anaesthesia has been induced. If per-operative radiology is needed (e.g. operative cholangiography) a request form is sent to the radiology department to book the procedure. Similarly, the pathology department is notified if an immediate pathology report will be needed on material removed at operation (e.g. frozen section examination of a biopsy).

The surgeon takes the opportunity to check that the patient has indeed understood the nature of the operation planned and its implications. The patient usually appreciates an outline of the procedures that will be undertaken prior to induction of anaesthesia, and should be forewarned about where he should expect to wake up, i.e. in a general ward, high dependency unit or intensive care unit. Reassurance should be given about the provision for pain relief and the patient should be alerted to the need for intravenous lines, catheters, tubes and monitoring equipment.

Implications for nursing staff

The nursing staff are responsible for removing and safeguarding dentures, rings and other jewellery, giving the premedication, testing the urine, and fixing a plastic band around the wrist which indicates name, religion, and dose and time of administration of premedication. To minimize the risk of aspiration of vomitus during anaesthesia, patients usually receive no food or fluids after 23.00 hours on the day before operation. If the operation is scheduled for the afternoon, a light breakfast is usually allowed.

An orderly is usually responsible for washing and shaving the operation site if this is required. A depilatory cream is less likely to give rise to wound infection but as it has to be applied for several days, it is not usually a practical alternative. Shaving is best performed as close to the operation time as possible, and can be carried out after anaesthesia has been induced. This is particularly important in patients who may receive an implant of foreign material, as shaving on the previous evening increases the risk of infection. Patients need not be shaved from 'nipple to knee' and a full pubic shave is rarely required, even for operations on the perineum. If possible, they should shower early on the morning of operation using 10% povidone iodine solution or 0.05% chlorhexidine solution, directing particular attention to washing the groin and axillae.

The drug chart is checked to ensure that essential medication has been prescribed. A fluid balance chart is commenced before all major operations, and in all patients with abnormal fluid and electrolyte balance.

Implications for anaesthetic staff

The anaesthetist should be alerted as early as possible to any condition likely to pose problems during anaesthesia and surgery. If there is real doubt about fitness for surgery, he should be consulted about the need for operation and its timing.

The aim of premedication is to sedate, relieve anxiety, and remove pain. It should be remembered that drugs are no substitute for explanation and reassurance. The commonest premedicants are benzodiazepines and opiates, the former having the advantage that they can be given by mouth. If stimulation of the mouth and pharynx is anticipated, an anticholinergic agent (usually atropine) is injected intramuscularly to prevent excessive secretion. Atropine has the added advantage that it blocks vagal influences on the heart and may prevent profound bradycardia. If atropine has not been given with the premedication, it is often injected at the time of induction of anaesthesia.

Many patients receiving drugs for long-standing medical conditions can take these early on the morning of anaesthesia if the anaesthetist agrees. Prophylaxis against deep venous thrombosis is administered according to the protocol of the surgical unit (usually 5000 units heparin subcutaneously three times a day for 5 days, commencing with the premedication). If prophylactic antibiotics are indicated, they are injected intravenously after induction of anaesthesia.

9

Anaesthesia and the operation

CONTENTS

The patient's name and identifying number must be clearly marked on all records and samples, and on a tag affixed to the patient, usually in the form of a wrist bracelet, which cannot be removed casually. At all stages in the hospital stay the staff must be satisfied that they are dealing with the correct patient. These precautions are particularly important if the patient is sedated, confused or unconscious. When there may be any doubt about the site of an operation (e.g. a right-sided breast lump or a left inguinal hernia), a mark is made on the skin with a felt pen or similar marker to indicate the site of the lesion or the proposed incision.

GENERAL ANAESTHESIA

The basic aims of general anaesthesia are reversible loss of awareness and temporary blocking of the gross response to stimulation (i.e. prevention of skeletal muscle movement and autonomic effects such as tachycardia, hypertension and sweating). At deeper levels of anaesthesia with inhalation agents, profound muscle relaxation may occur, facilitating access for abdominal surgery.

When anaesthesia was introduced in 1846–47 these aims were achieved with a single volatile agent,

either ether or chloroform. Inhalation proved an effective route to the blood and thence to the central nervous system (CNS). The problem with single-agent anaesthesia is that a relatively high concentration has to be given to achieve the desired effect. If the agent is very soluble in body tissues other than the CNS, as is the case with ether, recovery is very slow because a large mass of drug has to be eliminated. Chloroform is less soluble but is toxic to the heart and vomiting centre, factors which caused much morbidity when it was used as a single agent.

The ED_{50} of an inhalation anaesthetic is called the minimum alveolar concentration (MAC). This is the concentration (vol %) or, more precisely, the tension (kPa) which prevents half of the population given that agent from moving in response to a painful stimulus. As there is no synergism between anaesthetics, fractions of MAC can be added to each other.

Nitrous oxide has few unwanted side-effects but is poorly soluble and has MAC too high for it to be used as a single anaesthetic. If 66% nitrous oxide-in-oxygen is used as a carrier, a lesser concentration of a volatile anaesthetic can be used. Two-thirds of the anaesthetic effect is then due to nitrous oxide, but the side-effects of the volatile agent are kept to a minimum and recovery is more rapid than if it was used alone.

Although chloroform and ether are historically important, neither drug is much used in the UK today. Ether is still widely used in developing countries as it is the safest anaesthetic for non-professionals to use. Volatile anaesthetics used in the UK today are shown in Table 9.1. Halothane, enflurane and isoflurane are in current use whereas desflurane and sevoflurane may be used increasingly in future. Thus, probably the safest general anaesthetic given today is nitrous oxide with oxygen and one of the modern volatile agents, with the patient breathing spontaneously.

The anaesthetic machine

This is commonly referred to as Boyle's machine, after the London anaesthetist H.E.G. Boyle, who

Table 9.1 Some important features of volatile anaesthetics			
Drug	MAC (kPa)	Main advantages	Main disadvantages
Diethylether ('ether')	1.7	Inexpensive, wide availability of apparatus for safe use in developing countries	Flammable in air, explosive with oxygen-rich gas; slow uptake/recovery; vomiting
Chloroform	0.8	None	Cardiac arrhythmia; vomiting
Halothane	0.8	Huge successful international experience over 30 years	Cardiac arrhythmia (nodal rhythm); bradycardia; very rare hepatic necrosis alleged, especially if drug is repeated within 3 months (thought to be due to metabolite)
Enflurane	1.7	Less metabolized than halothane	Half potency of halothane; contraindicated in epilepsy or renal failure
Isoflurane	1.2	Less metabolized than enflurane	High cost; hypotension; possible problems in myocardial ischaemia
Desflurane	6.0	Virtually no metabolism. Very rapid recovery	Very expensive
Sevoflurane	2.0	Very rapid recovery	Some uncertainty about stability. Very expensive
MAC = Minimum alveolar concentration			

introduced trolleys on which were mounted gas cylinders and the means of vaporizing ether and chloroform. It is not named after the scientist Sir Robert Boyle, although his law relating pressure and volume is obeyed in the filling and emptying of gas cylinders. The anaesthetic machine has facilities for delivering and metering gases (oxygen, nitrous oxide, carbon dioxide and medical air) and accurate vaporizers for the volatile anaesthetics.

The patient's breathing system is connected to the main outlet from the machine. The minimum requirements of the 'circuit' are that:

- A reservoir of gas must be available that can supply the largest tidal volume and allow intermittent positive pressure ventilation of the lungs
- Resistance to breathing must be low
- The inspired gas concentrations must be known with accuracy.

Exhaled gas can only be rebreathed safely if carbon dioxide has been absorbed (by an incorporated soda lime absorber) and 'consumed' gases have been replaced. Alternatively, exhaled gas can be discharged by an appropriate arrangement of valves. This results in a higher consumption of gas and vapour and there must be an arrangement for scavenging so that gases can be discharged safely from the building.

The anaesthetic machine also serves as a convenient trolley for monitors and an automatic lung ventilator, and as a work surface for record charts and drug dispensing. Monitors include the electrocardio-gram (ECG) display, blood pressure measuring device, pulse oximeter (to measure pulse rate and oxygen saturation from a finger tip or ear lobe), neuromuscular block monitor, meters to measure gas concentration, and a spirometer. The varied design and complexity of these arrangements, as with modern cars, often reflects the needs and practices of the user and to some extent his personality. Record keeping is increasingly automated, rather like the 'black box' in aircraft (and with a similar purpose in mind).

Induction of anaesthesia

A normal person who has received no anaesthetic or CNS depressant is deemed to be fully conscious, whereas someone who receives an increasing overdose will eventually die. It is therefore important to recognize clinical signs at various depths of anaesthesia. The American, Arthur Guedel, proposed division of anaesthesia (for ether) into four stages:

Stage 1 spans full consciousness to loss of consciousness.

Stage 2 is a very unpleasant stage characterized by reflex hyperexcitability, breath-holding, risk of regurgitation and bladder emptying.

Stage 3 is characterized by return of a regular breathing pattern. As anaesthesia deepens through the third stage, the respiratory muscles fail increasingly, starting with the accessory muscles, and finally the diaphragm.

Stage 4 is respiratory arrest and soon leads to cardiac arrest unless oxygenation is maintained.

Thus, stage 3 is the depth of anaesthesia for surgery. It is subdivided into four planes of which plane 2 is the 'surgical plane'. This plane can be achieved by inhalation of the anaesthetic mixture, but depending on the speed of uptake, patients can be aware of the unpleasant effects of stage 2. Moreover, many patients do not like having a face mask applied while conscious, even when premedicated. The intravenous induction agents allow a rapid, pleasant drift into unconsciousness to the point where a face mask is tolerated and inhalation anaesthesia can be used without the unpleasant features of the second stage.

Sodium thiopentone (Pentothal) is an ultrashort-acting barbiturate which has enjoyed pride of place for intravenous induction for 50 years despite its appalling pharmacokinetic profile. Its long half-life (about 18 hours) makes it quite unsuitable for repeat administration or infusion, and it leaves a hangover effect. Attempts to replace it have been unavailing despite the regular emergence of new compounds.

Propofol (Diprivan) is a newer intravenous induction agent which has a short half-life and is suitable for repeat administration or infusion, and for continuous sedation during prolonged intensive care. It is difficult to dissolve in water and is presented as an emulsion.

Ketamine (Ketalar) produces a state of dissociative anaesthesia. In smaller doses than those required for induction it can be used as an analgesic. Unlike the other two intravenous anaesthetics, it has minimal cardiovascular effects but can cause bizarre hallucinations and other psychotic sequelae.

The concept of 'balance anaesthesia': the muscle relaxants

In the 1940s anaesthetists began to use smaller doses of intravenous tubocurarine ('curare') to produce partial neuromuscular blockade and muscle relaxation at lighter levels of anaesthesia. However, sensitivity to neuromuscular blockers varies enormously and in susceptible individuals difficulty in breathing necessitated assisted ventilation. It became clear that the best course was to increase the dose of tubocurarine, accept a greater degree of neuromuscular block in all patients, and ventilate the lungs with 'lighter' anaesthetic mixtures. This was one of the more important developments in modern surgery because:

- By reducing the risk of anaesthetic toxicity operations could be performed in patients who would previously have been regarded as unsuitable for general anaesthesia
- It allowed safer and more extensive surgery of the heart, lungs and brain
- It changed the practice of anaesthesia from an empirical art to a scientific discipline requiring specialist practitioners
- Experience in artificial ventilatory support was the springboard to the development of surgical intensive care units where such support is still the principal and most successful form of therapy.

A wide range of neuromuscular blockers is now used. Suxamethonium has a short duration of action (5–10 minutes) unless the patient has a deficient or abnormal cholinesterase (pseudocholinesterase) in which case blockade can be prolonged for up to 8 hours. It is the only *depolarizing* blocker used, and muscle fasciculation is usually seen shortly after injection.

Among the *non-depolarizing* (or 'competitive') blockers, tubocurarine, pancuronium and alcuronium are longer-acting than atracurium and vecuronium. The last two drugs have more rapid onset and offset of effect, accumulate less, and have fewer unpredictable side-effects such as change in heart rate and blood pressure. All non-depolarizing blockers can be antagonized with neostigmine, an anticholinesterase. This must be given with atropine to block the muscarinic effects of acetylcholine (e.g. bradycardia, bronchospasm, increased gut motility, and salivation) but retain the nicotinic effect on the neuromuscular junction and so restore normal conduction and allow return of spontaneous breathing.

The airway in anaesthesia

One of the major challenges in general anaesthesia is to protect the laryngeal inlet from foreign material and maintain a clear airway through the mouth and nose.

Protection of the larynx and trachea

The best guarantee against aspiration of gastric content is an empty stomach. Starvation helps greatly but gastric emptying rates vary. There is always the possibility that the starvation regimen may not have been adhered to rigorously, and in an emergency, there may not be enough time to await gastric emptying. Severe injury and opioids given to relieve pain can delay emptying further. When there is any doubt, a nasogastric tube should be passed to ensure that the stomach is empty.

Less common, but equally sinister, is tracheal soiling from blood in the upper airway or from cerebrospinal fluid (CSF) leakage following skull fracture.

The airway through the mouth and nose

The nasal airway is less likely to become obstructed than the airway passing through the mouth, but some patients do not have an effective nasal airway in the first place. The difficulty with the oral airway is that muscle relaxation induced by general anaesthesia causes loss of tone in the muscles related to the hyoid bone. The support which keeps the tongue in the normal conscious position is lost and it tends to fall back towards the posterior pharyngeal wall. This can very easily cause total airway obstruction and sudden death from asphyxia. Obstruction can be lessened by turning the patient on to his side (rather than leaving him supine) and inserting an oropharyngeal airway. However, the best guarantee of maintaining the airway during anaesthesia is to insert a tracheal tube. The orotracheal route is used most often, but naso-tracheal intubation is more appropriate if the operation is to take place within the mouth.

The endotracheal tube

Endotracheal tubes normally have an inflatable cuff to provide a seal between the outer surface of the tube and the tracheal lining. This helps to prevent ingress of material from the pharynx which could contaminate the trachea. The cuff also ensures that the airway passes *through* the tube rather than around it, so that once the anaesthetic breathing system is connected to the tube, only the planned anaesthetic mixture is inhaled.

The tube is easier to insert if the patient has received a neuromuscular blocking drug. If there is no urgency, a competitive blocker can be used; otherwise the very rapid block provided by suxamethonium allows intubation immediately after fasciculation has ended. It is not always necessary to maintain neuromuscular blockade throughout an operation. In some cases the patient may breathe the anaesthetic mixture through a face mask after an oropharyngeal airway has been inserted. Alternatively, an endotracheal tube may be inserted after suxamethonium has been given; after the 5 minutes or so that is needed to recover from suxamethonium, the patient breathes spontaneously although the tube remains in place.

The laryngeal mask

A newer method of airway maintenance is the laryngeal mask (Fig. 9.1). The device comprises a cylindrical oropharyngeal airway with an elliptical opening which sits over the laryngeal inlet in the laryngopharynx. A cushion or cuff surrounding the ellipse is inflated with air once the device is in place. The airway provided by the mask is more dependable than an oropharyngeal airway, but poorer than an endotracheal tube. Its attraction lies in the ease of insertion. The principle on which the device depends

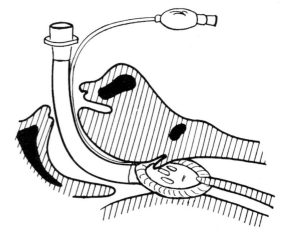

Fig. 9.1   The laryngeal mask airway.

is not fully understood, but the inflated cuff may keep the pharyngeal wall structures in their normal positions. The mask does not prevent regurgitation and aspiration, and so offers less protection to the trachea than a cuffed endotracheal tube. Nevertheless, it is usually effective in securing a good airway in patients breathing spontaneously. Some anaesthetists use the laryngeal mask for artificial ventilation and when difficulty in visualizing the larynx makes it difficult to insert a tracheal tube. Others consider that the mask is unsuitable for artificial ventilation. Propofol is preferred to thiopentone for the induction of anaesthesia when a laryngeal mask is to be used as the apnoea it induces greatly facilitates insertion.

LOCAL ANAESTHESIA

A local 'anaesthetic' blocks transmission of impulses along nerve fibres by altering membrane permeability. Used to block sensory nerves, it allows operations to be carried out painlessly in the area subserved, and can also be used to control postoperative pain. The anaesthetic can be injected into the operation site or injected proximally around the main trunks of appropriate nerves. Higher concentrations of anaesthetic block motor nerves; this can be a considerable advantage in situations such as spinal anaesthesia where profound muscle relaxation can aid surgical access.

A local anaesthetic must be non-irritant, rapid in action, completely reversible, and readily sterilized.

Lignocaine and bupivacaine are the local anaesthetics used most frequently. The total safe dose depends on the age and weight of the patient, site of injection, concentration of drug in solution, and whether adrenaline has been added. If absorbed systemically, local anaesthetics can stimulate the CNS and depress the myocardium. They should never be used without first consulting the data sheet and becoming fully familiar with the constraints on their use.

Topical anaesthesia

Local anaesthetic agents are absorbed through mucous membranes. Solutions and creams containing 0.5–4% lignocaine are used to anaesthetize the conjunctiva, the mucosa of the mouth, pharynx and larynx, urethra and bladder. They can be applied as sprays, gargles, soaked pledgets of cotton wool and gels. Anaesthesia develops rapidly and lasts for 30–60 minutes. As anaesthetics are absorbed very rapidly into the systemic circulation after topical use, care must be exercised in dosage. EMLA (entectic mixture of local anaesthetic) cream which contains lignocaine and prilocaine can be used as a topical anaesthetic for skin. It is particularly useful before venous cannulation in children.

Local infiltration

Lignocaine solutions can be infiltrated locally through a fine needle. They should not be injected into

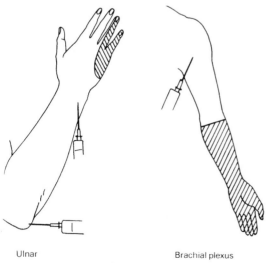
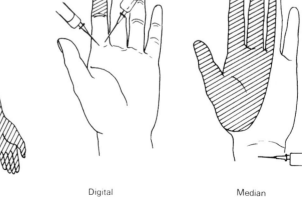

| Ulnar | Brachial plexus | Digital | Median |

Fig. 9.2 Common sites for nerve blocks.

inflamed tissues because systemic absorption may be rapid and the altered tissue pH affects their action.

Addition of adrenaline to local anaesthetic solutions in concentrations of up to 1 in 200 000 causes vasoconstriction and prolongs their action. Adrenaline-containing solutions are not used to anaesthetize digits and appendages because of the risk of critical impairment of blood flow. If local anaesthetic infiltration is used in combination with general anaesthesia, the solution should never contain adrenaline if the patient is receiving halothane (as adrenaline in these circumstances may increase myocardial irritability).

Nerve block

Lignocaine or bupivacaine (with or without adrenaline) can be injected around nerve trunks to achieve nerve block. The anaesthetist or surgeon must be aware of the course of the nerve, its surface markings, and the nature of the surrounding structures. As with all injections, the plunger of the syringe must be drawn back before injection so as to avoid intravascular injection. Common sites for nerve block are the brachial plexus in the axilla or root of neck, ulnar nerve at the elbow, anterior or posterior tibial nerves at the ankle, digital nerves at the roots of fingers and toes, and intercostal nerves below the ribs (Fig. 9.2). When multiple nerves supply a part (e.g. groin or scalp), a 'field block' can be achieved by a series of injections to block the nerves.

Regional intravenous anaesthesia (Bier's block)

Reduction of closed fractures and other simple surgical procedures on extremities can be performed under regional anaesthesia. This is induced by injecting a dilute solution of local anaesthetic into a vein while the limb is kept ischaemic by a tourniquet (Fig. 9.3). The principle is that the venous compartment of the occluded limb is filled with local anaesthetic solution which tracks into the vasa nervorum to block the nerves.

A blood pressure cuff is first applied to the upper arm or thigh, and an indwelling cannula is inserted into a distal vein. The limb is elevated, an elastic bandage applied to empty it of blood, and the cuff is then inflated to above systolic arterial pressure (usually to 250 mmHg). Bupivacaine and lignocaine should not be used for regional intravenous anaesthesia and the less toxic prilocaine (40 ml of 0.5% solution) is preferred. Anaesthesia lasts 30–60 minutes but the cuff becomes intolerable after half an hour. The cuff *must not be released before 15*

minutes have elapsed as sudden release of drug into the circulation may cause cardiac arrhythmia.

If the limb is painful, it may be impossible to apply an elastic bandage (e.g. when reducing a Colles' fracture); it may be sufficient to elevate the arm for 5 minutes before applying the cuff. The veins are emptied less effectively but the method usually succeeds.

Spinal and epidural anaesthesia

Local anaesthetic agents may be injected into the subarachnoid or epidural space to block spinal nerve roots as they pass from the cord to the intervertebral foramina. Spinal anaesthesia is performed through a lumbar puncture needle inserted between L3 and L4 (Fig. 9.4). Lignocaine or bupivacaine are used, and some anaesthetists prefer solutions which, by virtue of the addition of 6% dextrose, are heavier than CSF. The resulting 'heavy' solution gravitates, giving some control over the spread of the block when a subarachnoid injection has been made. Leakage of CSF may cause headache and the patient should remain recumbent in bed for up to 12 hours after spinal anaesthesia.

For epidural anaesthesia the needle is inserted into the epidural space which lies between the ligamentum flavum and the dura-arachnoid membrane (Fig. 9.5). The injection can be made at any level of the spinal column, including the caudal canal. The solution spreads upwards and downwards to create a band of anaesthesia. It is also possible to insert a fine catheter through the needle before it is withdrawn, allowing repeated injections to maintain anaesthesia for hours or even days. Thus epidural anaesthesia can be of value in controlling postoperative pain and the pain of labour.

The sympathetic outflow along the anterior nerve roots is also blocked by spinal and epidural anaesthesia. The resulting vasomotor paralysis can cause hypotension and bradycardia, effects which are particularly dangerous in hypertensive and arteriosclerotic patients.

Complications of local anaesthesia

The main complication of local anaesthesia is overdose. Excitability, apprehension, muscle irritability and convulsions result from stimulation of the nervous system. This is followed by depression and a shock-like state. Cardiovascular and respiratory depression occur and death from hypoxia may follow. The most important step is to oxygenate and if necessary, ventilate the patient's lungs. Diazepam

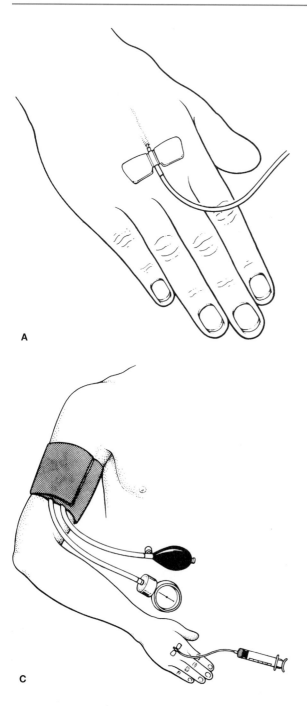

A

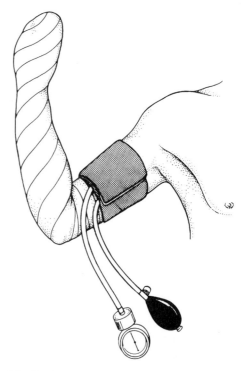

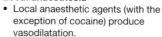

B

Fig. 9.3 Regional intravenous anaesthesia. After insertion of a cannula, the limb is elevated and exsanguinated using an elastic bandage. A sphygmomanometer cuff is then inflated and local anaesthetic is injected intravenously.

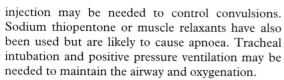

C

injection may be needed to control convulsions. Sodium thiopentone or muscle relaxants have also been used but are likely to cause apnoea. Tracheal intubation and positive pressure ventilation may be needed to maintain the airway and oxygenation.

Patients undergoing nerve block for operations such as herniorrhaphy may benefit from intravenous

Local anaesthesia
- Local anaesthetic agents (with the exception of cocaine) produce vasodilatation.

- Addition of adrenaline causes vasoconstriction and so slows the rate of absorption of the local anaesthetic with prolongation of its effect.

- Excessive vasoconstriction can cause ischaemic necrosis so that local anaesthetic solutions containing adrenaline must not be used when anaesthetizing digits.

- Concentration of adrenaline in local anaesthetics must not exceed 1 in 200 000.

- Adrenaline-containing local anaesthetic solutions must not be used in conjunction with the volatile anaesthetic, halothane, as this may increase myocardial irritability.

- When using regional intravenous anaesthesia in a limb (Bier's block), the occluding cuff must not be released within 15 minutes so as to avoid cardiac arrhythmias following release of local anaesthetic into the systemic circulation.

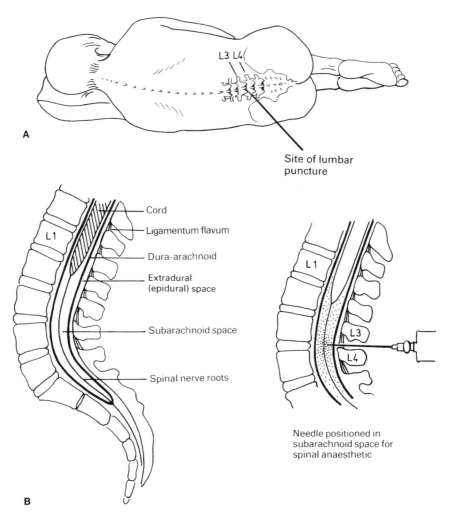

Site of lumbar puncture

Cord
Ligamentum flavum
Dura-arachnoid
Extradural (epidural) space
Subarachnoid space
Spinal nerve roots

Needle positioned in subarachnoid space for spinal anaesthetic

Fig. 9.4 Spinal anaesthesia. A Position of the patient. **B** Position of the needle in the spinal canal.

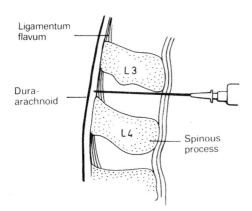

Ligamentum flavum

Dura-arachnoid

Spinous process

Fig. 9.5 Epidural anaesthesia.

sedation with a benzodiazepine such as midazolam. Sedation is a state of psychological relaxation, often with a mild hypnotic effect. The cough reflex and other protective reflexes are maintained. Sedation merges with anaesthesia at the stage where verbal contact is lost. This is an important distinction because the anaesthetized patient needs the full attention of an anaesthetist to monitor physiological status and manage the airway. The sedated patient does not pose this problem.

THE OPERATION

Apart from the dangers of anaesthesia, patients are

exposed to three main risks in the course of an operation: infection, the effects of trauma, and thromboembolic disease.

Infection

The wound may become infected from four sources: theatre air, instruments and materials, surgical and nursing staff and the patient.

Theatre air

The ventilation system of modern theatres ensures that frequent changes of air keep a low density of organisms. Fresh filtered air is blown into the theatre under pressure so that old air is expelled. The theatre air cannot be sterilized completely and there is always some 'fall-out' of organisms on to the operation site, wound drapes, and the floor. Laminar flow systems, which blow a current of filtered air over the operating table reduce, but do not abolish, this fall-out. They are used particularly in orthopaedic theatres where prosthetic devices are being implanted.

As an operating list progresses, the atmospheric bacterial count rises and infection is more common in patients undergoing long operations and in those placed at the end of a list. If more than four major operations are to be performed on one list, there should be a break of 1 hour after the fourth case to allow the count to fall.

Infection rates increase when 'clean' and 'infected' cases are treated in the same theatre. Ideally, infected cases should undergo surgery in a separate theatre. If this is not possible they should be treated after all 'clean' cases have been dealt with. Occasionally, a patient undergoing a 'clean' operation is found to have an abscess or other infective condition. After completion of such an operation, the list should be suspended for 1 hour while the theatre is cleaned.

Excessive movement of theatre personnel causes currents of air which may carry organisms to contaminate wounds and instruments. Excessive numbers of staff in theatre increase the risk of cross-infection.

Instruments and materials

In well-run theatres, the risk of infection from instruments and other materials is small. Sterilization equipment and procedures are checked routinely by a bacteriologist. At the end of each operation all contaminated materials are removed for re-sterilization or disposal.

If an instrument or swab is left inadvertently in the wound at the end of an operation, infection is inevitable. Standard counting procedures are used to keep a tally of swabs, packs, instruments and needles. The surgeon is responsible for ensuring that the count is correct and the nurse in charge of the case will account for all instruments and materials before completion of the operation.

Surgical and nursing staff

Humans harbour millions of organisms in and on their bodies. Organisms are numerous on the hands and perineal skin, and in the axilla, groin and other skin-fold areas. Bacteria shed from the hands include those of the resident commensal flora and those acquired transiently by contact with other potentially infective sites.

There is an abundant commensal flora in the oropharynx, terminal ileum, colon and genitourinary tract. Particular trouble can be caused by carriage of *Staphylococcus aureus* in the anterior nares or perineum, and by the presence of *Streptococcus pyogenes* in the throat of an asymptomatic individual. If a 'healthy carrier' of *Strep. pyogenes* is detected, or if a member of staff has a septic focus such as a boil (usually a staphylococcal infection), he or she is banned from theatre until the lesion has healed completely or carrier status has been eliminated by antibiotics. As nasal carriage of *Staph. aureus* is common, it is not practicable to regard this as grounds for permanent exclusion from theatre duty. However, a carrier traced as the likely source of infection in a patient should be withdrawn from the team and treated with a nasal antibiotic cream to eliminate the organism.

The hands. The 'scrub-up' technique is designed to remove surface organisms from hands and forearms. It cannot remove organisms from sweat glands and hair follicles. After routine cleansing the skin surface is recolonized in approximately 20 minutes. Excessive scrubbing should be avoided and many scrub-up areas are equipped with a stop-clock.

Recolonization is overcome in two ways. Firstly, by the use of sterile rubber gloves and gowns worn over a fresh laundered 'scrubsuit', and secondly, by using modern washing agents which combine a detergent with an antiseptic and remain active on the skin surface. Organisms arriving at the surface are killed for up to 2 hours after scrubbing with povidone iodine (Betadine) or chlorhexidine (Hibitane). Gloves are frequently punctured during operations so that after a 3-hour operation, 70% of gloves contain puncture holes. If a puncture is recognized, gloves must be changed. If the sleeve or any part of the gown becomes wet, thus creating a channel for transfer of organisms, the gown should be changed.

The body surface in general. Bacteria and skin flakes are shed continually from the body surface. Organisms from the perineum are particularly likely to be pathogenic. Shedding is reduced by wearing a theatre cap to cover the hair, and trousers gathered at the ankle may help to prevent dispersal from the perineum.

The upper respiratory tract. A mask is worn routinely in theatre to cover the mouth and nose and reduce the number of bacteria and bacteria-laden droplets expelled during breathing and conversation. Infection of a surgical patient is occasionally traced to a member of the theatre staff who is a nasal carrier of a pathogenic organism.

The patient

The patient is a potent source of 'endogenous' infection and the operation site may become infected in four ways:

- The patient may be an asymptomatic 'carrier' of pathogens, particularly if he has been in hospital for some time. Throat and perineal swabs may help to define such patients prior to operation so that appropriate antibiotic therapy can be prescribed.
- The patient may have intercurrent infection unrelated to his surgical problem (e.g. an infected skin lesion or rotten tooth) which should be treated before elective surgery. If operation cannot be postponed, the infection should be treated with antibiotics during and after surgery.
- The disorder for which the patient is undergoing operation may have produced local sepsis (e.g. an appendix abscess). When it is impossible to avoid entering the contaminated area, the wound is protected by measures such as local antiseptic solutions, antibiotics and delayed closure.
- The operation may have involved entry of a viscus such as the intestine which contains organisms. In elective surgery, this hazard is reduced by preparation of the intestine (see Ch. 29).

Effects of trauma

Tissue damage is inevitable in any operation. Its degree and extent affects the amount of blood loss, the risk of infection (dead or injured tissue is more liable to colonization), the extent of postoperative oedema and fluid sequestration, and the metabolic demands posed on the patient. A good surgeon handles tissues gently and protects all tissues outside the immediate field of operation.

Thromboembolic disease

In the majority of patients who develop deep venous thrombosis, the process starts during the operation itself. Emphasis is now placed on prevention, and measures taken during surgery include administration of low-dose subcutaneous heparin, avoidance of pressure on the calves while the calf muscles are relaxed, and the wearing of supporting socks or intermittent pneumatic calf compression (to assist venous return and avoid stagnation). Venous thrombosis is discussed in detail in Chapter 21.

THE RECOVERY PERIOD

Towards the end of operation, the level of anaesthesia is lightened and any neuromuscular block is antagonized. If an opioid has been given in large doses (to avoid or reduce the need for a volatile anaesthetic), it may be antagonized with naloxone. The aim is to restore spontaneous breathing and adequate alveolar ventilation, and ensure that competent laryngeal reflexes will prevent aspiration of material into the trachea. When conditions are judged to be correct, the cuff on the endotracheal tube is deflated, the mouth and pharynx are carefully sucked out, and the tube is withdrawn. Unless there is any contraindication (e.g. a limb in traction), the patient is safest in the semi-prone position to promote free drainage of pharyngeal material. If a nasogastric tube is in place, it should be allowed to drain freely into a suitable bag; it is dangerous to spigot the tube as this increases the risk of regurgitation of gastric contents around it.

The recovery room

The recovery room is an area where trained nurses look after the patient for the first 1–2 hours to ensure that the patient is awake, stable and comfortable before return to the ward. Care includes the following:

- Careful monitoring of vital signs (heart rate, blood pressure, respiration rate) and special attention to airway integrity
- Institution and maintenance of a satisfactory analgesic regimen
- Improvement of inspired oxygen concentration in all cases for at least the first hour. A controlled

oxygen mask delivering 28% oxygen is appropriate except in some patients with type 2 respiratory failure
- Early detection of haemorrhage
- Establishing a fluid balance regimen
- Instituting the postoperative chart.

The recovery room has continuity with the operating room so that the anaesthetist and surgeon remain aware of the condition of the patient and can move there quickly in the event of a problem.

The high dependency unit (HDU)

This area has a high level of trained nursing staff, although this is less than that of an intensive care unit. The HDU is an appropriate location in the first 24–48 hours for patients in whom cardiovascular status must be assessed carefully, oxygenation measured, and pain controlled by techniques such as extradural analgesia. It is not a suitable area for patients who are shocked or who need artificial ventilatory support. Good high-dependency care avoids some of the postoperative complications which would otherwise necessitate intensive care. As a working rule, a patient who is not well enough to be transferred to a conventional ward after 48 hours should probably be in an intensive care unit.

The intensive therapy unit (ITU)

A surgical ITU has continuity of experienced medical staff, a ratio of one trained nurse to each patient, a concentration of equipment needed for the care of the acutely ill, and effective links with other departments whose help may be needed at any time (e.g. radiology, haematology, bacteriology and nephrology). The unit is directed by a specially trained anaesthetist or surgeon who acts as a point of reference for the many specialists who may be involved. For example, a patient who has been severely injured in a road traffic accident may need the attention of a general surgeon, orthopaedic surgeon, neurosurgeon, ophthalmologist, faciomaxillary surgeon, and nephrologist.

Effective methods of continuous patient monitoring can be simple and inexpensive. An ECG monitor allows continuous measurement of pulse rate, blood pressure is measured readily by sphygmomanometry, and central venous pressure can be monitored by a simple saline manometer. Urine output can be measured by a calibrated reservoir and catheter. Electrolyte determinations and blood gas analysis are measured by automated laboratory equipment. More sophisticated monitoring which may be needed in some cases includes insertion of an arterial line to measure blood pressure, use of a pulmonary artery flotation catheter to measure pulmonary venous gas concentrations and pulmonary wedge venous pressure, and measurement of aortic blood flow by ultrasonic flow meter.

Equipment apart, the main value of an ITU is that it allows continuous care by trained personnel. Changes in skin colour, level of consciousness, and quality of pulse and circulation are still important guides to progress. Recognition of 'pattern changes' is still of the greatest significance and good nursing care remains the basis of intensive therapy. Given the patient population concerned, ITUs are not without their dangers, particularly in relation to cross-infection.

10
Postoperative care and complications

Following an operation there are three phases of patient care. After a short period of *immediate postoperative care* in a recovery room to ensure full return of consciousness, the patient is returned to *surgical ward care* unless there are indications for transfer to a high dependency unit or intensive therapy unit (see Ch. 9). On discharge from ward care, the patient may still require *rehabilitation and convalescence* before he is ready to resume domestic or other duties. This is provided by a period in a convalescent hospital or by a programme of graded activity in a rehabilitation centre.

The major life-threatening complications which may arise in the recovery room are airway obstruction, myocardial infarction, cardiac arrest, haemorrhage and respiratory failure. These complications can also arise during ward care, but except for haemorrhage and cardiopulmonary catastrophe, many of the problems arising in this phase do not threaten life and are often specific to the operation performed.

IMMEDIATE POSTOPERATIVE CARE

The recovery room has been discussed in part in Chapter 9. The remainder of this section is devoted to recognition and management of the major life-threatening complications which may arise in this period.

Airway obstruction

The airway must be kept clear at all times. The main causes of obstruction are as follows:

- *Obstruction by the tongue* may occur during unconsciousness. Loss of muscle tone causes the tongue to fall back against the posterior pharyngeal wall and may be aggravated by masseter spasm during emergence from unconsciousness. Bleeding into the tongue or soft tissues of the mouth or pharynx may be a complicating factor after operations involving these areas.
- *Obstruction by foreign bodies*, such as dentures, and by secretions and blood is a potent source of airway obstruction. Dentures must be removed before operation and precautions taken to guard against aspiration of gastric contents.
- *Laryngeal spasm* can occur at light levels of unconsciousness and is aggravated by stimulation.
- *Laryngeal oedema* may occur in small children after traumatic attempts at intubation or when there is infection (epiglottitis).
- *Tracheal compression* may follow operations in the neck and compression by haemorrhage is a particular anxiety after thyroidectomy.
- *Bronchospasm or bronchial obstruction* may follow inhalation of a foreign body or the aspiration of irritant material. It may also occur as an idiosyncratic reaction to drugs and as a complication of asthma.

Attention is directed at defining and rectifying the

cause of airway obstruction as a matter of extreme urgency. If the airway is clear, *hypoxia* is likely to be due to under-ventilation of areas of the lung with a mismatch between ventilation and perfusion. Blood gas analysis is undertaken and oxygen is given using a mask which delivers a known concentration of oxygen at given flow rates (e.g. the Ventimask which delivers 28% oxygen). The delivered concentration is marked on the mask itself. Mechanical ventilation via a cuffed endotracheal tube may still be needed if an adequate Pa_{O_2} or Pa_{CO_2} cannot be maintained.

Myocardial ischaemia

Postoperative cardiac failure is most likely to occur in the immediate recovery period. While in most cases there is a history of preceding cardiac disease, myocardial ischaemia or cardiac arrest can occur in an otherwise fit patient. Patients with ischaemia may complain of gripping chest pain but this is not invariable (particularly in the postoperative period) and hypotension may be the only sign. If ischaemia is suspected, electrocardiography is performed urgently and arrangements are made for cardiac monitoring. A sample of blood is withdrawn to estimate concentrations of cardiac enzymes.

Respiratory failure

Respiratory failure is defined as inability to maintain normal partial pressures of oxygen and carbon dioxide (Pa_{O_2} and Pa_{CO_2}) in arterial blood. Blood gas determinations are the key to its early recognition and should be repeated frequently in patients with previous respiratory problems. The normal Pa_{O_2} is over 13 kPa at the age of 20 years, falling to around 11.6 kPa at 60 years; respiratory failure is denoted by a value of less than 6.7 kPa. Severe hypoxaemia may result in visible central cyanosis.

Other special problems

Careful monitoring is needed for particular groups of patients. For example, those undergoing adrenalectomy require steroid replacement and careful monitoring of blood pressure and serum electrolytes, patients having neck surgery must be observed for the accumulation of blood in the wound which may cause rapid asphyxia, and those undergoing open-heart surgery require intensive cardiovascular monitoring.

CARE ON RETURN TO THE SURGICAL WARD

General care

On return to the ward, regular hourly or 2-hourly checks are made on pulse rate, blood pressure and respiratory rate. In some patients, hourly monitoring of nasogastric aspirate, urine output and wound drains are indicated. These measures are relaxed as the patient stabilizes.

Patients are normally visited morning and evening by the medical staff to ensure that there is steady progress. Anxiety, disorientation and minor changes in personality, behaviour or appearance are often the earliest manifestation of complications. The general circulatory state and adequacy of oxygenation are noted, and pulse, temperature and blood pressure are checked on the nursing chart. The need to retain tubes and catheters is checked, enquiry is made about urinary and bowel function, and full chest expansion and coughing is encouraged.

The chest is examined and all sputum inspected. The legs are checked for swelling, discolouration or calf tenderness. Fluid balance is reviewed, and serum electrolytes are measured daily in patients receiving intravenous fluids. Intravenous fluid therapy is discontinued once oral fluid intake has been established. Nutritional requirements are always borne in mind; a few days of starvation may cause little harm but enteral or parenteral nutrition is essential if starvation is prolonged.

Sleeplessness can be a troublesome and depressing problem after operation, and it is important to recognize and treat patients in need of quiet, rest and sedation.

Care after abdominal surgery

The abdomen is examined daily for evidence of excessive distension, tenderness or drainage from wounds or drain sites. The main abdominal complications are the slow recovery of intestinal motor function, anastomotic leakage, and bleeding or abscess formation. Return of bowel sounds and the free passage of flatus reflects recovery of peristalsis. If a nasogastric tube is in place it is kept open at all times (to serve as an air vent) and allowed to drain into a small plastic bag. Free drainage may be supplemented by continuous suction but is usually combined with intermittent manual suction. Many surgeons do not allow the patient to drink while a tube is in place, whereas others permit small measured amounts of fluid at regular intervals. Many surgeons retain the tube until a diminishing volume of hourly aspirate suggests that it can be removed. Nasogastric tubes are uncomfortable, and they should not be retained for longer than necessary.

Wound care

Bulky dressings are not normally used for incised wounds and the area can be inspected daily for signs of wound infection. Drains are often used to prevent accumulation of fluid or blood, and to allow egress of any infected material or leakage from anastomotic sites. Closed system drains employing mild suction (e.g. Redivac drains) are often preferred. The drain is normally removed once the amount of fluid recovered daily falls to a few millilitres.

Traditionally, skin sutures remained in place until the wound had healed soundly. Many surgeons now prefer early removal of sutures or staples to prevent unsightly 'crosshatching'. Sutures can then be replaced by adhesive strips (e.g. Steristrips) to prevent distraction and improve healing. At many sites, subcuticular sutures of absorbable or non-absorbable synthetic material are now preferred. If a wound becomes infected, it may be necessary to remove one or more sutures prematurely to allow egress of infected material.

COMPLICATIONS OF ANAESTHESIA AND SURGERY

General complications

Nausea and vomiting can be caused by operation and/or anaesthesia and an antiemetic of the phenothiazine group (e.g. prochlorperazine, 12.5 mg i.m.) can prove useful. Passage of a tracheal or nasogastric tube can traumatize the mucous membranes, particularly when the mouth is dry, and give rise to a troublesome but usually transient sore throat.

Damage to teeth

Patients with loose teeth or crown and bridge work may suffer dental damage during laryngoscopy, and tooth fragments can be aspirated into the respiratory tree. Such patients should be warned of the possibility of dental damage before operation.

Damage to the eyes

Corneal damage, leading in some cases to ulceration, can occur if the eyes remain open during anaesthesia; the complication is prevented by taping the eyelids.

Headache

Spinal anaesthesia may cause headache due to leakage of cerebrospinal fluid, and patients should remain recumbent for 12 hours after this form of anaesthesia. If headache persists it may be necessary to seal the injection site in the dura-arachnoid by a 'blood patch' (i.e. an extradural injection of the patient's blood which clots and so seals the leak).

Vascular complications and nerve injuries

Intravenous administration of irritant drugs or solutions can cause bruising, haematoma, phlebitis and venous thrombosis. Venous catheters, particularly those placed in large veins, should be securely sealed to guard against air embolism. Arterial cannulae and needle punctures are the commonest cause of arterial injury, and may lead to arterial occlusion and gangrene.

Nerve palsies can be caused by stretching or compression of nerve trunks and by extravascular injection of irritant solutions. The nerves most commonly affected are the ulnar nerve at the elbow, the radial in the upper arm, and the brachial plexus at the shoulder. Care must be taken to guard against nerve palsies when positioning patients on the operating table.

Muscle pain

Myalgia affecting the chest, abdomen and neck is a specific complication of suxamethonium administration and may last for up to a week.

Pulmonary complications

Once a patient has recovered fully from anaesthesia, the main respiratory problems are pulmonary collapse and pulmonary infection. Pulmonary embolism is a major complication of deep venous thrombosis which is considered elsewhere (p. 293).

Pulmonary collapse

Inability to breathe deeply and cough up bronchial secretions is the primary cause of pulmonary collapse after operation. Contributory factors include paralysis of cilia by anaesthetic agents, impairment of diaphragmatic movement, oversedation, abdominal distension, and wound pain. When there is complete obstruction of a major bronchus, air in the lung behind it is absorbed, the alveolar spaces close (atelectasis) and the affected portion of the lung contracts and becomes solid. The extent of collapse varies from closure of a small segment to collapse of a lobe, or when a main bronchus is obstructed, the entire lung. In most instances collapse occurs within 24 hours of operation.

The clinical signs of lobar collapse include rapid respiration, slight cyanosis and tachycardia. Breath sounds are diminished and there is dullness to percussion over the affected lobe. Arterial Pa_{O_2} is low and the chest X-ray shows areas of increased opacity. Massive collapse causes severe dyspnoea, the affected side of the chest is uniformly dull, and breath sounds are absent. The mediastinum is drawn over to the affected side and compensatory hyperinflation of the unaffected lung renders it hyper-resonant to percussion.

Postoperative pulmonary collapse is prevented by encouraging the patient to move around, breathe deeply and cough. Regular physiotherapy is of great value and coughing and deep breathing are encouraged after giving a small dose of analgesic while the abdominal wound is supported with the hands or by a temporary binder. Intermittent injection of local anaesthetic through an indwelling epidural catheter in the midthoracic region may alleviate pain. Bronchospasm is relieved by inhalation of salbutamol, and hypoxia is treated by giving oxygen by mask or nasal probes.

When treating established collapse, stimulation of the trachea by a catheter or the instillation of 1–2 ml of sterile saline encourages the patient to cough up secretions. Posture is important and the patient should be placed initially on the unaffected side so that he is forced to expand the collapsed lung. Bronchoscopy may be needed to suck out a plug of inspissated secretion, and antibiotic therapy is instituted after sputum specimens have been sent for culture and sensitivity determinations. When hypoxia is severe, endotracheal intubation, assisted ventilation and repeated bronchial aspiration may be needed.

Pulmonary infection

Pulmonary infection commonly follows pulmonary collapse or the aspiration of gastric secretions.

Pyrexia and a green sputum are typical. The chest signs are those of collapse with absent or diminished breath sounds, often in association with bronchial breathing and coarse crepitations from surrounding areas of partial bronchial occlusion. Chest X-ray usually demonstrates patchy fluffy opacities.

The patient is encouraged to cough and antibiotics are prescribed after sending sputum for bacteriological examination. Most pulmonary infections are caused by the respiratory commensals *Streptococcus pneumoniae* and *Haemophilus influenzae*, but *Staphylococcus aureus* and enterobacteria can also cause problems. Benzylpenicillin is the 'best guess' therapy for *Strep. pneumoniae* while *H. influenzae* is usually sensitive to ampicillin. Oxygen is given if there is hypoxia, and more intensive measures including bronchoscopy and assisted ventilation are instituted if respiratory function continues to deteriorate.

Cardiac complications

Although acute cardiac failure occurs most often in the immediate postoperative period, patients with ischaemic or valvular heart disease, arrhythmias or major surgical insult can also go into failure in the subsequent recovery period. Excessive administration of fluid in the early postoperative period is a common cause which can be avoided by monitoring central venous pressure. Treatment consists of avoiding further fluid overload, and the prescription of diuretics and cardiac inotropes.

Respiratory complications in surgery
- Respiratory complications are very common in abdominal and thoracic surgery.

- Important contributory factors include the effects of general anaesthesia (irritation of the airways and paralysis of cilia), failure to breathe deeply and cough, wound pain, abdominal distension and impaired diaphragmatic movement.

- Airway blockage by secretions leads to alveolar collapse which predisposes to infection (pneumonia).

- Common infecting organisms are the respiratory commensals *Strep. pneumoniae* and *H. influenzae*.

- Treatment consists of physiotherapy, oxygen, and antibiotics to treat infection. Bronchoscopy may be needed to remove plugs of mucus causing lobar collapse, and endotracheal intubation with assisted ventilation may be needed for respiratory failure.

Renal failure

Acute renal failure after surgery results from protracted inadequate perfusion of the kidneys. This may be due to hypovolaemia, sepsis or mismatched blood transfusion. Patients with pre-existing renal disease and jaundice are particularly susceptible to hypoperfusion and are more likely to develop acute renal failure.

The complication can largely be prevented by adequate fluid replacement before, during and after operation, so that urine output is maintained at 40 ml/hour or more. The importance of monitoring hourly urine output means that bladder catheterization is needed in all patients undergoing major surgery and in those at risk of renal failure. Early recognition and treatment of bacterial and fungal infections is also important in the prevention of renal failure.

Acute renal failure is characterized by oliguria associated with a dilute urine (specific gravity <1010; urea concentration <300 mmol/l). Oliguria in association with a concentrated urine suggests that the kidney is functioning but inadequately perfused, and is an indication to give more fluid. Rapid infusion of a litre of normal saline should increase urine output in such patients, and a careful check is advisable to exclude bleeding as a cause of hypovolaemia. If oliguria is associated with dilute urine and the patient appears well hydrated and has a stable circulation, a litre of normal saline is infused. If there is no renal response, 20–40 mg of frusemide is given intravenously; if there is still no response, treatment for renal failure is instituted on the basis that acute tubular necrosis has probably occurred.

Ischaemic renal lesions are usually reversible and the mainstays of treatment are replacement of observed fluid loss plus an allowance of 600–1000 ml/24 hour for insensible loss, restriction of dietary protein intake to less than 20g/24 hour, avoidance of hyperkalaemia and acidosis, and haemodialysis if conservative measures fail to prevent rapid rises in serum concentrations of urea and potassium.

Venous thrombosis and pulmonary embolism

These complications are discussed in detail in Chapter 21 but the essential details are summarized here for convenience.

Deep venous thrombosis (DVT)

Measures to prevent DVT include taking care to avoid compression of leg veins during and after operation, use of graded compression support stockings (*thrombo*embolism *de*terrent or TED stockings), and low-dose subcutaneous heparin (5000 units 12-hourly). Many surgeons use low-dose heparin in all patients over 40 who require a general anaesthetic.

DVT is frequently asymptomatic but may give rise to tenderness over the calf and swelling of the foot and leg. Bilateral ascending phlebography is used to confirm the presence and extent of thrombosis, and determine whether the clot occludes the vein. Thrombosis confined to the *calf veins* carries a low risk of embolism and mobile patients are simply given support stockings and encouraged to move around; if the patient is immobile then heparinization is considered. Thrombosis affecting the *iliofemoral segment* of the deep veins carries a significant risk of embolism, particularly when the clot is non-occlusive. The patient is anticoagulated (see below) and confined to bed for 48 hours with slight elevation of the foot of the bed. Thereafter the patient is given support stockings and mobilized. If there is suspicion of pulmonary embolism or the phlebogram shows a tail of non-occlusive thrombus, consideration is given to inserting a filter into the vena cava (see p. 298).

Anticoagulation is commenced with an intravenous bolus of heparin (5000 units) followed by a continuous intravenous infusion of 1000–2000 units/hour, the dose being adjusted to maintain a whole blood clotting time of two to three times the normal value. Heparinization is normally continued for 7–10 days and then gradually substituted by long-term oral anticoagulation using warfarin. The induction dose of warfarin is 10 mg/day, the dose being adjusted to maintain a prothrombin time (now reported as the International Normalized Ratio (INR)) at two to three times normal. The INR is measured daily until the ratio stabilizes.

Pulmonary embolism

Massive pulmonary embolus with severe chest pain, pallor and shock demands immediate cardiopulmonary resuscitation, heparinization and urgent pulmonary angiography. If the angiogram confirms that embolization has occurred, the catheter can be left in the pulmonary artery to monitor pressures. In some centres, suction is applied to this catheter while it is being withdrawn and so extract clot from the pulmonary arterial tree. Alternatively, fibrinolytic agents such as streptokinase can be infused intravenously to encourage clot lysis, or in extreme cases, the clot can be removed at open

---

Deep venous thrombosis

- Measures used routinely to prevent deep venous thrombosis (DVT) include low-dose subcutaneous heparin (5000 units 8 or 12 hourly) and graded compression (*thromboembolism deterrent* or TED) stockings.
- DVT is often asymptomatic and clinical assessment is notoriously unreliable.
- Bilateral ascending phlebography is the key investigation when DVT is suspected. Its objective is to determine whether:
  - DVT is present
  - thrombosis is confined to calf veins or affects the ilio-femoral segment
  - thrombus is occlusive or non-occlusive.
- Thrombosis confined to the calf veins carries a low risk of pulmonary embolism so that the patient is given TED stockings and mobilized.
- Ilio-femoral thrombosis carries a high risk of embolism (particularly when clot is non-occlusive) and bed rest and anticoagulation are prescribed.
- Anticoagulation is commenced with i.v. heparin (maintaining whole blood clotting time at 2–3 times normal) and within 7–10 days is transferred to oral warfarin (maintaining INR at 2–3 times normal).

---

pulmonary embolectomy under cardiopulmonary bypass.

If a small embolus is suspected in a patient complaining of chest pain, sometimes in association with tachypnoea, haemoptysis and a pleural rub and effusion, a perfusion-ventilation lung scan (V/Q scan, see Ch. 6) is the key investigation. A chest X-ray and electrocardiogram (ECG) are advisable, mainly to rule out alternative causes of pain and collapse. If the V/Q scan reveals lobar or segmental perfusion defects, the patient is heparinized and monitored carefully. In such cases it is also important to search for the source of the embolus; if phlebography reveals thrombus in the iliofemoral segments then a filter can be inserted into the inferior vena cava to prevent further pulmonary emboli.

Warfarin therapy is recommended in all patients who have sustained a pulmonary embolus, and therapy is normally continued for 3–6 months.

MANAGEMENT OF POSTOPERATIVE PAIN

There is great individual variation in pain threshold and tolerance. In general, surface wounds give rise to less pain than operations involving access to the chest and abdomen. It is important to discuss the likely pattern of pain with the patient before operation, providing reassurance and outlining the strategy that will be adopted.

Opiates remain the mainstay of pain avoidance and relief, and morphine remains the most-used analgesic. Intramuscular, intravenous and subcutaneous administration are used more commonly than the oral, rectal or transcutaneous routes. The aim is to achieve steady state tissue concentrations of drug, bearing in mind that the effective concentration may vary tenfold between individuals and that there may be peaks and troughs of need. These considerations explain the relative success of patient-controlled analgesia (PCA) in which the patient can press a button to deliver a pre-set intravenous dose of narcotic. PCA devices incorporate a safety cut-out to avoid overdosage and a computational system to monitor the dose administered. PCA not only achieves good pain relief when it is needed, but lessens the risk of pulmonary collapse seen with more traditional analgesic regimens.

Non-steroidal anti-inflammatory drugs (NSAIDs) effectively relieve less severe forms of postoperative pain. The drug can be given orally, rectally or parenterally, and it is often beneficial to give the first dose pre-operatively. NSAIDs occasionally cause side-effects (e.g. skin rashes, blood disorders, nausea and gastrointestinal discomfort), should not be given to patients with peptic ulcer (increased risk of bleeding) or asthma, and should be used cautiously in patients with renal, cardiac or hepatic impairment (risk provoking renal failure).

Other methods of pain relief include continuous maintenance of nerve blocks (e.g. epidural anaesthesia), and the use of the inhalation analgesic nitrous oxide in concentrations not exceeding 50%.

11
Special problems in surgical care

CONTENTS

The previous chapters dealt with the care of patients before, during and after operation who are generally fit for anaesthesia and operation. However special problems may arise in particular groups of patients; these are considered in this chapter.

THE EMERGENCY CASE

Time for detailed preparation may not be available when a patient admitted as a surgical emergency requires urgent operation. Priority must then be given to correction of a life-threatening condition and relief of pain. However, the following must not be disregarded.

• A detailed enquiry must always be made regarding conditions likely to affect anaesthesia, particularly cardiac, respiratory, metabolic and endocrine disease. The course of previous anaesthetics should be ascertained and a note made of any drugs taken over the past 3 months. In elderly men urinary problems are of particular importance, as chronic retention and uraemia may be troublesome during the postoperative phase.

• The cardiovascular and respiratory systems are always examined fully. Pulse rate and blood pressure are recorded, haemoglobin concentration is estimated, and a chest X-ray is obtained. An electrocardiogram (ECG) is necessary if there is any suspicion of cardiac disease and is advisable in all patients over 55 years of age. Arterial blood gas and pH determinations may be useful in patients who are shocked or who have respiratory disease.

• The state of nutrition and hydration is assessed, and blood urea and electrolyte concentrations are estimated in all patients. For all major procedures, a sample of venous blood is taken pre-operatively for blood grouping and cross-matching.

• Obvious deficiencies or illness are treated as far as possible before operation. Anaemia or blood loss should be corrected by transfusion; congestive cardiac failure by digitalization and diuretics; and dehydration by fluid and electrolyte replacement.

• A nasogastric tube is passed before anaesthesia in all patients who have vomited or who may have intestinal obstruction, peritonitis or a perforated ulcer. A 4–6-hour fast is desirable before operation. If this is not feasible, a nasogastric tube should be passed, the stomach emptied and the anaesthetist informed. In shocked patients a urinary catheter is passed to monitor urine volume. If large quantities of fluid or blood are being infused, a central venous line is inserted and pressure monitored.

• Consent forms must be signed (children under 16 years require parental consent). The site of the operation is marked, and the nursing staff should carry out their normal preparations. The type and dose of analgesic is determined only after discussion with the anaesthetist.

THE NEONATE

As the body of a newborn infant has a higher water content than that of an adult (700 mg/kg compared to 600 mg/kg), little fluid is normally required in the first few days of life. However, abnormal losses from the gastrointestinal tract can produce *dehydration* and *electrolyte depletion* within a few hours and an intravenous infusion is essential for all infants undergoing surgery. The neonate has a blood volume of 88 ml/kg, compared to 70 ml/kg in adults, and is very susceptible to *blood loss*. One unit of fresh blood should be cross-matched so that operative blood loss can be replaced rapidly, and 1 mg of vitamin K_1 (phytomenadione) is injected before operation to compensate for possible deficiencies in clotting factors.

Hypothermia can develop rapidly, particularly in premature or dehydrated infants. This is due to the relatively large surface area of the newborn and lack of subcutaneous fat. Hypothermia must be corrected rapidly or acidosis, hypoglycaemia and hyperkalaemia can occur. Heat loss is reduced by placing the infant on a warming pad during operation, and in an incubator set at 32°C postoperatively. Oxygen may be added to the air inflow, and humidity is maintained at 90–100% to reduce insensible water loss from the skin and to prevent crusting of bronchial secretions.

Hyperthermia may complicate anaesthesia in febrile infants with insufficient pre-operative fluid replacement. Rapid cooling is achieved by placing the patient in an ice-cooled alcohol bath.

Overhydration is readily produced postoperatively in premature babies. Provided operative blood losses are made good, postoperative intravenous infusion is unnecessary unless there are gastrointestinal losses.

Hypoglycaemia may complicate neonatal surgery and is treated by infusion of 10% glucose for several days. Every effort should be made to recommence oral feeding soon after surgery; otherwise parenteral feeding is required.

THE ELDERLY

Any surgical operation in the elderly carries a greater risk than in younger patients. Although the increased mortality is associated primarily with major operations, even the simplest procedure, e.g. hernia repair, may be hazardous. Because of structural and functional changes in the respiratory, cardiovascular and renal systems, and their altered metabolism, old people are less able to withstand the effects of operation than those who are young or middle-aged.

Respiratory system

With age, structural changes occur in the lungs and chest wall which reduce air space and restrict ventilation. Lung capacity, forced respiratory volume and compliance are reduced; gas exchange is less efficient and Pa_{O_2} falls. Rigidity of the pulmonary blood vessels produces an imbalance between ventilation and perfusion. Relatively unoxygenated blood 'shunts' from pulmonary artery to vein, further adding to hypoxia.

In elderly patients requiring elective surgery in whom respiratory impairment is suspected, a full investigation of the respiratory system should be carried out before operation. This includes estimation of forced vital capacity (FVC) and forced expiratory volume (FEV_1), and blood gas analysis. The sputum should be cultured and, if positive, an appropriate antibiotic given. Full oxygenation during and after operation is critical. Factors causing postoperative respiratory distress, such as pain and nasogastric intubation, are avoided. Intensive pre- and postoperative physiotherapy to the chest should be arranged.

Cardiovascular system

Atherosclerotic disease is common and thrombotic episodes are frequent. Many old people have ischaemic heart disease, and postoperative acute myocardial infarction may occur. A pre-operative ECG is advisable in all patients over 55 years of age. Fatal postoperative myocardial infarction is more common in those with previous infarcts, and pre- and postoperative cardiac monitoring is instituted in those with ischaemic changes. An elective operation should normally not be performed within 6 months of a proven infarct.

As vasomotor reflexes are defective, the elderly are intolerant to changes in blood volume. Hypovolaemia is avoided by monitoring blood pressure and ensuring good control of fluid and electrolyte balance.

The risks of postoperative deep venous thrombosis and pulmonary embolism increase with age. Prophylactic measures should be taken (see Ch. 21).

Renal system

The elderly are likely to have impaired renal function and are prone to develop acute tubular necrosis. Hypotension must be avoided. Urinary volume is monitored postoperatively so that oliguria can be recognized and treated promptly.

Metabolic effects

Body composition changes with age. Loss of cells, poor dietary intake, reduced caloric (energy) demands and endocrine hypofunction result in a chronic wasting state. Serum proteins must be estimated pre-operatively and any specific deficiencies treated.

Drug metabolism is altered in the elderly and dosage must therefore be carefully controlled. Oversedation should be avoided as it may cause disorientation and unnecessary immobilization.

THE PSYCHIATRIC PATIENT

All patients are anxious before operation. A calm and reassuring approach by ward staff and a truthful explanation of what lies ahead can do much to allay fear. Tranquillizers are rarely necessary. If pre-operative anxiety is excessive, operation should be postponed until a full psychiatric assessment has been made.

It must be remembered that psychiatric patients develop the same surgical diseases as 'normal' people. On the other hand, some hysterical patients produce a bewildering variety of symptoms in the hope of persuading a surgeon to operate. If careful investigation fails to elicit organic disease, a psychiatric opinion should be sought.

Patients with abnormal psychiatric behaviour or a history of psychiatric disorder need careful assessment by a psychiatrist during the pre- and postoperative periods. Drug therapy should be interrupted as little as possible during operation. Patients with suicidal and aggressive tendencies may require special supervision during their stay in a general hospital.

The management of postoperative mental disturbance requires recognition and treatment of precipitating factors, a sympathetic, calm and orderly approach to the patient, and if necessary sedation with diazepam (Valium; 15–30 mg daily in divided doses or 10 mg intramuscularly repeated in 4 hours), or with chlorpromazine (Largactil), starting with 25 mg orally three times a day, or 100 mg by suppository or 25–50 mg intramuscularly. Antidepressant therapy should not be given without psychiatric advice.

When treating mentally disturbed patients the following factors should be kept in mind.

- Old patients in a strange environment often become disorientated, particularly at night. Adequate light and a sympathetic approach may be all that is necessary to settle them.
- Disorientation may reflect hypoxia in which case it will resolve with oxygen and respiratory care.

- Acute retention of urine in the elderly may cause abnormal behaviour. Catheterization of a distended bladder will give relief.
- Mental changes ('toxic psychosis') occur in septicaemia and may be the first sign of septicaemic shock. Patients who become confused must be examined for evidence of chest, wound or urinary tract infection. If an intestinal anastamosis has been performed, leakage should be suspected.
- Postoperative disorientation can occur from withdrawal of alcohol. Excessive alcohol intake may not have been suspected pre-operatively or may be denied by the patient. If in doubt, his relatives should be consulted and treatment instituted.

THE JAUNDICED PATIENT

Operation in the presence of jaundice carries specific risks which are described in detail below.

Impaired coagulation

Bile salts in the intestine are necessary for the absorption of fat-soluble vitamins (A, D, E and K). In obstructive jaundice, bile salts are absent or present only in reduced amounts and absorption of vitamin K is impaired. Hepatic insufficiency may lead to diminished hepatic synthesis of factors II, VII, IX and X.

The prothrombin ratio (now reported as the International Normalized Ratio; INR) can be used to monitor levels of these factors. If the prothrombin time is prolonged, synthetic vitamin K_1 (phytomenadione) 10 mg/24 h is given intravenously or intramuscularly for several days before operation. If there is evidence of hepatocellular dysfunction, a full coagulation screen is required. Replacement of coagulation components may be necessary (see Ch. 4).

Acute renal failure ('hepatorenal syndrome')

The risk of renal failure in jaundiced patients is increased for several reasons.

- Dehydration is common and compounded by anorexia or vomiting.
- Infection in the biliary tree (cholangitis) commonly complicates biliary obstruction. Surgical manipulation and endotoxaemia can cause bacteraemia with toxic effects on the kidney.
- Patients with obstructive jaundice excrete conjugated bilirubin in the urine which may reduce glomerular perfusion and be toxic to tubular cells.

• Disordered coagulation increases the risk of haemorrhage and hypotension during operation, leading to reduced renal perfusion.

Assuming that coagulation defects have been corrected, the most important prophylactic measures are to ensure full hydration of the patient before operation and to monitor urine volume. The patient is catheterized, and sufficient intravenous fluids are given to ensure a urinary output of at least 40 ml/h during operation and for 48 hours thereafter. Some surgeons administer diuretic agents such as frusemide or mannitol (100 ml of a 20% solution commencing 1 hour before operation and given over 30 min) routinely during surgery but this is only necessary if adequate hydration fails to achieve adequate urine volumes. In patients with obstructive jaundice, the operation should be carried out under antibiotic cover to avoid bacteraemia.

Hepatotoxicity due to anaesthetic agents

Many drugs given in the peri-operative period are potentially hepatotoxic and care should be exercised when these are given to patients with liver damage. The anaesthetist will probably wish to avoid the use of halothane.

Jaundice and surgery
• Hepatic insufficiency may lead to diminished synthesis of coagulation factors II, VII, IX and X.

• Obstructive jaundice leads to absence of bile salts from the gut lumen and failure to absorb fat soluble vitamins (A,D,E and K). Failure to absorb vitamin K prevents manufacture of prothrombin and is reflected in prolongation of prothrombin time (now measured as international normalized ratio; INR).

• Renal failure is a common accompaniment of liver failure and the 'hepatorenal syndrome' is a potential risk in jaundiced patients undergoing surgery. Factors implicated in pathogenesis include dehydration, infection and endotoxaemia, diminished renal perfusion after blood loss, and toxic effects of bile pigments.

• Renal failure in jaundiced patients undergoing surgery is prevented by adequate hydration, monitoring urine output (with use of diuretics if appropriate) and antibiotic cover.

• Other factors which increase the risk of surgery in jaundiced patients include increased susceptibility to hepatotoxic drugs and anaesthetic agents, depressed defences against infection, and impaired healing due to malnourishment.

Hepatocellular injury is associated with delay in metabolism of drugs normally dependent on the liver for excretion.

Hepatitis virus

Jaundiced patients with serum hepatitis constitute a potential danger to medical and nursing staff. All jaundiced patients undergoing surgery must therefore have their serum tested for hepatitis B surface antigen so that adequate precautions can be taken if this proves positive.

THE MALNOURISHED PATIENT

Malnourishment presents special surgical hazards.

• As blood volume is reduced, any further reduction by haemorrhage is not well tolerated.
• Hypoproteinaemia leads to increased sequestration of fluid at the operation site and further reduces blood volume. The risk of pulmonary oedema following intravenous infusion of crystalloids is increased. If an intestinal anastomosis has been performed, local oedema may impair patency and delay return of normal intestinal function.
• Protein and vitamin deficiencies impair synthesis of collagen and delay wound healing. Wound dehiscence and anastomotic disruption are more common in patients who are malnourished.
• Resistance to infection is reduced by impaired production of antibodies.
• Protein reserves may be further depleted by the catabolic phase of the metabolic response.

The general nutritional state of these patients should be improved before operation if at all possible. If surgery cannot be delayed, full nutritional support must be given postoperatively.

Alimentary feeding

Pre-operative nutrition is best provided by the alimentary route using normal food. A daily intake of 3000–3500 kcal/100–120 g protein with added vitamins should be continued until body weight is within 15% of ideal.

If oral feeding is impracticable, e.g. in patients who cannot eat or who have an oesophageal or gastric obstruction, enteral feeding may be required (see Ch. 5). This can be given through a fine nasogastric tube or by gastrostomy or jejunostomy. The delivery of foodstuffs directly into the small intestine may cause diarrhoea, and hyperosmolar solutions should be avoided.

Intravenous feeding (parenteral nutrition)

If oral or enteral intake is not possible or inadequate, parenteral feeding (see Ch. 5) is the best method of supporting those who are malnourished. Solutions of synthetic amino acids and emulsified fats can be administered intravenously to provide a nutritionally balanced diet. Parenteral nutrition is particularly valuable in patients with excessive losses, e.g. from intestinal fistulas.

IMPAIRED HAEMOSTASIS

Haemostasis may be impaired by defective coagulation, disorders of the capillary endothelium, or platelet deficiency. The following are of surgical relevance.

Anticoagulant therapy

Heparin. Heparin interferes with platelet aggregation and has antithrombin and antithromboplastin actions. A single intravenous dose of 5000–15 000 units prolongs clotting time to two to three times normal for 2–5 hours. Rapid reversion to normal follows when therapy is discontinued.

Protamine sulphate combines with heparin to form a stable complex without anticoagulant activity and is used to counteract heparin if urgent operation is required. A dose of 1.0–1.5 mg antagonizes each 100 units of heparin. Protamine is given by *slow* intravenous injection. The quantity required decreases rapidly with the time elapsed after heparin injection: after 30 min only about 0.5 mg is required to antagonize each 100 units injected. As low-dose heparin therapy has been shown to prevent postoperative deep venous thrombosis, heparinized patients requiring surgery are best treated by subcutaneous injection of low doses (5000 units prior to operation followed by 5000 units twice or thrice daily thereafter).

Oral anticoagulants. Anticoagulants such as warfarin (coumarin) act as substrate competitors with vitamin K and depress manufacture of vitamin K-dependent clotting factors II, VII, IX, and X. As they take 36–48 hours to exert their full effect, heparin is used concomitantly when instituting therapy. The dose depends on the INR. Currently recommended ratios are 2–2.5:1 for prophylaxis of

deep vein thrombosis; 2–3:1 for treatment of deep vein thrombosis; and 3–4.5:1 for arterial grafts and prosthetic heart valves. Provided that the prothrombin ratio is not greater than 2:1, major surgery can be performed without excessive bleeding.

As these drugs are bound to albumin and there is negligible renal excretion, the duration of action is long. If liver function is adequate, 10–30 mg of synthetic vitamin K_1 (phytomenadione) given by intravenous or intramuscular injection will restore the INR to normal within 24–48 hours. More rapid restitution can be achieved by transfusion of factor concentrates or fresh frozen plasma (FFP).

In patients on long-term treatment with warfarin who are to undergo elective surgery, oral anticoagulants should be stopped 48 hours before operation and the INR ratio estimated daily. Heparin may be substituted if this falls to less than 2:1. In emergency situations where oral anticoagulants may predispose to haemorrhage, e.g. in acute pancreatitis, a similar regimen should be instituted on admission.

Haemophilia

Operations are potentially disastrous in haemophiliacs and close cooperation with a haematologist is essential. The level of anti-haemophilic globulin (factor VIII) must be maintained between 30 and 40% of normal by transfusion of concentrates of human anti-haemophilic globulin or, alternatively, fresh plasma. The adequacy of transfusion is monitored by sequential estimates of factor VIII (see Ch. 4); the prothrombin time is normal in haemophilia. Infection with human immunodeficiency virus (HIV), which has had disastrous effects in haemophiliacs, should no longer be a risk in view of the routine testing of donors for HIV-antibodies and heat-treatment of factor VIII.

The allied condition of Christmas disease (factor IX deficiency) is less common and usually less severe. Operation can be covered by transfusion of fresh frozen plasma or factor concentrate.

Thrombocytopenia

Thrombocytopenia may be 'idiopathic' or secondary to problems such as drug reactions, hyper-splenism, disseminated intravascular coagulation, or marrow destruction by radiotherapy or tumour. Patients receiving multiple transfusions of stored blood may also develop thrombocytopenia, as such blood does not replace platelet losses.

A platelet count of $40–50 \times 10^9/1$ is normally

adequate for haemostasis, and platelet transfusions should be used to attain this level in thrombocytopenic patients requiring surgery. This can be given by a 'bolus' infusion pre-operatively.

Disseminated intravascular coagulation (DIC)

The causes of this rare syndrome include major trauma, septicaemia, hypoxia, transfusion reaction, metastatic carcinoma and amniotic fluid embolism. An unusual cause is transfer of peritoneal fluid to the systemic venous system by an artificial shunt, as sometimes used in treatment of ascites. Coagulation systems are activated and platelet aggregation occurs within the vascular system, leading to thrombocytopenia, deficiencies of clotting factors and secondary activation of the fibrinolytic system. The level of fibrin degradation products (FDP) is raised.

In surgical patients, DIC is encountered most frequently in the postoperative period. Treatment is complex and may include steroids, heparin and epsilon-aminocaproic acid. A haematologist should be consulted.

Fibrinolysis

Primary fibrinolysis is occasionally seen in patients with liver disease and metastatic carcinoma and is quite distinct from the *secondary* fibrinolysis of the DIC syndrome. The plasma fibrinogen level is diminished, platelet count is normal, thrombin time is normal or only slightly prolonged, and there is an early increase in plasma levels of fibrin degradation products. Heparin is contraindicated; epsilon-aminocaproic acid acts as a fibrin substitute and is the treatment of choice. Its administration is controlled by a haematologist.

CARDIAC DISEASE

As already stated, a pre-operative ECG is obtained in all patients over 55 years and in those with cardiac symptoms to detect any arrhythmias and ischaemic changes, and to serve as a base for postoperative comparison. If cardiac disease is present, a cardiologist should be consulted pre-operatively.

Recent myocardial infarction seriously affects the response to surgery, and only emergency procedures are performed within 6 months of a proven infarct. Only after that time does the risk of a further infarct become acceptably low.

Cardiac disease and operation
- Pre-operative ECG is advisable in all patients over 55 and those with cardiac symptoms to detect arrhythmias and ischaemia, and provide a baseline.
- Non-urgent surgery should be avoided whenever possible in the first 6 months following myocardial infarction.
- Angina should be investigated before any non-urgent operation. Patients with severe 'crescendo' angina may benefit from coronary angiography and coronary artery bypass surgery before undergoing non-cardiac operations.
- Arrhythmias and cardiac failure should be corrected if possible before surgery.
- Antihypertensive therapy is usually continued except on the day of operation. Beta-adrenergic blockers may impair cardiac responses and cardiac function should be monitored carefully following operation.
- Patients on oral anticoagulants are usually transferred to heparin therapy until the risk of operation-related bleeding has diminished.
- Antibiotic prophylaxis is indicated in all patients with diseased or prosthetic valves or septal defects.

Patients with angina should be fully investigated before any operation. In mild cases of angina of effort, operation is safe provided anaemia is corrected, and full and continued oxygenation of the blood is achieved during and after operation. Respiratory depression must be avoided at all costs.

Wherever possible, operation is postponed in patients with severe angina, particularly when it is of the 'crescendo' type. In such patients coronary angiography and, if necessary, coronary artery revascularization has priority.

Cardiac arrhythmias are corrected before surgery if possible. Pre-operative digitalization may be required to control rapid atrial fibrillation, and lignocaine to suppress multiple ventricular ectopic beats.

Cardiac failure is an obvious risk factor, and in patients with acute congestive failure, operation should be delayed if possible until failure has been corrected by digitalization and diuretics. Elderly hypertensive patients must be examined carefully for evidence of congestive failure; this again should be treated pre-operatively if possible.

In patients with congestive failure particular care is taken with fluid replacement. Saline infusion is limited to 500 ml daily, urine volume is monitored, and diuretics are given as required. If large volumes of fluid or blood are required for resuscitation or correction of electrolyte deficiencies, monitoring of central venous pressure is essential.

Patients with valvular heart disease present a particular problem. They are liable to arrhythmias and cardiac failure, and may be taking drugs which can complicate the course of operation. Some patients may require replacement of the affected valve before any other surgery can be considered.

Patients with some types of artificial heart valve are likely to be receiving oral anticoagulants (e.g. warfarin). This therapy should be stopped pre-operatively and heparin substituted when the prothrombin ratio falls below 2:1. A low-dose heparin regimen is normally used. Vitamin K_1 should not be given to patients with a prosthetic heart valve as it may make them resistant to anticoagulant therapy for several days. Fresh frozen plasma (FFP) is preferred. The patient's normal anticoagulant regimen is reinstituted as soon as the risk of acute bleeding has passed. Postoperative arterial emboli indicate the presence of intracardiac thrombus, and emergency cardiac surgery may be required to avert a fatal embolic episode.

Drugs used to control hypertension are not normally withdrawn except on the day of operation. Beta-adrenergic blockers are commonly used for antihypertensive therapy. As they impair normal cardiac responses, cardiac function must be monitored carefully during anaesthesia and in the postoperative period.

CHEST DISEASE

Pre-operative assessment and management

All patients requiring general anaesthesia are screened for chest disease. This demands a careful history, physical examination and chest X-ray. Particular note is made of the patient's occupation and smoking habits, dyspnoea on exertion, and any history of previous chest infection.

When impaired pulmonary function is suspected, forced expiratory volume over a standard period of 1 second (FEV_1) and forced vital capacity (FVC) are measured by spirometry. In obstructive airway disease the FEV_1 may be less than 1 litre and the ratio of FEV_1 to FVC below the normal 80–65%. Arterial oxygen and carbon dioxide tension (Pa_{O_2} and Pa_{CO_2}), bicarbonate and hydrogen ion concentration are determined to provide a baseline for future comparison. Normal values are: $[H^+]$ 36–44 nmol/l; Pa_{O_2} 12–15 kPa; Pa_{CO_2} 4.4–6.1 kPa; and plasma bicarbonate 21–27.5 mmol/l.

If the patient has a productive cough, a specimen of sputum is sent for bacteriological examination. If the sputum is green and purulent, pre-operative antibiotic therapy is required; the choice of antibiotic depends on the results of culture and sensitivity determination.

Pre-operative physiotherapy helps clear the chest and is valuable training for deep breathing and coughing in the postoperative period. Smoking should be forbidden. If possible, the patient should stop smoking for at least 2 weeks before elective surgery. Bronchodilation with salbutamol by mouth or inhalation is useful in obstructive airway disease, and regular postural drainage should be instituted in patients with bronchiectasis or excess sputum.

Only life-saving operations should be undertaken in patients who are unable to maintain satisfactory ventilation and gaseous exchange at rest. Local or epidural anaesthesia should be considered as an alternative to general anaesthesia.

Postoperative care

Inhalation anaesthetics irritate the bronchial mucosa, inhibit ciliary action, increase bronchial secretions and reduce lung compliance. Wound pain impairs ventilation after thoracic and abdominal surgery. Sedation diminishes ventilation, and prolonged deep sedation is contraindicated in patients with chest disease. Frequent small doses of narcotics are preferred to infrequent large doses.

The patient should expand his lungs fully by deep breathing every 30–60 min and clear accumulated secretions by coughing. This is made easier if the abdominal wound is supported by a physiotherapist or nurse placing her hands around the lower chest. Regular physiotherapy is essential to encourage the patient to clear his chest of secretions. He must not be allowed to lie passively in bed taking shallow breaths. These fail to maintain lung expansion and allow accumulation of secretions, resulting in increasing atelectasis and bronchopneumonia. The chest is examined clinically twice daily and, in patients with chronic chest disease, a daily chest X-ray may be needed. Respiratory efficiency is monitored by blood gas estimations.

If the patient is not able to cooperate, tracheal suction is used to clear the airway and stimulate coughing. Bronchoscopy may be required if significant airway obstruction persists.

Oxygen therapy is indicated for arterial hypoxaemia; it should be given at a known concentration and its effect monitored by regular blood gas estimations. In patients with ventilatory failure necessitating artificial ventilation, the inspired oxygen is set to achieve the desired Pa_{O_2}. This should be at least 8–9 kPa. Individuals with chronic respiratory disease may live normally with a lower Pa_{O_2}, and in such patients only small increases in inspired oxygen (using a Ventimask or similar *controlled* oxygen therapy device) should be attempted.

Antibiotic therapy is continued postoperatively. Bronchodilators are continued in patients with obstructive airway disease. Intravenous fluid administration is monitored carefully, as even slight overload may precipitate pulmonary oedema.

Assisted ventilation

Patients with severe chest disease may require assisted ventilation for hours or days after general anaesthesia. The anaesthetist will not remove the endotracheal tube until spontaneous ventilation is adequate. Assisted ventilation is required if a steady increase in Pa_{CO_2} is accompanied by clinical deterioration and/or a rise in hydrogen ion concentration to above 44 nmol/l. Other indications for ventilatory support are a Pa_{O_2} of less than 8 kPa in a patient breathing 100% oxygen; failure to remove copious bronchial secretions; and a respiratory rate faster than 35/min.

There are two main types of ventilator: volume-limited and pressure-limited. In the volume-limited type a preset tidal volume is delivered. Pressure-limited ventilators cycle when the peak pressure in the trachea reaches a preset value.

A volume-limited respirator is preferred in patients with acute respiratory failure. Its high peak velocities compensate adequately for increased airway resistance and decreased pulmonary compliance. Oxygenation can be improved further by the use of positive end-expiratory pressure (PEEP), i.e. by adjusting the ventilator to deliver the desired air/oxygen mixture under positive pressure (5–10 cmH_2O) throughout the expiratory phase. This modification prevents alveolar collapse, decreases the diffusion distance for oxygen by thinning the alveolar wall, and encourages movements of fluids out of the alveoli and their adjoining interstitial space.

DIABETES MELLITUS

In the era before insulin become available, diabetic patients undergoing surgery were at considerable risk of developing fatal ketoacidosis. This risk is now reduced by meticulous attention to insulin and carbohydrate requirements and by regular testing of blood and urine. As a general rule, it is imperative to *avoid hypoglycaemia*; a degree of hyperglycaemia is acceptable provided that ketoacidosis does not occur.

Elective operations in diabetic patients

All diabetics must be admitted 2–3 days before operation to ensure that control is adequate. General anaesthesia can induce ketosis, and infection, starvation and trauma all increase the risk. Elective operations in diabetics are best carried out early in the day, with the patient placed first on the operating list. Specific management depends on the type of control of the patient's diabetes.

Patients controlled by diet alone require no particular action other than 4-hourly finger-prick blood glucose estimations and regular testing of urine for sugar and ketones. Insulin may be needed temporarily if the blood glucose rises and ketosis develops.

Patients whose diabetes is controlled by an oral hypoglycaemic agent should omit their tablets on the morning of the operation and restart as soon as oral feeding recommences. Otherwise management is as for patients controlled by diet alone.

Patients whose diabetes is controlled normally by insulin are easier to manage if soluble insulin rather than long-acting preparations are used. On the day before surgery the dose of depot insulin is halved and supplemented by soluble insulin later in the day. Hypoglycaemia is the major danger on the day of operation and *no* insulin is given prior to surgery.

Blood glucose concentration is estimated preoperatively. If it is less than 6.7 mmol/l, intraoperative hypoglycaemia is avoided by giving 25–50 g of glucose intravenously as a 10% solution. If it exceeds 11 mmol/l (and this is unusual) one-third of the daily insulin requirement is given as soluble insulin *once operation has been completed.*

Following minor surgery, the patient should be able to take carbohydrate orally. Drinks of 25 g glucose are given every 3–4 hours, each covered by 12 units of insulin.

After major operations, it may be some days before oral feeding is possible. Caloric (energy) requirements are supplied by intravenous infusion of glucose (100 g/l) covered by soluble insulin (0.5 units/g) and monitored by twice-daily estimates of blood glucose. Postoperative complications increase the tendency to ketosis. Each specimen of urine must be tested for glucose and ketones; ketonuria indicates the need to increase insulin dosage.

Arterial blood gases and hydrogen ion concentration are estimated to establish whether significant acidosis has developed. Electrolytes must be checked daily.

Once the patient is eating normally, he can revert to his usual insulin regimen. A temporary increase in insulin requirements is common after major surgery.

Emergency operations in diabetic patients

An intravenous infusion is established and blood glucose, arterial gases and hydrogen ion concentration are determined. The urine is tested for sugar and ketones. Glycosuria can usually be ignored *provided there is no ketosis.*

Ketoacidosis is an indication to defer surgery until acidosis and fluid and electrolyte abnormalities have been corrected by soluble insulin and intravenous fluids. Complete correction may not be possible until the precipitating surgical cause has been dealt with. Timely incision and drainage of an abscess may lead to marked improvement in the metabolic state. Considerable clinical judgement is required for optimal timing of surgical intervention. The operation is usually performed under cover of an infusion of 10% glucose to avoid hypoglycaemia. Postoperative carbohydrate and insulin requirements are determined by frequent testing of the blood and urine.

Diabetes mellitus and surgery
- In the 'pre-insulin era', fatal ketoacidosis was the major risk in diabetics.

- In the 'insulin era', hypoglycaemia is the major threat; some hyperglycaemia is acceptable provided that ketoacidosis does not develop.

- Diabetics should be admitted for 2–3 days before major surgery, and should be placed first on a morning operating list.

- Diabetics managed by diet alone merely require 4-hourly testing of blood glucose and urine testing for glucose and ketones.

- Diabetics managed by oral hypoglycaemic agents should omit therapy on the morning of operation, restarting therapy when oral intake is possible. Regular blood and urine testing may indicate the (temporary) need for insulin.

- Insulin-depended diabetics should be converted to soluble insulin rather than long-acting preparations. Hypoglycaemia is the major danger on the day of operation and they should not receive insulin prior to operation.

ALCOHOL ABUSE

Alcoholics are prone to malnourishment with hypoproteinaemia, chronic vitamin deficiency and poor liver function. Plasma proteins and liver function should be checked. Pre-operatively, the patient's nutritional state should be improved by ensuring an adequate caloric (energy) intake, and daily injections of a multivitamin preparation (e.g. Parentrovite, which supplies vitamins B and C). If liver function tests are abnormal, the prothrombin time should be estimated. If prolonged, 20 mg of synthetic vitamin K_1 is given daily by mouth or by intravenous or intramuscular injection.

Induction and maintenance of anaesthesia may require larger doses of anaesthetic than usual. The anaesthetist must be informed that the patient has a history of alcohol abuse.

Withdrawal symptoms can pose problems particularly in the postoperative period. These may take the form of autonomic disturbances, hallucinations, sleep disturbance, tremor and various affective states. Possible fatal complications include epileptiform fits, hypovolaemia, circulatory collapse and hyperthermia.

Management

The patient is nursed in quiet surroundings, isolated from the main ward. As alcoholic patients tend to be dehydrated and liable to hypoglycaemia and hypomagnesaemia, intravenous infusions of saline, glucose, vitamins and magnesium are recommended.

Sedation is required. *Chlormethiazole* (Heminevrin) is sometimes used. As the duration of the effects of alcohol withdrawal are not shortened by treatment, a full 9-day course must be given. The preparation is available in the form of capsules (each containing 192 mg chlormethiazole base) or as a syrup. Recommended doses are: 9–12 capsules on day 1, 6–8 capsules on day 2, and 4–6 capsules on day 3, given in divided doses three or four times daily. The dose is then reduced to the minimum amount which will control symptoms. In view of the risk of dependence, treatment with the drug should not be prolonged beyond 9 days. 5 ml of Heminevrin syrup can be substituted for each capsule, if desired.

If the patient will not swallow the capsules or syrup, or oral administration is impractical for other reasons, an 0.8% solution of chlormethiazole edisylate can be administered by slow intravenous infusion. The solution is administered at a rate of 60 drops/min (i.e. 4 ml/min) until the patient is drowsy and then at 10–15 drops/min (1 ml/min) to maintain sedation. Constant close supervision is necessary, and the infusion should be replaced by oral therapy with chlormethiazole capsules as soon as possible.

As chlormethiazole is metabolized by the liver, its action may be prolonged in patients with liver decompensation.

Diazepam (Valium) is now generally preferred to chlormethiazole. It is given initially by slow intravenous injection as an 0.5% solution, in a dose of 150–250 μg/kg body weight and at a rate not exceeding 5 mg/min. This is repeated if necessary after an interval of 4 hours or followed by an intravenous infusion to a maximum of 3 mg/kg over 24 hours. Treatment may be continued by oral medication (15–30 mg daily).

Facilities for reversing respiratory depression must be available when using either regimen.

THE CONTRACEPTIVE PILL

Thromboembolic episodes are increased in women taking oral contraceptives, particularly those which contain oestrogen. Current thinking favours discontinuing the 'pill' for 4 weeks before major elective surgery and all operations involving the legs. When discontinuation is not possible (e.g. trauma, emergency operation), consideration should be given to prophylaxis against deep venous thrombosis by prescribing subcutaneous heparin. If the pill is continued, full prophylaxis against deep vein thrombosis should be given (see Ch. 21).

PREGNANCY

Pregnancy may influence surgical diseases in several ways.

• Certain intra-abdominal conditions occur more frequently during pregnancy (e.g. urinary tract infection, cholecystitis and intraperitoneal haemorrhage).

• While acute abdominal inflammatory disease (e.g. appendicitis) is not more common in pregnancy, its course may be altered. The gravid uterus interferes with the normal walling-off of infective lesions by bowel or omentum, thus facilitating the spread of infection.

• The altered position of the viscera and laxity of the abdominal wall can modify the signs of acute abdominal disease and lead to delays in diagnosis. Although removal of a normal appendix during pregnancy should be avoided, it is equally important

not to allow appendicitis to proceed to the point of perforation.

• The need to avoid abdominal X-rays during the early months of pregnancy can increase diagnostic difficulties.

• The altered hormonal balance during pregnancy may influence the course of disease outside the abdomen. For example, breast cancer occurring during the second half of pregnancy can be particularly fulminating.

Elective surgery

Elective surgery should be avoided during pregnancy. Operation is particularly dangerous during the first trimester, when hypoxia, hypotension and drugs may cause developmental malformations in the fetus.

Essential surgery

If operation during pregnancy is mandatory, the anaesthetist must be forewarned. Drugs with teratogenic properties must not be given. As ovarian function is necessary for preservation of the fetus to the 16th week, ovaries should only be removed when there is no alternative.

Postoperatively the patient should be nursed in quiet surroundings. For most procedures the postoperative course is uneventful. If uterine pain, vaginal bleeding or vaginal discharge occur, an obstetrician must be notified immediately.

ENDOCRINE DYSFUNCTION

Pituitary-adrenal system

A particular problem is posed by patients with pituitary or adrenal disorders in whom any additional stress may impose demands which cannot be met by secretion of glucocorticoid or mineralocorticoid hormones. This is particularly important in patients whose pituitary and adrenal glands have been removed, or when therapy with steroid hormones has resulted in suppression of normal endogenous secretion. Any operation or acute illness places such patients in danger of acute adrenal failure.

Normally patients are aware of this problem and have been warned to increase the dose of maintenance steroids in such circumstances. In patients requiring a general anaesthetic, steroid cover is best provided by intravenous injection of 100 mg hydrocortisone (cortisol) sodium succinate at the start of the operation. This dose may be repeated during the operation and further doses given by intravenous infusion (100 mg/500 ml saline every 4–6 hours). Thereafter, intramuscular or oral administration of hydrocortisone in decreasing daily amounts will provide adequate steroid support.

Any surgical procedure is hazardous in patients with a catecholamine-secreting phaeochromocytoma of the adrenal medulla or paraganglionic tissue. Such patients have an extremely labile circulation and are prone to attacks of acute hypertension, hypotension and circulatory collapse. A history of paroxysmal adrenergic overactivity (hypertension, sweating, pallor, headache) or the discovery of hypertension in a young person should arouse suspicion. If there is no opportunity for a full pre-operative investigation, adrenergic blocking drugs and intravenous hydrocortisone sodium succinate should be available, and the blood pressure carefully monitored during induction and maintenance of anaesthesia.

Thyroid

It is also important to assess thyroid status in patients requiring surgery. Thyrotoxicosis is likely to precipitate serious cardiac and metabolic crises and must be controlled before any operation. Antithyroid drugs such as carbimazole are not suitable for this purpose, as it takes up to 10 days before they exert their full inhibitory effect. The beta-adrenergic blocking agents rapidly antagonize the peripheral effects of thyroid hormone, and propranolol 10–30 mg three times a day should be given to any thyrotoxic patient requiring emergency surgery. Postoperatively, the patient is sedated and antithyroid medication instituted.

Equally important is the recognition of hypothyroidism. Such patients may develop cardiac arrhythmias and arrest during anaesthesia, and hypothermia and electrolyte deficiencies may occur postoperatively. Careful administration of small doses of tri-iodothyronine, supplemented by hydrocortisone, is accepted treatment but must be carefully regulated.

Section 3
TRAUMA

12
Wounds and wound healing

CONTENTS

A wound is the disruption of the normal continuity of body structures. Trauma may be *penetrating* in that the surface epithelium is disrupted, or *non-penetrating* in that the integument remains intact while the force is transmitted to subcutaneous tissues or viscera. In both types of injury, inspection of the body surface may give little indication of the extent of underlying damage. Wounds may be classified according to the mode of damage:

Incised wounds are caused by a sharp instrument; if there is associated tissue tearing the wound is said to be *lacerated*.

Abrasions result from friction damage to the body surface and are characterized by superficial bruising and loss of varying thickness of skin and underlying tissue. Dirt and foreign bodies are frequently embedded in the tissues.

Crush injuries are due to severe pressure. Even though the skin is not breached there may be massive tissue destruction. Oedema can make wound closure impossible, and by increasing pressure within fascial compartments may cause ischaemic necrosis of muscle and other structures.

Degloving injury results from shearing forces causing parallel tissue planes to move against each other (e.g. when a hand is caught between rollers or in moving machinery). Large areas of apparently intact skin may be deprived of their blood supply by rupture of feeding vessels.

Gunshot wounds may be low velocity or high velocity. Bullets fired from high velocity rifles cause massive tissue destruction.

Burns are caused by heat, electricity, irradiation or chemicals (see Ch. 13).

PRINCIPLES OF WOUND HEALING

The essential features of healing are common to wounds of almost all soft tissues and result in formation of a scar. Epithelium, bone and nerve heal in distinct ways (see below). Soft tissue healing can be subdivided into three phases (Table 12.1) according to the development of tensile strength (Fig. 12.1).

Table 12.1   Phases of wound healing

Lag phase (2–3 days)
  Inflammatory response
Incremental or proliferative phase (approximately 3 weeks)
  Fibroblast migration
  Capillary ingrowth (granulation tissue)
  Collagen synthesis with rapid gain in tensile strength
  Wound contraction
Plateau or maturation phase (approximately 6 months)
  Organization of scar
  Slow final gain in tensile strength (80% of original strength)

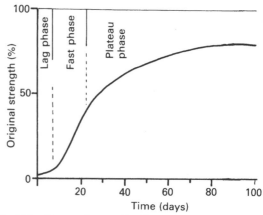

Fig. 12.1   Phases of wound healing.

Soft tissue healing

Lag phase

The lag phase is the delay of 2–3 days which elapses before fibroblasts begin to manufacture collagen to support the wound. It is characterized by the inflammatory response to injury in which capillary permeability increases and a protein-rich exudate accumulates. It is from this exudate that collagen is later synthesized. Inflammatory cells migrate into the area, dead tissue is removed by macrophages, and capillaries at the wound edges begin to proliferate.

Incremental phase

During the incremental or proliferative phase there is progressive collagen synthesis by fibroblasts and a corresponding increase in tensile strength. Fibroblasts arise from perivascular mesenchymal cells and migrate into the wound in response to the high lactate levels which result from ischaemia. Increased collagen turnover in areas remote from the wound suggests that there may also be a systemic stimulus for fibroblast activity. Collagen synthesis increases over a period of about 3 weeks during which the gain in tensile strength accelerates. Old collagen undergoes lysis while new collagen is laid down.

Proline and lysine are essential for collagen formation. They are hydroxylated by oxygen and ascorbic acid and incorporated into tropocollagen, which polymerizes to form collagen. The energy needed for collagen synthesis is supplied by oxygen and nutrients brought into the wound by ingrowth of capillary buds which form fragile capillary arches. In unapposed wounds, excessive formation of new capillaries mixed with fibroblasts, macrophages and leucocytes results in *granulation tissue*. To the naked eye, healthy granulation tissue is red, granular and friable, bleeding when touched.

In addition to making collagen, fibroblasts also synthesize the *mucopolysaccharide ground substance* which forms an ideal environment for alignment and approximation of the tropocollagen monomers prior to polymerization. Some fibroblasts known as myofibroblasts contain myofibrils which pull in the wound margins. This *wound contraction* reduces the size of the defect in unapposed wounds and must be distinguished from *contracture*, which can be the unfortunate result of healing when a wound crosses a joint and there is shortage of skin. The resultant scar restricts mobility.

The gain in tensile strength during the incre-

mental phase allows removal of skin sutures without wound disruption at times ranging from 4–5 days on the face and 10–14 days on the trunk and lower limb.

Plateau or maturation phase

After 3 weeks the gain in tensile strength levels off as the rate of collagen breakdown first approaches and then temporarily surpasses its synthesis. Excess collagen is removed during this final clearing-up process and the number of fibroblasts and inflammatory cells declines. Orientation of collagen fibres in the direction of local mechanical forces increases tensile strength for some 6 months but the original strength is never regained; skin and fascia usually recover only 80% of their original tensile strength.

At the time of suture removal the edges of the newly healed wound should be directly apposed and flat. Thereafter, for up to 3 months, the scar may become progressively raised, red and thickened. It can then remain static for a further 3 months before slowly improving to become narrow, flat and pale. These changes vary with age, race, direction of scar and degree of dermal damage. They are most marked in children, in whom scars take longer to resolve, while in the elderly they tend to mature and fade very quickly.

Hypertrophic scars are an exaggeration of the normal maturation process. They are very raised, red and firm but never continue to worsen after 6 months. They are particularly common in children and after deep dermal burns. They eventually resolve, often after several years, unless under tension. Resolution can be hastened by elastic pressure garments, steroid injections, or application of silicone gel; these scars should not be excised.

Keloids are similar to hypertrophic scars but continue to enlarge after 6 months and invade neighbouring uninvolved skin. They are most likely to occur across the upper chest, shoulders and ear lobes and are common in black patients. They are very difficult to treat successfully. If the measures described above fail, intralesional excision followed immediately by low-dose radiotherapy is sometimes effective.

Healing of specialized tissues

Epithelium

Epithelium heals by *regeneration* and not by scar formation. Epithelial cells at the edge of the wound lose their adhesion to each other and migrate across the wound until they meet cells from the other side. As they migrate, they are replaced by new cells formed by division of basal cells near the wound edge. The cells that have migrated undergo mitosis and the new epithelium thickens, eventually forming normal epithelial cover for the scar produced by the dermis. Wounds may heal by *primary intention* if the edges are closely approximated, for example by accurate suturing; epithelial cover is then quickly achieved and healing of the apposed deeper tissues produces a fine scar (Fig. 12.2).

If the wound edges are not apposed, the defect fills with granulation tissue and restoration of epidermal continuity takes time. The advance of epithelial cells across the denuded area is often hindered by infection. This is known as healing by *secondary intention* and usually results in delayed healing, excessive fibrosis and an ugly scar. If a wound has begun to

heal by second intention it may still be possible to speed healing by excising the wound edges and bringing them into apposition or covering the defect with a skin graft.

Bone

Torn blood vessels produce a haematoma between the fractured bone ends. An inflammatory response leads to ingress of fibroblasts, collagen formation and deposition of new bone. Any movement between the bone ends results in *callus* formation in which new bone is produced by subperiosteal and intramedullary osteogenic cells. Some cartilage may be formed in relatively ischaemic areas. The callus is at first spongy but gradually shrinks as the new bone becomes compact and bony union occurs. Strength returns gradually and, as with soft tissue injuries,

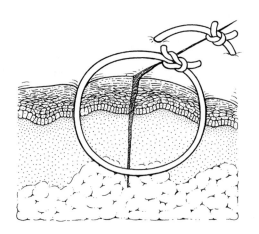
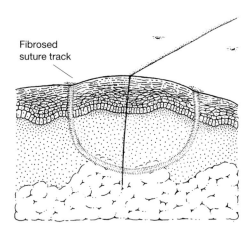

A. Healing by primary intention

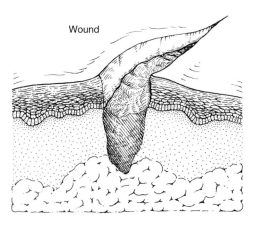
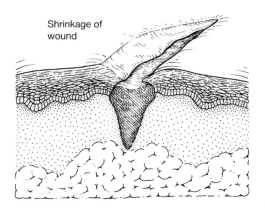

B. Healing by secondary intention

Fig. 12.2 Wound healing by A primary intention and B secondary intention showing shrinkage of the wound.

increases slowly over many months. Extensive remodelling finally obliterates the fracture site.

If the bone ends are fixed rigidly (e.g. by a compression plate), healing takes place without callus formation. The bone regains its normal appearance more quickly but takes longer to regain its strength.

Nerve tissue

Wounds of the nervous system involve both neural and connective tissue. Neural tissue in the central nervous system (CNS) cannot regenerate and fibroblasts derived from glial or perivascular cells replace nervous tissue with collagen.

If peripheral nerves are cut, axons degenerate distal to the injury but as long as the body of the nerve cell survives, axons from the proximal stump sprout and enter empty Schwann sheaths if the nerve ends are approximated. If the nerve ends are not approximated, fibroblasts fill the gap and the resulting collagen scar obstructs the sprouting axons. Not all axons find their way into a Schwann sheath. Some may end blindly in the surrounding tissue to form a 'neuroma' which can be very painful. Others may find their way into inappropriate sheaths, as when a sensory neurone enters a sheath leading to a motor end plate. Nevertheless, useful reinnervation is possible if nerve ends are accurately approximated with fine sutures to prevent excessive scarring. Regenerating axons can grow 4–5 mm a day but usually average 1–1.5 mm a day. If cut ends cannot be approximated without tension, the gap can be bridged with a nerve graft or substitute such as a

freeze-thawed muscle graft which can provide a conduit.

Intestine

Damage confined to gut mucosa is repaired by re-epithelialization without scarring whereas ulceration extending through to the submucosa and underlying muscle always leaves a permanent fibrous scar.

The stomach and small bowel have a plentiful blood supply, contain relatively few pathogenic bacteria and heal so well that leakage after anastomosis is uncommon. The oesophagus and large bowel have weaker walls and a poorer blood supply, and heal less well after surgery. In the distal colon, problems of healing are compounded by the large numbers of pathogenic luminal bacteria. Bacteria delay collagen synthesis and collagenase production can cause excessive lysis. Disruption of intestinal anastomosis is usually recognized clinically by the 4th–6th postoperative day.

Faulty surgical technique is a major determinant of leakage and infection after gastrointestinal anastomosis. The connective tissue of the submucosa is the strongest layer of the gut wall, and sutures or staples in this layer maintain apposition until tensile strength is regained.

FACTORS INFLUENCING WOUND HEALING

Many of the factors influencing healing are interrelated, e.g. the site of the wound, its blood supply, and the level of tissue oxygenation. While some adverse factors such as age cannot be influenced, others such as surgical technique, nutritional status and presence of intercurrent disease can be modified or eliminated.

Blood supply

Wounds of ischaemic tissues heal slowly, are prone to infection, and frequently break down. When this occurs, the ischaemic wound may not be able to sustain the metabolic demands of healing by second intention. Arterial oxygen tension (Pa_{O_2}) is a key determinant of the rate of collagen synthesis. Anaemia per se may not affect healing if the patient has a normal blood volume and arterial oxygen tension.

Poor surgical technique such as crushing tissue with forceps, approximating wound edges under tension, and tying sutures too tightly can render well-vascularized tissue ischaemic and lead to wound breakdown.

Infection

General factors. The risks of wound infection include age, presence of intercurrent infection, disordered nutrition, and cardiovascular and respiratory disease.

Local factors. These are of paramount importance. Bacterial contamination can be minimized by careful skin preparation and meticulous aseptic technique but some wounds are more likely to be contaminated than others (see below). Despite every precaution, bacteria may enter wounds from the atmosphere, from internal foci of sepsis, or from the lumen of transected organs. In some cases, contamination occurs in the postoperative period. Provided contamination is not gross and local blood supply is good, natural defences are usually able to deal with it and prevent overt infection. Devitalized tissues, haematoma and the presence of foreign material such as sutures and prostheses favour bacterial survival and growth. Common infecting organisms are staphylococci, streptococci, coliforms and anaerobes.

Overcrowding of wards and excessive use of operating theatres increase the bacterial population of the atmosphere and thus the risk of wound infection.

The role of prophylaxis. When wound contamination is anticipated, topical antibacterial chemicals or topical and systemic antibiotics can be used prophylactically. For example, lavage of the wound with the antibacterial povidone iodine reduces the incidence of wound infection after appendicitis. A short course of systemic antibiotics is normally used to prevent infection during colorectal surgery. In acute traumatic wounds, tetanus prophylaxis is routine but antibiotics are not normally necessary provided prompt and thorough surgical treatment is undertaken.

Age

Wounds in the elderly may heal poorly because of impaired blood supply, poor nutritional status or intercurrent disease.

Site of wound

Surgical incisions placed in the lines of least tissue tension are subject to minimal distraction and should heal promptly leaving a fine scar. In the face, these lines run at right angles to the direction of underlying muscles and form the lines of facial expression.

Wounds of the head and neck heal quickly so that sutures or skin clips can usually be removed within 3–5 days whereas sutures have to be left for some 14 days with wounds of the leg and foot. These differences reflect the importance of blood supply; warm vascular areas generally heal more quickly than cool extremities.

Nutritional status

When competing for resources, wounds have higher priority than unwounded tissue. Malnutrition has to be severe before healing is affected (see below). Protein availability is most important, and wound dehiscence and infection are common when the serum albumin is low. Healing problems should be anticipated if recent weight loss exceeds 20%.

Ascorbic acid is essential for proline hydroxylation and collagen synthesis. The number of fibroblasts is not reduced in scorbutic states. Zinc is a component of enzymes involved in healing and zinc deficiency retards healing. Supplements of ascorbic acid and zinc are effective in patients with known deficiencies, but do not improve healing in normal subjects.

Intercurrent disease

Healing may be affected by the disease itself or by its treatment. *Cachectic patients* with severe malnutrition (as seen in advanced cancer) have marked impairment of healing.

Diabetes mellitus impairs healing by reducing tissue resistance to infection and causing peripheral vascular insufficiency. Peripheral neuropathy with diminished peripheral sensation may add to the problem by allowing trauma to the healing wound.

Haemorrhagic diatheses increase the risk of haematoma formation and wound infection.

Obstructive airway disease lowers arterial P_{O_2} and so affects healing. Abdominal wound dehiscence is commoner in patients with respiratory disease because of the strain on the wound during coughing.

Corticosteroid therapy reduces the inflammatory response, impairs collagen synthesis and decreases resistance to infection. The effect of steroids on wound healing is most marked if they are given within 3 days of injury.

Immunosuppressive therapy impairs healing by reducing resistance to infection. Such patients are already compromised by their underlying disorder.

Radiotherapy greatly reduces the vascularity of the tissues, and healing of wounds in irradiated areas is often impaired.

Surgical technique

Skin incisions are placed where possible in the line of least tissue tension. Meticulous aseptic technique is essential to avoid wound infection and poor healing. Gentle tissue handling is mandatory. Crushing with tissue forceps, failure to achieve haemostasis, excessive use of diathermy and crude ligatures all contribute to wound devitalization.

Potentially infective sites (e.g. the gut lumen during colon surgery) should be isolated from the wound by additional sterile drapes, and spillage of contents avoided by correct use of occlusion clamps. Particular care must be taken in areas where there is reduced resistance to infection (e.g. bones and joints), where prosthetic implants are being inserted, or where infection would have particularly serious consequences (e.g. neurosurgery).

Accurate apposition of wound edges favours healing by first intention. Dead spaces in the depth of the wound are avoided, as bleeding and accumulation of exudate encourage infection. Correct suturing of the deeper layers often allows the skin edges to fall together without tension so that skin apposition can be achieved by superficial sutures or adhesive tape. Any potential dead space should be obliterated by deep sutures. If this is not possible, the space must be drained. Drains should also be used in contaminated wounds and those where a great deal of exudate is expected. They may be connected to a suction apparatus or allowed to drain by gravity.

Choice of suture and suture materials. The choice of suture materials is important. Foreign material in the tissues predisposes to infection. The finest sutures that will hold the wound edges together should be used. A wound must never be closed under tension.

Wounds are often subjected to stress postoperatively and while 5/0 or 6/0 sutures are appropriate for the face, stronger sutures (3/0 or 4/0) are needed for incisions near joints and still stronger ones for the abdominal wall. The suture should be strong enough to support the wound until tensile strength has recovered sufficiently to prevent breakdown. Absorbable materials are preferred for buried layers, but non-absorbable sutures may be needed in some situations, e.g. in the aponeurotic layer of an abdominal paramedian wound. Non-absorbable sutures should be inert, retain strength, and preferably be mono-filamentous, without interstices which might favour bacterial growth.

Suture materials are designed to pass through the tissues with as little trauma as possible. To this end, sutures are no longer threaded through a wide needle eye but are usually bonded to the needle without any increase in bulk (atraumatic suture). The needle may be round-bodied or triangular on cross-section. The round-bodied needle is used when tissue resistance is low (e.g. for intestinal suture), while a triangular needle is preferred when sharp cutting edges are needed to facilitate passage through tough tissues such as skin and aponeurosis.

To avoid wound devitalization, sutures should not be placed too close together or too near the wound margin, nor should they be tied too tightly. When closing the abdomen, many surgeons now use a mass closure technique in which a continuous suture of monofilament non-absorbable material (e.g. nylon) is placed through all layers of the abdominal wall except skin.

Factors affecting wound healing
- The site of the wound and its orientation relative to tissue tension lines is a major determinant of healing.

- Wounds with a good blood supply (e.g. head and neck wounds) heal well.

- Infection is a major adverse factor and the risk of infection is influenced by:
  - general factors such as the patient's age, presence of intercurrent infection, nutritional status, and cardiorespiratory disease.
  - local factors including bacterial contamination, antibacterial prophylaxis, aseptic technique, degree of trauma, presence of devitalized tissue, haematoma and foreign bodies.

- Intercurrent disease may impair healing – important factors include:
  - malnutrition
  - diabetes mellitus
  - haemorrhagic diatheses
  - hypoxia (e.g. obstructive airways disease)
  - corticosteroid therapy
  - immunosuppression
  - radiotherapy.

- Surgical technical factors which have a major influence on wound healing include:
  - gentle tissue handling
  - avoidance of undue trauma
  - accurate tissue apposition
  - meticulous haemostasis
  - appropriate choice of suture material.

PROBLEMS IN WOUND MANAGEMENT

Postoperative wound infection

Surgical procedures can be classified according to the likelihood of contamination and wound infection.

Clean procedures are those in which wound contamination is not expected and should not occur. An incision for a clean elective procedure should not become infected provided no infective focus is encountered and no viscus is entered which might contain pathogenic bacteria (e.g. colon). Subtotal thyroidectomy, parietal cell vagotomy and meniscectomy are examples of clean operations in which the wound infection rate should be less than 1%.

Clean-contaminated procedures are those in which no frank focus of infection is encountered but where a significant risk of infection is nevertheless present. Cholecystectomy, subtotal gastrectomy and prostatectomy are examples of operations in which wound infection occurs occasionally. Infection rates in excess of 5% denote breakdown in ward and operating theatre routine.

Contaminated or 'dirty' wounds are those in which gross contamination is inevitable and the risk of troublesome wound infection is high. Emergency surgery for perforated diverticular disease and drainage of a subphrenic abscess are examples of procedures in this category.

Clinical features

Postoperative wound infection usually becomes evident 3–4 days after surgery. Commonly the first signs are superficial cellulitis around the wound margins or swelling of the wound with some serous discharge from between the sutures. Fluctuation is occasionally elicited when there is an abscess or liquifying haematoma, and crepitus may be present if gas-forming organisms are involved. In some cases of deep infection there are no local signs although the patient may have pyrexia and increased wound tenderness. Systemic upset is variable, usually amounting to only moderate pyrexia and leucocytosis. Toxaemia, bacteraemia and septicaemia can complicate serious wound infection.

The differential diagnosis includes other causes of postoperative pyrexia, wound haematoma and wound dehiscence. Wound haematoma may result from reactive bleeding during the first 24–48 hours after operation. It causes swelling and discomfort but only minimal pyrexia and few systemic signs. As a haematoma is liable to become infected, it should be evacuated. Wound dehiscence is considered separately later in this chapter.

Prevention

The risk of wound infection is reduced by careful preparation of the patient, prophylactic use of antibiotics in high-risk patients and meticulous attention to good operative theatre techniques. To avoid cross-contamination, wounds should be dressed postoperatively in a separate treatment or dressing room and not in the general ward, and contaminated wounds should be left until last.

Severely contaminated wounds are sometimes best closed by *delayed primary suture*. For example, after emergency operation for perforated appendicitis or resection of gangrenous bowel in a strangulated hernia, the peritoneum and aponeurotic layer may be closed but the skin and subcutaneous tissues left open. Skin sutures may be inserted at this time but are not tied for several days, until it is clear that infection has been avoided.

Antibiotic therapy is essential for grossly contaminated wounds, the aim being to achieve high tissue concentrations as soon as possible. The choice of antibiotics is determined by the nature of the infection.

Antibiotics which achieve excellent concentrations in the wound include penicillin, flucloxacillin, ampicillin and cephalosporins. Gentamicin, carbenicillin and oxacillin achieve only modest concentrations and are used only when indicated by tests for bacterial sensitivity. These are often best given intravenously.

Following emergency surgery for faecal peritonitis, a combination of penicillin and gentamicin was commonly used to reduce the dangers of peritonitis, wound infection and septicaemia. For the destruction of anaerobes, metronidazole is now added routinely. Topical agents such as povidone-iodine may also be used to combat infection in contaminated wounds.

Although antibiotic treatment is a valuable and important part of management of the contaminated wound, it is no substitute for careful surgical management. Radical excision of the wound margins, thorough mechanical cleansing and delayed suture are the true foundations of success.

Treatment

Trivial superficial cellulitis can be managed expectantly. The area of redness is 'mapped out' with an indelible pen so that its extent can be monitored. Spreading cellulitis is an indication for antibiotic therapy.

Deeper and more serious infections can often be aborted by the removal of one or more skin sutures to allow free drainage of infected material from the suture track or wound. Failure to provide free drainage promotes infection in the hypoxic closed space and can lead to abscess formation. If removal of skin sutures does not result in free discharge of infected material, the wound should be probed gently with sinus forceps under aseptic conditions.

If pus is believed to be present but adequate drainage has not been provided, the patient should be returned to theatre for a full exploration of the wound under general anaesthesia. Following evacuation of pus and debris the wound is left open or packed lightly to prevent premature closure of the skin edges. Otherwise infection may persist in the depths of the wound.

Many infected wounds heal rapidly without further surgery, particularly if the original skin incision is placed in the line of least tissue tension. The problem is often to keep the wound open rather than to achieve closure. If it appears that spontaneous wound closure will take a long time, *secondary suture* or skin grafting can be considered to speed healing, but only once it is clear that infection has been eradicated. The presence of clean healthy granulation tissue in the wound is usually a good indication that closure can be undertaken.

In all infected wounds a wound swab or specimen of pus is sent routinely for bacteriological culture and sensitivity determination. Although antibiotics are not usually required when the infection is limited and free drainage has been established, they are indicated when there is spreading cellulitis, severe deep infection or persistent pyrexia. It is therefore important to know the sensitivity of the causative organism. In urgent cases a Gram-stain of a smear of material from the wound will give guidance as to the initial choice of antibiotic. If in doubt, a combination of a penicillin, a cephalosporin and metronidazole is reasonable.

Abdominal wound dehiscence

General surgical units should now have an overall incidence of abdominal wound dehiscence of less than 1%. Wound dehiscence is particularly troublesome in obese patients, and in those with chest complications, abdominal distension due to ileus or ascites, or a debilitating disease such as cancer. The risk can be minimized by careful pre-operative preparation, including chest care and cessation of smoking for at least 2 weeks before surgery, and by prompt treatment of any postoperative respiratory tract infection.

Signs of dehiscence are frequently delayed for 7–10 days after surgery. A profuse serosanguineous discharge of peritoneal fluid from the wound is often the first clinical sign and indicates dehiscence unless proved otherwise. The patient may be unaware that dehiscence has occurred, or may have felt 'something go' after a bout of coughing or sudden exertion. Although the surface of the wound may appear intact, disruption of the deeper layers can be demonstrated by contraction of the abdominal wall. This is best done by asking the patient to cough or to lift his head or straight legs from the bed. In some cases, protrusion of bowel or omentum through the wound makes it clear that dehiscence has occurred.

Immediate operative repair is mandatory when dehiscence is complete. Partial dehiscence of the deep layers can be treated conservatively, but only if operation is contraindicated by the patient's general condition. The patient is provided with an elastic or adjustable abdominal support which can be tightened by him during coughing or exertion. With careful management, the wound may then heal but an incisional hernia is inevitable and may require subsequent repair.

Surgical repair is carried out under general anaesthesia using 'through-and-through' sutures which pass through all the musculo-aponeurotic layers of the abdominal wall.

Traumatic wounds

These wounds are almost inevitably contaminated by bacteria. The state of immunity against tetanus is assessed and appropriate action taken (see Ch. 7). The wound is inspected carefully under good illumination to assess the extent of devitalization and injury to vital structures. It is important to appreciate that a small, apparently innocent wound may conceal extensive damage to deeper structures. Body cavities may have been penetrated, or tendons, nerves and blood vessels divided.

Damage to muscle, tendon or nerve is assessed by checking relevant motor and sensory function. If the injury involves a limb, the distal circulation is checked. Where appropriate, X-rays will help to establish whether peritoneal, pericardial or pleural cavities have been entered. A decision is made whether the wound can be dealt with under local (or regional) anaesthesia in the casualty department or whether there is any possibility of damage to deep structures requiring more extensive exploration under general anaesthesia in an operating theatre. Provided there is no obvious deep damage, small, relatively uncontaminated wounds should be treated under local anaesthesia on an outpatient basis. The wound margins are cleaned with a mild antiseptic such as cetrimide and the wound is irrigated copiously. Any devitalized tissue is removed, deep tissues are sutured with absorbable material and the skin margins are closed.

More extensive or severely contaminated wounds usually require inpatient treatment with exploration and debridement under general anaesthesia. The wound and its margins are cleansed, and pieces of grit, soil and other obvious foreign material are picked out. All devitalized tissue is trimmed back until bleeding occurs. This process is known as debridement. In areas of poor vascularity such as the leg, or if there is severe contamination, crushing or a fracture, the wound margins are formally excised

(Fig. 12.3). Bleeding from the wound margin is not a certain indication of its ultimate survival, as impaired venous drainage can lead to progressive necrosis, particularly after a crushing or degloving injury. If there if any doubt, the wound should not be sutured and a 'second-look' dressing change undertaken under anaesthesia after 48 hours.

Primary closure should also be avoided if there is significant delay in treating a grossly contaminated wound (i.e. more than 6 hours without antibiotic cover). If this is attempted, wound infection and breakdown are likely and there is a risk of anaerobic infection which may threaten both life and limb. It is also too late for formal excision, as bacteria will have penetrated the tissues, but foreign bodies and dead tissue should be removed in the usual way. The wound is dressed and antibiotics are started. The dressing is changed daily, and if the wound is clean in 2 or 3 days *delayed primary suture* may be carried out. If closure is delayed until granulation tissue has

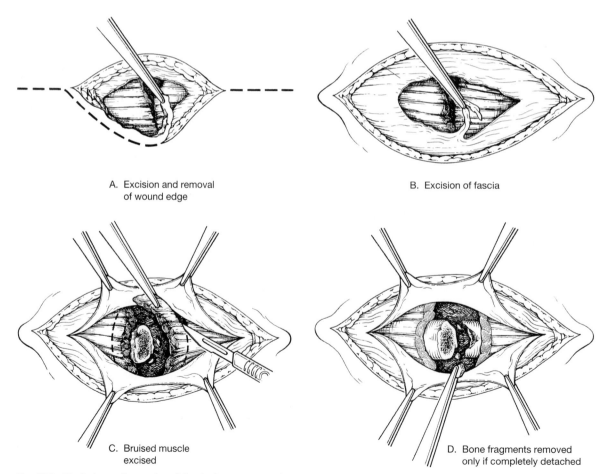

A. Excision and removal of wound edge

B. Excision of fascia

C. Bruised muscle excised

D. Bone fragments removed only if completely detached

Fig. 12.3 Technique of wound excision in the presence of a compound fracture.

formed, this is usually excised and *secondary suture* performed. If this is not possible, split skin grafts (see below) can be applied over the granulations.

Provided that surgical treatment is carried out early, prophylactic antibiotics (except those used for tetanus) are only required for deeply penetrating wounds such as dog bites or those caused by nails where adequate debridement may be impossible. However, the early use of antibiotics in situations where delay in surgical treatment is anticipated may allow primary suture of wounds after 8–12 hours, an interval that is normally considered safe.

Devitalized skin flaps

A common emergency problem is posed by the patient, usually an elderly female, who falls and raises a triangular flap over the surface of the tibia. In many cases the flap is blue-black in colour and obviously non-viable; in most, viability is uncertain. Similar injuries can occur elsewhere in the body.

The wound must be cleansed and all non-viable tissue excised. No attempt should be made to suture the flap back into place. Because of the post-traumatic oedema this would only be possible under tension and lead to death of the flap. If the defect is small, it can be treated conservatively on an outpatient basis. The wound is dressed, an elastic supporting bandage is applied to the leg and the patient is kept ambulant. The wound will normally take several weeks to heal. Alternatively, and this is essential if the defect is large, a split skin graft can be applied either immediately or as a delayed primary procedure. The patient must be kept in bed with the leg horizontal until the graft has taken.

Wounds with skin loss

The aim of wound care is to obtain skin cover and healing as soon as is safely possible, either by primary or by delayed primary closure. If skin has been lost as a direct result of trauma, or following excision of a tumour or necrotic tissue, direct suture will not be possible. If the skin defect is small and at a functionally or aesthetically unimportant site, it may be allowed to heal by secondary intention, but it is often better to speed healing by importing skin to close the wound. This may be by means of a *skin graft* (which requires a vascular bed as it has no blood supply of its own) or a *flap*.

Skin grafts

These may be *split skin* or *full thickness*. Split skin grafts are cut with a special, guarded freehand knife or an electric dermatome. The donor site heals by re-epithelialization from epithelial appendages in the dermis (the bases of hair follicles and sweat ducts) within 2–3 weeks, so that large sheets of skin can be taken. To cover very large areas the graft can be expanded by 'meshing'. The thinner the graft, the more easily it will take on a bed of imperfect vascularity, but the poorer the quality of skin, the more it will shrink. Split skin grafts are used to cover wounds after acute trauma, granulating areas and burns, or when the defect is large.

A full thickness graft leaves a donor defect (which needs to be sutured or grafted) as large as the one to be filled and requires a well-vascularized bed to survive. However, such grafts are strong, do not shrink and look better than a split skin graft. They are rarely advisable after acute trauma but are commonly used in reconstructive surgery to close small defects where strength is needed (e.g. on the palm of the hand) or a good cosmetic result is important (e.g. on the lower eyelid). An area where there is skin to spare is chosen for the donor site (e.g. the groin for the former and the area behind the ear for the latter).

Other tissues such as bone, cartilage, nerve and tendon can be grafted to restore function and correct deformity after tissue damage or loss.

Principles of management of contaminated traumatic wounds

- Contaminated wounds should be debrided under general anaesthesia.

- The contaminated wound and its margins must be cleansed thoroughly with removal of grit, soil and foreign bodies/materials.

- Devitalised tissue is formally excised until bleeding is encountered.

- Primary closure is avoided if there has been gross contamination and when treatment has been delayed for more than 6 hours. Inappropriate attempts to achieve primary closure increase the risk of wound infection and expose the patient to the risks of anaerobic infection (tetanus and gas gangrene).

- Wounds left open may be suitable for delayed primary suture after 2–3 days or for later excision and secondary suture (with or without skin grafting).

- Appropriate protection against tetanus must be afforded and the use of antibiotics should be considered.

Flaps

While grafts require a vascular bed to survive, flaps bring their own blood supply to the new site. They can therefore be thicker and stronger than grafts and can be applied to avascular areas such as exposed bone, tendon or joints. They are used in acute trauma only if closure is not possible by direct suture

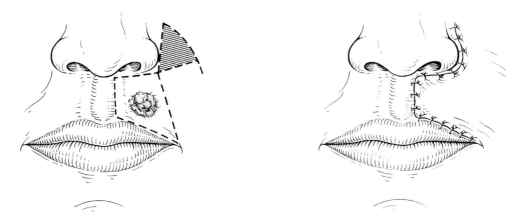

A   B

Fig. 12.4   Local skin flap used to repair a defect after the excision of a skin lesion.

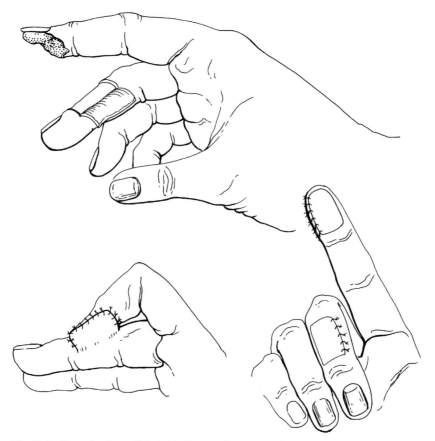

Fig. 12.5   Example of a pedicled skin flap used to cover a defect on the tip of the index finger. Once a blood supply is established, the pedicle is divided.

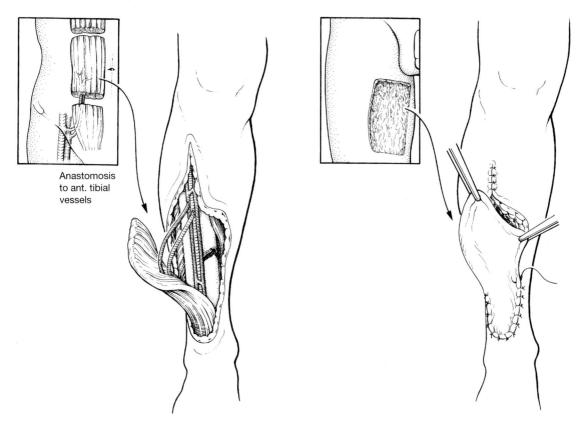

Anastomosis
to ant. tibial
vessels

Fig. 12.6   Example of free tissue transfer based on inferior epigastric vessels: A rectus abdominis muscle transferred to shin and its vessels (inferior epigastric vessels) anastomosed to anterior tibial vessels; **B** muscle covered by split-skin graft.

or skin grafting, and are more usually reserved for the reconstruction of surgical defects and for secondary reconstruction after trauma.

The simplest flaps use local skin and fat and are often a good alternative to skin grafting for small defects such as those left after excision of facial tumours (Fig. 12.4). If enough local tissue is not available, a flap may have to be brought from a distance and remain attached temporarily to its original blood supply until it has picked up a new one locally (Fig. 12.5). This usually takes 2–3 weeks, after which the pedicle can be divided.

Advances in our knowledge of the blood supply to the skin and underlying muscles have led to the development of many large skin, muscle and composite flaps which have revolutionized plastic and reconstructive surgery. One example is the use of the latissimus dorsi musculocutaneous flap for reconstruction of the breast.

The ability to join small blood vessels under the operating microscope now allows the surgeon to close defects in a single stage, even when there is no local tissue available, by *free tissue transfer* (Fig. 12.6).

Crushing and degloving injuries, gunshot wounds

Wounds of this type should never be closed primarily, as tissue destruction is always much greater than appears at first. After thorough irrigation and removal of any obviously dead tissue and foreign material such wounds should be lightly packed and dressed. Dressings are removed 48 hours later under anaesthesia and further excision is carried out if necessary. The wound is closed by suture, skin grafting or flap cover once it is clear that all dead tissue has been removed.

13
Burns

CONTENTS

STRUCTURE AND FUNCTIONS OF SKIN

While large burns have profound effects on most body systems, the skin is affected primarily. Skin consists of epidermis and dermis. The epidermis is a layer of keratinized, stratified squamous epithelium (see Fig. 13.1) which sends three appendages (hair follicles, sweat glands and sebaceous glands) into the underlying dermis. Because of their deep location, the appendages escape destruction in partial thickness burns and are a source of new cells for reconstitution of the epidermis.

The skin area ranges from 0.25 m^2 at birth to $1.5–1.9 \text{ m}^2$ in adults. Skin accounts for some 15% of lean body mass and is one of the largest organs in the body. It prevents excessive water loss, helps to control temperature and provides a barrier against infection.

TYPES OF BURN

Burn injuries range from the trivial to severe burns which pose a threat to life, involve long hospital stay, and carry risk of permanent disfigurement or impaired function. Most burns follow accidents in the home and could be prevented.

Burns may be caused by flames, hot solids, hot liquids or steam, or by physicochemical agencies such as irradiation, electricity or chemicals. Toddlers are particularly liable to scalding by hot liquids in kitchen accidents, and unguarded fires are a threat to all children. Severe disfigurement of the face and neck can result from clothing catching fire, although this has become less common with the use of less inflammatory clothing materials. Burns sustained in house fires are often accompanied by smoke inhalation with injury to the lungs. Alcohol is a common contributing factor in burn injury. Impaired mobility, poor co-ordination and diminished awareness of pain increase the incidence of burns in the elderly and infirm.

Sunburn is the commonest irradiation injury but is rarely serious. Industrial accidents account for most physicochemical burns, although accidental or deliberate ingestion of caustic or corrosive chemicals is still an occasional cause of domestic burns. The extent of injury caused by high-tension electrical cables is easily underestimated, as surface damage may be small despite extensive deep injury.

EFFECTS OF BURN INJURY

Local effects

The local effects result from destruction of the more superficial tissues and the inflammatory response of the deeper tissues (Table 13.1). Fluid is lost from the surface or trapped in blisters, the magnitude of loss depending on the extent of injury. Loss is greatly increased by leakage of fluid from the circulation

Table 13.1	Effects of burn injury

Destruction of tissue (depth depends on heat of causative agent and contact time)
    Loss of barrier to infection
    Fluid loss from surface
    Red cell destruction

Increased capillary permeability
    Oedema
    Loss of circulating fluid volume
    Hypovolaemic shock

Increased metabolic rate

(see below); instead of the normal insensible loss of 15 ml/m^2 body surface/h as much as 200 ml/m^2/hour may be lost during the first few hours. With deeper injuries the epidermis and dermis are converted into a coagulum of dead tissue known as *eschar*.

In its least severe form the dermal inflammatory response consists of capillary dilatation, as in the erythema of sunburn. With deeper burns, the damaged capillaries become permeable to protein, and an exudate forms with an electrolyte/protein content only slightly less than that of plasma. Lymphatic drainage fails to keep pace with the rate of exudation and interstitial oedema leads to a reduction in circulating fluid volume. An increase of 2 cm in the diameter of a lower limb represents accumulation of over 2 litres of interstitial fluid. Exudation is maximal in the first 12 hours, capillary permeability returning to normal within 48 hours.

Destruction of the epidermis removes the barrier to bacterial invasion and opens the door to infection. The burn surface may become contaminated at any time and wound care must commence when the patient is first seen. Sepsis delays healing, increases energy needs, and may pose a new threat to life just when the early dangers of hypovolaemia have been overcome.

General effects

The general effects of a burn depend on its size. Large burns lead to water, salt and protein loss, hypovolaemia and increased catabolism. Circulating plasma volume falls as oedema accumulates and fluid leaks from the burned surface. With large burns the effect is compounded by a generalized increase in capillary permeability with widespread oedema. Some red cells are destroyed by a full thickness burn, and many more are damaged but not destroyed immediately. However, red cell losses are small in comparison to plasma loss in the early period, and haemoconcentration is reflected in a rising haematocrit. Hypovolaemic shock ensues if plasma volume is not restored. The shifts in water and electrolytes are ultimately shared by all body tissues.

Large burns increase metabolic rate as water loss from the burned surface causes expenditure of calories to provide the heat of evaporation. In severe burns some 7000 kcal may be expended daily and daily weight loss of 0.5 kg is not unusual unless steps are taken to prevent it.

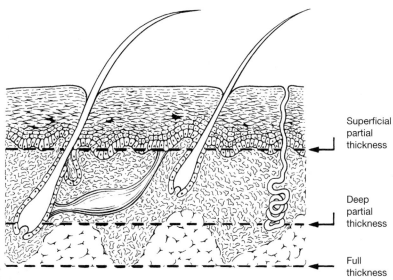

Fig. 13.1 Structure of skin.

Superficial partial thickness

Deep partial thickness

Full thickness

CLASSIFICATION OF BURNS

Burns are classified according to their depth as partial or full thickness skin loss (Fig. 13.1). In a partial thickness burn, epithelial cells survive to restore the epidermis. Full thickness burns destroy all of the epithelial elements.

Partial thickness burns

Superficial partial thickness burns involve only the epidermis and superficial dermis. Pain, swelling and fluid loss may be marked. New epidermal cover is provided from undamaged cells of the epidermal appendages and the burn heals in less than 3 weeks with a perfect final cosmetic result.

In *deep partial thickness* (or *deep dermal*) burns, the epidermis and much of the dermis are destroyed. Restoration of the epidermis then depends on intact epithelial cells within the remaining appendages. Pain, swelling and fluid loss are again marked. The burn takes longer than 3 weeks to heal as fewer epithelial elements survive, and often heals with production of ugly hypertrophic scars. Infection will delay healing and can cause further tissue destruction, converting the injury to a full thickness one.

Full thickness burns

A full thickness burn destroys the epidermis and underlying dermis, including the epidermal appendages. The destroyed tissues undergo coagulative necrosis and form an eschar which begins to lift after 2–3 weeks. Unless the raw area is grafted, epidermal cover can only occur through laborious inward movement and growth of cells from intact skin around the burn, and by contraction of its base. Fibrosis and ugly contracture are thus inevitable in all but small ungrafted injuries.

Determination of burn depth

There is no foolproof method for the early determination of burn depth; even experienced plastic surgeons may not be able to make an accurate assessment for days or even weeks after injury. However, a number of pointers are valuable.

Burn depth is proportional to the temperature of the causal agent and to the length of contact time. Scalds from liquids below boiling point usually produce partial thickness injury, whereas scalds from boiling water and burns due to prolonged contact with hot metal often produce full thickness damage. Flame burns can be of mixed depth but nearly always include areas of full thickness loss. Electrical burns are almost always full thickness and high tension electricity can cause devastating necrosis of muscles and other deep tissues.

Erythema denotes that epidermal damage is superficial, and blanching on pressure confirms that dermal capillaries are intact and that injury is partial thickness. A *dead white appearance* frequently indicates full thickness injury, although at least some of these burns prove to be deep dermal. A *dry leathery mahogany-coloured* eschar with visible thrombosed veins denotes full thickness destruction.

Intact cutaneous sensation implies that the epidermal appendages have survived as they lie at the same level as cutaneous nerve endings in the dermis. Superficial burns are thus very painful. In practice, anaesthesia to pinprick does not always indicate full thickness loss.

Blisters are accumulations of fluid superficial to the basal layer of the epidermis and suggest partial thickness injury. They are often broken by the time the patient is seen by a doctor but may continue to appear several hours after injury.

PROGNOSIS AFTER BURN INJURY

Prognosis depends on the following factors.

Age and general condition. Infants, the elderly, alcoholics and those ill from other disease fare less well than healthy young adults.

Extent of the burn. Extent can be calculated in the adult by using the 'rule of nines' (Fig. 13.2), but tables are available for more accurate calculations. The patient's hand with fingers together accounts for about 1%. The rule of nines cannot be used in children because of the relatively large size of the head (which accounts for about 20% of body surface at birth), whereas each lower limb accounts for only 13%. Hypovolaemic shock is anticipated if more than 15% of the surface is burned in adults, or more than 10% in a child. If the sum of an adult patient's age and percentage area of full thickness burn comes to more than 80, death is probable.

Depth of burn. Superficial burns of whatever size should heal without scarring within 3 weeks if properly treated. Deep dermal burns take longer and produce hypertrophic scarring. Full thickness burns inevitably become infected unless excised early, and in the case of large burns, infection may prove life-threatening.

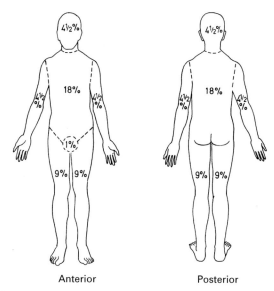

Fig. 13.2 **Rule of nines for calculating surface area of a burn.**

Table 13.2 First aid for burns
Arrest the burning process
Extinguish flames
Remove clothing
Cool with water
Ensure adequacy of airway
Avoid wound contamination
'Cling film'
Transfer for definitive treatment as soon as possible

Site of the burn. Burns involving the face, neck, hands, feet or perineum are particularly liable to threaten appearance or function. They require inpatient management.

Associated respiratory injury. This is now extremely common in house fires and usually results from inhalation of smoke from burning plastic foam upholstery. It is frequently fatal.

MANAGEMENT OF THE BURNED PATIENT

First aid

Prompt effective action prevents further damage, and may save life or prevent months of suffering. The key principles are to arrest the burning process, ensure an adequate airway and avoid wound contamination (Table 13.2).

Arrest the burning process. Burning clothing is extinguished by smothering the flames in a coat or carpet. The victim is laid flat to avoid flames rising to the head and neck with inhalation of smoke and fumes. Heat within clothing can continue to burn for many seconds after flames have been extinguished, so that clothing must be removed or doused in cold water. The same applies to clothing soaked in scalding water which will continue to cause damage until removed. Cool water is an excellent analgesic and dissipates heat but common sense must be applied. Immersing a child in cold water or covering a patient with cold soaks can cause hypothermia, and cooling counteracts the heat of a burn only if applied immediately after injury.

Chip pan fires are common. It is dangerous to attempt to remove the burning pan from the kitchen. The source of heat should be turned off and the pan covered with a lid, fibreglass firemat, or damp dishtowel to exclude air and extinguish the flames.

Chemical burns require copious irrigation for several minutes. If the eyes are involved, prompt and prolonged irrigation may save the patient's sight.

Electrical burning is arrested by switching off the current, not by pulling the patient free. If this is not feasible, the patient should be pushed free from the contact with a non-conductor such as a wooden chair.

Ensure an adequate airway. The patient must be moved as quickly as possible into a smoke-free atmosphere. Smoke and fumes can cause asphyxia, often contain poisons and can precipitate respiratory arrest. Mouth-to-mouth ventilation is commenced if necessary. If cardiac arrest follows electrocution, resuscitation is instituted.

Avoid wound contamination. The burn should be covered with a clean sheet or 'cling film'. Traditional 'household remedies' must be avoided. At best they are messy and interfere with subsequent care; at worst they are destructive, converting partial to full thickness injury.

Transfer to hospital

The patient should be transferred to hospital as quickly as possible, unless the burn is obviously trivial. Severe burns are best treated from the outset in a specialized burns unit. Hypovolaemia takes time to become manifest, and it is easy to misjudge the severity of injury, thus missing the opportunity for uncomplicated early transfer. Patients embarking on a journey expected to take more than 30 minutes should be accompanied by a trained person, and an intravenous infusion should be commenced if the burn is extensive. Transfer of patients with large burns between hospitals should be avoided between 8 and 24 hours after injury.

Full thickness burns are often relatively painless. Partial thickness injuries can be excruciating and opiates are usually needed. Analgesics must be given intravenously and the dose and route of administration noted.

Arrival in the accident and emergency department

Adequate ventilation

Maintenance of an adequate airway remains the first priority. Lack of respiratory symptoms on admission is no guarantee that the patient will remain free from airway problems. Every patient who has been exposed to smoke in a closed room should be admitted for observation. Respiratory tract injury is suggested by dyspnoea, cough, hoarseness, cyanosis, coarse crepitations on auscultation, and the presence of soot particles around the nostrils, in the mouth or in the sputum. Endotracheal intubation is advisable if there is anxiety about airway patency, and assisted ventilation may be needed. Tracheostomy is never undertaken lightly in view of the danger of infection of burned tissues around the stoma.

Initial assessment and management

Once airway patency is assured, the time of injury, type of burn and its previous treatment, and burn extent and depth are established. If the burn is over 15% in extent (or 10% in children), establishing an intravenous infusion takes priority over a detailed history and physical examination. Intravenous therapy may be needed for many days, but there may be few veins available and they must be treated with great respect. It is best to start with the most peripheral vein available in the upper limb, but in shocked patients with vasoconstriction, cannulation of the internal jugular or subclavian vein may be needed. Blood is withdrawn for cross-matching and determination of haematocrit and urea and electrolyte concentrations. Arterial blood gas analyses are performed if there is concern about the airway. Once an infusion has been established, the pulse rate, blood pressure and core/peripheral temperature difference are monitored; in patients with burns of

more than 20% a catheter is inserted to measure urine output hourly. Severe pain is relieved by intravenous injection of opiates. Tetanus can complicate burns and tetanus toxoid is given if the patient has not received it recently.

In general, patients with burns involving more than 5% of body surface should be admitted to hospital, as should all those with significant full thickness injury or burns in sites likely to pose particular management problems.

Prevention and treatment of burn shock

The aim of management is to prevent hypovolaemic shock by prompt and adequate fluid replacement (Table 13.3; see also Ch. 3). Opinions vary as to the relative amounts of colloid and crystalloid that should be used in resuscitation. Various 'formulae' are available to help calculate replacement needs but all are merely guides and the amounts of fluid given must be adjusted in the light of the patient's response. In a commonly used formula in the UK, the first 36 hours after injury are divided into six successive periods of 4, 4, 4, 6, 6 and 12 hours. The volume of colloid (e.g. purified protein solution (PPS)) to be infused in each period is calculated from the equation:

$$\frac{\text{Burn area (\%)} \times \text{body weight (kg)}}{2}$$

i.e. 0.5ml/kg for each percent burn. The need for fluid is greatest in the early hours, but excessive losses may persist for 36–48 hours.

Despite renal retention of sodium after injury, there is a tendency to hyponatraemia in the first 2–3 days due to secretion of antidiuretic hormone and sequestration of sodium in oedema. As inflammatory oedema is reabsorbed, the serum sodium concentration returns to normal, and unless water intake is maintained there is now a danger of hypernatraemia. Tissue destruction releases large amounts of potas-

Table 13.3 Hypovolaemic shock and burns
• Anticipate if burn more extensive than 15% (10% in children)
• Prevent by early intravenous resuscitation
• Control pain by adequate intravenous administration of opiates
• Fluid requirements assessed from patient's response 'Formulae' for fluid replacement provide rough guides only

sium into the extracellular fluid (ECF), but hyper-kalaemia is largely prevented by increased renal excretion as part of the metabolic response to injury (see Ch. 1). Once the first few days have passed, continuing potassium losses can produce hypo-kalaemia in a patient unable to eat and drink normally.

Water replacement. Daily water losses are replaced using 5% dextrose solution, taking care to avoid water intoxication in the first few days following injury. Excessive evaporation continues until the burn has re-epithelialized, and a high water intake must be maintained. Although most patients are thirsty, paralytic ileus may occur during the first 48 hours in those with very large burns so that giving oral fluids too soon can cause gastric distension, vomiting and aspiration. Most patients are able to drink normally after 48 hours and should be encouraged to do so.

Blood transfusion. Blood should not be given in the first 24 hours but may be needed thereafter in patients with large full thickness burns. Continuing red cell destruction in deep burns with bone marrow suppression can necessitate repeated transfusion, and haemoglobin concentration and haematocrit should be monitored.

Organ failure and burn shock

Organ failure and shock are discussed in detail in Chapter 3 and only those respiratory and renal problems specific to burn shock are considered here.

Respiratory complications

Inhalation of smoke and fumes can cause direct heat damage, carbon monoxide poisoning and damage from other chemicals, all of which predisposes to infection. Patients with head and neck burns are best nursed sitting up to encourage dispersal of oedema. Continued observation is mandatory and physio-therapy is essential to clear bronchial secretions. Chest X-rays and blood gas analyses are repeated regularly in patients with ventilation problems. Arterial hypoxaemia requires oxygen therapy, and early endotracheal intubation and assisted ventila-tion with positive end-expiratory pressure (PEEP) may be required. Antibiotics should be prescribed. Tracheo-stomy is occasionally unavoidable despite the pro-blems associated with its management. Encircling eschar impairing chest or abdominal expansion must be incised or excised.

Renal failure

Acute tubular necrosis may complicate extensive burns, especially in the elderly, those with pre-existing renal disease and those who develop haemo-globinaemia or myoglobinuria. These pigments appear in the urine after massive red cell destruction or extensive muscle damage (particularly after electrical injury) and can damage the tubules and obstruct urine flow by forming casts.

Hourly urine output should be maintained at 30–50 ml/hour in adults. Falling output reflects inadequate resuscitation or impending renal failure. Measurement of urine osmolality and the response to a test infusion will distinguish between them. Diuretics are used only if oliguria persists despite adequate fluid replacement, when 20% mannitol (1 g/kg) should be infused over 30 minutes.

Nutritional management

Evaporation from open wounds and sepsis are important causes of increased energy expenditure following a severe burn. Energy expenditure can be reduced by nursing in an environmental temperature of 30–32°C. A high caloric intake is impractical during the period of hypovolaemic shock, but is encouraged as soon as the patient can drink. The daily caloric intake in adults can be calculated as 20 kcal/kg body weight plus 70 kcal/percent burn, and it is essential to provide sufficient protein intake (1 g/kg body weight plus 3 g/percent burn).

In large burns, oral intake can usually be supple-mented at 48 hours by enteral feeding using a fine-bore nasogastric tube. If the patient's total calculated energy and protein requirements are supplied in this way, weight loss can be limited to less than 10%. Vitamin supplements and iron must also be provided. It is unusual to have to use parenteral nutrition in burned patients.

Sepsis

Septicaemia is a constant threat until skin cover has been fully restored. Resistance to infection is low, the wound provides a reservoir of infecting organ-isms, and catheters, cannulae and tracheostomy wounds are all potential sources of infection. Although the incidence of septicaemia has been reduced by topical antibacterial agents and early excision and grafting, the risk remains high with large burns. Regular monitoring by blood cultures is advisable. Systemic antibiotics are not prescribed routinely for fear of producing superinfection with resistant organisms; their use is reserved for invasive infection and for patients with positive blood cultures.

Curling's ulcer and gastric erosions

Acute duodenal ulceration (Curling's ulcer) and multiple gastric erosions may follow major burns. Early resumption of feeding reduces their incidence and H_2-receptor antagonists such as ranitidine are prescribed prophylactically.

LOCAL MANAGEMENT OF BURNS

Care of the burn wound commences at the time of injury and continues until epithelial cover has been restored. Infection poses the main threat to life once the first 48 hours have passed.

Initial cleansing and debridement

The wound is cleansed meticulously with a mild detergent containing antiseptic and saline as soon as possible after admission. Adherent clothing and loose devitalized tissues are removed. Cleansing must be carried out in an operating theatre or clean dressing room using aseptic technique. Blisters are

Consequences of burns
- The morbidity and mortality of burns depend on the site, extent and depth of the burn and on the age and general condition of the patient.

- Early consequences include:
  - hypovolaemia (loss of protein, fluid and electrolytes)
  - metabolic derangements (hyponatraemia followed by risk of hypernatraemia, hyperkalaemia followed by hypokalaemia)
  - sepsis which may be both local and generalized
  - haemolysis with anaemia and need for transfusion
  - hypothermia.

- Short-term consequences include:
  - renal failure (acute tubular necrosis due to hypovolaemia, haemoglobinuria and myoglobinuria)
  - respiratory failure (smoke inhalation, airway obstruction, ARDS)
  - catabolism and nutritional depletion
  - venous thrombosis
  - Curling's ulcer and erosive gastritis.

- Long-term consequences include permanent disfigurement, prolonged hospitalisation, psychological problems and impaired function.

punctured and serum expressed, and broken blisters are completely deroofed. General anaesthesia may be necessary, but in most cases pain can be relieved by intravenous opiates. In shocked patients, the wound is covered with a clean drape, and further local care is postponed until the circulatory state has stabilized.

Prevention of contamination

Destruction of the epidermis removes the normal barrier to infection, and in full thickness injury, thrombosis of cutaneous vessels impairs the normal response to infection. In large burns, both cellular and humoral immune mechanisms are depressed. Organisms readily colonize the burn wound and if dead tissue is present, multiply rapidly and invade the surrounding tissues.

Improved wound care and topical antibacterials have greatly reduced the risk of burn sepsis. Staphylococci remain by far the commonest infecting organism and *Pseudomonas aeruginosa* remains troublesome in most burn units. Haemolytic streptococci are feared because they can convert superficial into deep burns and can cause a severe systemic illness. Once contaminating organisms have been cleared, further contamination can be prevented in a number of ways. The methods described below are not mutually exclusive and more than one may be used as the patient's needs alter. All personnel coming into contact with burned patients must wear a cap and mask, and all dressings are applied using meticulous aseptic technique.

Exposure. After cleansing and debridement, burns of a single surface may be exposed to the air. Evaporation of the protein-rich exudate leaves a dry, adherent crust which is an effective barrier to bacteria as long as it remains intact. Exposure is particularly useful for burns of the face and neck, but can be used for burns of the trunk and extremities. The technique is difficult and should only be practised by units familiar with it; badly performed 'exposure' is a recipe for infection.

Evaporative dressings. These dressings prevent contamination, allow exudate to evaporate and provide comfortable support. After the initial cleansing, the wound is covered by a layer of sterile paraffin gauze, a layer of cotton gauze swabs, a bulky layer of cotton wool or Gamgee, and an outer retaining crepe bandage. The dressing is reviewed daily but left for 8–10 days unless exudate soaks through to the outside. The dressing is then changed down to the inner layer as bacteria traverse a soaked dressing in hours.

Semi-occlusive and occlusive dressings. 'Cling film' is useful in first aid but leaks and is too messy for use as a definitive dressing. OpSite is an adhesive film which is effective for small burns; it may also leak initially and should be covered with a well-padded dressing for 48 hours. Thereafter it can be patched or replaced as necessary. Many new dressings are now available; hydrogels and hydrocolloids absorb exudates but offer no particular advantages in acute management.

Commercial polythene bags of the 'snappy' type are cheap, sterile when taken from the roll, and useful for treating superficial hand burns. The hands are smeared with silver sulfadiazine cream or povidone iodine and the bags are kept in place with a bandage at the wrist. They must be changed daily after washing the hand and reapplying the antiseptic cream. 'Hand bags' prevent stiffness and allow the patient to continue to use the hand.

Topical antibacterial agents. Silver sulfadiazine cream (Flamazine) and povidone iodine (Betadine) are valuable local antibacterial agents for large burns. To be effective they must be reapplied daily. They are not necessary or cost-effective for minor burns given proper initial surgical debridement and use of evaporative dressings.

'Biological dressings'. Freeze-dried xenografts such as porcine skin can be reconstituted for use as temporary occlusive 'biological' dressings, but are very expensive. Amnion or stored homograft skin are now used rarely because of the danger of infection with human immunodeficiency virus (HIV), but skin from a close relative is used occasionally. Sheets of keratocytes grown in tissue culture are fragile and easily destroyed by infection, limitations which may be overcome in future by growing the cells on sheets of collagen or synthetic 'dermis'.

Relief of constriction (escharotomy)

The danger of progressive respiratory embarassment from encircling eschar has already been mentioned. Increasing oedema beneath encircling eschar in the limbs may imperil the circulation, and relieving incisions (escharotomy) which run from the top to the bottom of circumferential deep burns may be needed in the first few hours after injury.

Restoration of epidermal cover

Full thickness and deep dermal burns of less than 10% are suitable for primary excision of eschar and grafting under general anaesthesia within a few days of injury. *Tangential excision* is used for deep dermal burns; the dead outer layers of skin are shaved away down to the deep dermal layer and a split skin graft is applied immediately. More extensive burns can be partially excised and grafted soon after injury and the remaining areas of skin destruction treated by delayed grafting. Eschar begins to separate spontaneously after some 2 weeks, the process being accelerated by infection and delayed by topical antibacterial agents. As the slough separates, healthy granulation tissue should be revealed and when all the slough has gone (helped if necessary by the surgeon's scalpel), the burn should be ready for grafting. Haemolytic streptococci are a troublesome cause of graft lysis, and when such infection is present, grafting must be deferred until the patient has been treated with intravenous penicillin and barrier nursed until three successive wound swabs are negative.

Free skin grafts may be full thickness or partial thickness (split skin), but only split skin grafts are used to cover acute burns. The grafts may vary in thickness from epidermis only (Thiersch's grafts) to almost full thickness; medium thickness grafts are most commonly used. The donor site forms a new epidermis from residual islands of epithelium and more skin can be harvested after 14 days. Excess skin can be stored at 4°C for up to 3 weeks.

Full thickness grafts are used for secondary reconstruction in cosmetically important areas where contraction has to be avoided, or in areas such as the palm of the hands which are subject to repeated trauma. Avascular tissues such as bone, tendon or open joints may not provide sufficient nourishment for free grafts, and require cover with a vascularized flap.

A graft will not 'take' if there is movement between it and the recipient area, or if the graft is floated off by the accumulation of blood or serum. Large flat surfaces are covered by sheets or strips of skin which can be held in place by occasional sutures or staples. Accumulation beneath the graft is prevented by multiple small perforations. Grafts can be *meshed* in a machine which cuts small slits so that they can be expanded to cover an area nine times their original size (Fig. 13.3). In practice, expansion to more than three or four times is rarely used as the quality of the healed skin is poor. However, in very large burns when donor sites are scarce, widely meshed autograft skin care be covered with sheets of allograft; the latter provide temporary cover and as they are rejected, the autograft covers the surface by 'creeping substitution'.

Non-meshed grafts are exposed if feasible, but in many areas a bulky firm dressing is needed to protect

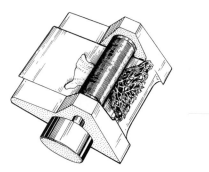

Fig. 13.3 Skin mesher for increasing the surface area of a split thickness graft.

the area. Meshed grafts need to be dressed to prevent the interstices from drying out. Shearing is prevented by leaving the sutures long and tying them over the dressing.

Functional and cosmetic result

With energetic treatment it is usually possible to restore skin cover to even the most extensive injury within 3 months, but wound closure is not the end-point. Skin grafts and donor sites must be kept soft and supple by applying moisturizing cream several times a day for many months. Splints may be needed to prevent contractures, and physiotherapy is essential to mobilize joints. Elastic pressure garments help to prevent the build-up of hypertrophic scars. In spite of all this care, reconstructive procedures may be required for many years to correct contractures or rebuild missing or distorted features. Severely burned patients often have a difficult time coming to terms with their disfigurement and limitations of their way of life. Long-term support with counselling from surgeon and supporting staff is invaluable.

14

Trauma and multiple injury

CONTENTS

EPIDEMIOLOGY OF TRAUMA

Trauma is the commonest cause of death between the ages of 1 week and 45 years, and is the third commonest cause of death irrespective of age. In the UK, approximately 500 000 patients sustain major injury each year, and of these, almost 25 000 will die. In the 'developed' world, road traffic accidents are the commonest cause of multiple injury, falls and interpersonal violence accounting for most of the remainder. Gunshot wounds are rare in Europe but not in the USA where in 1992, for the first time, there were more deaths from firearms than from road traffic accidents.

In most countries, the number of individuals dying annually in road traffic accidents is declining despite substantial increases in the number of vehicles and road users. This is due in part to improved design and construction of roads and vehicles, and in part to measures introduced to reduce the severity of injury (e.g. seat belts, crash helmets and air bags). Pedestrians, cyclists and motorcyclists remain at very high risk because of their relative lack of protection; the relative risk of injury for a motorcyclist is 20-fold greater than that for a car occupant.

Multiple injury exacts a huge toll in terms of pain and suffering, and the estimated cost to the Exchequer of an individual dying as a result of a road traffic accident in the UK is estimated at a staggering £750 000. Between 1% and 3% of the Gross National Product is consumed by accidents causing death or serious injury. As trauma principally affects the younger members of society, it leads to greater loss of working years of life than ischaemic heart disease and cancer combined. In the UK, individuals aged 15–24 years have a 1 in 75 chance annually of being killed or injured in a road traffic accident.

Alcohol and trauma

Alcohol is the single most important preventable cause of trauma. There is no 'safe level' for blood alcohol concentration in relation to its adverse effects on motor function or ability to concentrate. At a blood alcohol concentration of 80 mg% (the current legal limit in the UK) the risk of being involved in a road traffic accident doubles, and at 150 mg% it increases ten-fold. These risks are even greater in young inexperienced drinkers.

In road traffic accidents, one-third of all fatalities and 10% of all injuries involve alcohol consumption. Up to 60% of those injured by personal violence have been drinking, and alcohol is implicated in over 50% of deaths from burns, 50% of murders, 30% of cases of drowning, and 25% of fatal workplace accidents.

Intoxication increases the difficulty of assessment

and diagnosis, has deleterious effects on the normal protective pathophysiological response to trauma, and leads to greater morbidity and mortality following all forms of injury.

MECHANISMS OF INJURY

Traumatic injury is usually classified as 'blunt' or 'penetrating'. Blunt injury typically results from road traffic accidents and falls, whereas penetrating injury is often associated with interpersonal violence, either civilian or military. Blast injury is a third form of injury caused by explosions.

Blunt injury

Blunt injuries usually result from decelerating forces with crushing, shearing or torsion damage. The magnitude of injury reflects direct transfer of kinetic energy to the patient where the energy, $E = 1/2 \, mv^2$. Since the energy is directly proportional to the square of the velocities involved, the potential for injury increases dramatically with higher impact speeds. For example, death in a road traffic accident with an impact speed of 50 mph is 20 times more likely than in one occurring at 20 mph. Many of the methods used to reduce injury severity in motor vehicles (e.g. crumple zones, seat belts) act primarily by reducing the magnitude of velocity changes and hence the transfer of kinetic energy to the occupant.

Penetrating injury

In the UK as in much of Europe, knife wounds are the commonest penetrating injury. Few Accident and Emergency Departments experience a weekend without seeing this form of injury and it is particularly prevalent in males in the age group 15–24

years. Handgun injuries are uncommon outside the USA, and high-velocity injuries are extremely rare outwith military conflict and terrorism.

Damage in stab injuries and low-velocity firearm injuries is usually confined to the track of the weapon or missile. In low-velocity bullet wounds, the diameter of the track of tissue damage between the entrance wound and the exit wound (if present) is little larger than the diameter of the bullet. High-velocity missiles, such as those fired from modern weapons such as the AK 47 or Armalite rifle where the muzzle velocity exceeds 1000 m/second, produce cavitation and massive tissue disruption as the bullet passes through the body. The entrance wound is similar in size to the bullet but the exit wound (if present) is large, and the severity of tissue damage reflects the great dissipation of kinetic energy (Fig. 14.1). Bullets which 'tumble' or are deflected by structures such as bone, slow down even more and thus transfer even greater amounts of kinetic energy. Cavitation is due to compression and acceleration of surrounding tissues away from the bullet, and the sub-atmospheric pressure generated often sucks in foreign material resulting in major wound contamination.

Blast injury

These injuries occur as the result of fireworks, domestic or industrial explosions, and bombings. Bomb injuries combine the effect of shrapnel and flying debris with the damage caused by radiating shock waves and blast winds. Shock waves travel at just over the speed of sound, are reflected and multiplied by solid objects such as those found in confined spaces, and cause particular damage at gas/tissue interfaces (e.g. within the ear, respiratory tree and gastrointestinal tract). Blast winds set in motion by explosion may cause avulsion of the extremities.

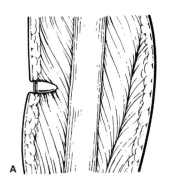 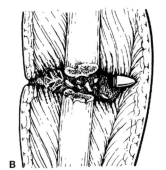 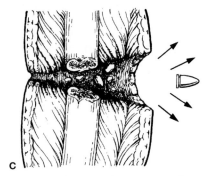

Fig. 14.1 High velocity missile with shock waves from track. Note that the exit wound is larger than the entry wound.

PATTERNS OF INJURY

Patients with multiple injuries often exhibit characteristic patterns of injury. Recognition of these patterns often allows injuries to be detected or suspected that might otherwise be missed on clinical examination. For example, an unrestrained car driver involved in a head-on collision may present with forehead lacerations from contact with the driving mirror or windscreen, an imprint on the chest from contact with the steering wheel, and injuries to the knee from contact with the dashboard. Head and neck injury, chest injury (possibly with myocardial contusion and a flail segment), and pelvic and posterior hip dislocation should all be considered in this scenario. Patients who land on their heels after a fall from a height may have fractures not only of their calcaneum, hips and pelvis, but also compression fractures of the lumbar or thoracic spine. The 'sandwich rule' states that if injuries are present in two separate anatomical areas, there is a high chance of injury to the areas between.

Pattern recognition is particularly important following trauma as patients are frequently unable to give a clear history because of altered consciousness, amnesia, or the effects of alcohol or drugs. Eye-witness accounts and descriptions of the scene of the accident from members of the emergency services are invaluable. Descriptions of the speeds involved and disposition of wreckage in road traffic accidents, of the nature of the landing surfaces when a patient has fallen from a height, and of the exact position in which an injured individual was found, may be of immense help when predicting and assessing the extent of injury.

TREATMENT PRIORITIES

Patients with multiple injury require a systematic approach from a team directed by an experienced clinician. The immediate priority is to identify and correct problems which endanger life, resuscitate the patient, and then determine the extent of other injuries and prioritize their management.

The ABC of trauma resuscitation

The initial stages of resuscitation are best remembered under the headings of *A*irway, *B*reathing and *C*irculation. In practice, these issues are not addressed sequentially but are handled simultaneously by a well-directed and efficient trauma team.

Airway

Establishment of a patent airway is of paramount importance. The spectrum of presentation varies from a fully conscious articulate patient to one who is deeply unconscious with an airway that is obstructed by anatomical derangement, or by blood, vomit or foreign bodies in the upper or lower respiratory tree. Although patients who are fully conscious and able to talk normally clearly have no airway problem, they must be reassessed frequently and monitored to ensure that this situation does not deteriorate.

The possibility of unrecognized cervical spine injury must always be considered, particularly when consciousness is altered or the history and examination suggest head and neck injury. A rigid cervical collar provides a degree of security by preventing excessive movement of the cervical spine; alternatively in-line stability of the neck may be maintained manually.

Some patients with altered consciousness and blunting of the reflexes which protect the airway can be managed by simply positioning the head and neck in the 'sniffing the morning air' position, and clearing blood, mucus, vomit or foreign material from the upper airway with a rigid (Yankauer) suction catheter. Dentures and plates must be removed. A smaller proportion of patients require other measures to maintain the airway. These include insertion of an oropharyngeal airway or passage of a cuffed endotracheal tube (Fig. 14.2). Tracheal intubation secures the airway and prevents aspiration of gastric contents or blood into the lungs. Intubation is a skilled procedure and is not without risks; these include inability to pass the tube, vagal stimulation, increased intracranial pressure, release

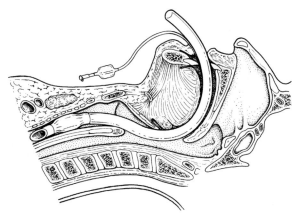

Fig. 14.2 Cuffed endotracheal tube in position. Inflation of the balloon prevents aspiration into the respiratory tract.

of catecholamines and exacerbation of cervical cord injury. Unless the patient is deeply unconscious, intubation requires induction of anaesthesia and the use of short-acting neuromuscular blocking drugs.

In certain situations, such as the presence of severe facial injury, endotracheal intubation may be impossible and a surgical approach is needed to ensure airway patency. Formal tracheostomy is a difficult and time-consuming procedure under these circumstances and needle cricothyroidotomy is used to 'buy time' in patients who are in extremis. A large-bore needle/cannula is inserted through the cricothyroid membrane and the patient is ventilated using a Y-shaped connector attached to an oxygen supply. Formal cricothyroidotomy can then be performed using a 2–3 centimetre horizontal incision (Fig. 14.3) to insert a cuffed tube into the trachea.

Breathing

Once the airway has been secured, oxygen delivery to the tissues depends on adequacy of the pulmonary and systemic circulations and normal pulmonary gas exchange. Hypoxia is easily overlooked in trauma patients as its typical features (pallor, sweating, agitation and signs of cerebral irritation) may be absent or attributed to other conditions. Cyanosis is rare as patients with acute blood loss seldom have the minimum concentration of deoxygenated haemoglobin (5 g/dl) needed for its detection. Injured patients must be given the highest possible concentrations of inspired oxygen to maximize tissue delivery. In practice, conscious patients are given

oxygen at high flow rates via a face mask while intubated patients are given 100% oxygen. Arterial blood gas sampling is required to ensure that hypoxia and/or hypercarbia are not developing.

A number of factors may impede normal pulmonary gas exchange and give rise to mismatching of ventilation and perfusion. Common problems include lung contusion, pneumothorax, aspiration and inhalation injury. Injury to the chest wall can compromise respiration by a variety of means. Pain can inhibit the depth and frequency of respiration leading to hypoxaemia. When ribs and/or sternum are fractured at more than one site, an unstable 'flail segment' may be created (Fig. 14.4) which can move paradoxically on respiration. This means that the segment is drawn inwards as the rest of the chest expands on inspiration, and pushed out as the rest of the chest moves inwards on expiration. The effect of this paradoxical movement is reduced

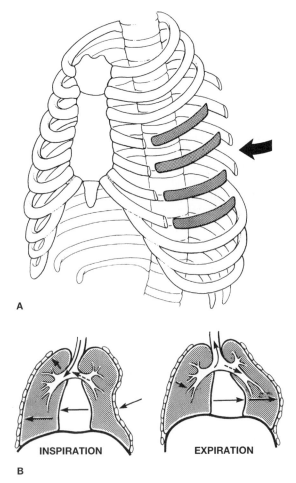

A

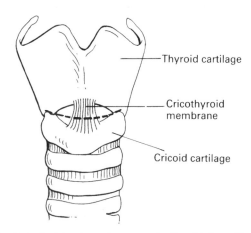

Fig. 14.3 Incision for emergency cricothyroidotomy. The gap between the thyroid and cricoid cartilage is easily palpable. The incision through the cricothyroid membrane is held open with a scalpel handle while a tube is inserted.

B

Fig. 14.4 Creation of a flail segment by multiple fractures.

ventilation in the underlying lung. Pneumothorax, the accumulation of air in the potential space between the visceral and parietal pleura, is often the result of lung puncture by fractured ribs. The loss of the normal intrapleural vacuum means that the lung does not fully inflate, with impairment of gas exchange. The pneumothorax may be difficult to detect clinically when small, but classically gives rise to reduced breath sounds over the affected side with a hyper-resonant note on percussion. Trauma may also result in bleeding into the pleural space (haemothorax) with compression of the lung and impairment of its expansion. Chest radiographs may help to demonstrate pneumothorax and haemothorax (Fig. 14.5), but the interpretation of radiographs taken in the supine position is often difficult.

Pneumothorax and haemothorax are treated by inserting a tube which will allow the air or blood to escape (see below). Tension pneumothorax is an even more dangerous form of pneumothorax in which the injured lung serves as a flap valve, allowing air to enter the pleural space during inspiration but not leave on expiration. Intrapleural pressure increases dramatically, the underlying lung collapses, and the mediastinum is pushed over to the opposite side, compromising the expansion of the other lung and impairing venous return to the heart. The affected chest is markedly hyper-resonant and breath sounds are inaudible. The trachea is often noted to be deviated away from the side of the tension pneumothorax. Tension may also develop in patients with an existing pneumothorax who undergo positive pressure ventilation before the pneumothorax has been drained.

A tension pneumothorax must be drained as an emergency without waiting for radiological confirmation. A wide-bore needle passed through the second intercostal space in the mid-clavicular line allows air to hiss out under pressure and temporarily relieves the situation. A thoracostomy tube must then be inserted through the fourth intercostal space in the mid-axillary line and the air is allowed to bubble out via an underwater seal drainage bottle (Fig. 14.6). Occasionally, patients present with an open sucking chest wound which communicates with the thoracic cavity; such wounds are occluded with a sterile dressing and a tube thoracostomy is performed.

Circulation

Control of bleeding and maintenance of circulating blood volume are aided by a number of simple

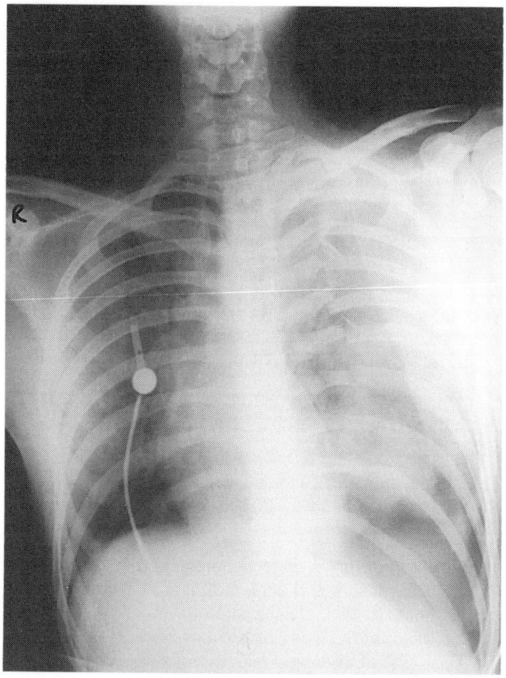

Fig. 14.5 Chest X-ray following road traffic accident. Blunt chest trauma has resulted in rib fractures and haemothorax.

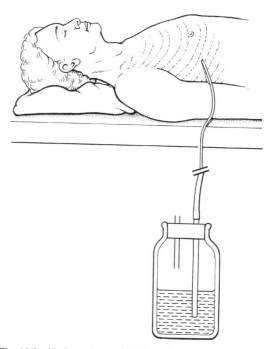

Fig. 14.6 Underwater seal drainage being used to drain air from a pneumothorax. The cannula has been inserted through the fourth intercostal space in the mid-axillary line.

measures. Gentle handling of the patient and avoidance of unnecessary movement ensures that bleeding into body cavities is not exacerbated. External bleeding is controlled by direct pressure rather than 'blind' clamping of vessels with artery forceps or the use of tourniquets. Bleeding from extensive scalp lacerations can be controlled temporarily by mass suture. Correctly applied pneumatic or traction splints can reduce blood loss from long-bone fractures by up to 50%, in addition to minimizing pain.

Prompt restoration of circulating blood volume is essential. Large-bore (12–14 gauge) cannulae are inserted percutaneously into the veins of both forearms, blood is taken for grouping and cross-matching, and fluid infusion is commenced. The choice of infusate is less important than the volume infused. In the UK a mixture of crystalloid (0.9% saline or Ringer lactate) and colloids (gelatins, dextrans or starches) is given in the first instance. Blood transfusion will normally be needed for patients who have lost more than 20% of their blood volume. Patients in extremis may be given Group O Rhesus negative blood while cross-matched blood is awaited.

The magnitude of blood loss is often underestimated. A fit young trauma patient can lose up to 20% of his blood volume before pulse rate or blood pressure change. By the time tachycardia and hypotension become apparent, losses of 30–40% are likely. In the absence of head injury or other reasons for loss of consciousness, altered consciousness due to blood loss denotes a deficit greater than 40% (i.e. more than 2000 ml of blood in a 70-kg adult).

The rate and amount of volume replacement are guided by estimates of the blood volume deficit, and the response and trends in vital signs during resuscitation. Regular measurement of pulse, blood pressure and urine output is essential, and while measurement of left and right heart filling pressure and cardiac output is valuable, such measures are seldom practicable outwith an intensive care unit. Red cell replacement aims to provide a haematocrit of approximately 30%, corresponding to a haemoglobin concentration of about 10 g/dl. Once the equivalent of one 'blood volume' (i.e. over 5000 ml in a 70-kg man) has been replaced, haemostatic problems may occur with oozing from wound and venepuncture sites and spontaneous bruising. These problems are due to dilution of haemostatic factors during resuscitation together with their consumption by the injury itself. Laboratory tests of coagulation will identify the specific defects so that platelets,

factor concentrates or fresh frozen plasma can be given as appropriate. Hyperkalaemia, hypocalcaemia and acid–base disturbances can arise when large amounts of stored blood are being transfused, and in-line blood warmers are essential to avoid or minimize hypothermia.

Clinical examination

Once the above priorities have been addressed, a detailed clinical examination is carried out. All of the patient's clothing must be removed and the entire body surface, including the back and perineum, is examined. All injuries are documented and the urgency of their management is assessed. The radiographic examination of all blunt trauma patients always includes radiographs of the chest and pelvis, and a lateral view of the cervical spine.

Immediate care of the injured patient

Airway – establish and maintain an unobstructed airway:
- clear blood, mucus and foreign material.
- insert an oropharyngeal airway or cuffed endotracheal tube.
- if intubation impossible/ineffective, establish patency by cricothyroidotomy.

Breathing – secure the delivery of oxygen:
- give the highest possible inspired oxygen concentration
- insert a thoracotomy tube with underwater seal drainage if required
- Remember that signs of hypoxia may be overlooked and that cyanosis is rare.

Circulation – control bleeding and maintain circulating blood volume:
- control external bleeding with direct pressure
- splint limb fractures (remember occult blood loss at fracture sites)
- Restore circulating blood volume:
  - crystalloids and colloids initially;
  - blood transfusion if > 20% of blood volume is lost.
- Remember that:
  - volume needed is often underestimated (pulse rate, blood pressure and urine output are valuable adjuncts to clinical assessment)
  - coagulopathy, hyperkalaemia, hypocalcaemia, acid-base disturbance and hypothermia are potential dangers.

HEAD INJURY

Head injury, alone or in combination with other injuries, is the commonest cause of death from trauma. Approximately 20 000 per million of the population attend hospital in any year because of head injury; some 25% of these patients will require admission and 1% will need neurosurgical intervention.

Primary brain damage

This occurs at the time of injury as a result of direct injury and/or displacement and distortion of brain tissue. Penetrating injury is much less common than closed head injury. The extent of primary brain injury depends upon the nature of the applied forces and its effects range from mild concussion with no loss of consciousness to severe brain damage with prolonged coma. The extent of primary injury is reflected in the state of consciousness and presence of focal neurological defects immediately after the accident. Diffuse brain injury can occur with little outward sign of damage. Because of the way in which the brain is suspended and tethered in the cranium, it can move relatively freely along an anteroposterior axis whereas lateral movement is restricted by the falx cerebri and falx cerebelli. Blows to the front or back of the head can therefore cause tearing or shearing of brain tissue. Diffuse shearing lesions in the white matter are commonly associated with tearing of the small vessels of the brainstem, resulting in ischaemia and interruption of neural pathways. *Concussion* is the state of altered consciousness caused by diffuse neuronal and axonal injury. As the magnitude of the injuring force increases, the brain substance may be contused or lacerated at the point of impact and at the opposite pole as the brain is set in motion and driven against the skull or dural septum ('contre-coup' injury, Fig. 14.7).

Secondary brain injury

This can occur at any time after the primary event and is commonly caused by hypoxia, hypercapnia, hypotension, intracranial bleeding and infection acting alone or in combination. In contrast to primary brain injury which cannot be influenced by treatment, secondary damage can be prevented or treated by avoiding or promptly eradicating the causal factors. Many of these factors cause secondary injury by raising intracranial pressure within the

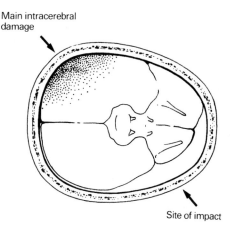

Fig. 14.7 Contre-coup injury. A blow to the head may result in injury to the opposite pole of the brain.

rigid and unyielding confines of the skull. This leads to cerebral compression and a critical reduction in cerebral blood flow. Pressure on the motor cortex causes progressive paresis on the contralateral side of the body, and eventually to extensor or 'decerebrate' rigidity. Further pressure rises may cause the temporal lobes to herniate through the tentorium cerebelli, compressing the ipsilateral oculomotor nerve (Fig. 14.8) and producing dilatation of the

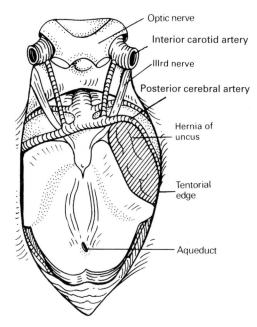

Fig. 14.8 Herniation of the temporal lobe through the tentorium may compress the oculomotor nerve causing irritation and palsy.

ipsilateral pupil. Continuing pressure effects may cause similar changes in the contralateral pupil.

Compression and ischaemia of the brainstem involves the cardiovascular and respiratory centres leading to increases in blood pressure, bradycardia and abnormal respiratory patterns. These are ominous prognostic signs and death follows swiftly unless pressure is relieved promptly.

The Glasgow Coma Scale (GCS)

The GCS (Table 14.1) is used internationally to assess conscious level in trauma patients. It uses three clinical parameters, namely the best verbal response, the best motor response and eye opening. A numerical score is given to each parameter and the sum is the GCS score. The maximum score in a fully conscious co-operative patient is 15. The GCS is a dynamic score and isolated readings are of less value than trends. A fall in the GCS with time indicates a deteriorating level of consciousness, either because of an intracranial event (e.g. an expanding intracranial haematoma) or extracranial factors such as hypoxia and blood loss. Continuing assessment of level of consciousness is a crucial factor in the early recognition of cerebral injury. For this reason, sedation is normally avoided in head-injured patients. Particular care is needed in patients who have taken drugs or alcohol as depression of

Table 14.1 Glasgow coma scale

Eyes open	spontaneously	4
	to verbal command	3
	to pain	2
	no response	1
Best motor response to verbal command	obeys verbal command	6
	localizes pain	5
	flexion withdrawal	4
to painful stimulus	abnormal flexion (decorticate rigidity)	3
	extension (decerebrate rigidity)	2
	no response	1
Best verbal response	orientated and converses	5
	disorientated and converses	4
	inappropriate words	3
	incomprehensible sounds	2
	no response	1
Total number of points (minimum 3, maximum 15)		—

consciousness may be wrongly attributed to these agents. When in doubt, assume that depression of consciousness is the result of brain injury.

Skull fractures

The presence of a skull fracture is less important in its own right than as an indication that life-threatening primary or secondary brain injury may be present or developing. Conversely, absence of a fracture does not exclude brain injury or compression, particularly in young children. When a skull fracture is present, intracranial haematoma is more likely, particularly when there is also depression of conscious level. For example, fully conscious (GCS 15) adults who have sustained a head injury without skull fracture have a risk of intracranial haematoma of approximately 1 in 6000. If a skull fracture is present this risk rises to 1 in 30, and when there is a skull fracture *and* a GCS score of less than 14, the risk is 1 in 4.

Although fractures of the vault are usually visible on plain radiographs (Fig. 14.9), their extent may not be clear, and they frequently extend to the base of the skull, traverse foramina and damage cranial nerves. The fracture may be compound because of involvement of the middle ear, air sinuses or cribriform plate. Depressed fractures are produced by indentation of the vault and are commonly compound because the scalp is breached. Basal skull fractures are rarely detected on standard radiographs but may be recognized by the presence of

Head injury
Primary brain injury:
• occurs at the time of injury and so *cannot* be influenced by treatment
• results from direct injury and displacement/distortion of brain tissue
• closed injury much more common than penetrating injury
• extent of primary injury is reflected in state of consciousness and presence of focal neurological defects *immediately* after the injury.

Secondary brain injury:
• occurs at any time after injury and *is* amenable to prevention/treatment
• commonly caused by hypoxia, hypercapnia, hypotension, intracranial bleeding and infection
• these causal factors commonly produce raised intracranial pressure
• as the skull is unyielding, raised intracranial pressure compresses the brain, reduces cerebral blood flow, and may lead to herniation.

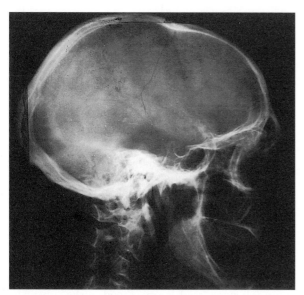

Fig. 14.9   Skull X-ray showing linear fracture of the cranial vault.

cerebrospinal fluid (CSF) rhinorrhoea or otorrhoea, the 'panda eyes' sign of anterior cranial fossa fractures, or bruising over the mastoid bone in middle cranial fossa fractures.

Management of specific head injuries

Scalp injury

Scalp injuries bleed profusely but heal well. Temporary haemostasis can be achieved by compression or mass suture, pending definitive repair after more pressing injuries have been dealt with. At definitive repair the surrounding area is shaved, and the wound is then debrided, cleaned and sutured (Fig. 14.10). Small wounds can be sutured or stapled in one layer. Larger wounds require a two-layer closure, the galea being approximated with absorbable sutures and the skin edges with interrupted non-absorbable sutures or staples.

Skull fractures

A computerized tomography (CT) scan is essential if the level of consciousness deteriorates despite optimal resuscitation. Other indications include a GCS of 8 or less following resuscitation, presence of a skull fracture with any depression of consciousness or focal neurological signs, or when general anaesthesia is needed for other surgical procedures in a patient who also has a head injury. The patient must remain absolutely still during scanning, and general anaesthesia may be needed in confused or restless patients. CT scanning provides information about brain swelling and will detect and define the extent of intracranial haematomas, particularly when contrast enhancement is used.

Four types of haematoma following intracranial bleeding may occur singly or in combination as a result of head injury:

Extradural haematoma.   This is usually the result of disruption of middle meningeal vessels by a fracture of the temporal bone. Primary brain damage is often minor and the classical history is one of transient loss of consciousness, a 'lucid interval' of apparent normality, and then a progressive deterioration of consciousness and development of 'coning' (which may be extremely rapid). It must be stressed that this pattern is far from invariable and that the 'lucid interval' has been overemphasized in the past. CT scanning reveals a lens-shaped haematoma which is convex on its inner surface (Fig. 14.11). Extradural haematomas are dealt with by creating a burr hole close to the fracture site, enlarging the opening by craniotomy, and evacuating the clot with

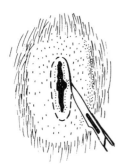
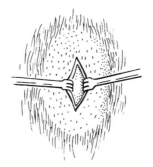
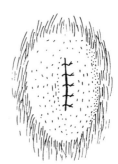

Fig. 14.10   Suture of a scalp wound. The edges of the wound are debrided and cleansed, followed by layered suture.

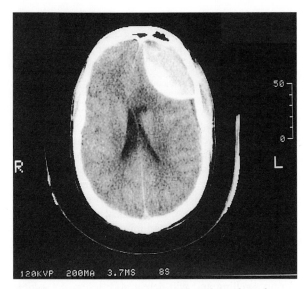

Fig. 14.11 CT scan of the head showing a lens-shaped extradural haematoma. The patient also had a fracture of the temporal bone, and required surgical evacuation of the clot.

achievement of absolute haemostasis prior to closure.

Subdural haematoma is more common than extradural haematoma. It results from laceration of brain substance and vessels (particularly the small cerebral veins). Blood accumulates in the subdural space (Fig. 14.12) and the haematoma has a distinctive appearance on CT scan, its inner surface being concave with respect to the underlying brain. Craniotomy is needed to remove the clot and arrest the source(s) of continued bleeding.

'Chronic' subdural haematoma can occur, particularly in the elderly and alcoholics, possibly because atrophy of the brain facilitates its displacement during trauma. Signs of cerebral compression may be delayed for weeks or months as the haematoma gradually enlarges due to absorption of tissue fluid by osmosis.

Subarachnoid haemorrhage. This is common following head injury. Blood in the subarachnoid space produces signs of meningeal irritation with headache, neck stiffness, photophobia and irritability. Conservative treatment is usual.

Intracerebral haematomas. Caused by trauma, these are found most often in the temporal

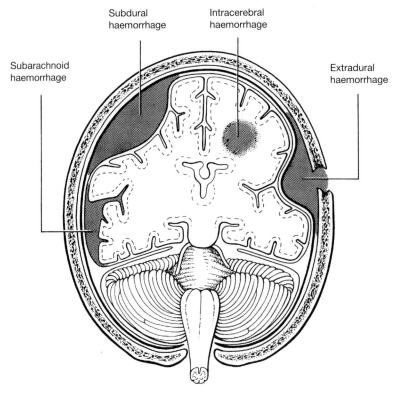

Subdural haemorrhage

Intracerebral haemorrhage

Subarachnoid haemorrhage

Extradural haemorrhage

Fig. 14.12 Sites of intracranial haemorrhage.

---

and frontal lobes. Large haematomas cause cerebral compression, produce localizing signs according to the area involved, and may rupture into the ventricular system. Surgery is usually only undertaken if compression develops or CT scanning shows a large expanding haematoma. The clot is evacuated at craniotomy and any devitalized brain tissue is removed.

Treatment of raised intracranial pressure (ICP)

Correction of hypoxia and hypercapnia and maintenance of an adequate circulating blood volume are the most important factors in preventing brain swelling and raised ICP. The injured brain is particularly susceptible to hypoxia and normal autoregulation in the cerebral circulation is disturbed, making the brain much less tolerant of hypotension or hypertension. ICP increases in a linear fashion with arterial P_{CO_2}, and controlled ventilation may be needed to keep Pa_{CO_2} between 3.5 and 4.0 kPa; reduction below 3.5 kPa is unnecessary and can lead

to paradoxical cerebral vasoconstriction. The use of an osmotic diuretic such as mannitol (given as a rapid intravenous infusion) is occasionally indicated to 'buy time' while arrangements are made to evacuate an intracranial haematoma.

Facial injury

The primary importance of facial fractures is their potential to obstruct the airway because of anatomical disturbance or profuse bleeding. Systematic palpation of the orbit, zygomatic arch and facial skeleton is vital. These fractures are easily overlooked as haematomas around the orbit can be wrongly attributed to basal skull fracture.

Fractures of the maxilla. These produce mobility of the facial skeleton which can be detected by gentle finger pressure on the hard palate. Anaesthesia in the distribution of the infraorbital nerve, dental malocclusion, diplopia and enophthalmos or exophthalmos may be present. Maxillary fractures can be classified using the Le Fort system (Fig. 14.13). A Le Fort I fracture involves only the maxilla and runs through the base of the maxillary antrum on either side and across the nasal floor through the septum. A Le Fort II fracture passes across the base of the nose through the posterior wall of the maxillary antrum and across the orbit. A Le

---

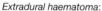

Intracranial bleeding following trauma

Extradural haematoma:
- usually the result of injury to the middle meningeal vessels

- the classical history of transient loss of consciousness at the time of injury followed by a lucid interval and then progressive loss of consciousness has been overemphasized; the pattern may vary considerably

- treatment consists of urgent open evacuation of clot and haemostasis.

Subdural haematoma:
- more common than extradural haematoma

- results from laceration of brain and tearing of vessels

- is treated by open removal of clot and arrest of bleeding

- a 'chronic' form may take weeks/months to become manifest in the elderly.

Subarachnoid haemorrhage:
- produces signs of meningeal irritation (e.g. headache, neck stiffness, photophobia and irritability)

- usually treated conservatively.

Intracerebral haematoma:
- temporal and frontal lobes most often involved

- may require open surgery if signs of compression develop and CT shows continued expansion of the haematoma.

Management of head injury
- ABC of Resuscitation must be applied

- Assess and monitor conscious level (Glasgow Coma Scale; GCS)

- GCS score and skull fracture influence the risk of intracranial haematoma:
  - GCS 15/no fracture   = 1 in 6000 risk
  - GCS 15/with fracture   = 1 in 30 risk
  - GCS < 14 with fracture   = 1 in 4 risk.

- Prevent/minimize increases in intracranial pressure by:
  - preventing hypoxia and hypercapnia
  - ensuring adequacy of circulating blood volume.

- CT scan essential if:
  - level of consciousness is depressed or GCS deteriorates despite optimal management
  - GCS < 8 following resuscitation
  - skull fracture is present with depressed consciousness or focal neurological signs or
  - general anaesthesia is needed for other surgical procedures.

- Debride, clean and suture scalp injuries in patients with no injuries of higher priority.

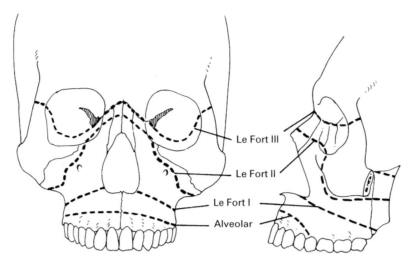

Fig. 14.13 Le Fort classification of maxillary fractures.

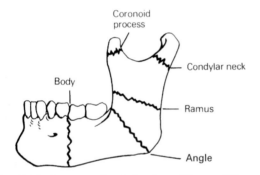

Fig. 14.14 Common sites for fracture of the mandible.

Fort III fracture separates the facial skeleton from the cranium, fracturing both zygomatic arches.

Mandibular fractures. Such fractures are usually easier to recognize. They are often compound because of associated laceration of the gums, and cause malocclusion and loosening of teeth. The common sites of fracture are the neck of the condyle or coronoid process, and the angle and ramus of the mandible (Fig. 14.14).

Facial fractures can usually be detected radiographically. Immediate management includes disimpaction of the fracture if the upper airway is blocked, and removal of blood, broken teeth, dentures or other foreign bodies from the airway. Major bleeding can follow fractures of the middle third of the face, and anterior and posterior nasal packs may have to be inserted.

Facial wounds require careful repair with fine (6–0) monofilament sutures. Complex injuries should be dealt with by specialists in plastic surgery.

All wounds are carefully explored to detect damage to underlying structures and the task of repair is kept as simple as possible by confining wound excision to the minimum necessary.

CHEST INJURY

Blunt injury

The severity of chest injury is easily underestimated. Clinical examination includes inspection of the chest wall and its movement to detect asymmetrical expansion or paradoxical movement. Signs of respiratory distress include 'grunting' respiration, tachypnoea, use of accessory muscles of respiration and indrawing of the intercostal muscles. Gentle palpation may reveal tenderness over fractures of the ribs and sternum, unstable segments of the chest wall, or the 'crackling' sensation of air in the tissues (surgical emphysema). Percussion may detect hyper-resonance due to a pneumothorax or dullness due to blood in the pleural space (haemothorax).

Arterial blood gas tensions are monitored to detect abnormalities and assess the response to treatment. A chest X-ray is essential to detect rib fractures, pneumothorax, haemothorax, tracheal or mediastinal shift, and mediastinal widening (indicating disruption of major vessels). Whenever the patient's condition permits, an erect or semierect film is preferred to reduce the risk of overlooking a small pneumothorax. Detection of rib fractures is important because of their association with damage to the lung, pneumothorax and haemothorax. However, up to 50% of rib fractures can be missed, even on careful examination of standard chest radiographs. Rupture of the diaphragm, which is more common on the left, may be suspected if stomach or bowel loops are visible in the chest, or the nasogastric tube ends above the diaphragm.

Traumatic pneumothoraces are always drained (p. 311) to allow the lung to re-expand and avoid the development of tension penumothorax. Haemothoraces can also impair ventilation by compressing the lung, and by the time they become apparent clinically or radiologically, over 1 litre of blood may be present with the patient showing evidence of hypovolaemia. Tube thoracostomy drains the blood and also treats any associated pneumothorax. Autotransfusion of the draining blood is sometimes undertaken if the bleeding is torrential.

Subcutaneous emphysema in the neck or chest wall is commonly due to laceration of the trachea or major bronchi. It may extend dramatically if positive pressure ventilation is used, resulting in a 'Michelin man' appearance.

Deceleration injury can cause myocardial contusion, often in association with fracture of the sternum or of the ribs anteriorly, and can simulate myocardial infarction and produce arrhythmias, cardiac failure and valve damage. Deceleration may also rupture the thoracic aorta (classically at the point where the arch joins the descending aorta) or other major vessels. Most patients with aortic rupture die within minutes, but in those who reach hospital, mediastinal widening on chest X-ray should signal the need for urgent arch aortography. Immediate direct suture or graft repair of the damaged vessel may then prove life-saving. The 'imprint' of the steering wheel on the sternum is a warning of deeper damage.

Penetrating chest injury

The great majority of penetrating chest injuries can be managed by tube thoracostomy, but if the penetrating object is still in place it should be left undisturbed until it can be removed in an operating theatre.

Penetrating cardiac injuries can lead to cardiac tamponade as blood escapes into the relatively inelastic pericardial sac. With each contraction of the heart, blood is forced into the pericardium, leading to compression of the heart, impaired filling and rapid progression to death. Tamponade is suspected by the combination of hypotension, tachycardia and raised central venous and jugular venous pressure. The chest X-ray is rarely helpful and time is rarely available for echocardiography. Immediate thoracostomy is usually advisable rather than attempts to decompress the pericardium by needle aspiration (pericardiocentesis). Once the pericardium has been opened, blood and clot within the sac are removed, and the wound in the heart can be controlled with a finger while formal suture closure is undertaken. Alternatively, a balloon catheter can be passed into the puncture wound, and after inflation of the balloon, traction is applied to stop the haemorrhage while the wound is repaired.

ABDOMINAL INJURY

Blunt injury

Clinical examination

Blunt trauma due to road traffic accidents is by far the commonest cause of abdominal trauma. Clinical assessment is difficult and unreliable as there may be few external signs. The history is often the best clue to the presence of internal injury but bruising, particularly of the 'pattern imprinting' type, is an important pointer when present. The anterior abdominal wall, perineum, urethral meatus, flanks and back must all be inspected; it is important to remember that the abdomen extends from the line of the nipples above to the level of the gluteal folds below. Abdominal palpation and percussion are usually unhelpful. Intraperitoneal bleeding may not be associated with guarding or tenderness while peritonism following rupture of a hollow viscus is often delayed. Palpation of the pelvic ring and lumbar spine may elicit local tenderness related to fractures. Undue importance has been accorded in the past to measurement of abdominal girth or listening for bowel sounds as these assessments are of no value in determining whether intraperitoneal injury is present.

Rectal examination is mandatory to assess sphincter tone (lost in spinal injury) and the position of the prostate in males (rupture of the urethra allows the prostate to ride upwards away from the anal canal). Blood at the urethral meatus implies urethral injury; this is much commoner in males because of the length of the urethra and frequently affects the junction of the membraneous and prostatic urethra. Urethral catheterization is contraindicated if there is any suspicion of urethral injury but in all other cases of major trauma, a catheter is inserted to detect haematuria and monitor urine output. Macroscopic haematuria indicates urinary tract trauma and the need for further investigation such as ultrasonography or intravenous urography (IVU).

Gastric distension is common in trauma patients because of air swallowing and paralytic ileus. It may compromise ventilation by raising and splinting the left hemidiaphragm, increase the risk of regurgitation of gastric contents and aspiration, and increase the frequency of acute gastric haemorrhage from erosions and gastritis. All patients with multiple injury should have a nasogastric tube passed so that the stomach can be kept empty. When fracture of the cribriform plate or anterior cranial fossa is suspected, the tube should be passed through the mouth rather than the nose to avoid introducing intracranial infection.

Adjuncts to clinical examination

Standard laboratory tests are of little value in assessing intra-abdominal injury. Leucocytosis and a low haematocrit are common but have little diagnostic or prognostic value. Hyperamylasaemia suggests pancreatic trauma but can also occur in bowel injury or infarction.

Plain X-rays are also of limited value in detecting blunt abdominal injury although the erect chest film may reveal gas under the diaphragm following gastrointestinal tract injury, or fracture of the lower ribs, raising the possibility of hepatic, splenic or renal injury. Fracture of the transverse processes of lumbar vertebra may give a clue to the presence of retroperitoneal or renal injury, while fracture of the pelvis raises the possibility of bladder or soft tissue injury.

In many patients the history and clinical examination alone indicate that the probability of intra-abdominal bleeding is sufficiently high to merit laparotomy. If the patient is haemodynamically unstable this should be undertaken without delay. If the patient is stable, further investigation may be helpful. Peritoneal lavage involves inserting a catheter through a small subumbilical incision under local anaesthesia so that a litre of warmed sterile saline solution can be run into the peritoneal cavity (Fig. 14.15). The fluid is then allowed to run back out under the influence of gravity. The presence of blood, bile or bowel content indicates the need for laparotomy. Ultrasonography and CT scanning may also prove useful if time permits and can detect free

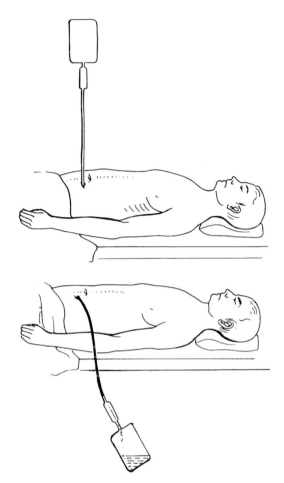

Fig. 14.15 Technique of peritoneal lavage for assessment of the need for laparotomy following abdominal trauma.

fluid, solid organ injury, and damage to the pancreas or retroperitoneal structures.

Principles of operation

Emergency laparotomy for blunt abdominal trauma is performed through a long midline incision. Blood is removed from the peritoneal cavity, and in the absence of contamination it can be autotransfused. In the initial appraisal, bleeding sites are clamped or compressed by packs, and open wounds of the intestine are occluded temporarily with light clamps. A full laparotomy is then performed and injuries are dealt with systematically.

Spleen. The spleen is the organ most often damaged by blunt trauma, particularly when it is already pathologically enlarged (e.g. malaria or infectious mononucleosis). The injury may range

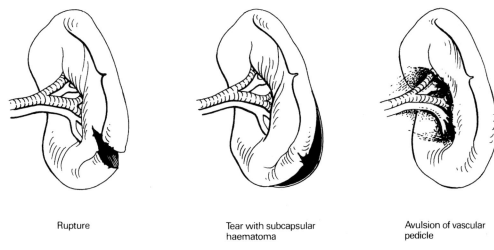

Rupture

Tear with subcapsular
haematoma

Avulsion of vascular
pedicle

Fig. 14.16 Types of splenic injury following blunt abdominal trauma.

from a minor subcapsular tear to complete shattering with avulsion of the spleen from its pedicle (Fig. 14.16). Occasionally, rupture of an expanding subcapsular haematoma can be delayed for weeks or even months after injury. Splenectomy is normally required for splenic injury but in view of the increased risk of bacterial infection (notably pneumococcal infection) after splenectomy, conservation can be attempted by suturing small tears or carrying out partial splenectomy. Alternatively, the damaged spleen can be wrapped in a haemostatic mesh or splenic tissue can be re-implanted elsewhere in the peritoneal cavity. The risk of overwhelming post-splenectomy sepsis is greatest in children and younger adults and prophylactic measures include the use of pneumococcal vaccines and penicillin, coupled with advice to seek treatment promptly for all infections.

Liver.   Blunt liver trauma may lacerate the liver surface, pulp the liver substance, cause intrahepatic haematomas and produce life-threatening bleeding (Fig. 14.17). Many liver injuries have stopped bleeding at the time of laparotomy or can be controlled by packing while other more pressing injuries are dealt with or the patient is transferred to a specialist centre. Suturing of the liver may be needed to achieve haemostasis, while more extensive injury may require lobectomy. In some instances, bleeding can be controlled by angiographic embolization.

Stomach.   The stomach can rupture if it was distended at the time of blunt trauma. Escape of gastric contents causes peritoneal irritation similar to that seen in perforated peptic ulcer. In most cases

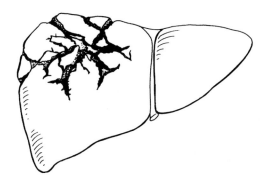

Fig. 14.17 Stellate laceration of the liver following blunt abdominal trauma.

the gastric wound can be excised and then sutured without the need for resection.

Pancreas.   The pancreas is at particular risk of blunt compression injury where it crosses the vertebral column (Fig. 14.18). The injury is often caused by handlebars in road traffic accidents and is particularly liable to occur in children. Associated duodenal injury is common, and as the rupture is retroperitoneal, it can be easily overlooked unless the duodenum is formally mobilized. Duodeno-pancreatic injury is particularly dangerous because of the proximity of large vessels and the dangers posed by leaking pancreatic enzymes. Control of haemorrhage is vital following full mobilization and inspection. Provided that the main pancreatic duct is intact, some injuries can be managed by external drainage alone. If the main duct is transected in the body or tail of the gland, distal pancreatectomy is indicated.

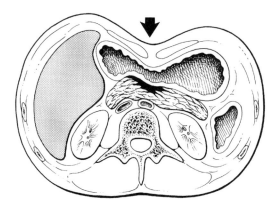

Fig. 14.18 Mechanism of pancreatic injury following blunt abdominal trauma. The pancreas is most liable to damage as it crosses the lumbar spine.

In extreme cases of injury to the duodenum and head of pancreas, pancreatico-duodenectomy (Whipple's operation, see p. 511) may have to be performed.

Penetrating abdominal injury

Patients with stab wounds and no other indications for laparotomy can be dealt with by exploring the wound locally in an operating theatre in the first instance. Laparotomy is only considered if the peritoneal cavity has been breached, and even then, a selective policy of careful observation can often avoid surgery if signs of peritonitis or hypovolaemia do not develop.

Patients with abdominal gunshot wounds must always undergo laparotomy.

URINARY TRACT INJURY

Blunt trauma to the loin, as in sports injuries, may cause contusion, laceration or rupture of the kidney. High-speed road traffic accidents can result in rapid deceleration with tearing or transection of the renal pedicle. Penetrating wounds of the kidney are relatively rare, but damage to the ureters, although extremely rare, is caused almost exclusively by penetrating injury.

The urinary bladder is particularly susceptible to blunt injury when distended, and associated pelvic fracture is common. The bladder may rupture intraperitoneally or extraperitoneally. Extra-peritoneal rupture results in extravasation of urine into the tissue planes with spread to the scrotum and anterior abdominal wall.

Urethral injuries in the male most commonly affect the prostatic and membranous urethra. The anterior urethra is injured less often but can be damaged by direct injury to the penis or perineum, classically as a result of 'straddle' injury. In contrast to bladder injuries, extravasation of urine is not prominent unless the sphincteric mechanism is disrupted.

Blood-stained urine, either voided spontaneously or obtained following urethral or suprapubic catheterization indicates significant urinary tract injury. In stable patients, further investigation is indicated. High-dose intravenous urography (IVU) and/or ultrasonography will assess renal injury and function, cystography can be performed to detect bladder rupture, and a urethrogram can be used to define urethral damage. Haematuria does not occur when the renal vascular pedicle is injured, and angiography is one way of assessing the severity of injury in these patients.

INJURY TO THE EXTREMITIES

The majority of patients with multiple injury also have injury to the extremities. These are rarely an immediate priority unless complicated by major haemorrhage and the trauma team must not be distracted from attention to Airway, Breathing and Circulation.

Penetrating wounds are cleansed, debrided and explored. Meticulous cleansing minimizes the risk of infection, debridement prevents tetanus and gas gangrene, and exploration uncovers unsuspected injury to major vessels, nerves and tendons. The principles of wound management are discussed in Chapter 12.

Splintage of injured limbs can reduce blood loss at fracture sites dramatically. As a rough guide, fracture of the humerus or tibia is associated with blood loss of some 500–1500 ml, a fractured femur leads to loss of 1000–2500 ml, while fracture of the pelvis may be associated with losses of 1000–4000 ml.

Vascular injury

Injury to major limb vessels may threaten life by haemorrhage or threaten limb survival by devascularization. Arterial injury may take the form of contusion, laceration or transection. The distal pulses must be assessed together with skin colour, temperature and capillary refill. A cold, pale, pulseless limb indicates interruption of the arterial supply and should not be misinterpreted as 'vessel spasm'. The peripheral circulation may be impaired progressively in shocked patients and repeated assessment during resuscitation is necessary. Haematomas are common after trauma, but arterial injury should be assumed if they are pulsatile or expanding.

Arterial contusion with occlusion to flow is due to intimal damage. Arterial lacerations usually continue to bleed as the intact portion of the vessel prevents retraction. When an artery is completely transected, the severed ends can retract with arrest of bleeding.

Venous injury may be due to penetrating trauma, and veins can be occluded by adjacent soft tissue damage or arterial injury. Oedema may then obstruct arterial inflow and lead to gangrene. Penetrating wounds can lead to an arteriovenous fistula.

Bleeding from vascular injury is controlled by direct pressure while the patient is resuscitated. The blood supply to the limb in question is then re-evaluated. Any evidence of ischaemia is an indication for urgent angiography unless there are nearby fractures or dislocations that should first be reduced, or any penetrating wounds that should be explored.

Fractures and dislocations

Unless they are complicated by neural or vessel injury, closed fractures and dislocations normally have a relatively low priority in management. Associated blood loss and pain can be minimized greatly by temporary splinting of fractures while more urgent injuries are dealt with.

Compound fractures are those which communicate with a body surface and are thus potentially infected. Fractures caused by bullets are regarded as compound regardless of the size of the entry wound. Compound fractures have a high priority once life-threatening conditions have been attended to as delayed or inadequate treatment predisposes to infection, non-union and osteomyelitis. The degree of soft tissue damage in open fractures is important in determining the outcome for the limb. The wound is managed by extensive debridement and meticulous cleansing. Primary skin closure is preferred unless the wound is grossly contaminated and there is doubt about tissue viability. The fracture is reduced and immobilized using internal or external fixation to achieve rigid stabilization of the fracture and promote wound healing. Antibiotics are always given routinely as is prophylaxis against tetanus. Early definitive management of long-bone fractures is important in reducing the frequency and severity of complications such as adult respiratory distress syndrome (ARDS), fat embolism and sepsis.

The development of the compartment syndrome may complicate limb injury, particularly in patients with long-bone fractures. As the injured limb swells, pressure in the unyielding osteo-fascial compartments may lead to ischaemia of the muscles within these compartments. The patient experiences increasing pain in the affected part (particularly on passive muscle stretching), paraesthesia and sensory deficit. It is vital to appreciate that compartment syndrome can develop in the presence of normal distal pulses, and intra-compartmental pressure can now be monitored to detect this complication. When the syndrome is suspected, all constricting bandages and casts must be removed and in the absence of immediate improvement, the enclosing fascia is incised widely (fasciotomy) to open the closed compartment.

Peripheral nerve injuries

These injuries are often the result of penetrating trauma but can be caused by fractures and dislocations.

Neuropraxia. This is the transient loss of physiological function after slight injury. There is no loss of continuity and no degeneration. The prognosis is excellent and recovery within 6 weeks is usual.

Axonotmesis. This follows compression or traction damage. Continuity of the nerve sheath is maintained but there is Wallerian degeneration of the nerve fibres beyond the point of injury. Recovery depends on axons regenerating and growing down the sheath (at a rate of 3–4 mm a day). Excessive fibrosis hinders growth and the final functional result is less than perfect. Passive exercises and careful splinting prevent contractures, and it is essential to protect the anaesthetic skin while the return of neural function is awaited.

Neurotmesis. This denotes division of a nerve with loss of cutaneous sensation and flaccid paralysis in the area supplied. Ingrowth of fibrous tissue frustrates attempts by the divided axons to grow distally and reinnervation of end-organs in unusual. Operative repair is needed if function is to be restored. Clean lacerations are repaired immediately by end-to-end suture of the sheath. If there is contamination, the nerve ends are marked with non-absorbable sutures and repair is undertaken after healing of the wound, usually within 2–3 weeks. The end-functional result is often disappointing as many axons fail to enter the appropriate neurilemmal sheath.

Limb replantation

It is now possible to replant an entire limb or one of its constituent parts using microsurgical techniques. For example, a digit can be replanted if it is sound while the big toe can be used to replace a severed thumb. The severed part is immersed in iced water, the arteries are perfused with a combination of low molecular weight dextran, heparin and saline, and the part is replanted as soon as is feasible.

Section 4
TRANSPLANTATION SURGERY

15

Organ transplantation

CONTENTS

To be successful, a transplanted organ must be accepted by its new host, and remain capable of normal function or at least enough function to support its new recipient. Since the time that clinical organ transplantation became a reality in the early 1960s, the number of vascularized organs which can be transplanted has progressively increased. Transplantable organs at the present time are kidney, liver, heart, heart/lung together, single lung and double lung. Minor success is being achieved with experimental intestinal transplantation but immunological and infective problems mean that this form of transplant is not yet in routine clinical use. At an intermediate stage between the well established and the not yet established, is pancreatic transplantation. The current position with this organ is that a few centres throughout the world carry out pancreatic transplantation with increasing success.

In this chapter the general principles of organ transplantation, particularly as applied to kidneys, will be discussed and briefer descriptions will be given of the current status of transplantation of liver, pancreas, and the intrathoracic organs. Bone marrow transplantation is now playing an increasing role in the treatment of haematological diseases such as aplastic anaemias, some types of lymphoma, and leukaemia. This is primarily a medical procedure and will be considered only briefly.

RENAL TRANSPLANTATION

Indications

Renal transplantation is the best treatment for chronic renal failure. The success of renal transplantation is due, at least in part, to the existence of ever improving dialysis which allows patients with renal failure to be kept alive and reasonably well until a donor organ becomes available.

Causes of renal failure

- *Congenital causes* include urethral valves and renal agenesis which often present as renal failure in the newborn. Polycystic kidneys may not produce evidence of renal insufficiency until adult life.
- *Trauma*. It is unusual for a patient to have both

kidneys injured at once, but a patient who has only one kidney may lose it through injury. Patients can be precipitated into acute and chronic renal failure from prolonged surgical shock and acute cortical necrosis of the kidneys.

- *Chronic pyelonephritis* is a very common cause of renal failure. It is sometimes associated with bilateral ureteric reflux, which can produce a hugely dilated collecting system, with stagnant infected urine.
- *Chronic glomerulonephritis* is an immunological condition in which a patient's immune system gradually destroys glomerular function of his own kidneys.

Methods of dialysis

Haemodialysis utilizes a dialysis machine. Blood is delivered from the patient to the machine. Dialysis occurs across the semi-permeable membrane within the machine and dialyzed blood is then returned to the patient. In order to maintain an adequate flow of blood of at least 200 ml per minute through the kidney machine, an arteriovenous fistula is created surgically between a peripheral artery and vein to allow the dilated veins to be cannulated twice or thrice weekly for dialysis. It is usual to insert one large needle into a vein to deliver blood to the machine and another to return it from the machine.

Alternatively, dialysis can be achieved by inserting a silastic cannula into the peritoneal cavity and using the peritoneum as the dialysis membrane. Dialysis fluid is introduced through the cannula into the peritoneal cavity, where it is left for 4–5 hours, during which time it extracts metabolic products and water from the circulation. The fluid is then drained from the peritoneal cavity, discarded, and the procedure repeated. This technique is continuous ambulatory peritoneal dialysis (CAPD).

Problems for dialysis patients

Access sites can thrombose or become infected and, for CAPD patients, peritonitis is a recurring problem. Dialysis patients do not enjoy the best of health. They are generally anaemic from loss of natural erythropoetin. They are lethargic and become easily tired. All clinicians treating patients with end-stage renal failure regard successful transplantation as the best management. It allows full restoration of health and relieves the patient of the burdens of dialysis. Transplantation is cheaper and

Table 15.1	Kidney transplants and waiting list	
	Kidney transplants	Waiting list
1983	1182	2693
1984	1552	2780
1985	1428	3443
1986	1586	3468
1987	1558	3564
1988	1612	3684
1989	1837	3705
1990	1870	3854
1991	1765	4113
1992	1717	4464
1993	1687	4564

frees dialysis places for the long-term support of patients who are either unsuitable for transplantation or for whom a donor organ cannot be found.

The need for transplantation

In the United Kingdom alone there are more than 4000 patients on the waiting list for a kidney transplant. Each year between 3000 and 4000 individuals present with end-stage renal failure and, to date, the maximum number of kidney transplants done in 1 year is approximately 1800. The requirement for donor kidneys is, therefore, not being met and the number of patients on the waiting list steadily increases each year (Table 15.1). This imposes a pressing need to establish good donor procurement programmes to allow more transplants to be done and better management protocols for recipients to minimize graft loss and thus reduce the need for retransplantation.

Since 1983 the number of kidney transplants done each year has slowly increased and yet the waiting list has almost doubled.

Renal transplantation
- The waiting list for renal transplantation in the UK has almost doubled in the past decade (to 4500 patients). Demand is outstripping supply in that less than 2000 transplant operations are performed annually.

- The operative mortality of renal transplantation is currently less than 5%.

- Graft survival rates are currently 80–90% at 1 year; the greatest risk to graft and patient is in the first 3 months.

- Renal transplantation greatly improves the *quality* of life, not just the duration of life.

Source of donor kidneys

Live-related donors

Since most people are born with two kidneys and only one is required, it is possible for one individual to gift a kidney to another. This clearly raises some ethical problems and imposes a grave responsibility on those who care for these donors. The best donor is either a parent or an adult sibling. There are occasional circumstances when the use of a more distant relative such as a grandparent, an aunt or an uncle may be justifiable.

Live-unrelated donors

When a spouse is blood-group compatible and wishes to be a donor, then it is ethically justifiable to carry out a physical and psychiatric assessment of overall suitability for donation. Other categories of unrelated live donors which may be considered are adults who were adopted as children and who wish to donate to one of their siblings by adoption. Similarly an individual who has been brought up within a family, as part of that family, may ethically be considered as a donor for a member of that family. In the UK all cases of genetically unrelated organ donation must by law receive the approval of the Unrelated Live Donor Transplant Regulatory Authority (ULTRA).

The greatest difficulties arise with the so-called 'emotionally related' donors because it is through the loophole of such donorship that unethical practices have passed. The use of bribery, coercion, or threat is completely unjustifiable in live donor transplantation and has recently been made illegal in the UK by the Human Organ Transplant Act 1989 (Fig. 15.1). This Act outlaws commerce in transplantation and specifically forbids the purchase of kidneys, either from live donors or from the families of cadaveric donors.

Cadaveric kidney donor

Of all kidneys transplanted in the UK 95% come from cadaveric donors. Currently, just under 2000 of these procedures are carried out annually. Donor suitability is summarized in Table 15.2.

Brainstem death

The traditional diagnosis of death is based on irreversible cessation of respiration and heart beat. It is now possible to maintain ventilation and the circu-

ELIZABETH II   c. 31

Human Organ Transplants Act 1989

1989 CHAPTER 31

An Act to prohibit commercial dealings in human organs intended for transplanting; to restrict the transplanting of such organs between persons who are not genetically related; and for supplementary purposes connected with those matters.

[27th July 1989]

BE IT ENACTED by the Queen's most Excellent Majesty, by and with the advice and consent of the Lords Spiritual and Temporal, and Commons, in this present Parliament assembled, and by the authority of the same, as follows:—

1.—(1) A person is guilty of an offence if in Great Britain he—

  (a) makes or receives any payment for the supply of, or for an offer to supply, an organ which has been or is to be removed from a dead or living person and is intended to be transplanted into another person whether in Great Britain or elsewhere;

  (b) seeks to find a person willing to supply for payment such an organ as is mentioned in paragraph (a) above or offers to supply such an organ for payment;

  (c) initiates or negotiates any arrangement involving the making of any payment for the supply of, or for an offer to supply, such an organ; or

  (d) takes part in the management or control of a body of persons corporate or unincorporate whose activities consist of or include the initiation or negotiation of such arrangements.

(2) Without prejudice to paragraph (b) of subsection (1) above, a person is guilty of an offence if he causes to be published or distributed, or knowingly publishes or distributes, in Great Britain an advertisement—

  (a) inviting persons to supply for payment any such organs as are mentioned in paragraph (a) of that subsection or offering to supply any such organs for payment; or

Prohibition of commercial dealings in human organs

Fig. 15.1 The Human Organ Transplant Act 1989.

Table 15.2 Suitability of kidney donors
Who may be a suitable donor?   • Age, 1 to 70+ years   • Brainstem dead and maintained on a ventilator. Will usually have suffered a severe head injury, an intracranial bleed, or cerebral ischaemia from a treated cardiac arrest.
Absolute contraindications to renal donation: • Major systemic sepsis   • Malignancy, except primary brain tumour   • Positive hepatitis surface antigen tests, or positive HIV antibody test   • Established renal failure in the donor.
Possible contraindications: • Prolonged hypotension in a donor with some evidence of renal insufficiency. In such circumstances the hypotension should be treated and renal function carefully observed to see if it improves. N.B.: if hypotension is corrected and renal output improved, an individual at first apparently unsuitable as a donor may become suitable.   • Some viral infections

Table 15.3   Requirements for diagnosis of brainstem death.

1. That pre-conditions are met, namely that
 • The patient is unresponsive and on a ventilator,
 • The cause of coma has been properly ascertained

2. That certain causes of potentially reversible apnoeic coma have been excluded, namely
 • Drug depression of the CNS
 • Very recent circulatory arrest with persisting shock and hypotension
 • Metabolic or endocrine disturbance
 • Primary hypothermia

3. Irreversibility of the loss of brainstem function is determined by the passage of time and by the failure of attempts to reverse the condition.
 The loss of brainstem function is ascertained by establishing absence of five brainstem reflexes.
 • *No pupillary response to light*
 • *No corneal reflex*
 • *No vestibulo-ocular reflex*
 • *No motor responses within the cranial nerve distribution in response to painful somatic stimulation. No gag reflex in response to tracheal stimulation*
 • The ultimate test is that for apnoea which is carried out according to strictly laid down criteria. After proper pre-oxygenation the patient is disconnected from the ventilator while diffusion oxygenation is maintained by a catheter down the endotracheal tube. The patient is then carefully observed to establish that no respiratory movements occur in response to a CO_2 concentration which should reach 6.65 kPa – a level sufficient to stimulate the respiratory centre if it is alive.

lation artificially. If, however, the brainstem is damaged so severely that it has died, the continued beating of the heart achieves nothing as brainstem death is irreversible. Cardiac arrest, despite mechanical ventilation, is inevitable. Death can be diagnosed by the irreversible cessation of brainstem function, i.e. brainstem death. Brainstem death should be diagnosed by two doctors as recommended by the Conference of Royal Colleges and set out in the current code of practice. Two doctors may carry out the tests together or separately and even if the tests confirm brainstem death, it is recommended that they be repeated. The interval between tests is a medical decision and will obviously vary depending on the primary diagnosis. The time of death is the time at which the tests were carried out for the final time. The requirements for diagnosis of brainstem death are summarized in Table 15.3.

When all the pre-conditions have been fulfilled and no response has been elicited to any of the tests, brainstem death may be diagnosed.

Donor nephrectomy

In the live-related donor this is a standard nephrectomy, usually through a loin incision, after the appropriate kidney has been selected by intravenous urography (IVU) and renal artery angiography.

In the cadaveric donor the procedure is as follows. Once brainstem death has been confirmed and permission for organ donation obtained from the family, cadaveric donor nephrectomy can commence. The donor is transferred to an operating theatre, ventilation is artificially maintained, and the cardiac output supported when necessary. The abdomen is opened through a midline incision and the intestines reflected from the posterior abdominal wall to leave the aorta, vena cava, and kidneys visible. The ureters are dissected leaving an adequate covering of adventitial tissue in which the blood supply runs. The kidneys are freed from their lateral and posterior attachments until they are attached to the donor only by the vessels and the ureter. The ureters are then divided as far distally as possible. Cannulas are inserted into the aorta and into the inferior vena cava, the aorta is clamped above the renal vessels and cold preservation solution instilled through the

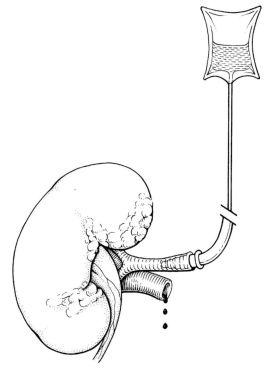

Fig. 15.2   The renal artery is cannulated. The kidney is perfused with cold preservation solution by gravity. External cooling is applied by immersing in ice-cold saline.

Diagnosis of brainstem death

The diagnosis of brainstem death requires that the following conditions are met:

- the patient is unresponsive and on a ventilator, and the cause of coma has been properly ascertained

- cause of potentially reversible apnoeic coma have been excluded (i.e. drug depression, very recent circulatory arrest, metabolic or endocrine disturbance, or primary hypothermia)

- irreversibility of the loss of brainstem function (i.e. no improvement with time or attempts to reverse the condition) as reflected in:
  - no pupillary reflex
  - no corneal reflex
  - no vestibulo-cochlear reflex
  - no motor response to painful stimuli in cranial nerve distribution (e.g. no gag reflex in response to tracheal stimulation)
  - apnoea (i.e. ventilator disconnected, oxygen made available by continued endotracheal insufflation, no respiratory movement despite rise in CO_2 concentration to 6.65 kPa).

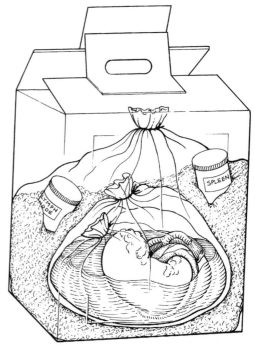

Fig. 15.3   Kidney is double-wrapped in two sterile plastic bags. These are placed in a third plastic bag containing crushed ice.

cannula until the kidneys blanch and become cold. The excess volume in the circulation is vented by the caval cannula. When the kidneys are well washed out, which is usually when between 1 and 2 litres of perfusion fluid have been instilled, they are removed in a single bloc with a segment of aorta and inferior vena cava.

The kidneys are transferred to a bowl of ice cold saline and the dissection and identification of individual vessels is completed. The ideal donor kidney is presented with a cuff of aorta on the renal artery or arteries and a cuff of inferior vena cava on the veins. Each renal artery is then cannulated and the kidney further flushed with proprietary preservation solution (Fig. 15.2). Each kidney is then separately placed in a sterile plastic bag to which has been added about 50 ml of preservation fluid. Each of these bags is re-wrapped in a further sterile bag, sealed, and placed in a large plastic bag containing a mixture of unsterile crushed ice and water. This is placed in a polystyrene container with a sample of spleen and lymph nodes for immunological testing (Fig. 15.3).

Preservation of donor kidneys

Live-donor transplantation

After removal, live-donor kidneys are cooled by flushing cold preservation solution through the renal

artery. The core temperature then falls to around 6°C and the kidney is placed in ice/saline solution where it will remain until the recipient vessels are prepared. Storage time for live-donor kidneys is normally less than 1 hour and immediate function of the kidney is expected when it is transplanted.

Cadaveric kidneys

In the early days of renal transplantation, attempts were made to preserve kidneys by circulating oxygenated perfusion fluid through them. However, expensive and elaborate equipment is not needed for preservation and kidneys are now stored cold in polystyrene boxes. The preservation procedure is initiated by flushing the kidneys out, cooling them, and packing them in cold conditions (0–4°C). In this way, kidneys can be preserved for 24–48 hours and, sometimes, for 72 hours.

Choosing a recipient

Since it is known that kidneys can be preserved safely for 24 hours and adequately for 48 hours, time is available to choose the best recipient and to transport the kidney to that recipient. Most countries having large renal transplant programmes also have organ sharing systems between the transplant centres which take account of tissue matching of the donor and recipient. Sharing systems have evolved because it is known that when donor and recipient match closely at the HLA, A, B, and DR loci, the chances of a successful outcome are better. Since the possible permutations of tissue antigens which an individual can possess are enormous, the chances of good matches are low, but can be improved when there is a large recipient pool to choose from. Thus it is normal for a transplant centre which retrieves two kidneys from a donor, to allow one of them to go to another centre if it has a well-matched recipient. Some of the criteria used to allocate kidneys are as follows:

- A kidney recipient must be blood group ABO-compatible with the donor.
- It is preferable that he should be ABO identical.
- A young and otherwise fit recipient has preference over an older and less fit one.
- Time spent on dialysis is taken into account.
- Clinical urgency: a patient running short of access sites for dialysis would be accorded higher priority.

When recipients have been chosen, they are admitted to the appropriate hospital and the kidneys are transported to that hospital.

Recipient assessment

Each recipient requires a complete clinical assessment plus electrocardiogram (ECG) and, when indicated, chest X-ray, to ensure fitness for major surgery. It is important to check that there is no active focus of infection. A blood count is done to assess the degree of anaemia present and the urea and electrolytes measured to ensure that the patient is adequately dialyzed. Two units of blood are cross-matched and a serum sample from the potential recipient is tested against donor lymphocytes extracted from the lymph node or spleen samples to ensure that the recipient's serum contains no pre-formed antibodies against donor antigens. This cross-match test takes about 4 to 5 hours and only when it is negative may the transplant proceed.

The transplant operation

The kidney is transplanted extra-peritoneally low in the abdomen. It is traditional to put the right kidney into the left side and vice versa but this is not an absolute necessity. The vessels can be made to lie comfortably on either side and the only requirement is to ensure that the ureter is pointing downwards. The renal vein is connected to the external iliac vein end-to-side and the renal artery is connected to the internal iliac artery end-to-end or to the external iliac artery end-to-side (Figs 15.4, 15.5). Great care is required not to tie the knots too tight and so constrict the anastomosis. In child recipients who have small vessels, the common iliac vein and artery are used or even the inferior vena cava and aorta. The clamps are released by removing the venous one first and, if no marked bleeding is noted, the arterial one. The kidney will become pink and often urine can be seen draining from the cut end of the ureter. The ureter is connected to the bladder either by a submucosal pull-through technique or by a direct ureterocystotomy. Some surgeons like to leave a self-retaining stent through the anastomosis. If this is done, it may be removed at cystoscopy 2 to 12 weeks later. The bladder is drained for 5 days by an indwelling urethral catheter or, in small children, by a suprapubic cystotomy.

Ischaemic injury and early renal function

The cadaveric kidney sustains a series of injuries which may inhibit its early function.

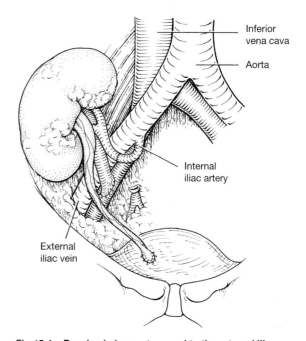

Fig 15.4 Renal vein is anastomosed to the external iliac artery end-to-side. The right internal iliac artery in the recipient has been ligated distally and the proximal end anastomosed end-to-end to the donor's renal artery. The ureter is anastomosed to the bladder by the on-lay technique.

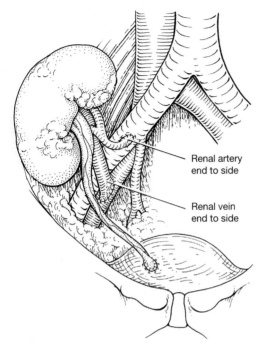

Fig. 15.5   The renal artery is anastomosed end-to-side to the external iliac artery.

Agonal injury

This is injury sustained by the kidney in the time between the donor's fatal event and removal of the kidney; it may be severe, as when a donor is hypotensive and acute tubular necrosis occurs.

First warm ischaemic time

This is the interval between the time at which the circulation is cut off from the kidney and the kidney is cooled. When the donor is a beating heart cadaver, the first warm ischaemic time is zero as the kidney is cooled in situ before its blood supply is interrupted. Where kidneys are removed after cardiac arrest, the first warm ischaemic interval may be up to 1 hour. Most kidneys will recover from a warm ischaemic period of 30 minutes; between 30 and 60 minutes the injury can be sufficiently severe that it prevents the kidney from working; more than 60 minutes is unacceptable for transplantation.

Cold ischaemic time

This is the period when the kidney is packed in ice saline and stored at a temperature of between 0°C and 4°C. If the first warm ischaemic period is negligible this storage time can be up to 48 hours and sometimes up to 72 hours.

Second warm ischaemic time (anastomosis time)

This is the time when the vascular connections are made at operation and circulation is restored to the kidney. Although the kidney may be surrounded by cold swabs during the creation of the anastomoses, it nevertheless does warm up slowly. The second warm ischaemic time is usually less than 30 minutes.

Early function of the kidney is determined by the combination of ischaemic injuries together with early immunological factors when it is exposed to the host's immune system. Approximately two-thirds of all kidneys transplanted work immediately and much research is being directed at securing early function in the remainder. The main direction of this research is to minimize storage injury and to administer calcium channel-blocking agents such as nifedipine to the recipient immediately after transplantation to improve perfusion of the graft.

Immune suppressive treatments

Without immune suppressive treatment, all allografts would be rejected. Drugs, given singly or in combination, are the mainstay of immune suppression.

Cyclosporin A (CyA)

This is the major immune suppressant in current use. It is effective, less toxic, and easier to manage than some of the earlier drugs. Its most important side-effect is that it is nephrotoxic and there were concerns that long-term treatment would produce increasing injury to the transplanted kidney. CyA has now been in use for more than 15 years and these fears appear to be groundless. It has additional troublesome side-effects of causing hirsutism and gingival hypertrophy. Many believe that cyclosporin alone is the best immune suppressive treatment while others believe that it should be combined with oral steroids.

Oral steroids

Steroids have long-term metabolic effects, causing connective tissue defects, a Cushingoid appearance, osteoporosis, and gastrointestinal bleeding. It is now customary to combine oral steroids with H_2-receptor antagonists in order to prevent peptic ulceration.

Azathioprine

Until approximately 10 years ago this was the main immune suppressant drug. It was gradually replaced by cyclosporin but is beginning to make a come-back in combination with cyclosporin and, sometimes, steroids. The rationale behind combination therapy is that it permits a reduced dose of each of the drugs individually and may, therefore, minimize the side-effects of any one drug.

Antibody therapy

Proprietary preparations of polyclonal antibodies such as antithymocyte globulin which destroy all T-cells and monoclonal antibodies which can be targeted against specific T-cells, are extremely potent but difficult to use. They are associated with an increased risk of viral infections in the recipient.

Risks of immune suppression

Infection

Insufficient immune suppression may lead to rejection of the allograft. Over-suppression so damages the immune system that infections supervene. The most dangerous infections are fungal and viral infections such as herpes and cytomegalovirus. Bacterial infections can usually be prevented by prophylactic antibiotic treatment at the time of transplantation.

Neoplasia

Follow-up studies of transplant recipients have shown an increased incidence of neoplasia in long-term recipients. This particularly applies to skin cancers which can usually be treated, and lymphoid tumours which are much more difficult to treat. It seems likely that the incidence of other forms of neoplasm is also increased.

Monitoring the transplant recipient

Blood pressure, central venous pressure (CVP) and pulse rate must be carefully monitored in the early hours after transplantation. A drop in blood pressure may result in under-perfusion of the transplanted organ causing acute tubular necrosis or, in more serious cases, vascular thrombosis and immediate graft loss.

Until satisfactory renal function is established, the patient is still in renal failure and fluid intake and output must be carefully monitored. Urine output is perhaps the single most important observation and it must be remembered that some patients in renal failure pass urine from their own kidneys. A small urine output, therefore, may not necessarily indicate early transplant function. Daily measurement of serum electrolytes and creatinine is required, and particular attention is paid to the serum potassium level which can sometimes rise sharply after transplantation, especially if blood transfusion has been needed, and early postoperative dialysis may be required. A fall in the serum creatinine without dialysis indicates the onset of function in the transplant.

Monitoring a renal transplant recipient is more difficult if renal function has not been established. In this situation the clinician does not have the valuable help of urine output and falling creatinine to assess progress. Causes of primary non-function are graft infarction due to arterial or venous thrombosis, ureteric obstruction, acute tubular necrosis, cyclosporin nephrotoxicity or acute rejection.

Postoperative complications: diagnosis and management

Vascular thrombosis

This may be arterial or venous. It can be suspected if a transplanted kidney suddenly stops functioning. If the vein has thrombosed the graft will become swollen and tender. If the artery has thrombosed these signs are absent. Diagnosis may be confirmed by Doppler ultrasound or isotope scanning of the kidney. Angiography of the kidney can also give the diagnosis, but is rarely required. When the kidney is shown to be infarcted it should be removed at the next available opportunity. All donor tissue should be excised and the iliac vessels repaired.

Ureteric leak

This may occur for technical reasons or more frequently from ischaemic necrosis of the lower ureter. There is usually a drop in urine output associated with severe discomfort in the back or lower abdomen from extravasated urine. It should be noted that if the kidney transplant did not function at once, then sometimes the first evidence of function is the development of pain due to leakage of extravasated urine. When this diagnosis is suspected there is little to be gained from elaborate investigation. The wound should be re-opened and the graft explored. It is usually possible to re-implant the ureter into the bladder, but if a length of the ureter has necrosed it may be necessary to anastomose the patient's own ureter to the renal pelvis of the graft.

Ureteric obstruction

This manifests itself by a drop in urine output and by a swollen and tender kidney. It can be confirmed by ultrasound scan or isotope scan. If the obstruction is incomplete then an expectant policy should be adopted since the cause may be oedema at the ureterocystotomy and this may resolve spontaneously. Severe, early obstructions should be treated by re-operation. Late obstructions can sometimes be treated by percutaneous stenting but further surgery may be needed.

Acute rejection

About two-thirds of all kidney transplant recipients experience at least one episode of acute rejection. This presents with flu-like symptoms, blood pressure may rise, body temperature rises, urine output drops and the graft becomes tender. If the serum creatinine has been falling, it will start to rise. The diagnosis can usually be made clinically and if there is doubt, can be rapidly confirmed by percutaneous needle biopsy of the grafted kidney.

First episodes of acute rejection should be treated by intravenous methyl prednisolone 500 mg/day for 3 days. A second acute rejection requires a further course of methyl prednisolone followed by oral steroids in a dose of 200 mg of prednisolone a day declining to a maintenance dose of 10 mg per day, over approximately 2 weeks. Third acute rejections would be treated by antithymocyte globulin (ATG) or one of the monoclonal antibodies.

Cyclosporin nephrotoxicity

This diagnosis is made when a transplanted kidney's function diminishes and when the other causes of diminished function have been excluded. Elevated cyclosporin blood levels are often noted, but some patients experience cyclosporin nephrotoxicity with blood levels within the normal range. Management consists of reducing the dose of cyclosporin and (occasionally) substituting an alternative immune suppressive drug.

Acute tubular necrosis

This is the commonest cause of primary non-function in a transplant kidney and is due to the injury sustained by the kidney during the death of the donor, the operation of nephrectomy, the storage and the re-implantation. Management of the condition is to suspect its existence on the basis of the history, exclude other causes of primary non-function, and then await spontaneous recovery.

Progress after transplantation

A straightforward transplant recipient would expect to be out of hospital within 10–14 days after grafting. Daily follow-up with measurement of serum creatinine is required for a short period thereafter and then the follow-up interval is gradually increased so that at 2 years, the patient attends at intervals of approximately 3 months.

Success rates of renal transplantation

The operation of renal transplantation does carry a small mortality risk, especially if high-risk patients are accepted as candidates for transplants. However, most good centres have an operative mortality of less than 5%. Graft survival is around 80% at 1 year and in some centres it exceeds 90%. The greatest risk period for graft and patient is during the first 3 months. After that graft loss is sometimes due to chronic vascular rejection and some patients die of cardiovascular causes with a functioning renal transplant.

The greatest measure of the success of renal transplantation is the fact that the recipient is usually able to undertake a very active life, including heavy work and sport. There is also a marked return of fertility, particularly in young women who seldom conceive while on dialysis, but frequently do so after transplantation. Appropriate contraceptive advice should be offered.

LIVER TRANSPLANTATION

Indications

The commonest indications for hepatic transplantation in adults are primary biliary cirrhosis, post-hepatitis cirrhosis, and acute hepatic coma. An increasing number of patients with alcoholic cirrhosis are receiving transplants provided they have stopped drinking and some patients with primary biliary tumours are being grafted. In children the usual causes are biliary atresia and disorders of

Overview of organ transplantation
- The number of transplants performed in the UK in 1993 were as follows:
  - kidney – 1687 (approximately half the perceived need)
  - liver – 545 (programme now probably expanding to cope with need)
  - heart – 401 (less than half of the perceived need).
- Lung transplantation may involve unilateral/bilateral lung transplantation or combined heart lung transplantation. The lung is in direct contact with the external environment, infection and rejection are major problems, and 1 year survival rates are only about 70%.
- Pancreas transplantation is usually restricted at present to severely diabetic patients with end-stage renal failure. Islet transplantation may offer a viable alternative to organ grafting in future.
- Small bowel transplantation is in the early stages of clinical application. The bowel is susceptible to ischaemic injury, is a major source of infection, and contains large amounts of lymphoid tissue (which may trigger the graft versus host reaction).
- Bone marrow transplantation is limited by problems with immunosuppression and graft versus host disease; recurrence of the original disease or fatal complications develop in up to half of the patients treated.

hepatic metabolism. Great judgement is required as to the timing of hepatic transplantation. Many of the conditions progress very slowly and patients can survive well for years with badly damaged livers. It is therefore important not to transplant them too early, but it is also important not to wait until their general health is so poor that they are unfit for this major surgical operation. In acute hepatic failure due to conditions such as fulminant hepatitis and paracetamol overdose, immediate transplantation is necessary if a suitable donor can be found. It should be remembered that in hepatic failure there is no equivalent to the dialysis available for the treatment of renal failure and these patients will die unless transplanted.

The need for liver transplantation

There is only a small waiting list for hepatic transplantation because organ supply comes close to meeting demand and because patients in acute hepatic failure survive only a short time unless they are grafted. In the UK 545 patients received a liver graft in 1993.

Source of donor livers

These livers are almost always retrieved from brain-dead cadaveric donors. Suitability of liver donors is summarized in Table 15.4. A few live-related liver transplants have been performed by resecting a hepatic lobe from a volunteer donor and grafting it into the recipient. This is a high-risk operation for the donor and the ethics of undertaking it are debated.

Donor hepatectomy

The abdomen is opened through a midline incision and if the procedure is combined with donation of thoracic organs, a full-length sternal split is also performed. The liver is dissected free taking particular care to isolate its arterial supply from the coeliac axis. The inferior vena cava above and below the liver is freed and the portal vein dissected. The common bile duct is isolated just above the duodenum. The liver is cooled in situ by infusing cold preservation fluid via the aorta through its arterial circulation and also through the portal circulation by cannulation of the splenic vein. The preservation solution currently used is the University of Wisconsin (UW) solution and 3–4 litres of fluid are flushed through the liver, the excess volume being vented from the lower vena cava. The liver is then removed, placed in ice/saline and further preservation fluid is flushed through the hepatic artery. The liver is packed in ice/saline in sterile bags (as for the kidney), and transported in an insulated box.

The use of UW solution has allowed hepatic preservation times up to 18 hours.

Choosing a recipient

A liver recipient must be blood group ABO compatible. The size of the liver should be appropriate for the size of the recipient, although nowadays it is possible to transplant livers reduced in size by removing the left lobe and indeed it is sometimes possible to implant the left lobe into one recipient and the right lobe into another.

Table 15.4   Suitability of liver donors

Indications of a suitable liver donor
Less than 65 years old with no lower age limit
Brainstem dead and maintained on a ventilator.
Contraindications
As in the cadaveric renal donor except that a patient in renal failure may still be a liver donor.

Tissue matching

Tissue matching is not a requirement of liver transplantation and it is not normal to carry out a preoperative cross-match test.

The liver transplant operation

The liver is usually transplanted orthotopically, that is to say the recipient's own liver is removed and the new liver implanted in its place. The upper abdomen is opened with a large bilateral subcostal incision, to which a vertical extension is frequently added (the Mercedes incision; Fig. 15.6). The recipient hepatectomy may sometimes be difficult because of co-existent portal hypertension and the presence of many dilated veins. Vascular clamps are applied to suprahepatic vena cava, infrahepatic vena cava, the hepatic artery, and the portal vein. The supraduodenal common bile duct is divided, after which the main vessels are divided and the liver is removed (Fig. 15.7). The donor liver is then implanted by carrying out the suprahepatic vena cava anastomosis first, followed by the infrahepatic vena cava, the hepatic artery anastomosis and the portal vein anastomosis, at which point the clamps may be released and the liver re-vascularized. The donor and recipient common bile ducts are anastomosed end to end (Fig. 15.8).

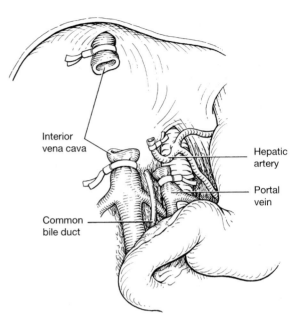

Fig. 15.7 The recipient's liver has been removed. The hepatic artery, portal vein, and the supra- and infrahepatic vena cava are shown clamped and divided. The common bile duct has been divided and the liver has been removed.

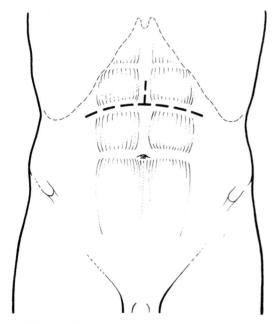

Fig. 15.6 The Mercedes incision.

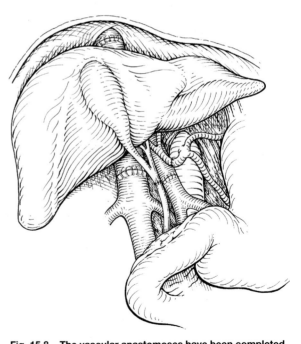

Fig. 15.8 The vascular anastomoses have been completed and the donor and recipient common bile duct anastomosed. This anastomosis is sometimes performed over a T-tube inserted through the recipient's common bile duct.

Immune suppressive treatments

These are very similar to the ones employed in renal transplantation. Acute rejection is less of a problem in liver transplantation than in renal transplantation and will usually respond to intravenous methyl prednisolone.

Postoperative problems

Bleeding

The recipient has had an extensive major surgical procedure with four vascular anastomoses. The hepatectomy may well have been difficult and some blood loss may have occurred, necessitating the transfusion of a large amount of third-party blood and resulting in deficiencies in the clotting mechanisms. These deficiencies are exacerbated if the donor liver functions poorly and does not produce clotting factors.

Vascular thrombosis

The vessel most often affected is the hepatic artery. The diagnosis can be made by Doppler ultrasonography or angiography and hepatic artery thrombosis is an indication for early re-transplantation.

Bile leak

This relatively common complication normally requires re-operation and may require biliary reconstruction with implantation of the donor bile duct into a Roux-en-Y segment of jejunum.

Results

The results of modern liver transplantation are very good. One-year patient survival rates of 70% are commonplace and results better than this can be achieved, particularly in young children with metabolic liver disorders in whom long-term graft survivals in excess of 80% can be expected. When it is remembered that the conditions being treated are uniformly fatal, it can be seen how excellent these results are. A successful liver transplant recipient may expect to return to a completely normal way of life.

CARDIAC TRANSPLANTATION

Transplantation of the heart now has an established place in the treatment of end-stage cardiac failure. Half the recipients have ischaemic heart disease and most of the rest have cardiomyopathy, usually idiopathic but occasionally post-viral. Children can be treated as successfully as adults, and increasing numbers of young patients are being transplanted. The cardiac donor obviously has to have a normal heart with good function at the time it is removed. The coronary arteries are flushed with ice-cold solution to produce rapid cooling for myocardial preservation. The ischaemic time has to be kept as short as possible and certainly less than 6 hours, so that the operation in the recipient is well underway before the donor heart is brought to the operating theatre. Using cardiopulmonary bypass to support the rest of the body, the recipient's heart is removed leaving most of both atria behind, as well as lengths of pulmonary artery and aorta (Fig. 15.9). The atrial remnants are sewn to the corresponding parts of the donor heart and the great vessels anastomosed end-to-end. The four suture lines take only 20–30 minutes to complete.

Postoperative care is the same as for any patient after open-heart surgery with 24–48 hours in the Intensive Care Unit followed by rapid mobilization in the ward. Immune suppression usually consists of a combination of cyclosporin, azathioprine, and prednisolone, although some surgeons discontinue steroids after 3 months. The heart is regularly biopsied using miniature forceps passed into the right ventricle via the internal jugular vein. With this surveillance, rejection can be detected at an early stage and can usually be treated successfully.

Survival rates after cardiac transplantation are very good with about 85% of patients living for at least a year and 75% reaching 5 years. As with other transplanted organs, there is an inexorable loss of grafts with time due to chronic rejection. The continued low-grade immunological attack on the donor heart causes damage to the coronary artery endothelium with subsequent cylindrical narrowing of the vessels. The patient does not experience symptoms of coronary artery disease such as angina because the heart is denervated. However, if severe coronary artery disease is detected at surveillance angiography, re-transplantation may eventually be required.

The patient with a transplanted heart may live a completely normal life, undertaking a full range of activities, including sports. Unfortunately, there is a tremendous shortfall in the number of donor hearts

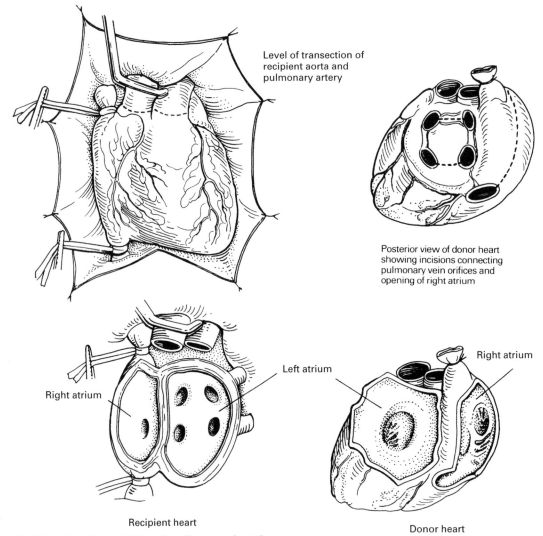

Level of transection of
recipient aorta and
pulmonary artery

Posterior view of donor heart
showing incisions connecting
pulmonary vein orifices and
opening of right atrium

Right atrium

Left atrium

Right atrium

Recipient heart

Donor heart

Fig. 15.9 Technical principles of cardiac transplantation.

available. With current indications, the need is for 20 heart transplants per million of the population, but in the UK only five to seven per million are transplanted and 401 of these transplants were carried out in 1993.

PULMONARY TRANSPLANTATION

Transplantation of the lungs has developed along three different routes over the last 10 years since clinical success was first achieved. The combined heart and lung transplant is required for patients with pulmonary vascular disease and co-existent heart failure. Such patients have very high pulmonary artery pressures which may be the result of primary pulmonary hypertension or secondary to congenital heart disease in the Eisenmenger syndrome. Patients with septic lung disease, predominantly those with cystic fibrosis, require replacement of the two diseased lungs but they are able to retain their own hearts in the bilateral or double lung transplant procedure. Finally, patients with good cardiac function and no infection usually suffer from emphysema or pulmonary fibrosis and a single lung transplant may be used.

The lung is a particularly fragile organ and the

permitted ischaemic time is only about 6 hours. It is very liable to sustain damage in the donor and only about 25% of cardiac donors have transplantable lungs.

The heart/lung transplant requires cardiopulmonary bypass and is performed through a median sternotomy incision. Bilateral and single lung transplants are performed through a lateral thoracotomy and may be done without bypass. The airway anastomosis is particularly fragile and may be wrapped with flaps of pericardium to minimize the risk of anastomotic leaks.

Following transplantation, immunosuppression is achieved with triple therapy using cyclosporin, azathioprine, and steroids. The lung is particularly prone to rejection and transbronchial biopsies performed through the bronchoscope are now used for routine monitoring. Infection is a severe problem. The lung is the only transplanted organ in direct contact with the outside world and many patients, for example those with cystic fibrosis, will have previous infection in their airways. For these reasons the early success rate of lung transplantation is not as good as that achieved with cardiac transplantation and survival rates of 70% at 1 year are achieved. Chronic rejection is a serious problem and causes scarring and narrowing of the small airways. However, if successful, the functional results are excellent and these patients can return to all forms of activity.

PANCREAS TRANSPLANTATION

This transplant procedure still has a high complication and failure rate which means that it is usually offered to severely diabetic patients with end-stage renal failure from diabetic nephropathy. These patients undergo combined renal and pancreatic grafting from the same donor. There is a great need for pancreatic transplantation alone for the thousands of diabetic patients who have not yet developed one of the severe complications of diabetes mellitus.

A few years ago the standard operative procedure consisted of transplanting the tail of the pancreas by anastomosing its blood vessels to the iliac vessels on the opposite side to the kidney implant. Considerable problems were caused by the escape of pancreatic exocrine secretion from the transected pancreatic duct and methods to occlude this duct with resin or anastomose it to various viscera were only partially successful. Nowadays, the usual procedure is to transplant the entire pancreatic gland with a cuff of duodenum containing the orifice of the pancreatic duct. This duodenal cuff is anastomosed to the bladder and the pancreatic fluid escapes with the urine. Results of pancreatic transplantation are improving and experienced centres achieve graft survival rates of around 70% at 1 year. The results, however, are not yet good enough to justify using pancreatic transplantation alone in diabetic patients.

Immune suppression is identical to that used for the renal transplant recipient. Monitoring of the graft can be difficult but some guidance can be obtained from the status of the simultaneously transplanted kidney. However, severe rejection may be present in the pancreas with minimal rejection in the kidney.

In the field of pancreatic transplantation there is great debate whether the ultimate solution for diabetic patients will be solid organ transplantation of the pancreas or whether it will be infusion of isolated islets of Langerhans. These can be isolated, preserved, and even cultured at present. They can be infused into the portal system where they embolise in the liver and can function for a short time. However, the isolated islets are very vulnerable to rejection and long-term survival of functioning islet allografts has not yet been achieved in man.

SMALL BOWEL TRANSPLANTATION

It is over 30 years since Lillehei and his colleagues in Minneapolis demonstrated that transplantation of the gut was technically feasible. However, intestinal transplantation has not advanced much beyond the experimental stage. The small bowel is susceptible to ischaemic injury. The major problems are those of transplanting a highly infected tissue into a patient who needs to be immune suppressed and of transplanting a considerable amount of donor lymphoid tissue in Peyer's patches which can mount an immune reaction against the recipient (i.e., graft-versus-host disease). Improvements in immune suppression and the appearance of the new agents undergoing clinical testing, such as FK506, has meant a resurgence of interest in this form of treatment. Intestinal transplantation would be used in the relatively small number of young patients who have lost their entire small bowel from injury, volvulus, or inflammatory bowel disease. The alternative of a lifetime of total parenteral nutrition is not attractive and provides a great incentive to the development of small bowel transplantation. A small

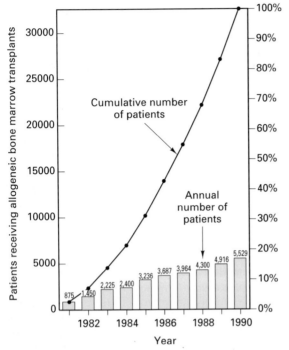

Fig. 15.10   Numbers of bone marrow transplants performed.

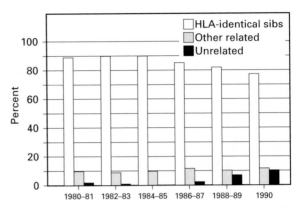

Fig. 15.12   Donors of bone marrow.

number of cases are now recorded in which small bowel transplantation has resulted in grafts surviving for more than 2 years after operation.

ALLOGENEIC MARROW TRANSPLANTATION

Worldwide, allogeneic marrow transplantation has developed extensively for treatment of a number of

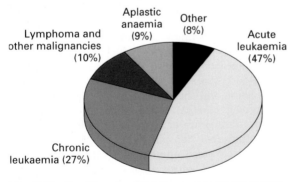

Fig. 15.11   Conditions for which bone marrow transplant is carried out.

haematological problems. Data from the International Bone Marrow Transplant Registry has shown the extent to which this treatment is now used and the range of conditions for which it is indicated (Figs 15.10 and 15.11).

The majority of transplants are from HLA identical matched donors (Fig. 15.12). Success rates vary according to the disease treated and the stage of the disease at which marrow transplantation is performed. The best results are seen in patients under 30 years treated during the first remission of their disease. The problems with immune suppression are even greater than in vascularized solid organ transplantation and are compounded by the ability of the donor bone marrow to mount a severe immunological attack on the recipient (graft-versus-host disease). Allogeneic marrow transplant, even from matched donors, remains a difficult treatment to administer and recurrence of disease or death due to complications still occurs in some 40 to 50% of patients in most treatment groups.

CONCLUSION

Transplantation of solid organs represents one of the greatest medical advances in the last three decades and conditions which only a short time ago had mortality rates of 100% now have survival rates of 80% or better with patients experiencing a quality of life that is very close to normal. An inadequate supply of donor organs prevents many patients from receiving these life-saving treatments.

Section 5
SURGICAL ONCOLOGY

16
Principles of surgical oncology

THE NATURE OF A NEOPLASM

A neoplasm or new growth consists of a mass of cells which proliferate in an atypical and uncontrolled way, and serve no useful function. The mechanism by which this abnormal activity is induced is not known; a prime event is the induction of change in nuclear DNA by a virus, radiation, or chemical carcinogen. Such changes can lead to activation or over-expression of certain genes (oncogenes) which lead to neoplastic transformation and therefore initiate the first step in the formation of a neoplasm. Equally, inactivation of tumour suppressor genes may also lead to the development of neoplasia. Changes within the cellular genome may occur frequently but as a result of endogenous DNA repair mechanisms, normality is restored. Similarly, neoplastic transformation of cells does not necessarily result in a tumour. Transformations occur continuously, but because of immune surveillance or simple wastage, i.e. loss of cells from the surface, mutant cells are destroyed before they proliferate. For persistence of growth these protective mechanisms must break down to allow the neoplastic cells to reproduce within the tissues of their host. It may

also be that for the formation of a tumour the stem cells must be transformed so that they can constantly replicate in mutant form (Fig. 16.1).

The host's internal environmental may also have a role in the 'promotion' of tumour growth. Good examples are the 'hormone-dependent' cancers of the breast, prostate, and endometrium, which require a 'correct' balance of hormonal secretion from the endocrine glands of the host for their continued growth (Fig. 16.2).

Types of neoplasm

Neoplasms may be benign or malignant. The essential difference is the capacity to invade and metastasize. The cells of benign tumours do not invade surrounding tissues but remain as a local conglomerate. Malignant tumours are invasive, and their cells enter blood and lymphatic channels to be deposited in remote sites. These deposits form

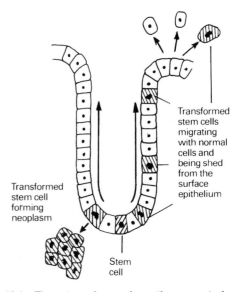

Fig. 16.1   The nature of a neoplasm; the concept of cells transforming and either being released to the surface or forming a tumour.

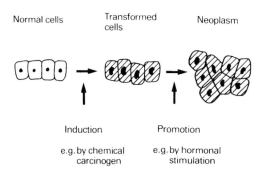

Normal cells   Transformed cells   Neoplasm

Induction   Promotion

e.g. by chemical carcinogen   e.g. by hormonal stimulation

Fig. 16.2 Induction and promotion of tumour growth.

'secondary' or 'metastatic' tumours similar in cell type to the original 'primary' site. Malignant tumours are fatal because of their ability to metastasize. Malignant tumours are sometimes detected in a pre-invasive stage known as carcinoma in situ. Although many of these tumours progress to an invasive phase there is evidence to suggest that this does not always happen.

The distinction between simple and malignant tumours is fundamentally clinical, but must be confirmed by histopathological examination. Tumours can also be classified according to their:

- Tissue of origin, e.g. skin, gastrointestinal tract, breast, or nervous system
- Gross appearance, e.g. ulcerating, proliferating, fungating, cicatrizing
- Microscopic appearance and cellular origin.

Tumours arising from epithelial cells are known as adenomas if benign and as carcinomas if malignant; those from mesenchymal or connective tissues are named after their tissue of origin, e.g. lipoma, fibroma, myoma, angioma if benign, and liposarcoma, fibrosarcoma, myosarcoma, angiosarcoma if malignant.

Tumour progression

It is now evident that many tumours start as benign lesions but as a result of cumulative genetic change (e.g. point mutations or chromosomal loss/translocation) associated with over-expression of certain oncogenes and loss of expression of tumour suppressor genes, may progress to frank malignancy. Furthermore, the aggressiveness of a malignant tumour can also be related to such progressive change. It is important, however, to appreciate that this apparently logical sequence of events may not occur in all cases. The concept of tumour progres-

sion also allows hope that if early benign lesions are removed, this may prevent patients developing invasive disease. Screening for such benign lesions in high-risk groups (e.g. adenomatous polyps in patients with first-degree relatives with a history of colon cancer) is likely to form one of the main platforms for cancer prevention in future. Furthermore, elucidation of the genetic changes associated with development of a more aggressive tumour phenotype may provide new targets for the induction of tumour differentiation and hence tumour control.

Mechanisms of spread

Traditionally, a malignant tumour was believed to spread initially by local permeation, i.e. by direct centrifugal extension along tissue spaces, and then by embolization of lymphatics to the regional lymph nodes. Metastasis to these regional lymph nodes was regarded as the first step in the dissemination of a malignant process which for the moment was contained as a regional disease. The second step, that of dissemination by the bloodstream, was thought to follow after a discrete interval (Fig. 16.3). It was this theory which led to the belief that cancer was 'curable' provided that it had not spread beyond the regional nodes, and to the development of 'curative' radical operations designed to eradicate all malignant cells in the region occupied by the primary tumour and its related lymph nodes.

This theory is no longer tenable. It is now believed that even at the earliest stage, tumour cells can invade both the lymphatics and the blood vessels and so be transported to regional and distant sites to form widespread micrometastases. Regional lymph node involvement is no longer regarded as a *stage* in the progression of the disease but is often simply an *indicator* that widespread dissemination has occurred (Fig. 16.4). It is this realization which has led to a reappraisal of the role of local treatment, and to recognition of the need for systemic treatment for long-term control of the disease. There remains a group of patients, however, who have only local disease with or without regional lymph node metastasis and in whom adequate local treatment can still achieve cure.

The mechanisms which control invasion and metastasis are obscure. Malignant cells secrete a number of factors which may determine their biological behaviour and promote growth at both primary and metastatic sites. Examples are 'angiogenesis factor', which stimulates surrounding capillary

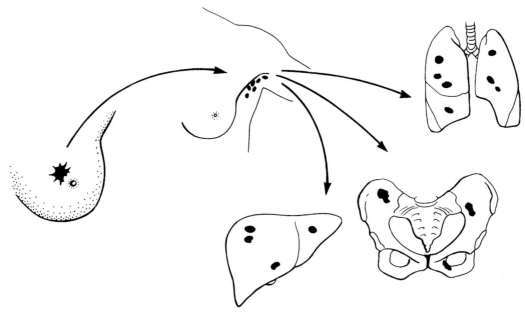

Fig. 16.3 Traditional concept of progressive dissemination of cancer.

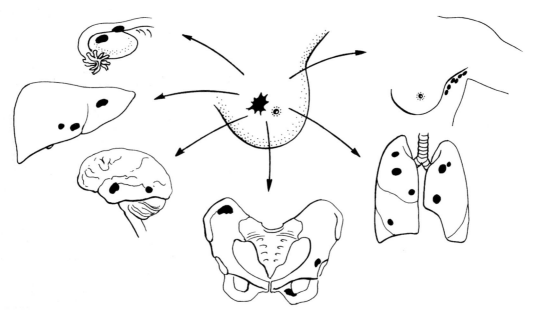

Fig. 16.4 'Explosive' concept of dissemination of cancer.

growth; proteolytic enzymes, which digest surrounding fibrous tissue; and prostaglandins, which induce osteolysis and allow development of skeletal deposits. Tumour cells may also induce host cells to secrete products which may aid invasion and promote metastasis.

The natural history of a tumour is also related to its growth rate which, in turn, is determined by the balance between cell division and cell death. Some tumours are slow-growing and years may pass before deposits reach a size which threatens normal tissue function. Other tumours grow rapidly as a result of a high rate of cell proliferation while some grow rapidly with a relatively normal rate of cell proliferation if cell death is slow to occur. Since the selectivity of conventional cytotoxic chemotherapy frequently depends on a high rate of neoplastic cell proliferation, the latter scenario may explain some of the lack of success of such therapy. The reason for the differences in tumour growth rate is ill-understood but the degree of differentiation of the tumour cells is one factor. Tumours which histologically are composed of primitive 'anaplastic' cells are more aggressive than well-differentiated tumours.

Natural history and estimate of cure

Benign tumours rarely threaten the life of the patient; they are usually self-limiting but may cause functional abnormalities. On the other hand, malignant tumours invade and metastasize and relentlessly replace normal tissues, destroy supporting structures, disturb function, and eventually cause death. Calculations based on an exponential model of growth suggest that three-quarters of the lifespan of a tumour is spent in a 'preclinical' or occult stage (Fig. 16.5) and that the clinical manifestations of the disease are limited to the final quarter. The number of cell divisions (or 'doublings') which can take place is finite. The 'doubling time' determines the total duration of a tumour's lifespan, assuming that this time remains constant. It is estimated that 45 doublings are required for a single cell to produce a tumour of 1 cm in diameter, and that a further 15 doublings will result in a tumour of 1kg (1 billion cells), which is likely to be fatal. The faster the cell cycle, i.e. the shorter the time between each doubling, the more rapid is the course of the disease and the shorter the survival.

These estimates of tumour growth do not take account of the variations which may occur as a result of periods of accelerated or retarded growth. Nor do they take account of the variable longevity of cells. It is now believed that a more appropriate mathematical model for tumour growth is not exponential but 'Gompertzian' (Fig. 16.6).

Definition of cure and survival

For cure every malignant cell must be eradicated. Not only should there be no recurrent tumour during the patient's lifetime, there should also be no evidence of residual tumour at death. This rigid definition of curability can rarely be applied. A normal duration of life without further clinical evidence of disease is generally accepted as evidence of cure even though microscopic deposits of tumour may still be present.

'Cure' rates of individual cancers are assessed by survival rates at various times after treatment. Conventionally, 5- and 10-year intervals are used. Cumulative survival curves (life-tables) can be constructed for individual cancers and compared with those of age-matched healthy subjects of the same population (Fig. 16.7). Divergence of these two curves indicates that patients with cancer are dying faster than their normal counterparts, while parallel curves indicate that patients with the disease are dying at no greater rate than their age-matched controls. The point at which these two curves become parallel is the time at which cure can be assumed.

Cure rates vary according to the aggressiveness of the disease and the success of treatment. In some cancers, e.g. those of the stomach and lung, metas-

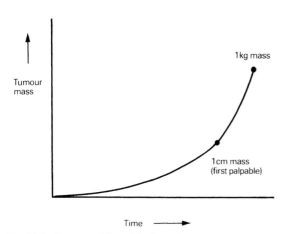

Fig. 16.5 Exponential model of tumour growth.

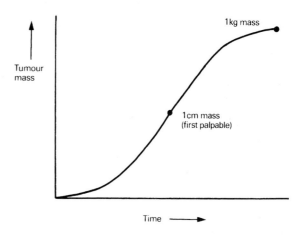

Fig. 16.6 Gompertzian model of tumour growth.

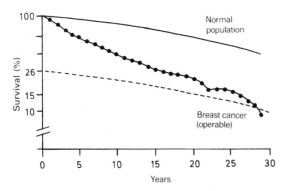

Fig. 16.7 Cumulative survival curve in operable breast cancer (•–•). At 20 years the curve begins to parallel that of the normal population. (From Brinkley & Heybittle 1981, Yorkshire Breast Cancer Group Symposium.)

tases grow rapidly and cause death within a few years of clinical presentation. In others, e.g. cancer of the breast and melanoma, many years may elapse before metastatic spread becomes evident and even when metastases have occurred, life may be long (Fig. 16.8). It is for this reason that five-year survival rates cannot provide a satisfactory estimate of cure for all tumours.

Many regard the treatment of a malignant tumour as a matter of extreme urgency. When one considers the natural duration of a cancer, a week or two spent in careful investigation, counselling and planning of treatment is good practice. However, this period must not be unduly delayed as patients with cancer are naturally worried and wish to have their initial treatment completed within a reasonable time.

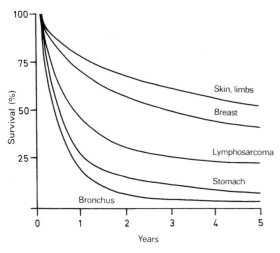

Fig. 16.8 Survival curves for different malignant neoplasms.

THE MANAGEMENT OF CANCER

It is important to appreciate that management of cancer patients is usually conducted on a multidisciplinary team basis (Table 16.1). Good communication with the patient and between team members forms the basis of optimal patient care. There are several steps in the management of the patient with cancer:

- Diagnosis of the disease
- Determination of its extent (staging)
- Planning and administration of treatment
- Provision of prognosis and counselling.

The exact sequence of events may differ from one patient to the next. For example, it may be necessary to remove the tumour to obtain full information on staging and the presence or absence of functional biological markers before an adequate treatment plan can be evolved.

Diagnosis of disease

Benign tumours often remain unrecognized during life or may cause symptoms due to local or general effects. Malignant tumours vary in their clinical effects. Some cause rapidly progressive and debilitating illness; in others local effects predominate; while yet others remain subclinical and are only discovered as an incidental finding.

Local effects

A tumour which lies on the body surface or within a hollow viscus may bleed or discharge mucus or pus. With tumours of the gastrointestinal tract, diarrhoea is often a manifestation.

Table 16.1 Multidisciplinary team involved in cancer care	
Medical staff	Surgeon
	General physician
	Medical oncologist
	Radiotherapist
	Hospice physician
Nursing staff	Ward nurse
	Chemotherapy nurse
	Nurse counsellor
Paramedical staff	Oncology dietician
	Physiotherapist
	Occupational therapist
	Clergy

A hollow viscus or duct may be obstructed. Bronchial obstruction and pulmonary collapse can be caused by a tumour of the lung, intestinal obstruction by a tumour of the bowel, and jaundice by tumour of the bile ducts or pancreas.

A tumour within a closed space may cause pressure symptoms. For example, increased intracranial pressure may complicate intracerebral tumours, and paraplegia may result from a tumour of the spinal cord. Invasion of an organ by tumour may compromise its normal functions and cause organ failure. Invasion of tissues such as the pancreas, bone or nerves can cause severe pain. A cancer can also mimic the pain of benign disease. For example, cancer of the stomach can produce dyspeptic symptoms similar to those of a benign ulcer.

Systemic effects

The majority of cancer patients with progressive disease will eventually lose weight and a proportion become so emaciated that they appear to die of starvation. This syndrome is known as cancer cachexia and is clinically characterized by anorexia, severe weight loss, lethargy, anaemia and oedema. The cause of weight loss in cancer is multifactorial and usually results from a combination of reduced food intake and increased metabolic rate. The mechanisms which underlie the anorexia and hypermetabolism are not clearly understood. Secretion of proteins or peptides (e.g. cytokines) either by the tumour or host cells (e.g. macrophages) may be

significant factors. Sensible dietary advice and elimination of factors likely to contribute to anorexia (e.g. pain, constipation) remain the mainstay of treatment.

The secretory products of some tumours produce characteristic clinical syndromes. These products may be appropriate to the organ of origin (Fig. 16.9). Thus, a tumour of the adrenal cortex may secrete excess corticosteroid and cause Cushing's syndrome; a parathyroid tumour may secrete excess parathormone and cause hypercalcaemia; while an islet cell tumour of the pancreas may secrete excess insulin and cause hypoglycaemia. On the other hand, secretory products may be inappropriate to the site of a tumour (Fig. 16.9). Such 'ectopic' secretion occurs predominantly in tumours of neuroendocrine origin and produces a variety of endocrine syndromes.

Clinical signs

A tumour on the surface of the body is obviously visible; those within a body cavity or hollow viscus may be seen through an endoscope. Tumours of subcutaneous tissues or superficial organs, e.g. the breast, may form a visible swelling but are more likely to be found by palpation.

Many tumours lie deep within the body and do not produce clinical signs. Simple radiology may demonstrate a soft tissue tumour, e.g. of the lung or bone, but for tumours of the stomach or intestine, contrast studies are necessary. For some deep-seated tumours, e.g. of the pancreas or brain, other methods of imaging are needed. These include angiography, radioactive scintiscans, ultrasonography (US), computerized tomography (CT) and magnetic resonance imaging (MRI).

Tumours may also cause functional disturbances which can often be demonstrated by the resultant physical (e.g. electroencephalographic) or biochemical abnormalities. For example, abnormal liver function may indicate invasion of the liver by tumour.

Presymptomatic diagnosis

It is now recognized that by the time a tumour becomes clinically apparent it may already be far advanced. This has led to 'screening' of normal populations, with the result that many tumours are now diagnosed at a presymptomatic stage. For example, contrast studies and endoscopy can be used to detect mucosal cancers of the stomach; mammography can detect impalpable breast cancer; cytological examination of urinary deposits can

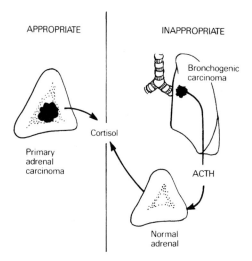

APPROPRIATE   INAPPROPRIATE

Bronchogenic carcinoma

Cortisol

Primary adrenal carcinoma

ACTH

Normal adrenal

Fig. 16.9 Examples of appropriate and inappropriate tumour secretion.

detect cancer of the bladder; and cytological examination of vaginal secretions can detect cancer of the cervix. Screening is expensive and its effectiveness in relation to cost must be critically evaluated before routine use. In the United Kingdom, cervical cytology and mammographic screening are available as a national service.

Confirmation of the diagnosis

Neoplastic disease can be detected cytologically, e.g. by the demonstration of malignant cells in secretions, in washings from hollow viscera or in needle aspirates. However, a definitive histological diagnosis is required in most cases of suspected cancer. No major mutilating procedure for cancer should ever be carried out without cytological or histological proof of malignant disease. The suggestion that a preliminary biopsy can facilitate the spread of cancer is not supported by fact, and punch, needle and drill biopsies are now established techniques (see Ch. 6). Initial cytohistological diagnosis allows further investigation and treatment of the disease to be planned on the basis of a proven diagnosis.

Staging

The aim of 'staging' is to define the extent of the disease and assess its likely prognosis. The International Union against Cancer (UICC) has described a system of staging (TNM) in which three components are assessed. These are the extent of the primary tumour (T), the presence and extent of metastases in regional lymph nodes (N), and the presence of distant metastases (M). The addition of numbers to each component indicates the extent of malignant disease.

In the initial TNM system only clinical, radiological and endoscopic investigations were used (Table 16.2). Such clinical staging is still important in defining the extent of local disease, but its value in detecting the extent of metastatic spread is limited. For example, the palpability of regional lymph nodes is a poor indicator of their involvement by tumour. Impalpable nodes may still contain metastases, while palpable nodes may be the seat of reactive hyperplasia (sinus histiocytosis) rather than tumour. Lymphangiography may aid the detection of metastases in regional nodes in some types of cancer, but, in general, histological assessment is the only certain method. Similarly, small deposits of tumour in viscera and bones cannot be detected by routine radiology. Even the resolution of radioisotope

Table 16.2 TNM pre-treatment classification (post-treatment histopathological classifications have also been defined)		
T — Primary tumour		
Tis	Pre-invasive carcinoma (carcinoma in situ)	
T0	No evidence of primary tumour	
T1, T2, T3, T4	Evidence of increasing degrees of size and/or local extent of primary tumour	
TX	The minimum requirements to assess the primary tumour cannot be met	
N — Regional lymph nodes		
N0	No evidence of regional lymph node involvement	
N1, N2, N3	Evidence of increasing degrees of involvement of regional lymph nodes	
N4	Evidence of involvement of juxtaregional lymph nodes (where applicable)	
NX	The minimum requirements to assess the regional lymph nodes cannot be met	
M — Distant metastases		
M0	No evidence of distant metastases	
M1	Evidence of distant metastases	
	Pulmonary: PUL	Bone Marrow: MAR
	Osseous: OSS	Pleura: PLE
	Hepatic: HEP	Peritoneum: PER
	Brain: BRA	Skin: SKI
	Lymph nodes: LYM	Other: OTH
MX	The minimum requirements to assess the presence of distant metastases cannot be met	

scintiscans, ultrasonograms, CT and MRI scans is insufficient to detect small deposits. Many patients who on clinical and radiological grounds appear to have localized disease (M0; see Table 16.2) have in fact unrecognized widespread microscopic tumour deposits. For this reason the TNM system has now been modified to include not only a pre-treatment clinical classification but also a post-surgical histopathological classification denoted as pTNM. Excision of regional lymph nodes is one way to provide such information. In some melanomas and skin tumours, and in cancer of the bladder and large bowel, histological assessment of the depth of tumour penetration provides important information about the extent and prognosis of the disease.

Biochemical 'markers' which reflect functional abnormalities following invasion of organs or tissues are seldom helpful. Although metastases in the liver may cause elevation of liver enzymes, and metastases in bone an increase in urinary excretion of collagen breakdown products (hydroxyproline), such tests are rarely of value in detecting occult metastatic disease. Of more importance are specific markers of tumour burden (Table 16.3) which can also be used to detect residual tumour after removal of the primary

Table 16.3	Some 'specific' tumour markers
Marker	Likely tissue of origin
Human chorionic gonadotrophin	Chorion Testis
Acid phosphatase	Prostate
Prostate-specific antigen	Prostate
Carcinoembryonic antigen	Colon and rectum Breast Liver Bronchus Pancreas
α Fetoprotein	Liver Testis
CA 125	Ovary

lesion. These are available for prostatic cancer (prostate-specific antigen), chorionic carcinoma (human chorionic gonadotrophin; HCG) and to some extent for cancer of the colon (carcinoembryonic antigen; CEA) and liver cancer (alphafetoprotein; αFP). CEA and αFP are two of the so-called 'oncofetal antigens' secreted by fetal tissues and some tumours. Other markers reflect the turnover of nucleoproteins, e.g. the levels of polyamines and methylated nucleosides in the urine. The main value of biological markers is not in the detection of early disease but in monitoring the progress of recurrent disease.

Prognosis is also affected by the biological characteristics of a tumour. For example, its size, degree of nuclear and cellular anaplasia and the extent of lymphocytic infiltration all influence outcome.

Breast cancers which contain cytoplasmic protein with a high affinity for binding oestrogen (oestrogen receptors) are more likely to respond to hormonal measures and have a better prognosis than those which do not.

Tumours associated with marked reactive changes in regional nodes (sinus histiocytosis) fare better than those associated with inactive lymph nodes. This reactive change may represent a host–tumour response.

Treatment

Benign tumours

Provided sufficient surrounding tissue is excised to ensure its complete removal, a benign tumour is cured by local excision. Some benign tumours, e.g. pleomorphic adenomas of the parotid, extend beyond their apparent macroscopic limits. Removal of the involved segment of the gland or organ is then the only sure way to cure.

Malignant tumours

A radical cancer operation implies complete or nearly complete removal of the organ or tissue bearing the tumour together with the regional lymph nodes and such intervening tissue as is necessary to achieve a monobloc resection. Sometimes it is not possible to remove all the local disease. Moreover, early systemic dissemination may have occurred. Thus for many patients treatment is multimodal and an adjuvant to surgery is needed to provide both local and systemic control. For example, adjuvant chemotherapy may help prevent both local recurrence and distant metastasis. However, surgical excision must be adequate and adjuvant radiotherapy or chemotherapy must not be regarded as a safety net for careless surgical practice.

Local treatment of malignant tumours

Some malignant tumours grow slowly, have little tendency to recur and may be cured by local excision. In many cancers, however, local treatment is used primarily to control local disease and prevent local and regional recurrence. Reduction of tumour burden may also contribute to the success of systemic treatment, which is aimed at controlling the disease as a whole (e.g. ovarian cancer).

The extent of the local treatment required for a malignant tumour depends on its natural history, in particular the likelihood of local recurrence and multifocal deposits. Anatomical considerations are also important, particularly with a view to ease of surgical reconstruction. Achieving a balance between relief of symptoms and the morbidity induced by radical cancer therapy is often difficult, and it is important to remember that the quality of life is as important as the duration of survival.

During any operation for cancer care is taken to try and avoid spillage of malignant cells. In some sites (e.g. testis, large bowel) it is usual to ligate the main vessels draining the area before the tumour is mobilized so that malignant cells are not shed into the circulation. Before handling a tumour of the bowel, a ligature is placed around the bowel proximally and distally to prevent spillage of cells into the lumen which may cause recurrence at the anastomosis. Many surgeons now irrigate the wound or body cavity with dilute cetrimide or betadine to destroy 'free floating' cells and thus reduce the likelihood of local recurrence. However, the evidence that this is of value is limited.

Radiotherapy is sometimes a useful alternative to surgery (Fig. 16.10). The development of high-

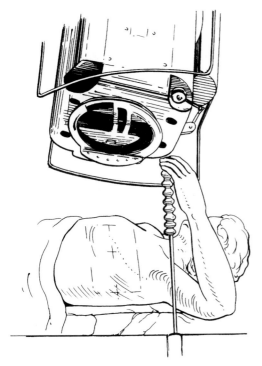

Fig. 16.10 Radiotherapy for cancer of the breast.

energy irradiation with megavoltage X-rays or accelerated electrons permits more effective irradiation of the tumour with less damage to the skin and surrounding tissues. Although techniques to increase tumour sensitivity to X-rays have been studied extensively (including hyperbaric oxygenation and radio-sensitizing drugs) results have not been impressive. Many tumours are relatively resistant to radiation.

As mentioned previously, radiotherapy can also be used to increase the local control achieved by surgery. For example irradiation of the pelvis may be valuable in rectal carcinoma. When tumours are relatively radiosensitive, radiotherapy can reduce the need for radical cancer surgery and a more cosmetically acceptable conservative operation is then possible (e.g. lumpectomy and radiotherapy as opposed to mastectomy in breast cancer).

Treatment of regional lymph nodes

The management of regional lymph nodes depends on the site and type of the tumour. With some tumours, e.g. those of the gastrointestinal tract or breast, regional lymph nodes are routinely resected or irradiated irrespective of their involvement. In others, e.g. malignant melanoma or head and neck cancer, regional lymph nodes are treated only if it is proved that they contain metastatic growth. This difference in treatment has arisen from considerations of technique and morbidity rather than from any logical plan of management. In general, nodes which can readily be removed in continuity with the primary tumour are treated by primary block excision. Removal of uninvolved nodes has no therapeutic advantage. By contrast, removal of involved nodes is a rational way to reduce tumour burden and prevent progression of regional disease. Prior sampling of lymph nodes for histological examination is indicated particularly in sites where node dissection causes severe morbidity, e.g. the neck and groin.

Radiotherapy may also be used to treat regional lymph nodes and so prevent continued growth of lymphatic deposits. This is routinely done in some radiosensitive tumours, e.g. seminoma of testis.

Systemic therapy

'Adjuvant' systemic therapy is now advised for many types of cancer. Its aim is the control of occult metastatic disease but effective agents are still lacking, particularly for solid tumours. Controlled trials to assess the value of chemotherapeutic agents are an essential prerequisite to their routine clinical use. Chemotherapy is toxic; morbidity and quality of life must always be considered before advising this form of treatment.

The recognition that different chemotherapeutic agents act at specific points in the cell cycle has led to the use of combinations of cell cycle-dependent and independent drugs. These compounds, which may be administered for months or even years, have revolutionized the treatment of lymphomas but are as yet of little proven value in solid tumours except those of the testis and ovary and, to a lesser extent, the breast and colon.

Other methods of systemic therapy, e.g. suppression of circulating hormones or stimulation of the immune system, are under study. For example, the anti-oestrogen tamoxifen may be beneficial when used as adjuvant therapy in primary breast cancer.

Follow-up

Most cancer patients attend follow-up clinics in hospital where their clinical condition is kept under review. In general, it is wasteful to use sophisticated investigations to try to detect metastatic disease in asymptomatic patients. In most solid tumours amenable to surgical treatment it is more important to check that there is no local recurrence of disease and that the patient is symptom-free.

Palliation of advanced cancer

The terminal stages of malignancy can be prolonged, and pain and other distressing symptoms are common. Effective palliation is achieved by:

- Local and/or systemic therapy to induce tumour regression
- Non-specific treatment which does not affect tumour growth but relieves symptoms.
- Psychological and social aspects of care both for the patient and family.

Specific therapy

Tumour regression can be induced by local radiotherapy or by systemic hormone therapy or chemotherapy according to tumour type. Surgery has a small but significant role in the palliation of advanced malignant disease. Local excision of an ulcerating or fungating tumour may prove worthwhile, and palliative resection of gastric or rectal tumours often spares considerable discomfort. Surgery may also relieve functional upsets caused by tumours despite the presence of advanced disease. For example, in carcinoma of the oesophagus the distressing symptoms of dysphagia may be overcome by resection, bypass, intubation, or endoscopic laser ablation of tumour. When a palliative operation is performed the patient and his relatives should understand that its object is to prevent additional suffering and not to attempt cure.

Symptomatic care

Pain relief. A wide range of analgesic and narcotic drugs are available to relieve pain. The choice depends on the type of pain, its severity and the stage of the illness. The aim is to achieve complete analgesia without impairing mental clarity or inducing side-effects. It is essential never to let the patient 'wait' for his or her next dose of analgesic. Schedules of administration are planned to prevent rather than treat pain. When pain is severe, narcotic drugs should be used; fear of addiction is irrelevant in this context.

Treatment should start with simple analgesics for mild pain (e.g. paracetamol or coproxamol) and move to more potent agents if the pain is not readily controlled (e.g. dihydrocodeine, mefanamic acid or

buprenorphine). For severe pain, slow release morphine sulphate tablets (MST) are usually administered 12-hourly and can be combined with morphine elixir or dextromoramide for occasional breakthrough pain. For persistent pain, the dose of MST should be increased rapidly. Sometimes patients have difficulty swallowing and morphine elixir is used. However, in this situation, a subcutaneous or intravenous infusion of morphine given via a portable syringe pump is often the best form of therapy. It is important to remember that potent opiate analgesics almost inevitably cause constipation and a laxative (e.g. lactulose) must be given concomitantly. Pain due to intracerebral or nerve root compression can often be helped by dexamethasone (8–16 mg daily in divided doses). Pain may also be reduced by neurosurgical procedures (see Ch. 37).

Pain from bony metastases can be very distressing. If the disease is localized (e.g. to a single vertebra) then a 'single shot' course of radiotherapy can be very effective. For more disseminated bony disease, a trial of chemotherapy or hormone therapy may be appropriate (e.g. in breast cancer). Finally, a non-steroidal anti-inflammatory agent (NSAID) (e.g. ibuprofen) can act synergistically with opiate analgesics so that the dose of the latter may be dramatically reduced.

Supplementation of analgesics with antiemetics (e.g. prochlorperazine and Stemetil 5–10 mg) and tranquillisers (e.g. chlorpromazine and Largactil 25–50 mg) prevents nausea and relaxes the patient. In specific cases use of a transcutaneous nerve stimulator may be useful.

Vomiting may be caused by mechanical obstruction of the stomach or intestine, by drug toxicity, or by anxiety and fear. Reassurance, attention to diet, and prescription of sedatives and/or antiemetics may help. Obstructive vomiting may require surgical relief.

Dyspnoea can be helped by a bronchial dilator, e.g. salbutamol or aminophylline. Diffuse lymphangitic permeation of the lungs can cause severe respiratory distress which may be relieved by prednisone (10–15 mg three times daily). Purulent sputum may indicate the need for antibiotic therapy. Episodic bouts of acute dyspnoea terrify the patient, particularly at night, and adequate sedation is essential. Excessive bronchial secretion can be controlled with atropine.

The majority of patients with terminal cancer develop a monilial infection (thrush). Nystatin suspension usually leads to considerable improvement in appetite and well-being. Sucking a slice of fresh pineapple is a good way to clean the mouth.

The smell of a fungating lesion is distressing, and may be minimized by nursing the patient in a well-ventilated cubicle and using deodorant aerosols or fumigators and frequent applications of chlorhexidine or metronidazole-soaked dressings.

Adequate sleep is essential. Nitrazepam (Mogadon) is best, except for the elderly in whom chlormethiazole (Heminevrin) is preferred.

Prognosis and counselling

Honesty is the basis of the doctor–patient relationship and it is almost always best to tell patients that they have cancer. However, in doing so one should reveal as much of the truth as the patient wishes to have or can withstand. When therapy is undertaken with curative intent it is most important to emphasize that this is the goal in mind. Radical cancer surgery followed by radiotherapy or chemotherapy can be very arduous and maintenance of morale is essential. When palliation is the objective it is important not to remove the patient's hope for 'the end of hope is the beginning of death'. A diagram is often useful in explaining the site of the tumour and the nature of treatment. It is usually best to speak to patients in a quiet, private room with one of the nursing staff present.

Care of the dying

Death from malignant disease is usually a gradual process of withdrawal. A sympathetic doctor can greatly help the patient and his relatives. A dying patient must never feel abandoned in a surgical ward and doctors and nursing staff must be prepared to spend time to help the patient to die with dignity. It is often useful to alert the local hospice early so that if a patient wishes to receive such care then it can be organized. It is not usual to tell a patient that he or she is dying from malignant disease, but relatives must be kept informed. In some cases, a frank but kind discussion with the patient and his relatives can do much to restore confidence and prepare everyone for the inevitable outcome.

The attention of a doctor must not cease after the death of a patient. Words of sympathy from a member of the surgical staff can give great comfort to the bereaved relatives.

Section 6
SYSTEMATIC SURGERY

17

Skin, connective tissues and soft tissues

CONTENTS

and flattened as they migrate to the surface to be shed. The basal layer also contains pigment cells (melanocytes) which synthesize melanin from tyrosine and phenylalanine and pass it to the keratinocytes. The melanin forms a pigment layer which protects the cells of the basal layer from ultraviolet light.

The junction between epidermis and dermis is undulating. Dermal papillae push upwards into the epidermis, and the intervening ridges of epidermis are known as rete pegs.

Three types of epidermal appendage extend into the dermis, and in some sites, into the subcutaneous tissues. The *hair follicles* produce hair, the colour of which is due to pigment produced by melanocytes within each follicle. The *sebaceous glands* secrete sebum into the hair follicles to lubricate the skin and hair. The *sweat glands* are coiled tubular glands lying within the dermis. *Eccrine* sweat glands secrete salt and water on to the entire skin surface, whereas *apocrine* glands secrete a musty-smelling fluid in the axilla, eyelids, ears, nipple and areola, genital areas and the perianal region.

The *nails* are flat horny structures composed of keratin. They arise from a matrix of germinal cells which can be seen as a white crescent (lunula) at the base of the nail. If a nail is avulsed, a new nail grows from this matrix. If the matrix is destroyed and nail regeneration is impossible, the layer of epidermal cells covering the nailbed thickens to form a keratinized protective layer.

Structure of skin

The skin of an adult covers an area of 1.5–1.9 m². It is thinnest on the eyelids and glans penis, and thickest on the palms, soles and back. Skin has two layers (Fig. 17.1). The *dermis* is composed of collagen, elastic fibres and fat and supports blood vessels, lymphatics, nerves and the epidermal appendages. The *epidermis* is a keratinizing stratified squamous epithelium and is avascular. Its basal germinal layer produces keratin-producing cells (keratinocytes) which become increasingly keratinized

Diagnosis of skin swellings

Three questions should be asked when examining a surface swelling.

1. *Is the swelling in the skin or the subcutaneous tissues?* This is determined by 'pinching up' the overlying skin to see whether it can be moved independently.

2. *Is the swelling epidermal or dermal?* An epithelial swelling causes roughening of the skin surface, papiliform growth or ulceration even while still small. The stretched but otherwise normal epidermis over-

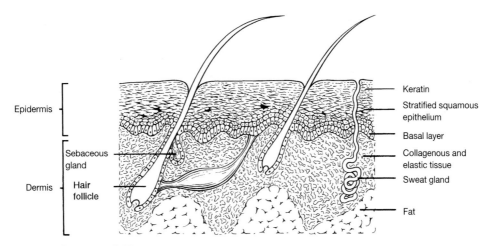

Fig. 17.1 Structure of skin.

lying a dermal swelling can look glossy but remains smooth (although it may ulcerate eventually from pressure necrosis when the swelling becomes large).

3. *Is the swelling pigmented?* Melanin produces black to brown pigmentation and, in general, such pigmentation is characteristic of melanocytic activity (although lesions, such as basal cell carcinoma, can also have melanin within constituent epidermal cells). Warty growths are prone to bleed, and the breakdown of blood to haemosiderin produces reddish brown to yellow pigmentation. Such pigmentation is also a feature of vascular malformations (haemangiomas).

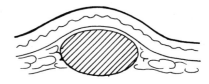

> **Key questions when examining skin swellings**
> - Is the swelling located in the skin or in the subcutaneous tissues, i.e can the overlying skin be pinched up and moved independently of the swelling?
> - Is the swelling epidermal or dermal? Epithelial swellings create irregularity of skin surface when small whereas dermal swellings do not.
> - Is the swelling pigmented? Pigmentation most often (although not always) indicates melanocytic activity.

CYSTS

Sebaceous cysts

Sebaceous (or epidermoid) cysts lie *within* the skin and are dermal swellings covered by epidermis (Fig. 17.2). The cyst has a thin wall of flattened epidermal cells and contains cheesy white epithelial debris and sebum. Sebaceous cysts are common in hair-bearing areas and are thought to arise from blockage of a hair follicle. They form soft smooth hemispherical swellings over which the skin cannot be moved. A small surface punctum is often visible, and marks the site of the involved hair follicle. If infection supervenes, the cyst becomes hot, red and painful.

Uninfected sebaceous cysts are removed under local anaesthesia if they are unsightly and causing problems (e.g. when combing the hair). A small elliptical incision is made in the skin, and the ellipse of attached skin is used as a retractor while the cyst is

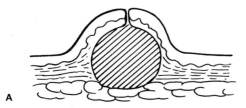

Fig. 17.2 Types of cyst. A Sebaceous (epidermoid) cyst; **B** dermoid cyst

dissected free from the surrounding dermal and subcutaneous structures (Fig. 17.3).

Infected cysts are incised to allow the infected material to escape. Excision is deferred until the inflammation has settled; in some cases the inflammation destroys the cyst lining so that excision is not necessary.

Dermoid cysts

Dermoid cysts (Fig. 17.2) arise from nests of epidermal cells which have been sequestered in the dermis during development or implanted as a result of trauma. *Congenital dermoid cysts* are found at sites of embryonic fusion, notably on the face, base of the nose, forehead, and occiput. External angular dermoid is the commonest congenital dermoid cyst and lies at the junction of the outer and upper margins of the orbit in the line of fusion of the maxilla and frontal bone. *Implantation dermoid cysts* are found at injury sites, notably the plantar surface of the hand and fingers.

These cysts are lined by squamous epithelium and contain sebum, degenerate cells, and in some cases, hair. A soft rubbery swelling forms deep to the skin. The cyst may be fixed deeply, particularly when situated on the face.

Implantation dermoids can be removed under local anaesthesia. Congenital dermoids usually require formal dissection under general anaesthesia as they may extend deeply. For example, external

angular dermoids can extend within the cranium and their excision should be preceded by a skull X-ray and tomography (CT) scan.

TUMOURS OF THE SKIN

Skin tumours may arise from the epidermis or dermis (Table 17.1). Epidermal tumours are common and can arise from basal germinal cells or melanocytes. Dermal tumours arising from connective tissue elements are rare, although a dermatofibroma can occasionally produce a hard collagenous nodule of the lower limb which merits removal. The remainder of this section will be devoted to the commoner epidermal neoplasms.

EPIDERMAL NEOPLASMS ARISING FROM BASAL GERMINAL CELLS

Papillomas

Papillomas (or warts) are common benign skin neoplasms.

Infective warts. These papillomas are common (hence the term verruca vulgaris) and are the result of viral infection. They are found most commonly on the hands and fingers of young children and adults, are spread by direct inoculation, and are often multiple. They form greyish-brown, round

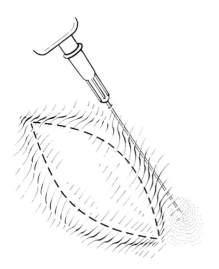

A

Fig. 17.3 Removal of a sebaceous cyst. After infiltration of local anaesthetic **A**, an elliptical incision is made in the skin overlying the cyst **B**, and used as a retractor while the cyst is dissected free.

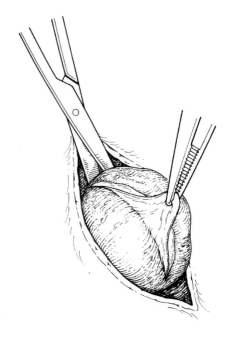

B

Table 17.1 Classification of skin tumours

Cell/tissue of origin	Type of tumour

Epidermal neoplasms (common)
  From basal germinal cells
	Papillomas
	  Infective warts
	  Senile warts
	  Pedunculated papilloma
	Keratoacanthoma
	Premalignant keratoses
	Carcinoma in situ
	Epidermoid cancer
	  Basal cell cancer
	  (rodent ulcer)
	  Squamous cell cancer

From melanocytes	Benign pigmented moles
	  Common mole
	  Giant hairy mole
	  Blue naevus
	  Halo naevus
	Malignant melanoma
	  Melanotic freckle
	  (lentigo maligna)
	  Superficial spreading
	  melanoma
	  Nodular melanoma
	  Other forms of
	  melanoma

Dermal neoplasms (rare)	Fibroma Lipoma Neurofibroma

or oval, elevated lesions with a filiform surface and keratinized projections (Fig. 17.4), and may be studded with spots of blood. These warts often regress spontaneously but can be removed by caustics (acetic acid) or freezing (liquid nitrogen or CO_2 snow).

Plantar warts (verruca plantaris) are particularly troublesome infective warts acquired in swimming pools and showers. They are found under the heel and metatarsal heads, are flush with the surface (Fig. 17.5), and are intensely painful. If persistent, they are treated by curettage or freezing.

Infective warts in the perineum and on the penis may be of venereal origin, and are found in syphilis, human immunodeficiency virus (HIV) infection and lymphogranuloma. Infective warts are also common in immunosuppressed patients.

Senile warts. These basal cell papillomas occur in the elderly. They form a yellowish-brown or black greasy plaque (syn. seborrhoeic keratosis) with a cracked surface which falls off in pieces and has been likened to the end of a dirty paint brush. Senile warts are often multiple, commonly affect the upper back and trunk, and are best treated by curettage.

Pedunculated papilloma. These simple non-infective papillomas form a flesh-coloured spherical warty mass on a stalk of normal epithelium. If small, they can be dealt with by tying a thread around the pedicle (so that it necroses and the papilloma falls off); if large, the papilloma and its pedicle are removed formally with an ellipse of normal skin.

Keratoacanthoma (*molluscum sebaceum*)

This lesion can be confused with squamous cancer as it can develop at an alarming rate; it is in fact a benign self-limiting lesion. It occurs most commonly on the face as a hemispherical nodule with a friable red centre crusted with keratin (Fig. 17.6). The lesion is infective in origin and is found mainly in those over 50 years of age. It heals after shedding its central core but can also be eradicated by curettage.

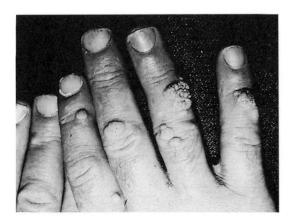

Fig. 17.4 Verruca vulgaris. Infective warts affecting the hands.

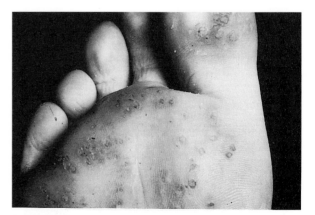

Fig. 17.5 Verruca plantaris (plantar warts) affecting the sole of the foot.

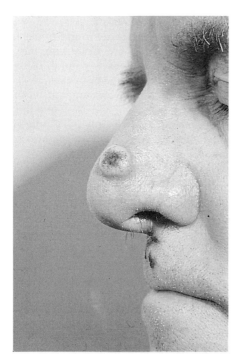

Fig. 17.6 Keratoacanthoma affecting the nose of an elderly man.

Premalignant keratoses

Actinic (solar) keratosis is characterized by small, single or multiple, firm warty spots on the face, back of the neck and hands. Such keratoses are particularly common in older, fair-skinned people who have been exposed excessively to sunlight. The scaly lesions drop off periodically to leave a shallow premalignant ulcer. The keratoses should be biopsied to exclude frank malignancy and then treated by freezing.

Intraepidermal cancer (carcinoma in situ)

This non-invasive form of skin cancer forms a discrete, often solitary, raised brown or red fissured plaque which is keratinized. Histologically there are hyperplastic and atypical epithelial cells but no evidence of invasion. Intraepidermal skin cancer is also known as Bowen's disease and, when it affects the penis or vulva, as erythroplasia of De Queyrat.

Epidermoid cancer

Skin cancer occurs primarily on exposed areas and in those with poor natural protection against sunlight. Albinos and patients with xeroderma pigmentosa (a congenital defect leading to undue sensitivity to sunlight) are at particularly high risk whereas skin cancer is rare in negroes and the yellow-skinned races. Chronic skin irritation by chemicals (e.g. arsenic, tar and soot), chronic ulceration (e.g. old burns or varicose ulcers), and excessive exposure to irradiation are also established causes. Epidermoid cancer is particularly common in men over 50 years of age. There are two distinct pathological forms: basal cell and squamous cell cancer.

Basal cell carcinoma (rodent ulcer)

Rodent ulcers are very slow-growing, only locally malignant and hardly ever metastasize. They almost all arise in the skin of the middle third of the face, typically on the nose, inner canthus of the eye, forehead and eyelids (Fig. 17.7). The earliest lesion is a hard pearly nodule, dimpled in its centre and covered by thin telangiectatic skin. Cystic degeneration may make the lesion raised and translucent. Microscopically, club-shaped projections of basal epidermal cells extend into the dermis and are surrounded by an inflammatory reaction.

Over a period of years the rodent ulcer repeatedly scales over and breaks down. Spread is extremely slow and is often of the 'field fire' variety in which the edges spread while the centre appears to be 'burned out'. Occasionally the tumour is highly invasive and can burrow deeply despite little apparent surface activity.

All suspicious lesions must be biopsied. Surgical excision or radiotherapy can be used for definitive treatment, but the latter is contraindicated if the lesion is close to the eye or overlies cartilage. Complex reconstructive surgery may be needed in patients who present late.

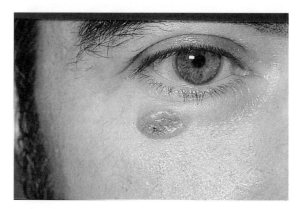

Fig. 17.7 Basal cell carcinoma (rodent ulcer). Note the raised pearly edge.

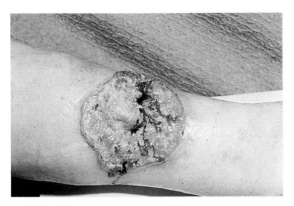

A

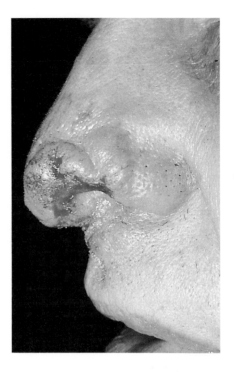

B

Fig. 17.8 A Squamous cell carcinoma at the site of long-standing leg ulceration. **B** Squamous cell carcinoma of the nose.

Squamous cell carcinoma

This tumour may affect any area (Fig. 17.8) but is particularly common on exposed parts such as the ear, cheeks, lower lips and back of the hands. It commonly develops in an area of epithelial hyperplasia or keratosis. In mucosa, such as the lips, the analogous change is leukoplakia. The lesion starts as a hard erythematous nodule which proliferates to form a cauliflower-like excrescence or ulcerates to form a malignant ulcer with a raised fixed hard edge. The cancer grows more quickly than a rodent ulcer but more slowly than a keratoacanthoma. Histologically, it consists of atypical squamous cells which infiltrate the dermis to form concentric 'pearls' or 'nests'. The regional nodes can be involved early and become enlarged, hard and fixed.

The choice of treatment (surgery or radiotherapy) depends on the tumour size, site and aggressiveness. Palpable lymph nodes are best excised by block dissection, unless they are fixed and more suitable for radiotherapy. Bleomycin and other chemotherapeutic agents are of limited value.

EPIDERMAL NEOPLASMS ARISING FROM MELANOCYTES

Benign pigmented moles

The number of melanocytes is relatively fixed (approximately 2000 million) regardless of the colour of the individual, but the amount of pigment produced varies between individuals. As a developmental abnormality, conglomerates of melanocytes may migrate to the dermis or epidermis to form a melanocytic naevus or 'mole' (shapeless mass). The naevus cells can cause a variety of pigmented spots and swellings (naevi) according to their site and activity (Fig. 17.9).

Moles showing melanocyte activity at the junction of epidermis and dermis (junctional change) are common in childhood; all moles on the sole and palm are of this type. Migration of sheets of naevus cells to the dermis produces a dermal naevus; migration to both dermis and epidermis produces a compound naevus.

Common moles. The common mole is a flat or slightly raised brown-black lesion covered by normal epidermis. It has a period of active growth during childhood due to junctional activity, but usually becomes quiescent at puberty and may later atrophy. If naevus cells migrate to the dermis, the lesion becomes firm and raised, and there is often aberrant hair growth. The epidermis remains smooth if it remains uninvolved, but can become soft and roughened in a compound naevus.

As only 1 in 100 000 moles become malignant they need not normally be removed in the absence of cosmetic reasons. Active growth in childhood need not cause concern, but growth after puberty demands removal. Increase in pigmentation, scaliness, itching and bleeding also give rise to anxiety about malignancy and indicate the need for excision. Any mole which develops these characteristics should be removed with at least 3 mm of surround-

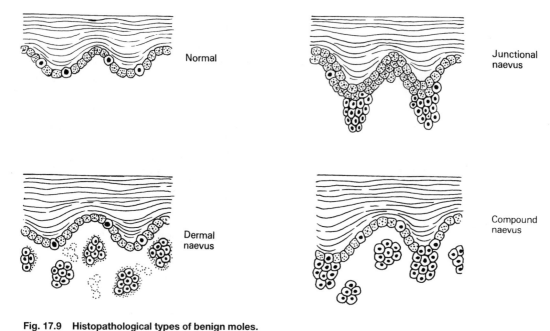

Fig. 17.9   Histopathological types of benign moles.

ing normal skin. Further treatment depends on the histological appearances (see below).

Giant hairy mole.   Unlike the common mole, this lesion is present at birth. It occupies a wide area which may correspond to a dermatome. Typical sites are the bathing trunk area and face. The risk of malignant change is small but such moles should be kept under observation, and in some cases there may be cosmetic indications for excision and skin grafting. Histologically, the lesion is highly cellular,

the cells containing abundant pigment and being confined to the dermis. Neural elements are often present and these moles are often associated with neurofibromas.

Blue naevus.   This deep intradermal naevus can appear blue because the melanin-containing cells are deep in the dermis. It can develop at any time from birth to middle age. Variants include the beauty spot (a blue-black papule on the face and arms), and the Mongolian spot (a brownish transient birthmark in the skin overlying the sacrum of dark-skinned races).

Halo naevus.   This pigmented naevus is surrounded by a white circle of depigmentation associated with lymphocytic infiltration. It is thought to be an immune response.

Malignant melanoma

Malignant melanomas affect predominantly fair-skinned people. They are rare in negroes but can occasionally affect depigmented areas such as the palms, soles and mucosa. Exposure to sunlight is the major precipitating factor. In Scotland the incidence is 8 per 100 000 individuals per year, compared to 40 per 100 000 in Queensland, Australia. The incidence has increased worldwide and in Scotland there has been a 100% increase over the last 10 years. Malignant melanomas are commoner in females due to a higher incidence on the lower leg of women.

Epidermal neoplasms arising from melanocytes

- A mole is due to a conglomeration of melanocytes.

- Melanocyte activity at the junction of epidermis and dermis (i.e. junctional activity) is common in childhood.

- Migration of melanocytes into the dermis produces a dermal naevus while migration to both dermis and epidermis produces a compound naevus.

- Only 1 in 100 000 moles become malignant so that the presence of a mole is not in itself an indication for removal. Active growth in childhood need not cause concern but growth thereafter should.

- Excision is indicated if a mole shows an increase in pigmentation, scaliness, itching or bleeding. A 3-mm excision margin is adequate in the first instance.

About half of all malignant melanomas are thought to arise in pre-existing naevi. The average individual has 14 melanocytic naevi and the risk of any one of them becoming malignant is very small. However, the greater the number of moles, the greater the risk, particularly in those with a family history of malignant melanoma.

The essential feature of malignant melanoma is invasion of the dermis by proliferating melanocytes with large nuclei, prominent nucleoli and frequent mitoses. Three distinct clinico-pathological types of malignant melanoma are common.

Melanotic freckle (lentigo maligna). One in ten malignant melanomas arises in a melanotic or senile freckle. These occur most commonly on the face of elderly women (Fig. 17.10), beginning as a brown-red patch which grows slowly, advancing and receding over the years. The edge of the lesion appears serrated or map-like but its margin with normal skin is abrupt. Kaleidoscopic pigmentation of the surface is typical. This premalignant phase may last for 10–15 years, during which conglomerates of large round melanocytes extend laterally in the basal epidermis. The first sign of malignancy is a brownish-red papule which develops eccentrically within the freckle and which indicates vertical extension of melanocytes into the dermis.

Superficial spreading melanoma. This is the commonest type of malignant melanoma (Fig. 17.11). It occurs on the trunk and exposed parts, and is most common in middle age. During a pre-invasive phase which lasts for at most 1 or 2 years, malignant cells spread outwards in the epidermis in all directions. In contrast to the malignant freckle, the surface is slightly raised and the outline indistinct. Pigment-

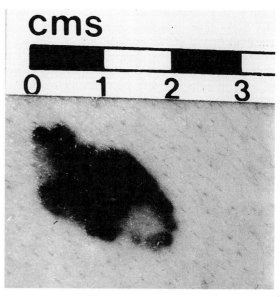

Fig. 17.11 Superficial spreading melanoma.

ation is patchy and there may be a wide range of colours. Vertical invasion of the dermis occurs while the lesion is still relatively small and produces an indurated nodule which soon ulcerates or bleeds. A few long white hairs often appear at the site of dermal invasion.

Nodular melanoma. These elevated deeply pigmented melanomas can occur at any site and at any age, but are particularly common in females on the lower leg (Fig. 17.12). They may occur at the site of a pre-existing benign naevus. Nodular melanomas are vertically invasive from the start, and there is no initial intraepidermal spread and therefore no surrounding pigmented macule. The total

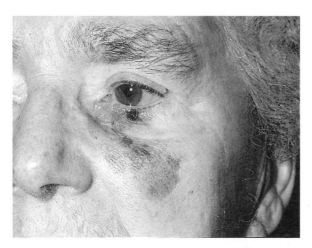

Fig. 17.10 Melanotic freckle on the face of an elderly female.

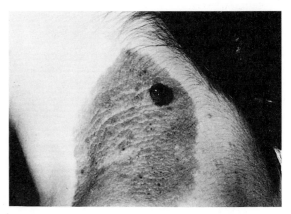

Fig. 17.12 Nodular melanoma arising in a pigmented naevus.

width of the lesion rarely exceeds that of two or three rete pegs. The nodule enlarges steadily, both centrifugally and on the surface. Surface spread is detected by destruction of normal skin lines. The lesion darkens progressively, and the surface over the area of active growth becomes jet black and glossy. Bleeding may follow trivial injury, and is noted as spots of blood on clothes. Crusting, scab formation, itching, irritation and ulceration are typical, and satellite nodules may form around neglected lesions.

Other types of malignant melanoma. Not all melanomas are deeply pigmented. *Amelanotic melanomas* are rare, pale pink lesions which can grow rapidly.

Acral lentiginous melanoma is uncommon in Caucasians but is seen on the soles and palms in darker-skinned races (Fig. 17.13). It resembles superficial spreading melanoma in its behaviour, although the thick skin of the affected regions may mask some of the features and cause late presentation with nodularity and ulceration.

Subungual melanomas affect the thumb or great toe of the middle-aged and elderly, causing chronic inflammation beneath the nail ('melanotic whitlow'). Pigmentation is not usually visible in the early stages

and the lesion is often misdiagnosed as a paronychia or ingrowing toenail.

Spread of malignant melanoma

Malignant melanomas (particularly nodular melanomas) spread readily by the lymphatics and bloodstream. 'In transit' metastases may develop in the subcutaneous or intracutaneous lymphatics and form painless discoloured nodules in the line of the lymphatics between the primary lesion and the regional nodes. Lymph node metastases often present as firm enlargement of a node which remains untethered and mobile. The disease then spreads to adjacent regional and central nodes. Blood-borne metastases can occur at any site but are common in the brain, liver, lungs, skin and subcutaneous tissues. Extensive metastatic growth may be associated with excretion of melanin or its precursor (5-S-cystine L-dopa) in the urine. In about 5% of cases, metastases are present in the absence of a recognizable primary site.

Clinical and pathological staging

Three clinical stages are recognized and staging has major prognostic implications (Table 17.2). For lesions in clinical stage I, the most reliable prognostic indicator is the depth of the lesion (Fig. 17.14); the more superficial the lesion, the better the prognosis (Table 17.2). Depth can be measured by reference to the normal layers of skin (Clark) or by a micrometer gauge (Breslow). As the skin layers may be distorted by the tumour, the Breslow system is usually preferred. Mitotic activity also influences prognosis, and tumours can be graded according to the number of mitotic figures in each field.

Melanotic freckles and superficial spreading melanomas tend to remain superficial and so have a better prognosis than nodular melanomas.

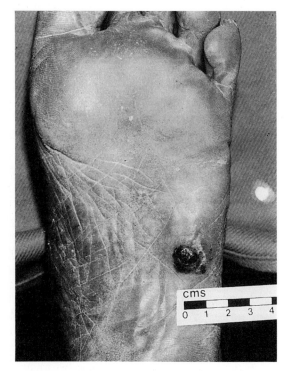

Fig. 17.13 Acral lentiginous melanoma arising on the sole of the foot.

Table 17.2 Prognosis in relation to the stage and depth of malignant melanoma	
Clinical stage	5-year survival rate (%)
I Primary lesion only	70
Breslow depth (mm)	
<1.5	93
1.5–3.5	60
>3.5	48
II Primary lesion + regional lymph node or satellite deposit	30
III Metastatic disease	0

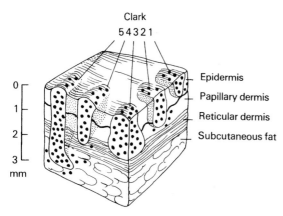

Fig. 17.14   Methods of grading malignant melanoma according to depth of invasion.

Treatment of malignant melanoma

A *biopsy* is essential to confirm the diagnosis. Thereafter, the depth and stage of the disease are assessed to define the most appropriate form of treatment. Small pigmented lesions are excised with a margin of 3 mm of normal skin, usually under local anaesthesia. Larger lesions can be sampled by incision biopsy without detriment.

Surgical excision is used to treat stage I lesions. Wide excision with a margin of normal skin of at least 5 cm was once routine, but has been shown to be unnecessary, particularly for the more superficial melanomas. Breslow depth is now used as the determinant of clearance margin, using a formula of 1 cm of clearance for every millimetre of depth. A smaller margin may be acceptable to avoid mutilation, for example on the face.

The tumour and surrounding skin is excised down to the deep fascia so that the entire depth of subcutaneous fat can be removed. Smaller defects can usually be closed primarily after undermining the wound edges. Large defects have to be covered with a split skin graft or flap (Fig. 17.15).

A block dissection of regional lymph nodes carries significant morbidity and is no longer carried out routinely. However, if the nodes are involved (clinical stage II) or the primary tumour is close, block dissection is performed.

There has been recent interest in perfusion of involved limbs with cytotoxic agents, but this is usually reserved for patients with advanced or recurrent local disease.

Treatment of metastatic disease

The treatment of metastatic melanoma remains unsatisfactory. Occasional short-lived remission has been achieved with chemotherapy (using agents such as nitroso-ureas and dacarbazine). Immune stimulation (with bacille Calmette-Guérin (BCG), C. parvum or vaccinia virus) or injection of irradiated melanoma cells offered promise but is without proven benefit. Newer approaches include the use of high-dose interleukin-2, given alone or in conjunction with activated immune cells or other lymphokines. Although this approach can reduce the

---

Malignant melanoma
- Malignant melanomas are predominantly but not exclusively a disease of fair skinned individuals.
- Exposure to sunlight is the key aetiological factor.
- The lesion is commoner in females, reflecting the higher incidence of malignant melanomas of the lower leg.
- 50% of all malignant melanomas arise in a pre-existing naevus.
- The essential feature of malignancy is invasion of the dermis by proliferating melanocytes (which show large nuclei, prominent nucleoli and frequent mitoses).
- Malignant melanoma spreads rapidly by the lymphatic system and the bloodstream. 'In transit' metastases may develop in the lymphatics of the skin and subcutaneous tissues.

Management of malignant melanoma
- The depth of the lesion is a key prognostic factor and can be assessed by micrometer (Breslow) or by reference to normal layers of the skin (Clark). Superficial spreading melanomas and melanotic freckles have a better prognosis than nodular melanomas.
- A biopsy is essential to confirm malignancy, assess depth and stage, and define the optimal method of treatment.
- Once malignancy is confirmed, an excision margin of 1 cm for every 1 mm of Breslow depth is advised. The lesion is excised down to the deep fascia to remove all subcutaneous fat. Skin grafting may be required to close the defect.
- Lymph node or satellite deposits reduce 5-year survival rates from 70% to 30%, while patients with distant metastases are not expected to survive for 5 years.
- Block dissection of regional lymph nodes is no longer practised routinely but may be indicated if the nodes are obviously involved or located close to the primary lesion.

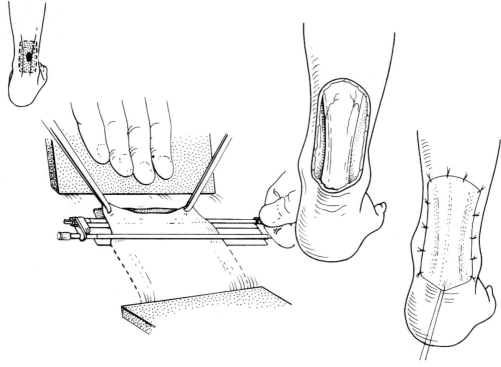

Fig. 17.15   Excision of nodular melanoma with split-skin grafting.

size of metastatic deposits, its role in management remains uncertain.

VASCULAR NEOPLASMS (HAEMANGIOMAS)

The histological classification of haemangiomas is complex and they are best differentiated by their clinical behaviour (i.e. whether they regress or persist).

Involuting haemangiomas

These true neoplasms arise from endothelial cells. They appear at or within weeks of birth, and affect predominantly the head and neck. Superficial involuting haemangiomas form a bright red raised mass with an irregular bosselated surface (strawberry naevus); deeper lesions form a soft, blue-black tumour covered by normal skin.

Active growth continues for about 6 months. The tumour then remains static until the child is 2 or 3 years of age, when it shrinks and loses its colour. The lesion usually disappears before the child is 7 years of age and should be left alone.

Non-involuting haemangiomas

These hamartomas are due to abnormal formation of blood vessels and are of two main types.

Port wine stain

This bright red patchy lesion often overlies the area of distribution of a peripheral nerve. Microscopically there are enlarged capillaries in the dermis. The lesion neither grows nor involutes and good cosmetic results can be achieved by laser therapy.

Cavernous haemangioma

This bluish-purple elevated mass appears in early childhood. It empties on pressure and then refills, and histologically consists of mature vein-like structures. It is treated by excision. *Cirsoid aneurysm* is a variant in which the mass of vein-like structures is fed directly by arterial blood and becomes tortuous, dilated and pulsating. The scalp is a common site and the mass may erode the skull. Penetrating channels may connect the scalp lesion with a similar malformation in the extradural space. Angiography is essential to show the extent of the lesion and outline its arterial supply. Angiographic emboliza-tion may be useful prior to ligation of the feeding vessels and excision of the lesion.

TUMOURS OF NERVES

Neurilemmoma

This is an encapsulated solitary benign tumour which originates from the Schwann cells of a nerve sheath and forms a subcutaneous swelling in the course of the nerve. It is laterally mobile but fixed in the direction of the nerve (Fig. 17.16). It may cause radiating pain in the distribution of the involved nerve. Most neurilemmomas occur superficially in the neck or limbs. They grow slowly, have no malig-nant potential, and are readily treated by excision.

Neurofibroma

This is regarded as a hamartoma of nerve tissue. Such lesions may be solitary but more commonly they are multiple in von Recklinghausen's disease (neurofibromatosis). This autosomal disorder is present at birth or becomes apparent in early child-hood. Multiple dermal and subcutaneous nodules arise from peripheral nerves in association with patches of dermal pigmentation ('café-au-lait' spots). The tumours cause bony deformities particu-larly of the spine. The tumours are potentially malig-nant. Increase in size of existing swellings or appearance of new swellings suggests malignant change.

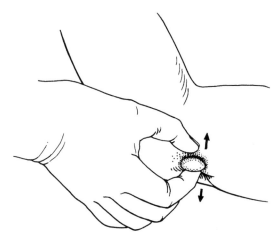

Fig. 17.16 Neurilemmoma showing characteristic lateral mobility.

TUMOURS OF MUSCLE AND CONNECTIVE TISSUES

Lipoma

A lipoma is a slow-growing benign tumour of fatty tissue which forms a lobulated soft mass enclosed by a thin fibrous capsule. Large lipomas rarely undergo sarcomatous change.

Although lipomas can occur in the dermis, most arise from the fatty tissue between the skin and deep fascia. Typical features are their soft fluctuant feel, their lobulation and the free mobility of overlying skin.

Lipomas may also arise from fat in the intermus-cular septa, where they form a diffuse firm swelling under the deep fascia which is more prominent when the related muscle is contracted. They may cause discomfort.

As lipomas are radiolucent, soft tissue X-rays can be diagnostic, but are only indicated when the diagnosis is in doubt and removal may pose problems. Unless small and symptomless, a lipoma should be removed.

Liposarcoma

Liposarcoma is the commonest sarcoma of middle age. It may occur in any fatty tissue but is most common in the retroperitoneum and legs. Wide surgical excision is recommended but can be difficult for retroperitoneal tumours, and postopera-tive radiotherapy and chemotherapy are advised but of doubtful worth. Most liposarcomas grow slowly, and recurrence may take a long time to develop.

Fibrosarcoma

This tumour arises from fibrous tissue at any site but is most common in the lower limbs or buttocks. It forms a large deep firm mass. Wide excision is the initial treatment of choice; radiation therapy may be indicated in the palliation of recurrence.

Rhabdomyosarcoma

This greyish-pink soft fleshy lobulated or well-circumscribed tumour arises from striated muscle. The tumour is more common in children, is highly malignant, and requires treatment by radical excision and/or radiotherapy. Amputation of a limb may be unavoidable.

MISCELLANEOUS CONDITIONS

DISORDERS OF SWEAT GLANDS

Hidradenitis suppurativa

This is a chronic infection of apocrine glands in the axilla, perineum or groin. It is precipitated by shaving, poor hygiene and the use of chemical deodorants. Multiple intradermal abscesses lead to sinus formation, fibrosis and a painful diffuse chronic infection of the skin.

As the apocrine glands discharge into the hair follicles, the condition is resistant to local antiseptics. Long-term tetracycline therapy may be successful. If not, excision of the axillary skin with skin grafting is required.

Hyperhidrosis

This disorder of the eccrine sweat glands most commonly affects the axillae of young women. Initial treatment consists of the application of a solution of aluminium chloride. In severe cases the eccrine glands can be scraped away from the undersurface of the skin by inserting a sharp curette through a small incision.

If excessive sweating of the hands or feet causes serious problems, sympathectomy may be indicated.

GANGLION

This common cystic swelling arises from the fibrous capsule of a joint or a fibrous tendon sheath. It contains mucoid material within a fibrous capsule and was once considered to be due to herniation of synovial membrane. It is now thought to result from degeneration of collagen.

A ganglion most commonly appears as a smooth tense hemispherical subcutaneous swelling on the dorsum of the wrist or foot (Fig. 17.17). Other sites include the palm of the hand, the palmar surface of a finger over the distal interphalangeal joint, and the lateral side of the knee over the superior tibiofibular joint. Those on the dorsum of the foot are often bluish in colour due to the thin overlying skin. So-called 'mucous cysts' arising from the small joints of the hands in older people are believed to be of similar origin. A ganglion should be differentiated from a bursa, which is a fluid-filled fibrous swelling overlying a bony exostosis.

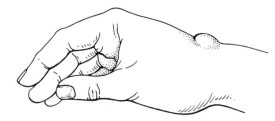

Fig. 17.17   Ganglion in a typical site.

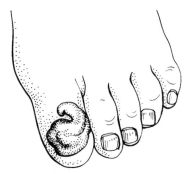

Fig. 17.18   Onychogryphosis.

Excision under general or regional anaesthesia is preferred. A tourniquet is applied to provide a bloodless operating field for careful and complete removal of the ganglion.

DISORDERS OF THE NAILS

Onychogryphosis (hooked nail)

This overgrowth of nail resembles an ox or goat horn. The big toenail is most commonly affected (Fig. 17.18). Simple avulsion of the nail does not

---

Ganglion
- A ganglion usually takes the form of a smooth tense hemispherical swelling, most commonly on the dorsum of the wrist.

- It arises from the fibrous capsule of a joint or tendon sheath.

- The ganglion itself has a fibrous capsule and contains mucoid material which may result from degeneration of collagen.

- Ganglions causing symptoms or cosmetic problems are best excised under general or regional anaesthesia so that a tourniquet can be applied to create a bloodless field.

prevent recurrence and excision of the nailbed is required. A flap of skin is reflected from the base of the nail and the germinal layer removed. Care must be taken to excise the edges of this layer completely or troublesome spikes of nail continue to grow. An alternative to excision of the nailbed is to cauterize it with phenol.

Ingrowing toenail

This is due to the sharp edges of the nail impinging on the surrounding skin folds (Fig. 17.19). The skin is split and infection follows. The condition is painful and made worse by misguided attempts to cut the nail back at the corners.

The patient usually comes for help once infection has occurred. An attempt is made to 'lift out' the ingrowing portion of the nail with a pledget of gauze soaked in antiseptic. The patient is then instructed to cut the nail square, or shorter in the centre than at the edges, and to avoid wearing narrow shoes.

Once infection has spread under the nail, or the nail has become deeply embedded, it is best to avulse it under general anaesthesia. Antiseptic footbaths then allow the infection to resolve rapidly. The patient is instructed on the correct way to cut the new nail.

If the condition recurs, the nailbed must be ablated surgically or with phenol (Fig. 17.20). Wedge excision of the lateral portion of the nail and underlying nailbed is no longer advised.

Nailfold infections (paronychia)

Pain, redness and swelling at the side and base of a nail are the first signs. This may extend around the nail to produce a horseshoe swelling of the nailfold. Extension under the nail and into the underlying pulp space may occur (Fig. 17.21).

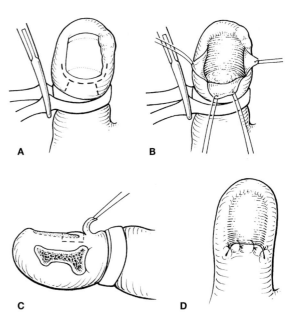

Fig. 17.20   Operation for ablation of the nailbed. A skin incision; **B** nail avulsed and skin flaps raised; **C** excision of nailbed; **D** skin flaps sutured.

A minor paronychia will usually resolve spontaneously, but if the infection is spreading, an antibiotic (penicillin) should be given. The development of a tense shiny swelling indicates suppuration and the need for surgical drainage. A single unilateral incision may suffice, but if the infection extends under the nail, a flap of skin should be reflected from the nailbase, which is then excised to allow free drainage (Fig. 17.22). A simple vaseline gauze dressing is applied.

Failure of an acute paronychia to resolve leads to chronic thickening of the nailfold. Fungal infection is a common cause of chronic paronychia and nail scrapings are essential for diagnosis. The possibility

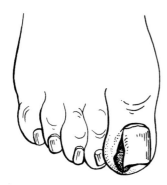

Fig. 17.19   Ingrowing toenail.

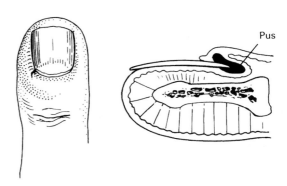

Fig. 17.21   Paronychia. The longitudinal section shows relation of pus to the nailbed.

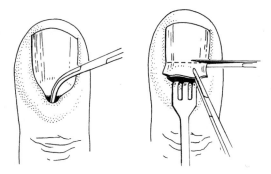

Fig. 17.22   Surgical treatment of paronychia.

of a subungual melanoma must always be kept in mind.

FIBROSING AND CONSTRICTING CONDITIONS OF THE HAND

Contraction of fibrous tissue occurs in many parts of the body. In the hand, this may restrict free movement.

Dupuytren's contracture

The palmar aponeurosis is a triangular fibrous structure which covers the tendons in the palm of the hand and prevents their forward dislocation (Fig. 17.23). It originates from the tendon of palmaris longus and/or flexor retinaculum and is inserted into the proximal and middle phalanges of the fingers. Thickening and contracture of this aponeurosis is called Dupuytren's contracture. A similar condition can affect the plantar fascia of the sole of the foot but, because of constant stretching of the plantar fascia by weightbearing, this often goes unnoticed.

The aetiology of Dupuytren's contracture is obscure. Some cases are familial, while others are associated with alcoholism, chronic ill health, and epilepsy (accounted for by the use of phenytoin).

The first sign is usually a small fibrous nodule or cord just distal to the distal palmar crease in the line of the fourth finger. The medial half of the palmar fascia gradually contracts so that the ring and little fingers become drawn towards the palm of the hand (Fig. 17.24). This causes a hook-like deformity so that an object once grasped cannot be released. Other fingers progressively become involved. The skin of the palm may fuse with the underlying fascia and become raised and rock hard, or it may become puckered and indrawn. Vessels, nerves and tendons remain free from the fibrotic process.

If the patient is seen at an early stage, he is advised to keep stretching the aponeurosis by passively extending his fingers, e.g. by sitting on the backs of his hands. Once the disease has given rise to contracture this is no longer helpful. If the contracture is

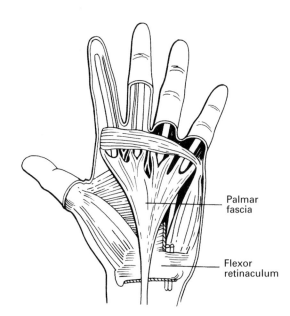

Fig. 17.23   Flexor retinaculum and palmar fascia.

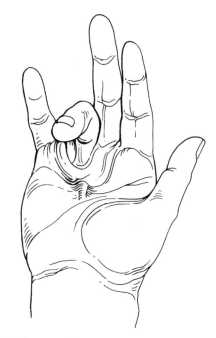

Fig. 17.24   Dupuytren's contracture.

localized to a single finger and the overlying skin is still freely mobile, the taut bands of the palmar aponeurosis may be divided by subcutaneous fasciotomy. If several fingers are involved, complete excision of the palmar aponeurosis is required. In severe and long-standing cases the capsules of the metacarpophalangeal and proximal interphalangeal joints become permanently contracted. Capsulotomy is then indicated. Amputation of a severely affected single finger is sometimes necessary.

Stenosing tenosynovitis

Stenosing tenosynovitis is caused by a fibrous stricture in a tendon sheath, usually at the site of a 'pulley' or tunnel through which the tendons pass when changing direction. The tendons predominantly affected are those of the thumb at the level of the radial styloid and those of the finger in the distal part of the palm.

De Quervain's synovitis. This is the name applied to stenosing tenosynovitis affecting the fibrous sheath of the tendons of the thumb (the abductor pollicis longus and extensor pollicis brevis) as they run through the tunnel at the tip of the radial styloid process (Fig. 17.25). There is pain and tenderness over these tendons which is exaggerated by active or passive stretching of the tendons. Simple domestic tasks such as wringing clothes or lifting a teapot may cause severe pain.

Trigger finger. This is the more common condition and is due to thickening of the fibrous flexor tendon sheath at the metacarpophalangeal joint (Fig. 17.26). Pain and tenderness occur on active or passive movements of the affected finger. As the tendon is drawn through the narrowed portion of the sheath it develops a fibrous bulge which may prevent its ready return and 'lock' the finger in flexion. Attempts to extend the finger may require passive assistance which will cause the tendon to 'snap' through the strictured area.

In infants and young children, mainly the thumb is affected. Since the child usually does not know how to extend the thumb passively, it remains flexed and may be mistaken for a congenital anomaly. A palpable nodule at the base of the thumb is the clue to the true diagnosis.

These conditions can be corrected permanently by surgical decompression of the fibrous tendon sheath.

Repeated stress injury (RSI). This is a condition in which there is pain and weakness in the wrist

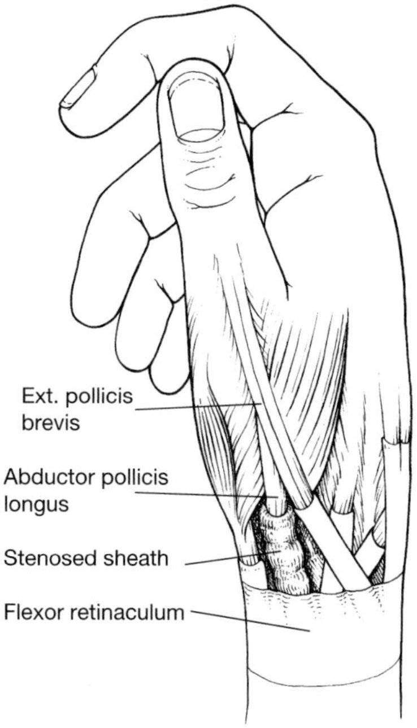

Ext. pollicis brevis

Abductor pollicis longus

Stenosed sheath

Flexor retinaculum

Fig. 17.25   De Quervain's tenosynovitis.

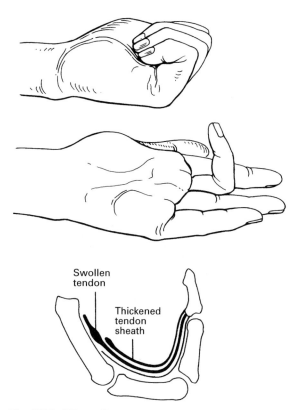

Swollen tendon

Thickened tendon sheath

Fig. 17.26   Trigger finger.

and forearm of keyboard operators. The cause is not understood. RSI is now classed as an industrial disease for which compensation may be claimed.

Nerve compression syndromes

Nerves can be compressed where they run within fibrous or rigid compartments. Examples are compression of the median nerve as it passes under the pronator teres in the forearm, the ulnar nerve as it runs in the groove of the medial condyle of the humerus or around the hook of the hamate, and the lateral cutaneous nerve as it enters the thigh.

The commonest form of nerve compression is the *carpal tunnel syndrome*, in which the median nerve is compressed as it runs below the flexor retinaculum at the wrist (Fig. 17.27). It affects primarily middle-aged women, is a complication of pregnancy, myxoedema and acromegaly, and may be precipitated by local oedema leading to increased tension under the retinaculum. Symptoms include pain, particularly at night, in the thumb and lateral three fingers, disturbance of sensation, and wasting of the muscles supplied by the median nerve (first two lumbricals, abductor and flexor pollicis brevis, opponens pollicis).

Splinting of the wrist at night relieves the pain and is a useful diagnostic test. Relief may also be obtained by injection of hydrocortisone succinate under the retinaculum in the line of the nerve. Surgical decompression is required if there is muscle wasting or when conduction studies demonstrate a nerve block at the site of the retinacular tunnel. This simple operation can be performed through a small incision using a tenotome (Fig. 17.28).

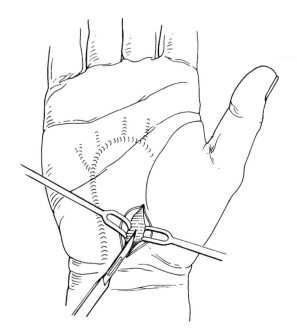

Fig. 17.28   Relief of carpal tunnel syndrome.

INFECTIONS OF THE HAND

The hand is particularly prone to minor injury. Even the most trivial puncture wound must be treated with respect; otherwise infection may enter the anatomical spaces within the hand. The commonest infecting organism is *Staphylococcus aureus*, and

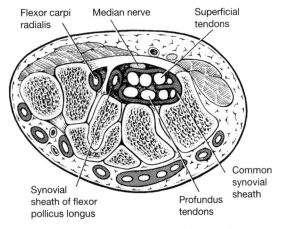

Flexor carpi radialis   Median nerve   Superficial tendons

Synovial sheath of flexor pollicus longus   Profundus tendons   Common synovial sheath

Fig. 17.27   Anatomical relationships of the carpal tunnel.

Carpal tunnel syndrome
- The syndrome is produced by compression of the median nerve as it passes beneath the flexor retinaculum at the wrist.

- The syndrome is commoner in middle-aged females, and in pregnancy, myxoedema and rheumatoid arthritis.

- The patient complains of altered sensation and pain in the thumb and lateral three fingers (particularly at night) and has wasting of the muscles of the thenar eminence (abductor and flexor pollicis brevis, and opponens pollicis) and the lateral two lumbricals.

- Splinting of the wrist at night relieves pain and may help to confirm the diagnosis.

- Injection of steroids may also bring relief but surgical incision of the flexor retinaculum is indicated if symptoms persist or muscle wasting develops.

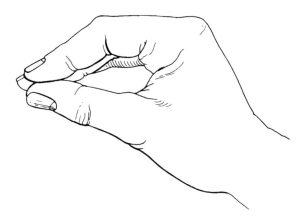

Fig. 17.29 Position of function of the hand.

prompt and effective therapy is necessary to prevent serious consequences.

In general, the principles of management of a hand infection are to give systemic antibiotics, elevate the limb and immobilize the hand in the position of function, i.e. with the thumb and fingers semiflexed (Fig. 17.29). The choice of antibiotic depends on the likely source of infection. In view of the common frequency of staphylococci, flucloxacillin, which is not inactivated by penicillinase, is usually the first choice. If streptococcal infection is suspected on account of rapidly spreading lymphangitis, large doses of benzylpenicillin are given. If rapid resolution does not occur, the antibiotic should be changed, e.g. to erythromycin or a second-generation cephalosporin (cefuroxime), and consideration given to draining the infection. Anaerobic or mixed infections of the hand (e.g. from bite wounds) demand urgent attention.

Collar-stud abscess

When a blister becomes infected, a subepithelial abscess forms. If the overlying skin is callous, the abscess spreads by pointing through the dermis into the subdermal fat, forming a so-called 'collar-stud'

abscess (Fig. 17.30). Such abscesses may track deeply into the anatomical spaces of the finger and hand. Early surgical treatment by deroofing the superficial compartment and dilating the dermal tract to allow free drainage of underlying pus is advised.

Pulp space infection

The pulp space lies anterior to the distal phalanx and is divided into loculi containing fat and fatty tissue by septa running from the front of the phalanx to the skin (Fig. 17.31). Infection within the unyielding loculi rapidly builds up painful tension and interrupts the blood supply to the distal phalanx, predisposing to septic necrosis of the bone.

Surgical decompression is performed as soon as an abscess is suspected, i.e. if the pulp is tense, swollen or red, or if the patient complains of throbbing pain. As it is important not to damage digital nerves and vessels, incisions are placed longitudinally over the point at which the abscess points, or in the midline anteriorly. Such incisions must not cross the flexor crease over the distal interphalangeal joint for fear of entering the flexor tendon sheath or joint capsule. The spaces over the middle and proximal phalanges may also be infected directly, but this is less common.

Web space infection

The web spaces contain loose areolar tissue and provide a path of least resistance for pus tracking from an infected blister situated distally in the palm or from the lumbrical canals to the fingers. The skin anterior to the web becomes thickened, red and glazed, but swelling is mainly dorsal. If there is a collar-stud abscess in the distal palm, the space is decompressed through this. Otherwise it is best opened through a small dorsal incision.

Midpalmar and thenar space infection

These potential spaces lie in the palm between the anterior surface of the metacarpals and interossei

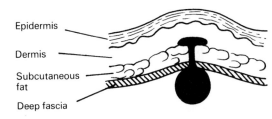

Epidermis

Dermis

Subcutaneous fat

Deep fascia

Fig. 17.30 Collar-stud abscess.

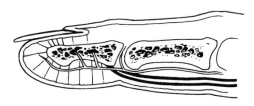

Fig. 17.31 The pulp space.

(midpalmar space), and the adductor pollicis and flexor tendons (thenar space). They may become infected by spread from a web space or tendon sheath, or by direct puncture.

Because the palmar aponeurosis restricts swelling anteriorly, swelling of the hand is disproportionately great on the dorsum, which becomes grossly ballooned. Maximum tenderness is felt anteriorly over those parts of the spaces which are least covered by overlying tissues (Fig. 17.32).

Surgical decompression is achieved by incisions placed over the site at which the infection points. Damage to vital structures is avoided by blunt dissection through the deeper tissues. If there is no obvious site of pointing, the spaces may be opened from the medial or lateral side of the hands.

Acute tenosynovitis

To allow free and frictionless movement of the hand, the flexor tendons are enclosed in two layers of synovium separated by fluid and surrounded by a fibrous sheath (Fig. 17.33). Infection may gain access to these synovial spaces by spread from

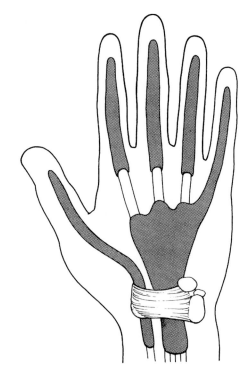

Fig. 17.33   The flexor tendon sheaths of the hand.

contiguous infection or by direct puncture, and then spreads rapidly within them.

Most commonly, acute tenosynovitis affects the flexor sheath of a finger, which becomes grossly swollen and semiflexed. Any attempt to move the tendon, either actively or passively, causes severe pain. Such passive movements must be tested gently. Tenderness is maximal just proximal to the crease over the metacarpophalangeal joint where the digital tendon sheath projects into the palm.

Infection of the flexor sheath of the thumb spreads into the radial bursa on the lateral side of the palm. Infection of the sheath of the little finger may involve the common flexor sheath, in which case there is gross oedema of the whole hand, especially the dorsum. The fingers are held in a semiflexed position and any attempt at moving or stretching the flexor tendons is painful. There is diffuse tenderness over the palm which is maximal on the medial side and may also be elicited in the forearm above the flexor retinaculum.

If there is no immediate response to intensive conservative therapy, surgical decompression of the affected sheath is indicated. Otherwise necrosis of the tendon may occur. Normally two small incisions

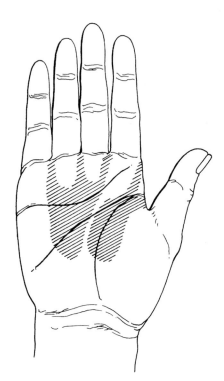

Fig. 17.32   Midpalmar and thenar spaces.

are made through which pus can be evacuated and soft catheters inserted to allow irrigation and instillation of an appropriate antibiotic.

Vibration white finger

This industrial condition occurs in those using vibrating tools e.g. in shipyards or metalworks. The fingers and thumb became white and cold and intensely painful, causing the worker to stop using the tool. Most often no other physical signs are present, the digital arteries being patent on ultrasonography. The affected worker is eligible for compensation.

18

The breast

CONTENTS

ANATOMY AND PHYSIOLOGY

The breast is an appendage of skin and is a modified sweat gland. It is composed of glandular tissue and fat, its secretions draining on to the surface of the nipple through 5–7 main duct orifices. Although often described as being segmented like an orange, the glandular tissue and ducts interweave to form a composite mass. The primary secreting unit is a group of saccular alveoli draining into a ductule, the 'terminal duct-lobular unit'. In the resting state this unit secretes watery fluid which is thought to be reabsorbed through the walls of the larger ducts (Fig. 18.1), although secretions can be obtained by nipple suction in some 75% of premenopausal women.

The alveoli and ducts are lined by a single layer of epithelial cells, the last centimetre of the main ducts by stratified squamous epithelium. Contractile myoepithelial cells surround the ducts and move secretions along them.

The shape of the female breast is due to the fat contained within fibrous septa, and not to the glandular tissue. With aging, the glandular and fibrous tissue atrophy, the skin stretches, and the breast sags.

The breast lies between the skin and the pectoral fascia to which it is loosely attached. It extends from

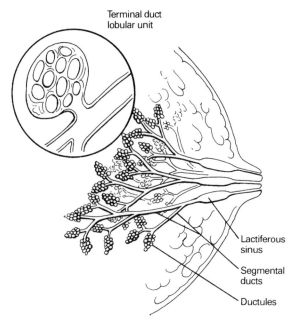

Fig. 18.1   Structure of the breast and its secreting unit.

the 2nd to the 6th rib and from the lateral border of the sternum to the midaxillary line. The axillary tail of the breast runs upwards between the pectoral muscles and latissimus dorsi to blend with the axillary fat. The excellent blood supply of the breast comes laterally from the lateral thoracic artery and perforating branches of the intercostal vessels, and medially from perforating branches of the internal mammary artery. The profuse lymphatics drain medially to the internal mammary nodes and later-ally via the pectoral and subscapular nodes (Fig. 18.2) to the central and apical axillary nodes and the subclavian trunk. A few lymphatics drain to nodes between the pectoral muscles and some pierce the pectoral fascia to enter the chest with the perfo-rating vessels. Although lymph from the medial part of the breast may drain medially, lymph from all parts drains laterally to the axillary nodes, the main route of lymphatic spread of breast cancer.

Development of the breast

Early in intrauterine life two 'milk ridges' form on a line from midclavicle to groin. These consist of ectodermal cells which form buds, the number of which varies from species to species. In women there are two pectoral buds from which solid cords extend into the subcutaneous tissues and develop into the alveoli and ducts of the breast. Accessory buds of breast tissue may be found elsewhere on the milk lines.

Hormonal control of breast development and function

In the newborn, circulating maternal hormones may cause one or both breasts to enlarge temporarily and secrete a colostrum-like fluid ('witches' milk') from the nipple. The breast then normally remains dormant until puberty when the onset of cyclical hormonal activity stimulates growth, branching of ducts, and formation of ductules and primitive terminal duct-lobular units.

In the resting state, terminal duct-lobular units can be recognized microscopically, but lobular development only becomes marked during pregnancy. There is good evidence that oestrogen, adrenocortical steroids and growth hormone promote duct development, that prolactin is essen-tial for alveolar formation, and that a tetrad of oestrogen, progesterone, prolactin and growth hormone are needed for the full development seen in late pregnancy. The placenta is an important source of these hormones in pregnancy.

During pregnancy, ovarian and placental steroids inhibit lactation. Delivery reduces the amount of circulating oestrogen and so increases the sensitivity of the breast epithelium to the lactational complex (prolactin, growth hormone and cortisol). Suckling stimulates the release of prolactin and oxytocin, and oxytocin stimulates the myoepithelial cells to eject milk into the terminal ducts. These effects are reversed by weaning.

Normal and abnormal growth of the breast

With the approach of puberty, a firm 'button' of breast tissue develops beneath the nipple. At first this may be unilateral and can be mistaken for a cyst or fibroadenoma. Surgical interference with the developing breasts can seriously distort their eventual form and is avoided unless there is unequiv-ocal evidence of malignancy. Malignancy in this age group is extremely rare but is suggested by skin fixation and ulceration.

During the menstrual years the cyclical changes in the breast can cause heaviness, discomfort and increasing nodularity, particularly in the latter part of the menstrual cycle.

Excessive growth of one or both breasts can cause so much discomfort and embarrassment that reduc-tion mammoplasty is required. The operation must be deferred until the breasts are fully grown, and is designed to restore a small youthful shape by removing a portion of the breast and transposing the nipple to a new site. Small breasts can cause enough

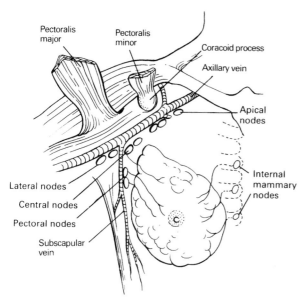

Fig. 18.2 Axillary and internal mammary nodes.

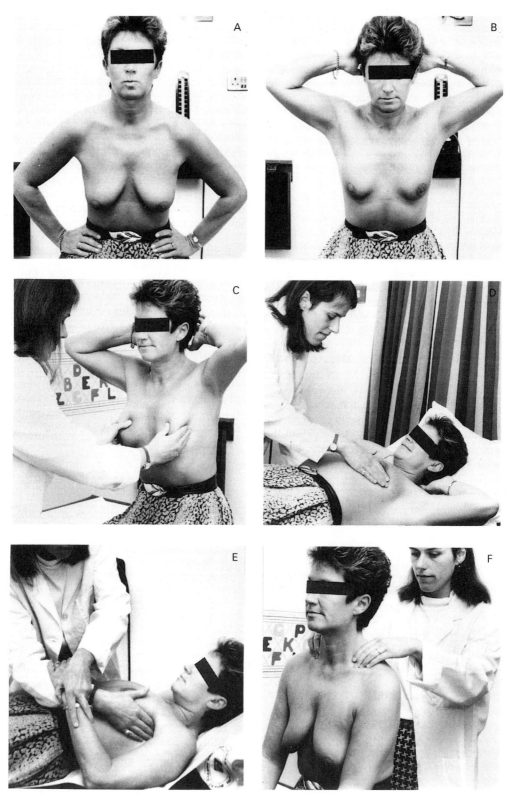

Fig. 18.3 **Examination of the breast: A** & **B** positions for inspection; **C** & **D** positions for palpation of the breast; **E** examination of the axilla; **F** examination of the supraclavicular area.

embarrassment to justify surgical augmentation (see below).

Complete failure of development of both breasts may be due to ovarian agenesis. In Turner's syndrome this is associated with infantilism, short stature, webbed neck and cubitus valgus. Failure of development can be associated with absence of the pectoral muscle (Poland's syndrome). Breast construction or reconstruction depends on tissue availability and the size of the opposite breast (if present). In its simplest form it consists of inserting a silicone prosthesis, but achievement of symmetry may necessitate the use of a tissue expander or a myocutaneous flap (see p. 226).

EVALUATION OF THE PATIENT WITH BREAST DISEASE

History

The patient is asked particularly whether she has noticed any discrete abnormality or areas where the texture differs from normal. Any premenstrual discomfort, nipple discharge, or recent nipple retraction or distortion is noted. It is important to establish whether the patient has had previous breast complaints, attended a breast clinic, and had a mammogram or biopsy. Marital status, number of children (and whether breast fed), age at first pregnancy, menstrual status, and date of last period are always recorded. It is essential to enquire whether there is a family history of breast disease.

Physical examination

The patient undresses to the waist and sits facing the examiner (Fig. 18.3). The breasts are inspected from in front while the patient's arms are placed by her side, then raised above her head, and finally placed upon her hips. The examiner looks for asymmetry, visible lumps, flattening, skin tethering, abnormal fixation of the breast, and retraction or alteration in the axis of the nipple. The patient is then asked to lean forwards, and the breasts are again inspected and then gently palpated. The fingers are slid behind the lateral border of pectoralis major, seeking enlarged pectoral nodes.

Further palpation of the breast is best carried out with the patient lying down. If the arm is raised so that the hand is tucked beneath the head, the breast 'flows' over the chest wall. The patient is asked to point to any abnormality and this area is examined first. Thereafter each quadrant is examined by gentle palpation between the fingers and the underlying chest wall.

Palpation is repeated with the patient's arms at her side. The axilla is palpated for lymph nodes while the arm is supported to relax the axillary muscles. Subscapular and supraclavicular nodes are best palpated from behind.

If a lump is felt, its position, size (as measured by callipers), consistency, discreteness and fixation are carefully recorded. It is particularly important to decide whether a lump is smooth, irregular or nodular, and whether it is separate from the surrounding breast tissue or integrated within it. Fixation to skin is sought by pinching up the skin over the mass, while fixation to the pectoral muscles is assessed by moving the mass while the pectoral muscles are first relaxed and then contracted by asking the patient to place her hands on her hips and press in.

If the patient complains of nipple discharge, an attempt is made to reproduce the discharge, determine whether it arises from one or several ducts, and test it for blood. Pressure is applied to the areolar margin with one finger, and on 'moving round the clock' one observes whether the discharge can be reproduced and whether a dilated duct or nodule can be felt (Fig. 18.4). If this manoeuvre fails, the breast tissue immediately beneath the nipple is picked up and gently compressed.

Any discharge is tested for blood with a Clinitest strip and a smear is made for cytological examination. If the discharge emanates from one duct, note should be made of the position of that duct and whether its orifice is dilated.

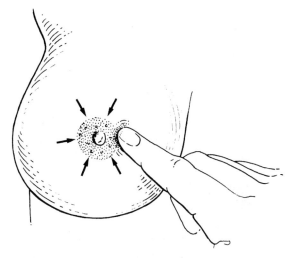

Fig. 18.4 Method of differential palpation.

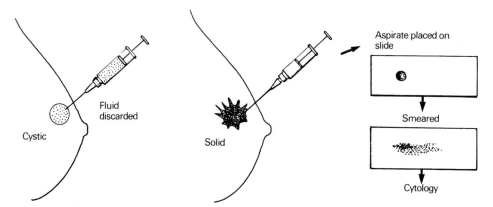

Fig. 18.5   Needle aspiration of a breast mass.

Ancillary investigations

Needle aspiration and cytology

Needle aspiration of a breast lump is performed in the clinic using a 10- or 20-ml syringe and 21-gauge or smaller needle. A special handle is available which allows the operator to apply constant suction with one hand while steadying the mass between finger and thumb of the other hand. The consistency of the mass can be assessed while inserting the needle; the sudden relief of resistance on entering a cyst, the tough rubbery feel of fibrocystic tissue, and the grittiness of cancer are typical.

A cyst is emptied of fluid. If the lesion is solid, an aspirate is taken by applying constant suction and advancing and withdrawing the needle several times through the centre of the tumour. Suction pressure on the syringe is then released and the needle is removed so that its contents can be expressed on to a slide to prepare smears for staining and examination (Fig. 18.5).

Mammography

Mammography uses high-resolution film and X-rays of low penetrating power so that the radiation dose is

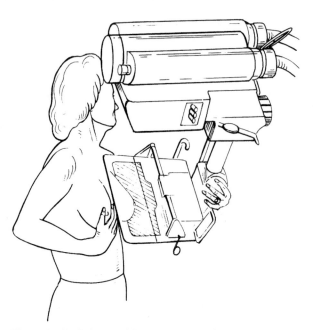
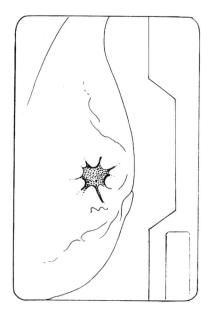

Fig. 18.6   Mediolateral oblique mammography.

kept as low as possible (0.5–1.5 mGy per film). An oblique view (Fig. 18.6) is now standard and includes the whole breast on the film. A cranio-caudal view can also be obtained, although the oblique view usually suffices for population screening of asymptomatic women. In symptomatic patients, mammography is usually reserved for those over 35 years of age unless a definite lesion is discovered clinically.

In some clinics, xeromammograms are preferred as they highlight changes of density, show calcifications clearly and can be read in reflected light. Xeromammography requires a larger dose of radiation than mammography, an important factor when screening populations of well women.

Breast biopsy

Specimens for the histological examination of breast lesions were at one time obtained by surgical excision biopsy, often with immediate examination by frozen sections. The need for biopsy to diagnose malignancy has been largely overcome by the advent of mammography and fine needle aspiration cytology. If biopsy is needed, a core of tissue is usually obtained by a closed technique employing a Tru-cut needle (or biopsy gun).

Surgery is still used to remove benign lesions. If the lesion is superficial, biopsy can be performed under local anaesthesia; if not, a general anaesthetic is used. Incisions should be transverse, follow the curve of the breast, and avoid distortion of contour.

Removal of mammographically visible but impalpable lesions can pose problems. Some surgeons simply perform a wide local or segmental resection, but it is better to localize the lesion radiologically before operation by a hooked needle (Fig. 18.7) or injection of a radio-opaque and visible dye. Following excision the specimen must be X-rayed to confirm that it contains the lesion. Frozen section examination of such small lesions is not advisable and considerable experience and expertise may be needed for their pathological assessment.

THE PAINFUL BREAST

Pain, discomfort and heaviness in the breasts are particularly common and, if severe, can interfere with the quality of life (including the patient's sex life) and cause irritability and depression. Breast pain can be cyclical, occurring predominantly in the premenstrual phase, or non-cyclical (i.e. without

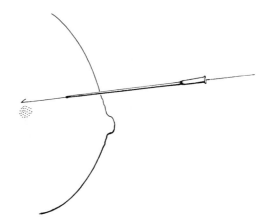

Fig. 18.7   Localization of non-palpable mammographic lesion.

relationship to the menstrual cycle). Cyclical breast pain is often associated with tender nodularity and fullness, particularly in the upper and outer quadrants of the breast, and is generally assumed to have a hormonal basis. Non-cyclical pain may be associated with inflammatory disease or duct ectasia (see below), and can be a symptom of neurosis. Pain is an uncommon symptom of cancer.

Following clinical examination, a mammogram is obtained in women over 35 years of age. Most patients have no local disease and can be firmly reassured. If cysts are present they should be aspirated, and tender fibrous nodules occasionally require excision. If cyclical symptoms are severe, bromocriptine (an antiprolactin), danazol (a gonadotrophin inhibitor) or tamoxifen (an anti-oestrogen) can be prescribed. Non-cyclical pain is not helped by these measures and if reassurance fails to bring relief, psychiatric support may be needed.

INFLAMMATORY DISEASE OF THE BREAST

Acute and chronic mastitis

Although inflammation of the breast can accompany systemic infection (e.g. mumps, tuberculosis and actinomycosis), the common form of acute mastitis results from local staphylococcal infection. Acute mastitis occurs most frequently during the puerperium and infection usually gains access through a cracked nipple. Improved hygiene has done much to reduce its incidence.

Acute mastitis starts as a localized painful, tender,

red and indurated area. It may resolve spontaneously or spread through the breast which becomes hot and swollen. Fever and toxicity develop. Necrosis and pus formation cause a multilobular abscess. If the abscess is superficial, fluctuation may be elicited and the overlying skin becomes thin and glazed.

Antibiotics can abort the infection if given early in adequate doses. Needle aspiration can be used to obtain a specimen for culture and sensitivity determinations. Cessation of breast feeding and firm breast support may be all that is needed or bromocriptine (2.5 mg twice daily) can be prescribed.

An established abscess is drained surgically. The abscess cavity is entered through a curved transverse incision. All loculi are broken down to form a single cavity, a biopsy is taken from the abscess wall, and a tube drain is brought out through the wound or through a stab incision in the dependent part of the breast. A specimen of pus is always sent for bacteriological culture and sensitivity determinations and antibiotics are continued for some 5 days.

An alternative to surgical drainage is repeated aspiration of the abscess using a 19-gauge needle in conjunction with antibiotic therapy. Suppression of lactation is not needed but the patient is reviewed at least twice weekly until signs of infection have resolved totally. Ultrasonography can be used to monitor the size of the abscess.

Inadequate antibiotic therapy can retard pus formation but increase fibrosis. The breast becomes chronically thickened and honeycombed with pus, and can resemble an inflammatory cancer. Treatment consists of multiple incisions, biopsies, and drainage.

Non-lactational mastitis

A segment of breast may become inflamed in young non-lactating women, forming a red tender periareolar swelling. Initial treatment consists of antibiotic therapy and as anaerobes are frequently involved, metronidazole is often prescribed with flucloxacillin. If a periareolar abscess forms, a small circumareolar incision is used to drain pus, even if this results in formation of a mammary duct (see below).

Granulomatous mastitis

This rare granulomatous disease of unknown aetiology is characterized by recurrent chronic inflammatory masses in the breast with sinus formation, usually at some distance from the nipple. It can be confused with cancer.

Mammary duct fistula

This condition affects young women and is more common in smokers. It may be caused by blockage of a lactiferous sinus by a keratin plug. The sinus becomes dilated, its epithelium undergoes squamous metaplasia, and infection leads to a periareolar abscess. The abscess then bursts spontaneously or is incised, and a fistula forms with its external opening at the areolar margin.

Recurrent attacks of inflammation lead to intermittent discharge of pus. Treatment consists of surgical excision of the wall of the lactiferous sinus, its related cavity, and in some cases, the affected segment of breast. Alternatively, the lactiferous sinus can be unroofed from the fistula opening to the point at which the duct opens on the nipple. The lining is excised and the wound is left to granulate or is dealt with by delayed primary closure. Antibiotic cover is advisable.

Paraffin and silicone granulomas

Liquid paraffin was at one time injected into the breast for augmentation, but caused inflammation and the formation of abscesses and chronic sinuses. Organic polymers of silica (silicones) with glue-like consistency were then used for injection into the submammary space. Pure silicones are inert but additives used to prevent migration caused multiple painful lumps (silicone granulomas) and sinus formation in some patients. Silicone gels are still used for augmentation but are now enclosed in an envelope of silicone elastomer. Although generally held to be safe, there are still anxieties about the long-term safety of these prostheses and the possible local and systemic effects of silicone gels if the enclosing envelope bursts.

BENIGN EPITHELIAL TUMOURS

Fibroadenoma

This is the commonest breast tumour of young women and arises from aberrant development of a lobule. It is *not* a neoplasm. The fibroadenoma forms a well-demarcated painless smooth firm swelling which is characteristically mobile, hence the term 'breast mouse'. Fibroadenomas may be multiple. Mammography may not show the lesion or reveal a rounded density with a radiolucent halo from compression of surrounding fat.

Fibroadenomas consist of fine connective tissue

('fibrosis') and abnormal multiplication of ducts and acini ('adenoma') in varying proportions. About one-third of clinically diagnosed fibroadenomas are really areas of fibrocystic change.

Fibroadenomas typically take some 6–12 months to double in size and usually stop growing when about 3 cm in diameter. If untreated the lesion may undergo hyalinization and merge with surrounding tissues to form a hard calcified mass. Most surgeons recommend removal of fibroadenomas to avoid these long-term changes and relieve anxiety that a neoplasm is present. Fibroadenomas occasionally disappear spontaneously, and provided aspiration cytology reveals no malignant cells, removal may be deferred in favour of continued follow-up in women under 35 years of age. Fibroadenomas may grow during pregnancy but malignant change is extremely rare.

Soft fibroadenoma. A softer, more rapidly growing variant, it can affect older women; it is cured by surgical excision and must be differentiated from a phyllodes tumour (see below).

Giant fibroadenoma. A rare variant found in adolescent females, particularly in some African countries. The lesion appears a few years after puberty and the girl complains that one breast has enlarged rapidly. The breast is distended by a soft lobular tumour in which clefts can be palpated. The skin is thin and distended veins are visible, yet the tumour is not fixed to skin or deeper tissues. Mammography reveals a large well-defined opacity. These tumours are quite benign and are cured by *complete* local excision.

Phyllodes tumour

The classical term 'cystosarcoma phyllodes', once applied to these tumours, derives from the leaf-like masses of tumour tissue which project into cystic cavities and the 'sarcomatous' appearance of the stroma on microscopy. It is a misnomer and the term 'phyllodes tumour' is now preferred, although sarcomatous degeneration of the stroma and metastasis occur in 10% of cases. The tumour is fibroepithelial and some believe that it originates in a fibroadenoma.

Clinically the tumour presents as a rapidly growing unilateral breast mass in women aged 40–50 years. Advanced tumours have an irregular bosselated surface, palpable deep clefts and shiny stretched skin through which distended veins can be seen (Fig. 18.8). Lymph node enlargement is rare.

Small tumours are removed with a wide margin of normal breast while total mastectomy with axillary

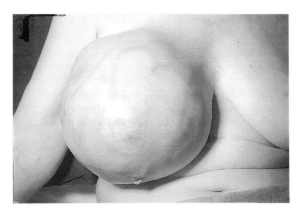

Fig. 18.8   Clinical appearance of a phyllodes tumour.

node sampling is advised for larger tumours. As the overlying skin must be widely removed, replacement using a myocutaneous flap may be necessary. Radiotherapy is of no value.

CYSTIC DISEASE AND EPITHELIAL HYPERPLASIA

Definition of terms

Cystic disease. This is a disease of breast lobules in which acini dilate and breast acini coalesce; *duct ectasia* denotes dilatation of the duct system. The two conditions may co-exist. Cystic disease is common in late premenopausal and menopausal women but, unlike cancer, its incidence does not increase with age and it is rare after the menopause. The cysts retain an epithelial lining which may show metaplastic transformation to apocrine (pink-cell) type. If the outflow duct is also obstructed, a large *tension cyst* may form which is full of clear yellow, green or brownish fluid.

Benign epithelial hyperplasia. The term 'adenosis' may still be used to denote non-neoplastic change in the breast in which the glandular elements are increased in number while the epithelial cells maintain a normal relation to the basement membrane. The terms 'epitheliosis' and 'papillomatosis' should now be discarded, having been replaced by the generic term of 'benign epithelial hyperplasia'. This is a focal increase in the number of epithelial cell layers to three or more instead of the usual two. The change may be mild, moderate or florid depending on the extent of filling of the lobule or duct spaces; and of normal or atypical type depending on cytological appearance and pattern.

Atypical hyperplasia is believed to represent the border-line lesion between benign epithelial hyperplasia and carcinoma-in-situ.

If adenosis is accompanied by marked proliferation of fibrous tissue it is termed 'sclerosing adenosis'; the epithelial elements may be so distorted and strangled by this fibrous proliferation that microscopically the lesion resembles scirrhous carcinoma.

Clinical presentation and diagnosis

Diffuse cystic disease may affect the whole breast which becomes heavy, thickened and lumpy. Pain and discomfort are common, particularly in the premenstrual phase of the cycle. On mammography the breast parenchyma is dense and ductal and vascular shadows are obscured. The edges of cysts and fibrotic nodules form so-called 'curvilinear shadows'.

Localized thickening is caused by aggregation of small cysts or by fibrosis. The patient notices that a segment of breast has a different texture, particularly at the end of the menstrual cycle, and that the thickening does not resolve and soften between periods. The area feels rubbery, thickened and nodular on clinical examination, and is more easily palpated with the fingers than with the flat of the hand. Provided that mammograms do not show a discrete opacity or microcalcification, the patient can simply be kept under review. If the mammogram does show such changes or if there is clinical suspicion of a discrete nodule, fine-needle aspiration cytology (or biopsy) is mandatory.

Sclerosing adenosis produces a firm mobile nodular mass which may suggest malignant disease. On needle aspiration it feels tough and rubbery rather than hard and gritty. Biopsy is the only safe course of action, but skilled pathological examination is necessary to avoid misdiagnosing the lesion as cancer.

Tension cysts form a firm hard mass which may be well demarcated, smooth and mobile, or integrated into an area of fibrocystic disease, when its surface feels irregular. Clinical differentiation between tension cyst and cancer is not always easy but absence of skin fixation is a helpful guide. Aspiration of clear yellow, green or brown fluid confirms that the lesion is a cyst. No further treatment is indicated unless a residual mass can be felt after aspiration, there is a significant amount of blood in the aspirate, the mammogram shows any suspicious areas, or the cyst refills on more than one occasion. Cytological examination of cyst fluid is not of value.

Risk of malignancy

Retrospective studies suggest that the risk of developing breast cancer is increased by two to three times in women with cystic disease. This association awaits confirmation.

BENIGN DISEASES OF THE DUCTS

Nipple discharge

Discharge may emanate from one or more ducts. It may be clear and straw-coloured, or yellow, green or dark brown. The discharge may contain blood. Particular attention is paid to the periareolar area on palpation, and the discharge should be examined for red blood cells and malignant cells. Mammography is requested and ductography (X-ray following injection of water soluble contrast medium into the affected duct) considered.

Non-bloody discharge from a single duct is not normally an indication for surgery, provided that the mammogram is clear and the patient is not unduly anxious.

Bloody discharge from a single duct is characteristic of duct papilloma (see below), while multiple duct discharge containing blood is most often due to duct ectasia. Rarely it occurs during pregnancy. Provided mammography does not show localized disease and cytology is negative, no action is normally required. If the discharge is profuse or if the patient is concerned, surgery is indicated. A circumareolar incision allows the nipple and areola to be retracted so that the reponsible duct can be excised (microdochectomy) with the related breast segment. If multiple ducts are affected, a core of central breast tissue containing the main ducts is removed close to the undersurface of the nipple; the nipple is then everted and its contour maintained by inserting a purse-string suture.

Duct ectasia

This condition is characterized by dilatation of the major ducts which fill with inspissated creamy secretion, and by periductal inflammation in which round cells predominate (Fig. 18.9). It is not known whether duct dilatation occurs first with leakage of secretion and a resulting inflammatory response, or whether primary periductal inflammation destroys

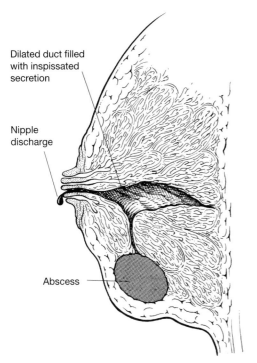

Fig. 18.9 Duct ectasia and associated breast abscess and nipple discharge.

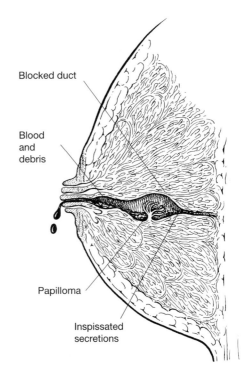

Fig. 18.10 Duct papilloma.

duct elasticity and causes duct dilatation. Duct ectasia may be asymptomatic or produce one or more of the following:

- Bloody, serous or creamy nipple discharge from one or more ducts
- Nipple retraction or inversion due to duct shortening
- Acute inflammation in a breast segment which may lead to a non-lactational abscess or mammary duct fistula
- Chronic inflammation of a localized area or breast segment (so-called plasma cell mastitis) in which a hard craggy area may mimic cancer, particularly as there may be associated skin tethering and dimpling and nipple retraction.

Duct ectasia is treated by excising the involved ducts and surrounding breast tissue; nipple inversion may require plastic surgery to restore contour.

Duct papilloma

Papillomatous growths can arise from the epithelium of the main ducts (Fig. 18.10), usually within 1 cm of the nipple. Bleeding from a single point on the nipple is characteristic and the involved duct often has a dilated slit-like orifice. The papilloma can sometimes be felt as a small nodule at the areolar margin. Pressure at that point reproduces the discharge. The lesion may be visible on mammography or ductography as a filling defect in a dilated duct. Treatment consists of surgical excision of the involved duct.

CANCER OF THE BREAST

Aetiology of breast cancer

Breast cancer is the commonest cancer of women in economically developed countries. In the United Kingdom, at least 7% of women will develop breast cancer; it is estimated that 150 000 women are living with the disease and that one will die from it every 30 minutes.

The cause of breast cancer is not known, but its differing incidence in various countries (Japanese have one-sixth the incidence of Europeans) and the fact that migration from low-risk to high-risk areas increases incidence in the migrants, suggests a strong environmental effect. Some believe that dietary factors, and particularly fat intake, are important. Within any country, the incidence of breast disease is correlated with higher social class.

Breast cancer is predominantly a disease of females and functioning ovaries are undoubtedly related to its initiation. Duration of reproductive life is important in that early menarche and late menopause increase risk, as does nulliparity, while the younger a woman is at first pregnancy, the less likely she is to develop the disease.

The risk of breast cancer increases with age, but because the number of women at risk diminishes, its peak prevalence is in the age group 50–60 years. There is some reduction in risk during the menopause (Fig. 18.11) giving rise to speculation that there are two types of breast cancer, affecting premenopausal and postmenopausal women respectively.

Breast cancer is more common when there is a history of the disease in a first-degree relative. In part this may be an environmental effect but some women belong to families in which susceptibility to breast cancer is inherited as an autosomal dominant trait. Attention is currently focused on the likelihood of a breast cancer gene being present on the long arm of chromosome 17. A history of breast biopsy is also associated with an increased risk of breast cancer, particularly when there has been atypical hyperplasia of the epithelium. These factors have been used alone and in combination to try to define a high-risk population of women who might benefit from selective screening. They are also being used to define a population of women in whom the prophylactic value of the anti-oestrogen tamoxifen is being assessed.

Types of breast cancer

Carcinoma in situ

Non-invasive cancers of the breast are confined to the ducts and acini and have not penetrated the basement membrane of the epithelium. Lobular carcinoma in situ, usually an incidental finding in biopsy specimens in postmenopausal women, is now regarded only as an indicator of increased cancer risk in one or other breast. Intraduct carcinoma is now usually detected as microcalcifications on mammography. It has a long natural history and a good prognosis, but if untreated may lead to the development of an invasive cancer.

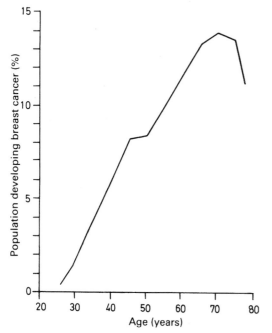

Fig. 18.11 Incidence of cancer of the breast related to age.

Invasive cancer

Ductal cancer.   About 90% of all invasive cancers are ductal in type, and the great majority have no special histological features. Ductal cancers with specific features include medullary, tubular and mucoid cancer. *Medullary cancer* accounts for 5% of invasive cancers and is a sharply circumscribed tumour composed of syncytial sheets of large neoplastic cells. The cancer shows diffuse infiltration by mononuclear lymphoid cells and has a better prognosis than other ductal cancers. *Tubular cancer* is a well-differentiated tumour which accounts for 3% of invasive cancers and also has a better than average prognosis. It is characterized by small tubular-like structures haphazardly arranged in a loose cellular stroma, and can be confused with sclerosing adenosis. *Mucoid cancer* is a rare circumscribed tumour with a copious matrix of mucinous tissue. It also has a relatively good prognosis.

Lobular   cancer. Lobular invasive cancer accounts for up to 10% of breast cancers. It is typified by the bland homogenous nature of its small cells and histological variants include cribriform, solid and tubular types.

Biological behaviour of breast cancer

Spread of breast cancer

Invasive breast cancer spreads by the lymphatics and the bloodstream (Fig. 18.12). The regional nodes most commonly affected are those in the lower axilla, from which cancer may spread to the apical axillary and supraclavicular nodes. Tumours in all parts of the breast can spread to not only the axillary nodes but also to the internal mammary nodes, particularly when the axillery nodes have became involved. Only rarely are the internal mammary nodes the sole group of involved regional nodes, and then in medial tumours.

Internal mammary node involvement is a bad prognostic sign and usually indicates spread to the mediastinal nodes and pleural cavities. It was once believed that haematogenous spread only took place after the regional nodes were involved; it is now appreciated that tumour cells can bypass the node 'filter' and that both forms of spread can occur from the start. Systemic spread may involve any site but metastases are particularly common in the skeleton, lungs, liver, brain, ovaries and peritoneal cavity.

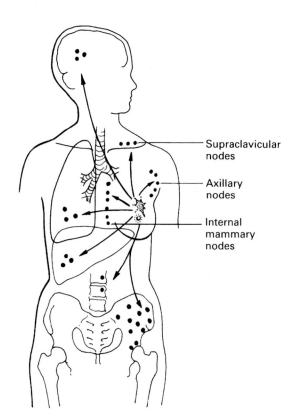

Fig. 18.12 Common sites of spread of breast cancer.

Supraclavicular nodes

Axillary nodes

Internal mammary nodes

Breast cancer grows slowly and metastases may develop many years after apparently successful local treatment. The larger a tumour and the more extensive its local spread at presentation, the worse the prognosis. Similarly, the more lymph nodes involved, the worse the prognosis. Only a third of women with four or more involved axillary lymph nodes survive beyond 5 years.

Factors influencing prognosis

Biological factors which affect tumour aggressiveness include the type of tumour and its relationship with its 'host', and are summarized in Table 18.1. For example, tumours which have a smooth contour, are well-differentiated, exhibit elastosis or marked lymphocytic infiltration, and evoke reactive hyperplasia in regional nodes have a better prognosis than poorly differentiated lesions with a spiculated contour, no lymphocytic infiltration and no reaction in regional nodes. Similarly, tumours which express differentiation antigens, have a high oestrogen receptor (ER) activity and a greater proportion of diploid cells have a more favourable prognosis than undifferentiated aneuploid tumours which are ER-negative.

Curability of breast cancer

Long-term follow-up of series of women treated by local surgery and radiotherapy indicates that 'cure' (defined as survival for a normal life-span with freedom from recurrent disease) is achieved in less than 40% of patients with 'operable disease' and in

Table 18.1 Factors influencing the prognosis of breast cancer

Tumour
  Size
  Contour

  Histological type
  Grade of differentiation
  DNA ploidy
  Degree of elastosis
  Presence of necrosis
  Lymphocytic infiltration

  Oestrogen receptor concentration

Lymph nodes
  Involvement by tumour
  Number of nodes involved
  Reactive changes

Distant metastases

less than 20% of all cases (see Ch. 16, Fig. 16.8). Even after 30 years, women with breast cancer have an excess mortality from metastatic disease.

Diagnosis of breast cancer

Clinical examination

Breast cancer usually presents as a lump which is painless or at most associated with tingling discomfort. It is most commonly located in the upper outer quadrant of the breast and may have given rise to recent nipple retraction. A dry scaling or red weeping appearance of the nipple with bleeding on contact may signify infiltration of malignant cells from an underlying breast cancer and is known as Paget's disease. Visible signs of tumour fixation include asymmetry of the breast and flattening of its contour, dimpling or puckering of the overlying skin, and retraction or alteration in the axis of the nipple. These signs are more evident when the patient sits with her hands raised above her head, or when she places them on her hips and pushes out the chest. During inspection and palpation it is vital that both breasts are examined; this allows comparison between the two sides and may detect unsuspected cancer in the opposite breast.

Palpation classically reveals a hard irregular mass which merges into the surrounding breast tissue. In a fatty breast the cancer can appear deceptively soft due to 'packaging' by surrounding fat and can be mistaken for a lipoma. It is important to appreciate that *any* discrete lump, no matter how small or mobile, can be a cancer. This is particularly important in young women with a glandular breast in which cancer can be difficult to distinguish clinically from a fibroadenoma.

Some patients present with advanced local disease and have skin ulceration, infiltration, oedema or fixity which can contract the whole breast to the chest wall.

The axillae and supraclavicular areas are examined to determine whether nodes can be palpated, and if so, whether they are soft, hard, mobile, matted or fixed to surrounding structures.

Fine-needle aspiration

When dealing with a breast mass fine-needle aspiration allows distinctions between a solid lesion and a cyst. If no fluid is obtained, an aspirate of the tumour is prepared for cytological examination as described on page 64. The demonstration of malignant cells provides unequivocal evidence of cancer but does not distinguish between in situ and invasive cancer.

Mammography

In expert hands, mammography is an accurate means of diagnosing cancer and has a sensitivity of 95%. A cancer appears as a dense opacity containing clustered microcalcifications and has an indefinite outline from which irregular spicules jut out into the surrounding breast (Fig. 18.13). Secondary signs of tumour include thickening of the overlying skin,

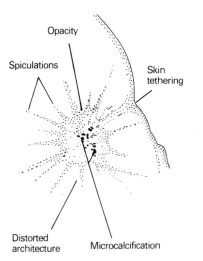

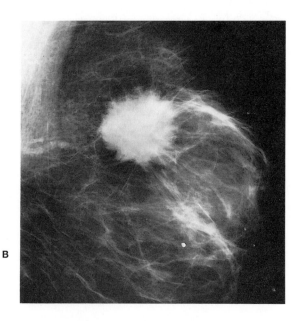

Fig. 18.13 A: Some mammographic signs of breast cancer. B: Mammogram showing large breast cancer with spiculation.

duct distortion, vascularity and distended veins. Mammography is less accurate in younger women as the density of the lesion may differ little from that of the surrounding parenchyma. As with clinical examination, it is important to examine both breasts.

Tru-cut biopsy

The final diagnosis of cancer rests on histopathological examination. The availability of fine-needle aspiration and Tru-cut biopsy means that it is no longer necessary to rely on frozen section examination at the time of definitive surgery. In many cases, the diagnosis of cancer is made with sufficient certainty by mammography and fine-needle aspiration that definitive treatment can be planned without formal biopsy but histological proof of malignancy is usually obtained before a mastectomy is performed.

Staging of breast cancer

The TNM system of *clinical* staging (Table 18.2) traditionally determined curability by local treatment. It was once thought that if a growth was confined to the breast and axillary nodes, it could be eradicated by mastectomy and axillary node clearance or a combination of surgery and regional radiotherapy. While this is no longer accepted, clinical staging still allows comparison of series of patients treated in different centres and identifies patients with local disease unsuitable for surgical treatment. Its two main drawbacks are the fact that palpable axillary nodes are not necessarily involved by tumour, and that clinical methods are not sufficiently sensitive to detect 'micrometastases' in viscera and bones.

The first drawback has been resolved by removing and histologically examining some or all of the axillary nodes, thus permitting *pathological* TNM staging. The second problem remains in that even sophisticated tests of organ function and newer methods of radiology frequently fail to detect occult metastatic disease. At present, routine examination for metastatic disease is usually restricted to chest X-ray, haematological examination and liver function tests. A bone scan is performed in some centres, particularly those undertaking therapeutic trials, but its yield is relatively low.

Screening for breast cancer

Recognition of the fact that breast cancer frequently presents at an incurable stage has led to immense interest in earlier detection. Programmes of education and self-palpation have encouraged women to seek advice if they detect the smallest abnormality. With mammography it has become possible to detect cancers of less than 1 cm in diameter (see p. 214) months or even years before they become palpable. Controlled studies indicate that regular mammographic screening of women over 50 can reduce mortality from breast cancer by 20%. A UK national programme now offers mammography, using a single mediolateral oblique view, every 3 years to women aged 50–64 years. As radiation is a potential cause of breast cancer, its dose is kept low by using sensitive film-screen combinations.

Efficient screening programmes require skilled teams to carry out clinical examination, high-quality mammography (including magnification views), ultrasonography, and fine-needle aspiration to differentiate solid from cystic lesions. Stereotactic equipment is available to guide a fine needle into impalpable lesions to obtain material for cytological examination. If biopsy of impalpable lesions is indicated, the techniques described on page 215 are employed.

As screen-detected cancers are small, they are well-suited to methods of treatment which conserve the breast, and are best managed by surgeons and radiotherapists with particular experience of these techniques.

Table 18.2   The TNM classification of breast cancer

Primary tumour

Tis	Preinvasive carcinoma (carcinoma in situ) Paget's disease (no tumour)		
T0	No evidence of primary tumour		
T1	Tumour < 2 cm	a)	no fixation to underlying pectoral fascia/muscle
T2	Tumour 2–5 cm	b)	fixation to underlying pectoral fascia/muscle
T3	Tumour > 5 cm		
T4	Any size with direct extension to chest wall or skin		
	a) fixation to chest wall		
	b) oedema, lymphocytic infiltration, skin ulceration, satellite nodules		
	c) both of the above		
	d) inflammatory carcinoma		

Regional lymph nodes

N0 No regional node metastases
N1 Metastases to movable ipsilateral axillary nodes
N2 Fixed ipsilateral nodes
N3 Metastases to ipsilateral internal mammary nodes

Distant metastases

M0 No evidence of distant metastases
M1 Evidence of distant metastases (including metastases to supraclavicular lymph nodes)

TREATMENT OF OPERABLE BREAST CANCER

In situ breast cancer

Ductal carcinoma in situ (Tis, N0, M0) localized to a small area of the breast is treated by excision of the area with a cuff of surrounding breast tissue. The role of adjuvant radiotherapy and tamoxifen is being investigated.

Widespread or multifocal in situ cancer is best treated by mastectomy; this can be followed by breast reconstruction if requested.

Operable breast cancer

Operable tumours are those restricted to the breast (T1,2,3, N0, M0) or associated with *mobile* axillary nodes on the same side (T1,2,3, N1, M0). As discussed earlier, the realization that radical treatment of breast and axilla cured only a minority of patients led to the concept that many of these patients have micrometastases and so require both local and systemic therapy.

Local therapy

There are two currently accepted methods of local therapy:

Wide excision and radiotherapy. This involves excising the tumour with at least a 1-cm margin of macroscopically normal breast. The approach is unsuitable for tumours which are multicentric, associated with carcinoma in situ, and large in relation to the size of the breast. If extensive carcinoma in situ or inadequate clearance margins are revealed on histological examination, further excision or mastectomy is required. The axillary nodes are either cleared surgically or sampled (by removing at least four nodes) and dealt with by radiotherapy if their involvement is confirmed. Wide local excision is followed by radical radiotherapy, using megavoltage equipment to deliver a high dose of radiation (50 Gy) to the breast, chest wall and nodal regions (if indicated). Fractionation techniques are used to minimize skin reactions, and the dose given to the tumour bed can be boosted by an external electron beam or 'afterloading' iridium[90] wire into plastic tubes left in the area at operation.

Mastectomy. This is the alternative method of local treatment (Table 18.3). It is indicated for cancers that are multifocal or large in relation to the size of the breast, and when radiotherapy is

Table 18.3 Local treatment of operable breast cancer		
Option	*Advantages*	*Disadvantages*
Wide local excision	Breast conserved	Radiotherapy needed
		Unsuitable for multifocal disease
		Unsuitable for large tumours
Modified radical mastectomy	Radiotherapy not needed	Mutilating
	Can treat multifocal disease	
Simple mastectomy	Surgery less demanding	Radiotherapy needed if nodes positive
	Can treat multifocal disease	Mutilating

contraindicated (e.g. poor respiratory function) or unavailable. Some patients prefer mastectomy to wide local excision because they regard it as a more complete operation. The operation may take the form of mastectomy with axillary node sampling (and radiotherapy if the nodes are involved), or mastectomy with axillary node clearance. The classical mastectomy described by Halsted removes

---

Operable breast cancer — local treatment

Ductal carcinoma in situ
- Small area treated by wide local excision (adjuvant tamoxifen/radiotherapy under investigation)
- Widespread areas treated by mastectomy ± breast reconstruction

Invasive carcinoma (T1,2,3 N0,1 M0)
Local therapy may consist of breast conservation or mastectomy:
- Breast conservation implies:
  – Wide excision of the cancer (unsuitable for multicentric/large tumours or widespread in situ disease; further excision/mastectomy needed if initial excision proves unsatisfactory)
  – 50 Gy megavoltage irradiation of breast, chest wall and tumour bed
  – Axillary node clearance or 4-node sampling (50 Gy to region if nodal involvement confirmed histologically)

- Mastectomy needed for multifocal/large cancers, when radiotherapy is contraindicated, or when the patient so chooses. It may take the form of:
  – Simple mastectomy with axillary node sampling (followed by nodal irradiation if nodes involved histologically)
  – Modified radical (Patey) mastectomy with axillary node clearance

the breast, pectoralis major and minor muscles, and the axillary nodes; it is mutilating and now seldom performed. The 'modified radical mastectomy' described by Patey is less mutilating in that the axillary nodes are removed without resecting the pectoralis major muscle. Radiotherapy is used after radical mastectomy only if the tumour involves the pectoral fascia or when metastatic nodes cannot be adequately cleared.

Systemic therapy

The aim of systemic therapy is to eradicate micrometastases or at least inhibit their growth. A recent overview of controlled trials indicates that recurrence rates and survival are improved significantly when anti-oestrogen treatment or multi-agent chemotherapy is given as an adjunct to primary local surgery.

In premenopausal women, ovariectomy (or ovarian irradiation) and a minimum of 6 months' chemotherapy (cyclophosphamide, methotrexate and 5-fluorouracil) appear to be equally effective as adjuvant therapy. Recent information suggests that ovarian ablation may be more effective for oestrogen-receptor rich tumours, whereas chemotherapy is more effective for those without receptor activity.

In older women, the anti-oestrogen tamoxifen (given for 2 years or more) and chemotherapy both significantly reduce relapse rates and improve survival. In this age group the influence of oestrogen-receptor status is less certain in determining the response to tamoxifen.

It is important to appreciate that adjuvant systemic therapy is effective both in patients with involved and uninvolved axillary nodes, but because of their poorer survival the gains may appear greater in those with involved nodes. For this reason, particularly when using chemotherapy, many surgeons use systemic therapy only in patients with positive nodes and those with other poor prognostic factors (e.g. large anaplastic cancers, lymphovenous invasion and oestrogen-receptor negative cancers).

Trials are underway to determine whether the combination of anti-oestrogen therapy and chemotherapy is better than either alone, and whether there are benefits to using systemic therapy *before* local treatment.

Complications of treatment

Radiotherapy. Following radiotherapy the skin must be kept dry during the erythematous reaction

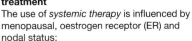

Operable breast cancer — systemic treatment
The use of *systemic therapy* is influenced by menopausal, oestrogen receptor (ER) and nodal status:
- Premenopausal women:
  - with ER-rich tumours should have ovarian ablation (i.e. oophorectomy or ovarian irradiation)
  - with ER-poor tumours should have at least 6 months' CMF chemotherapy

- Older women should have tamoxifen for at least 2 years or 6 months' CMF chemotherapy (ER status less reliable indicator in this age group)

- Systemic therapy known to be beneficial in patients with uninvolved nodes as well as those with involved nodes (but chemotherapy often used only in those with positive nodes ± other poor prognostic factors)

which often lasts 5–6 weeks. The patient is advised not to wash and a light talc is applied. If moist desquamation occurs, zinc and castor oil ointment is applied. The patient must avoid direct sunlight on the area for several years or serious sunburn will result.

Lymphoedema of the arm. Troublesome lymphoedema is often a complication of surgery and radiotherapy but can result from malignant infiltration of axillary lymphatics. Removal of axillary nodes interrupts lymphatic drainage and the effect is compounded by radiotherapy or postoperative infection. Axillary vein thrombosis may also occur, and in combination with lymphoedema results in massive arm swelling.

Oedema involves the hand and then spreads up the arm. If untreated, the whole arm becomes swollen, tense, brawny, hard, heavy and painful. Infection from minor injuries results in attacks of cellulitis and lymphangitis, usually of streptococcal origin. In rare cases, small tumour nodules appear in the skin; although these could be due to angiosarcomatous changes they are usually metastatic deposits of breast cancer.

Surgical treatment of lymphoedema is unsatisfactory and it is best treated by intermittent compression with an inflatable sleeve which encloses the entire limb, and by a supportive elastic arm stocking. The patient must avoid minor trauma to the limb and must wear gloves when carrying out rough work or gardening. Occasionally lymphoedema becomes so severe that the limb becomes an intolerable burden and forequarter amputation is required.

Psychological effects of mastectomy. Following mastectomy, one-third of patients have anxiety and depression that is severe enough to require psychiatric help. The symptoms include intolerance of body image, concern about effects on husband and family, and anxiety about relationships with other people. The patient may withdraw from normal social relationships and radically alter her domestic and sexual activities. While many of these problems are related to the mutilation of mastectomy, fear for the future is equally important, and patients treated by local excision and radiotherapy may also be affected.

Counselling is essential and most specialist units employ nurse counsellors who keep the patient fully informed about the nature of her disease and its treatment, advise on prosthetic support, and are trained to recognize and support patients with significant psychiatric upset.

The mutilation of mastectomy can be offset by reconstructing the breast immediately or subsequently. The simplest procedure consists of inserting a silastic prosthesis in a pocket created behind the pectoral muscle. The size of implant that can be used is limited and it tends to ride higher than the normal breast; the technique is particularly useful after bilateral mastectomy when symmetry is easier to obtain.

The tissue expansion technique involves inserting an expandable bag behind the pectoral muscle. Small amounts of fluid are injected regularly through a subcutaneous injection port over a period of months until a suitable space is created for a prosthesis.

Where loss of tissue or postradiation fibrosis is marked, it may be necessary to advance a myocutaneous flap to provide a new skin covering for the prosthetic breast. A latissimus dorsi flap (Fig. 18.14) is usually preferred to a flap based on the rectus abdominis as it is more reliable.

Follow-up

After treatment for primary breast cancer, patients are reviewed 3-monthly for 2 years, 4-monthly for the next 3 years, and annually thereafter. Attention centres on local control. In those treated by mastectomy, the chest wall and regional node areas are carefully examined. In those treated by breast conservation, detection of recurrence in the breast is not easy and annual mammograms are advisable (although postirradiation lymphoedema may make mammography less than satisfactory). A routine search for metastatic disease is a waste of time in asymptomatic patients. Because of the incidence of cancer in the other breast (1% per year), annual mammography of the contralateral breast is advisable.

TREATMENT OF LOCALLY ADVANCED BREAST CANCER

A breast cancer is locally advanced (T4) when it extends beyond the breast parenchyma to ulcerate the skin, becomes fixed to the chest wall, or infiltrates dermal lymphatics to produce satellite nodules or skin oedema (peau d'orange). Inflammatory breast cancer is a form of locally advanced disease in which the overlying skin becomes red and oedematous due to involvement of subdermal lymphatics and capillaries. Involvement of the axillary nodes to the extent that they become matted, fixed to surrounding tissues, or cause arm oedema also constitutes locally advanced disease.

Even though there is no clinical evidence of metastatic disease, primary surgical treatment is inappropriate and the disease is regarded as inoperable. Conventional treatment consists of systemic chemotherapy or anti-oestrogen therapy, in combination with local radiotherapy. However, more effective control may be achieved by giving intensive chemotherapy for 3–6 months and carrying out local surgery once the tumour has been 'de-staged'. Primary systemic therapy is also now being used for large operable (T3) tumours, partly with the objective of reducing the extent of local surgical treatment.

TREATMENT OF ADVANCED BREAST CANCER

Advanced breast cancer can cause distressing symptoms such as discomfort from ulcerating and fungating chest wall lesions, dyspnoea from lung and pleural involvement, and pain from bony metastases. The main aim of treatment is to relieve symptoms and improve the quality of life; one must not prolong life at the expense of increasing misery. As control of disease is important in reducing symptoms, measures to effect tumour regression are normally instituted as soon as metastatic disease is recognized. These include local surgery or radiotherapy, and systemic treatment by hormones or chemotherapy.

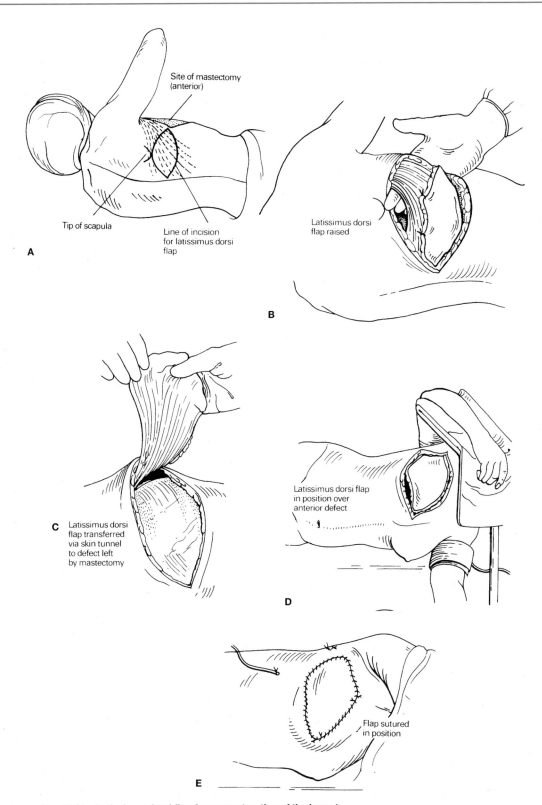

Fig. 18.14 **Latissimus dorsi flap for reconstruction of the breast.**

Assessment of the patient

When treating metastatic disease it is essential to measure progress if ineffective treatment is not to be prolonged and cause more problems than the disease itself. *Tumour response* is assessed by serial clinical or radiological measurement of deposits, recognizing that it is sometimes difficult to be certain whether a tumour is regressing or progressing. Measurement of *symptomatic response* is even more difficult and relies on self-assessment scales (to grade severity of symptoms such as pain, breathlessness and fatigue) or activity ratings (in which ability to perform day-to-day activities is expressed numerically). *Treatment morbidity* is assessed by using structured questionnaires to monitor side-effects.

Any form of treatment takes time to exert benefit and in general, 3 months should be allowed to elapse before therapy for advanced breast cancer is regarded as ineffective.

Systemic treatment

Endocrine therapy

Some breast cancers are hormone sensitive (Fig. 18.15). Oestrogens are the main hormones implicated in promoting the disease. In premenopausal women, the ovaries are the main source of oestrogens and synthesize them from C-19 steroids under the control of pituitary gonadotropins. After the menopause and ovarian atrophy, oestrogen synthesis depends on the conversion of C-19 precursors of adrenal origin by aromatizing enzymes in fat, muscle, liver and the breast itself.

The action of oestrogen on target tissues depends on its binding to specific receptor protein, the resulting complex acting on the genome to stimulate protein synthesis and cell proliferation. Some 60% of breast cancers possess ER activity, and this can be measured by radio-immunoassay or enzyme-linked immunoassay (on cytosol preparations), or by immunohistochemical staining of tissue slices or aspirates.

A variety of methods are available to reduce the levels of circulating oestrogen or inhibit its action:

Surgical ablation. In premenopausal women, removal or irradiation of the ovaries effects remission in about one-third of patients with advanced disease. The average duration of remission is 18 months.

In older women with non-functioning ovaries, oophorectomy is of no value but the source of C-19 precursors can be removed by bilateral adrenalectomy. Alternatively, production of all adrenocortical steroids can be abolished by removing or ablating the pituitary (by inserting radioactive yttrium) and so arresting adrenocorticotrophic hormone (ACTH) production (see Ch. 19). These surgical procedures result in a life-long need for cortisone replacement and have been superseded by pharmacological approaches.

Pharmacological ablation. A variety of agents can be used to prevent oestrogen synthesis or interfere with its peripheral actions.

Gonadotropin-releasing hormone (Gn-RH) analogues. Pituitary gonadotropin secretion is normally stimulated by pulses of Gn-RH of hypothalamic origin. If the pituitary is bombarded continuously with large amounts of Gn-RH, it becomes desensitized and gonadotropin secretion is inhibited. Analogues of the natural hormones can now be used to induce 'medical castration' and are given as a nasal spray or as delayed-release capsules which are implanted subcutaneously into the abdominal wall. Early results are encouraging.

Aromatase inhibitors. Aminoglutethimide is an anticonvulsant which inhibits aromatase activity. In postmenopausal women it reduces oestrogen synthesis, but because it acts on hydroxylating enzymes in the adrenal cortex, it also inhibits cortisol synthesis. It must therefore be given with hydrocortisone (40 mg/day) and a dose of 0.5–1 g daily gives similar remission rates in advanced breast cancer to surgical adrenalectomy (30%). Side-effects such as lethargy, skin rash, gastrointestinal upset and thrombocytopenia/leucocytopenia can be troublesome,

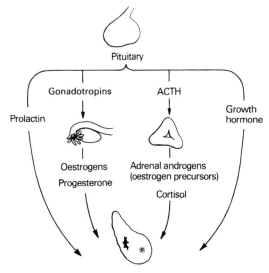

Fig. 18.15 **Hormones which may influence breast cancer.**

and smaller doses may have to be used or the drug reserved for 'second-line' use. Newly synthesized aromatase inhibitors such as 4-hydroxyandrostene-dione are free of such side-effects.

Tamoxifen. This drug binds to the oestrogen-receptor protein, forming an ineffective complex which prevents access of oestrogen to its receptor. A dose of 20 mg daily produces a remission rate equal to that achieved by other endocrine means (30%). Tamoxifen has few side-effects, although thrombo-cytopenia, jaundice and vaginal bleeding occasionally occur, and is without doubt the endocrine treatment of choice in postmenopausal women. In premenopausal women it is not clear whether it is as effective as ovarian ablation or the use of Gn-RH analogues.

Other agents. High doses of oestrogen, androgen and progesterone were once used to treat advanced breast cancer and occasionally caused remission. Progestogens (medroxyprogesterone acetate and megestrol acetate) are still used as 'second-line' therapy. Prolactin inhibitors (levodopa and bromocriptine) and the gonadotropin inhibitor, danazol, have also been used by some.

Chemotherapy

Single-agent chemotherapy is less effective in breast cancer than combination therapy using cell cycle-dependent and independent drugs. Doxorubicin (Adriamycin) is the most effective drug and is now included in most regimens although its dose is limited by cardiotoxicity. Cyclical combination chemotherapy produces remission in 60% of patients, the duration of remission averaging 6 months.

Selection of therapy

Treatment of advanced breast cancer has been rationalized by ER assay. Receptor-rich tumours have a 50% chance of responding to endocrine therapy, whereas receptor-poor tumours are generally refractory.

In premenopausal women with receptor-positive tumours, ablation of ovarian function should still precede other forms of endocrine treatment. This is the most effective method of reducing oestrogenic influences, and patients who respond positively are likely to benefit from other agents (e.g. aminoglutethimide or progestogens) when their tumour subsequently relapses. Those who fail to respond are likely to be unresponsive to further endocrine

measures. Gn-RH analogues, which have a profound but reversible effect, now offer a useful alternative to oophorectomy.

In postmenopausal women, a 3-month trial of tamoxifen is usual. Some surgeons reserve this drug for patients with ER-rich tumours, whereas most use the drug regardless of ER status, knowing that a small proportion of patients with ER-poor tumours will gain worthwhile benefit. In a responding patient the drug is continued until relapse, when 'second-line' treatment is initiated with aminoglutethimide (plus hydrocortisone) or high-dose progestogen.

For women with ER-negative tumours and those who fail to respond to endocrine therapy, chemotherapy is the only alternative. In some life-threatening situations (e.g. severe bone marrow depression or pulmonary lymphangitis) immediate chemotherapy is the preferred option regardless of tumour receptor status.

General support

Care of the patient with advanced breast cancer requires more than control of the tumour, and includes control of all symptoms, particularly when

---

Treatment of advanced breast cancer

Locally advanced disease (T4)
- Conventional treatment consists of systemic chemotherapy or anti-hormonal therapy in combination with local radiotherapy

- Intensive chemotherapy for 3–6 months may 'downstage' the tumour sufficiently to allow local surgery

Systemic disease
- The aim is to relieve symptoms and improve the quality of life.

- Endocrine therapy is useful in ER-rich tumours and may consist of:
  - ablation of organs producing oestrogen (i.e. oöphorectomy, ovarian irradiation, adrenalectomy, pituitary irradiation or hypophysectomy)
  - pharmacological prevention of oestrogen synthesis (i.e. Gn-RH analogues or aromatase inhibitors)
  - pharmacological interference with peripheral actions of oestrogen (i.e. ER blockade using tamoxifen)
  - 'second-line' therapy with agents such as progestogens

- Systemic therapy with combination of cell cycle-dependent and independent drugs is useful, particularly in patients who do not have hormone-sensitive tumours.

there is no response to chemotherapy or endocrine treatment (see Ch. 16).

Treatment of special problems

Pleural metastases. Pleural effusions are regarded as malignant until proved otherwise in patients with a history of breast cancer. Severe dyspnoea demands urgent aspiration and a small chest drain is inserted through the 8th or 9th space in the midaxillary line and connected to watersealed drainage to which suction is applied. Fluid is sent for cytology.

Pleural effusions usually respond to systemic therapy but if they do not, a cytotoxic agent such as bleomycin can be instilled through the drain. The tube is then clamped while the patient lies supine, prone and on either side. The clamp is removed after 24 hours and the tube connected to watersealed drainage to empty the pleural cavity completely.

Lung metastases. Discrete lung metastases do not cause severe symptoms but lymphangitis carcinomatosa (in which the lung lymphatics are infiltrated by tumour) can cause severe dyspnoea and bronchospasm. This may be relieved by steroids (prednisolone 30 mg daily) and bronchodilators such as salbutamol. Chemotherapy is the preferred treatment.

Hypercalcaemia. Transient hypercalcaemia occurs in 40% of patients with bone metastases, and is severe (serum calcium exceeding 3 mmol/l) in 10%. Symptoms include nausea, constipation, thirst, polyuria, personality change, muscle weakness and bone pain. Hypercalcaemia can develop rapidly in patients receiving hormone or diuretic therapy.

Persisting severe hypercalcaemia must be reversed. Saline infusions correct dehydration, and with a loop diuretic are used to promote a diuresis and calcium excretion. The bisphosphonate, pamidronate disodium, given by slow intravenous infusion is now the preferred treatment for severe hypercalcaemia, the dose being dictated by the calcium levels. The cytotoxic agent plicamycin is also effective but is now seldom used in view of its unpredictability and marrow toxicity.

Bone metastases. These are usually osteolytic and often cause severe disabling pain. Systemic therapy is essential but local radiotherapy (20 Gy over 5–7 days) can relieve pain and promote healing. Recalcification of weight-bearing bones can prevent pathological fracture, vertebral collapse and paraplegia. If fracture occurs, orthopaedic reinforcement may be needed, and can include hip replacement. Oral phosphates can confer additional benefit.

Spinal cord compression. Compression of the cord by extradural tumour must be recognized early and treated promptly; patients with back pain who develop neurological symptoms are surgical emergencies. Magnetic resonance imaging (MRI) replaces myelography as a means of determining the site and extent of cord compression. The spinal cord is decompressed surgically (see Ch. 37) and radiotherapy arranged.

Brain metastases. Rising intracranial pressure and neurological dysfunction can be caused by intracerebral metastases. Once cerebral secondaries are suspected, steroids (dexamethasone 10 mg i.v. followed by 4 mg i.m. at 4-hourly intervals) are prescribed and a computerized tomography (CT) scan is arranged. Treatment can be continued with oral dexamethasone (2 mg three times a day), and whole head irradiation (30 Gy over 3 weeks) may be worthwhile despite hair loss. Surgical excision is rarely indicated but can provide striking palliation in patients with a single metastasis.

Liver metastases. Progressive liver failure and jaundice can result from infiltration of the liver by metastases. Endocrine treatment occasionally induces dramatic shrinkage but chemotherapy is usually indicated. Steroid therapy can improve well-being.

Special problems in metastatic breast cancer
- Pleural effusions may be treated by aspiration and instillation of cytotoxic agents such as bleomycin.

- Lung metastases are often asymptomatic but dyspnoea and bronchospasm may be relieved by steroids, bronchodilators and chemotherapy.

- Hypercalcaemia causes nausea, constipation, thirst, polyuria, weakness, pain and personality change, and is treated by rehydration/biphosphonates.

- Bone metastases may require local radiotherapy, systemic chemotherapy, oral phosphates, and orthopaedic reinforcement if giving rise to symptoms.

- Spinal cord compression can be treated by surgical decompression, or steroids and radiotherapy.

- Brain metastases may benefit from steroids and irradiation. Surgery can be used for isolated metastases.

- Liver metastases can be treated by steroids (and chemotherapy) if giving rise to pain.

MISCELLANEOUS TUMOURS OF THE BREAST

Connective tissue tumours

Benign tumours such as lipomas, angiomas and neurofibromas are rare. A lipoma forms a soft lobulated mass which on mammography is radiolucent, and can be confused with a 'pseudolipoma', the soft fatty mass which may surround a small scirrhous cancer.

Malignant tumours such as angiosarcoma and fibrosarcoma are all rare. Sarcomas present as a rapidly enlarging mass, spread by the bloodstream, and are dealt with by radical local surgery. They are radioresistant.

Lymphoma

The breast is occasionally the site of a lymphomatous deposit which forms a smooth, discrete and firm mass resembling a fibroadenoma. Axillary nodes are typically rubbery and discrete.

Secondary tumours

Metastases from tumours elsewhere (e.g. bronchus, thyroid, melanoma or the opposite breast) produce a well-defined mass clinically and on mammography.

THE MALE BREAST

Gynaecomastia

Enlargement of the male breast is increasingly common. Histologically the swelling consists of duct and fibroepithelial elements; alveolar formation is rare. Although the condition appears clinically to be unilateral, mammography usually shows hypertrophy of both breasts. Irritation and tenderness of the nipple may be present.

Gynaecomastia must be differentiated from cancer. Whereas cancer is usually eccentric in

Table 18.4   Drugs commonly associated with gynaecomastia

Amphetamines	Oestrogens
Adrenocorticosteroids	Phenothiazines
Androgens	Radioactive iodine
Bendrofluazide	Reserpine
Cimetidine	Salbutamol
Digoxin	Spironolactone
Marijuana	

relation to the nipple, stony hard and fixed, gynaecomastia is more often concentric and firm, lacking skin fixation or ulceration.

Gynaecomastia which results from excessive hormonal stimulation is often bilateral, and can be 'physiological' at puberty or the 'male menopause'. Increased levels of circulating oestrogen resulting from therapeutic administration (e.g. in cancer of the prostate) or excessive production (e.g. in testicular feminization or oestrogen-secreting adrenal tumours) can also cause gynaecomastia. Failure to metabolize steroid hormones in chronic liver disease can cause gynaecomastia in association with testicular atrophy.

Drugs other than steroids are an important cause of gynaecomastia (Table 18.4). Spontaneous resolution is common and treatment does not need to be discontinued unless pain and tenderness are severe or the patient is unduly perturbed.

If surgical treatment becomes necessary, the gynaecomastic breast is removed through a subareolar incision, preserving the nipple and overlying skin.

Cancer

Breast cancer is one hundred times less common in men and occurs at an older age than in women. Due to the lack of breast tissue, the cancer rapidly becomes fixed to the chest wall and commonly ulcerates. The treatment is similar to that of breast cancer in women. The tumour is often hormone sensitive and excellent regression can follow orchidectomy or tamoxifen therapy. Aminoglutethimide can be used as 'second-line' treatment.

19
Endocrine surgery

CONTENTS

THYROID GLAND

Surgical anatomy and development

The thyroid gland develops from the thyroglossal duct which grows downwards from the pharynx through the developing hyoid bone. The duct bifurcates on the front of the trachea and fuses with elements from the 4th branchial arch, from which the parafollicular C-cells which secrete calcitonin are derived. The duct is normally obliterated in early fetal life but can persist in part to produce a thyroglossal cyst. The upper end of the duct is marked in extrauterine life by the foramen caecum at the junction of the anterior two-thirds and posterior third of the tongue. Arrest of descent of the duct may result in an ectopic thyroid (e.g. lingual thyroid).

There are two pairs of parathyroid glands. The superior pair arise from the 4th branchial arch and are applied to the back of the thyroid, just above the inferior thyroid artery and at the level of the cricoid cartilage. The inferior glands arise from the 3rd arch (in association with the thymus) and are less constant in position. They are usually applied to the back of the inferior poles of the thyroid, but can lie within the gland, some distance below it, in the upper mediastinum or within the thymus.

The right and left lobes of the thyroid lie on the front and sides of the trachea and larynx at the level of the 5–7th cervical vertebrae (Fig. 19.1). The two lobes connect by a narrow isthmus overlying the 2nd and 3rd tracheal rings. The thyroid normally weighs 15–30 g, and is invested by the pretracheal fascia which binds it to the larynx, cricoid cartilage and trachea (Fig. 19.2). The strap muscles (sternohyoid and sternothyroid) lie in front of the pretracheal fascia, and must be separated to gain access to the gland.

The superior thyroid artery runs down to the upper pole of the gland from the external carotid while the inferior thyroid artery runs up to the lower pole from the thyrocervical trunk (a branch of the subclavian artery). As it nears the gland, the inferior

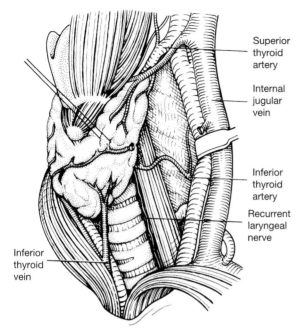

Fig. 19.1   Anatomy of the thyroid gland. The middle thyroid vein has been divided to allow forward rotation of the left lobe of the gland.

artery usually passes in front of the recurrent laryngeal nerve, but may branch around it. Blood from the thyroid drains through superior, middle and inferior thyroid veins to the internal jugular and innominate veins (Fig. 19.1), while lymph drains laterally to the deep cervical chain and downwards to pretracheal and mediastinal nodes. The recurrent laryngeal nerve is a branch of the vagus which passes upwards in the groove between the oesophagus and trachea to enter the larynx and supply its intrinsic

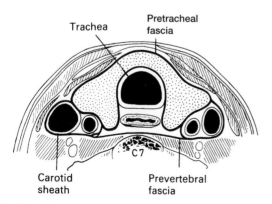

Fig. 19.2   Transverse section of the neck at the level of the seventh cervical vertebra to show the arrangement of the deep cervical fascia.

muscles, while the superior laryngeal nerve (also a branch of the vagus) runs down with the superior thyroid vessels and supplies the cricothyroid muscles which tense the vocal cords. Both nerves can be damaged during thyroid surgery (p. 240).

Thyroid function

The thyroid follicles secrete tri-iodothyronine (T3) and thyroxine (T4). T3 is the active hormone and T4 is converted to T3 peripherally. Synthesis involves combination of iodine with tyrosyl groups to form mono- and di-iodotyrosine, which are then coupled to form T3 and T4. The hormones are stored in follicles bound to thyroglobulin and, when released, circulate free or bound to plasma proteins.

Secretion of T3 and T4 is controlled by thyroid stimulating hormone (TSH) secreted by the anterior pituitary. TSH release is in turn controlled by thyrotropin releasing hormone (TRH) from the hypothalamus (Fig. 19.3). Circulating levels of T3 and T4 exert a negative feedback effect on the hypothalamus and anterior pituitary.

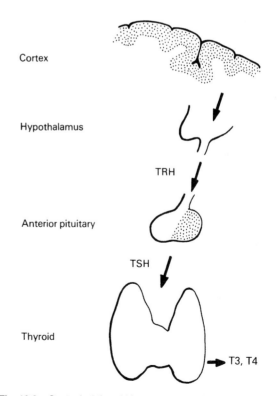

Fig. 19.3   Control of thyroid hormone secretion.

Assessment of thyroid disease

Thyroid function is assessed by T3, T4 and TSH assay. Pregnancy or oestrogen administration increases the level of thyroid binding globulin so that estimation of the ratio of free:bound hormone may be needed. TRH and TSH stimulation tests are used to determine the site of failure of production of thyroid hormones.

The thyroid can be imaged by plain films, ultrasonography or radio-isotope scan (^{99m}Tc-sodium pertechnetate behaves like iodine and is 'trapped' by the gland). The main value of scanning is to differentiate between 'hot' (actively functioning), 'cool' (normally functioning) and 'cold' (non-functioning) thyroid nodules. Total isotope uptake also reflects thyroid activity.

Fine-needle aspiration cytology is used to determine the nature of thyroid nodules, while detection of thyroid antibodies by red-cell agglutination techniques is used to diagnose autoimmune thyroiditis.

ENLARGEMENT OF THE THYROID GLAND (GOITRE)

A goitre is a visible or palpable enlargement of the thyroid. The swelling appears in the lower part of the neck and retains the shape of the normal gland (thyreos–Greek for shield). The swelling characteristically moves upwards on swallowing, and careful observation usually detects the movement during a spontaneous swallow. Patients in consultation are often nervous and have a dry mouth, and to ask them to swallow repeatedly is unnecessary.

'Physiological' enlargement

Transient enlargement may occur during puberty or pregnancy.

Non-toxic nodular goitre

This common disease occurs endemically in areas of iodine deficiency but can be sporadic or a reaction to drugs. It is more common in females. In the past, lack of iodine in the diet was a common cause of thyroid enlargement but 'endemic goitres' in areas such as Wales and Derbyshire are now rare because table salt is iodized. In areas of the world where iodine intake cannot be guaranteed, iodized oil emulsion can be injected.

In iodine deficiency, the gland initially enlarges diffusely and the follicles fill with colloid. Later multiple nodules develop, some of which contain abundant colloid while others show degenerative change with formation of cysts, areas of old and new haemorrhage, and even calcification. The goitre varies greatly in size from little more than normal to a gland weighing several hundred grams. The whole gland may be involved or the changes may be confined to one lobe.

Clinical features

Most multinodular goitres are asymptomatic. Others cause tracheal compression and dyspnoea, particularly when the goitre extends behind the sternum. Oesophageal compression can cause dysphagia. Very rarely, bleeding into a nodule may cause pain and rapid enlargement, and in the case of retrosternal goitre, respiratory distress. The thyroid is visibly enlarged and multiple nodules are usually palpable (Fig. 19.4). Sometimes only one nodule is palpable, giving the erroneous impression of a solitary nodule.

Plain films of the thoracic inlet may reveal tracheal compression or deviation in the case of retrosternal goitre (Fig. 19.5). Thyroid function is established by T3, T4 and TSH assay. Isotope scans are usually unhelpful.

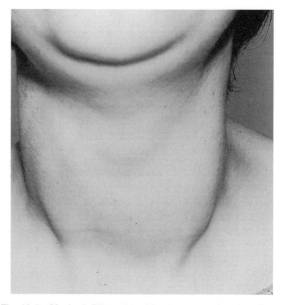

Fig. 19.4 Marked diffuse thyroid enlargement in a female patient with multinodular disease.

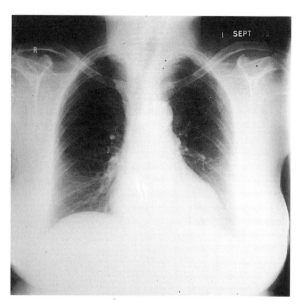

Fig. 19.5 X-ray of the thoracic inlet showing a retrosternal goitre with marked deviation of the trachea to the right.

Treatment

Administration of thyroxine occasionally prevents further enlargement by suppressing TSH secretion, but regression of the goitre is unusual. Large goitres and those causing symptoms of compression require subtotal thyroidectomy. Some patients request surgery for cosmetic reasons. As the gland is not functioning normally, the risk of hypothyroidism following operation is greater than after resection for thyrotoxicosis. Thyroxine may be used after operation to suppress TSH secretion and prevent enlargement of the residual gland.

Thyrotoxic goitre

Diffuse thyroid enlargement can result from stimulation by TSH or TSH-like proteins, resulting in increased production of T3 and T4 and thyrotoxicosis. However, most goitres occur in euthyroid individuals.

Thyroiditis

Subacute thyroiditis (De Quervain's disease)

This rare condition is associated with a 'flu-like' illness during which there is painful diffuse swelling of the gland. Thyroid antibodies may appear in the serum. The disease may be due to a viral infection

and usually resolves, although occasionally it runs an intermittent course.

Autoimmune thyroiditis (Hashimoto's disease)

This condition is believed to be due to destruction of thyroid follicles by immunocompetent lymphocytes. Antibodies are detected in the serum against thyroglobulin, thyroid cell cytosol and microsomes. Histologically there is marked lymphocytic infiltration around destroyed follicles. The patient is usually euthyroid, but thyrotoxicosis can occur. In the long term the patient becomes hypothyroid.

Post-menopausal females are most commonly affected (female-to-male ratio 10:1). The thyroid is diffusely enlarged and firm. A nodular form may be confused with multinodular goitre.

Diagnosis depends on demonstrating high titres of circulating antithyroid antibodies, particularly to microsomal components of the follicle cells. Biopsy helps to confirm the diagnosis. Lymphoma may occur in a thyroid which has been affected by long-standing Hashimoto's disease.

Thyroxine causes regression of small goitres, but subtotal thyroidectomy is needed when a large goitre is causing compression symptoms. Surgery can be difficult because of the firm nature of the gland and inflammation of surrounding structures, and there is a higher than normal risk of damage to the recurrent laryngeal nerves or parathyroids.

Riedel's thyroiditis

In this very rare condition, the thyroid is replaced by dense fibrous tissue, resulting in a firm painless swelling and tracheal compression. The cause is unknown. Surgical decompression of the trachea may be required.

Solitary thyroid nodules

Slow-growing and painless 'solitary' nodules are common, although 50% of them are in reality a conspicuous palpable nodule in a gland affected by multinodular goitre. Of true solitary nodules, half are benign adenomas and the rest are cysts or differentiated cancer.

The pivotal test is fine-needle aspiration cytology, complemented by ultrasonography, isotope scans and thyroid function tests (Fig. 19.6). Tru-cut biopsy can cause bleeding or nerve damage and is no longer used. Cysts can be aspirated, and provided that they do not refill and that cytology is negative, they need not be removed. Very rarely a cyst

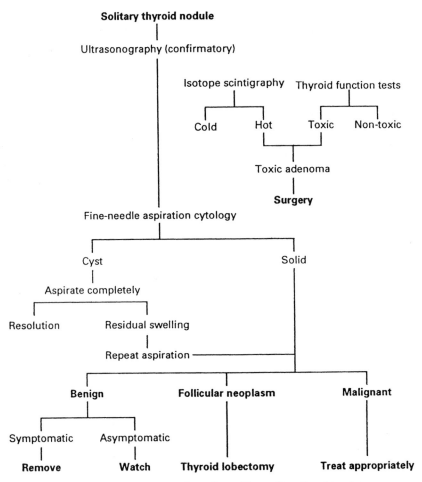

Solitary thyroid nodule
|
Ultrasonography (confirmatory)

Isotope scintigraphy   Thyroid function tests

Cold   Hot   Toxic   Non-toxic

Toxic adenoma
|
Surgery

Fine-needle aspiration cytology

Cyst   Solid

Aspirate completely

Resolution   Residual swelling
|
Repeat aspiration

Benign   **Follicular neoplasm**   **Malignant**

Symptomatic   Asymptomatic

Remove   **Watch**   **Thyroid lobectomy**   **Treat appropriately**

Fig. 19.6 Algorithm for management of a patient with a solitary thyroid nodule.

contains a carcinoma (often papillary) within its wall, and blood staining of the aspirate or a residual swelling after aspiration should raise the suspicion of malignancy. Cytology cannot distinguish between a follicular adenoma and follicular carcinoma, and surgery is needed if aspiration reveals a follicular neoplasm. Intra-operative frozen section does not always provide a definitive diagnosis but demonstration of carcinoma means that radical surgery is needed. In some cases, carcinoma is only revealed on definitive histopathological examination, and more radical re-operation is then indicated.

Other forms of neoplasia

All forms of cancer can produce a goitre, especially if the neoplasm arises from C-cells (medullary carcinoma) or lymphocytes (lymphoma).

HYPERTHYROIDISM

Thyrotoxicosis results from overproduction of T3 and T4; because of the feedback mechanism, serum TSH levels are reduced or undetectable. The three conditions which may produce thyrotoxicosis are primary thyrotoxicosis (Graves' disease), toxic multinodular goitre and toxic adenoma.

Primary thyrotoxicosis

This condition accounts for 75% of cases. It is an autoimmune disease in which TSH receptors in the thyroid are stimulated by circulating thyrostimulating immunoglobulins (TSI). The gland is uniformly hyperactive and very vascular, and is usually symmetrically enlarged. Histologically there

---

Goitres

- Physiological enlargement of the thyroid gland may occur during puberty or pregnancy.

- Non-toxic nodular goitre is associated with iodine deficiency and drug reactions; it is usually asymptomatic but can cause compression symptoms.

- Thyrotoxic goitre results from stimulation of the gland by TSH or TSH-like proteins, resulting in excessive production of T3 and T4. About 25% of cases of thyrotoxicosis are due to a toxic multinodular goitre (in which a longstanding non-toxic goitre develops one or more hyperactive nodules which function independently of TSH levels).

- Thyroiditis can produce diffuse painful swelling which may be subacute (de Quervain's disease) or autoimmune (Hashimoto's disease). Riedel's thyroiditis is a very care cause of painless thyroid swelling and tracheal compression where the gland is replaced by fibrous tissue.

- A solitary thyroid nodule often proves to be a conspicuous palpable nodule in a gland affected by multinodular goitre. True solitary nodules may be adenomas, cysts or cancers, conditions which are distinguished by fine-needle aspiration cytology, ultrasonography, isotope scans and function tests.

- Thyroid cancers can produce a goitre, particularly in the case of medullary carcinoma of the thyroid and lymphoma.

---

is marked epithelial proliferation with papillary projections into follicles devoid of colloid. TSI can cross the placental barrier so that neonatal thyrotoxicosis can occur.

Clinical features

The patient is usually a young female (sex ratio 8:1), and the condition can be familial. The thyroid is usually moderately and diffusely enlarged and soft, and because of its vascularity, a bruit may be audible.

High circulating levels of T3 and T4 increase the basal metabolic rate and potentiate the actions of the sympathetic nervous system.

Metabolic effects. The patient feels hot at rest and is intolerant of warmth. The skin is moist and warm because of peripheral vasodilatation and excess sweating. Weight loss is the rule despite increased appetite. Cardiac output is increased to meet the metabolic demands.

Sympathetic effects. Tachycardia is present, even during sleep. Palpitations can be troublesome and cardiac irregularities and arrhythmias (especially

atrial fibrillation) are common in older patients. The hands have a fine tremor, the upper eyelids are retracted (levator palpebrae superioris has some non-striated muscle which is innervated by the sympathetic nervous system) and there is lid lag, gastrointestinal motility is increased and there is general hyperkinesia. Anxiety and psychiatric disturbance may occur.

Other features. Exophthalmos is usual but not invariable. Ophthalmoplegia, pretibial myxoedema, proximal muscle myopathy, and finger clubbing are sometimes present. Menstrual irregularity and relative infertility can occur.

Diagnosis

The diagnosis is usually obvious clinically, although in patients with anxiety, distinction from neurosis can be difficult. Raised T3 and T4 levels coupled with low TSH levels are confirmatory. The TSH response to intravenous injection of TRH is absent owing to atrophy of the TSH-producing cells of the pituitary.

Treatment

Antithyroid drugs. These drugs block iodine incorporation into tyrosine and so prevent synthesis of T3 and T4. Carbimazole given in full blocking doses (30–60 mg daily in four divided doses) can render the patient euthyroid within 4–6 weeks. Maintenance doses (5–15 mg daily) can then be used. If full blockade has to continue, T3 (liothyonine sodium 10–20 µg daily, increasing at weekly intervals to 60 µg daily in divided doses) is added to provide hormone replacement. As primary thyrotoxicosis is likely to remit, carbimazole is normally stopped after 12–18 months. However, 60–70% of patients relapse within two years of stopping treatment, compliance may be low, and sensitivity reactions (skin rash, gastrointestinal upset and agranulocytosis) can occur. This means that radioactive iodine therapy or surgery is usually considered.

Radioactive iodine. Many consider that this is the treatment of choice, given that the risks of genetic damage are minimal in the patients and their offspring as long as it is not used in pregnancy. Patients require thyroxine replacement but can lead an otherwise normal life with little risk of recurrence.

Surgery. Subtotal thyroidectomy is a good form of treatment for many patients, especially those in younger age groups. Operative mortality and morbidity is low in experienced hands; 70% of patients are cured by surgery and recurrence is usually due to insufficient removal of glandular tissue. Hypothyroidism occurs in 20–25% of patients and low T3 and T4 levels with high TSH levels persisting for more than 6 months signals the need for lifelong thyroid hormone replacement.

The patient is rendered euthyroid before surgery with antithyroid drugs. Iodine is no longer given before surgery to reduce vascularity. Beta-adrenergic blocking drugs are commenced in the week before operation to counter sympathetic activity and make the gland less vascular, provided there is no cardiac failure, obstructive airways disease and diabetes (where they may mask hypoglycaemic symptoms). Propranolol is given in a dose of 40–80 mg every 6 hours, the aim being to reduce the pulse rate below 80 beats per minute. Long-acting preparations may be preferred. The drug is continued on the morning of operation and for 7 days thereafter to avoid 'thyroid storm' or 'thyrotoxic crisis'; excessive sweating or tachycardia after operation is an indication to increase the dose.

Toxic multinodular goitre and toxic adenoma

A toxic multinodular goitre is responsible for thyrotoxicosis in about 25% of patients. There is usually a long-standing non-toxic goitre in which one or more nodules become hyperactive and function independently of TSH levels. A single functioning adenoma is a rare cause of thyrotoxicosis (1–2% of patients). The adenoma secretes thyroid hormones autonomously, TSH secretion is completely suppressed and the remainder of the gland is nonfunctional.

Clinical features and diagnosis

Toxic multinodular goitre is commoner in older women, and cardiac complications such as arrhythmias are particularly frequent although exophthalmos is rare. Patients with a toxic adenoma hardly ever have exophthalmos, ophthalmoplegia or myopathy.

Isotope scans demonstrate one or more areas of increased uptake in toxic multinodular goitre, whereas in toxic adenoma, the nodule is 'hot' and the remainder of the gland is 'cold'.

Treatment

Treatment consists of removal of the hyperfunctioning glandular tissue by subtotal thyroidectomy (multinodular goitre) or lobectomy (toxic adenoma).

MALIGNANT TUMOURS OF THE THYROID

Thyroid cancer accounts for less than 1% of all forms of malignancy. As with all thyroid disease, females are more often affected (sex ratio 3:1). The three main types of thyroid carcinoma are papillary (50%), follicular (10–25%) and anaplastic (25–40%) cancers; the remainder are medullary carcinomas and lymphomas. The incidence of thyroid cancer is increased by exposure to ionizing radiation.

Papillary carcinoma

This tumour is rare after the age of 40 years. It presents as a slow-growing solitary thyroid swelling which is not particularly hard. Enlarged lymph nodes are palpable in one-third of patients and may be the only finding in some patients with a microscopic primary (a situation once misinterpreted as a 'lateral aberrant thyroid'), but distant metastases are rare. Occasionally, papillary carcinoma is discovered as an incidental finding in a gland removed for other reasons. Histologically, complex papillary folds lined by several layers of cuboidal cells project into what appear to be cystic spaces.

Treatment

The disease is commonly multifocal so that total or near-total thyroidectomy is indicated. Involved lymph nodes are removed but radical neck dissection is not necessary. Hormone replacement therapy (T3, 20 μg four times a day) is monitored by TSH estimations. Widespread metastases are rare but may be amenable to radioactive iodine therapy. The disease has an excellent prognosis with 10-year survival rates approaching 90%.

Follicular carcinoma

This disease typically presents as a solitary thyroid nodule in patients aged 30–50 years. Lymph node metastases are much less common than haematogenous spread and 20% of patients have deposits in the lungs, bone or liver. Histologically, malignant cells are arranged in solid masses with rudimentary acini. Venous invasion is common.

Treatment

Treatment consists of total thyroidectomy with preservation of the parathyroids. All palpable lymph nodes are removed and if tumour is present within them, a modified radical neck dissection is carried out. If a postoperative radioisotope scan reveals increased uptake in the skeleton or neck, therapeutic doses of radio-iodine are given. T3 is administered routinely to suppress TSH secretion. Plasma thyroglobulin levels should be undetectable after surgery and radio-iodine, and can be monitored as a marker of recurrent disease.

The disease is more aggressive than papillary carcinoma and the 10-year survival rate is 50%.

Anaplastic carcinoma

These rapidly growing highly malignant tumours tend to occur in older patients. Local invasion may involve the recurrent laryngeal nerve(s) and cause hoarseness, compress the trachea and cause dyspnoea and stridor, and compress the oesophagus and cause dysphagia. Invasion of the cervical sympathetic nerves may cause Horner's syndrome (contraction of the pupil, enophthalmos, narrowing of the palpebral fissure and loss of sweating on the face and neck). Pulmonary metastases are common.

Treatment

Resection is rarely possible but surgery can relieve tracheal compression. Radiotherapy or chemotherapy is of marginal value. The prognosis is poor and 70% of patients die within a year of diagnosis.

Medullary carcinoma

This tumour arises from the parafollicular C-cells which secrete calcitonin. There is hard enlargement of one or both thyroid lobes and cervical lymph nodes are involved in 50% of cases. The tumour may occur sporadically or as part of a multiple endocrine neoplasia (MEN) syndrome type II (Sipple's syndrome).

Calcitonin levels are elevated although the serum calcium remains normal. Calcitonin assay can be used to monitor progress and to screen relatives.

Treatment

Treatment consists of total thyroidectomy and dissection of the lymph nodes in the central compartment of the neck. Medullary carcinoma in MEN IIb syndrome is particularly aggressive and those affected rarely live beyond 30–40 years of age.

Lymphoma

Primary lymphoma of the thyroid is a rare complication of autoimmune thyroiditis. It is amenable to treatment by radiotherapy and chemotherapy.

THYROIDECTOMY

Technique

The gland is exposed through a transverse skin-crease incision placed midway between the sternal notch and thyroid cartilage. The deep cervical fascia is divided longitudinally in the midline and the strap muscles are separated. Each lobe is mobilized by dividing first the vessels supplying the superior pole, then the middle and inferior thyroid veins, and finally the inferior thyroid artery. Many surgeons first expose the recurrent laryngeal nerves so that

---

Thyroid cancer

- Thyroid cancers may arise from the epithelium (papillary 50%, follicular 10–25%, anaplastic 25–40%), parafollicular C cells (medullary carcinoma) or lymphoreticular tissue (lymphoma).

- Papillary cancers are rare after 40, are often multifocal, and spread to lymph nodes but rarely disseminate widely. Total or near-total thyroidectomy with removal of involved nodes is followed by T3 replacement therapy. 10-year survival rates approach 90%.

- Follicular carcinoma occur in the age group 30–50, spread preferentially by the bloodstream, and are treated by total thyroidectomy. Involved nodes require radical neck dissection, and residual neck or skeletal radio-isotope uptake signals the need for radio-iodine therapy. T3 is used routinely to suppress TSH production. The 10-year survival rate is 50%.

- Anaplastic carcinoma occurs in older patients, spreads locally and frequently gives rise to pulmonary metastases. Curative resection is rarely possible, radiotherapy/chemotherapy are of little value, and 70% die within 1 year.

- Medullary carcinomas secrete calcitonin, may involve both lobes and involve neck nodes in 50% of cases. They may be sporadic or part of MEN II. Treatment consists of total thyroidectomy and node dissection, and prognosis is frequently poor.

they can be protected from harm. The amount of thyroid tissue removed depends on the indication for operation. Care is taken to preserve the parathyroid glands. Haemostasis must be meticulous and drains are no longer used in closure. The layers of the neck are reconstituted with interrupted absorbable sutures and the skin is approximated with skin clips which are removed on the second postoperative day.

Complications of thyroidectomy

Haemorrhage

Early secondary haemorrhage should not occur if meticulous haemostasis is achieved before closure. If bleeding does occur, it can compress structures in the thoracic inlet leading to venous engorgement, tracheal compression and asphyxia. The wound must be reopened urgently, and the patient is intubated and taken back to theatre for exploration of the wound, removal of haematoma and control of bleeding.

Nerve damage

The external branch of the *superior laryngeal nerve* may be damaged during ligation of the vascular pedicle of the upper pole of the thyroid. Inability to tense the vocal cord results in a weak, hoarse deep voice. Anaesthesia of the mucous membrane of the upper larynx allows foreign bodies to enter the larynx more readily.

Damage to the *recurrent laryngeal nerve* is even more serious. Traction on a nerve causes temporary paralysis of a vocal cord in 5% of patients undergoing thyroidectomy, but recovery within 3 months is the rule. Division of a nerve paralyses the cord in the 'cadaveric' position (i.e. midway between the closed and open position). The normal cord on the other side compensates by crossing the midline in phonation, but the voice is altered in timbre and weak.

Bilateral nerve injury results in stridor and ineffective coughing when the endotracheal tube is withdrawn at the end of the operation. The tube is reinserted immediately and tracheostomy may be needed if there is no improvement within 10 days. The paralysis is originally flaccid but fibrosis draws the cords together and even if tracheostomy has been avoided, increasing dyspnoea on exertion may be troublesome. Laryngoplasty may be needed to reconstitute the cords; if this fails, permanent tracheostomy may be unavoidable.

The vocal cords must be examined to document their position and movement before and immediately after thyroid surgery for medicolegal reasons. All patients must be fully counselled about the risks of thyroid surgery beforehand; a forewarned patient is much less aggrieved than one who has not had the risks of surgery explained.

Hypothyroidism

Thyroid function is monitored after surgery in case replacement therapy is needed. The risk of hypothyroidism depends on the type of disease and extent of surgery.

Hypoparathyroidism

Damage to the parathyroids may lead to tetany, so that calcium levels and neuromuscular irritability are monitored after total or subtotal thyroidectomy).

Scar complications

A hypertrophic or keloid scar can develop, particularly when the incision has been placed low in the neck. Recurrent keloid is common after excision of the scar (with or without steroid infiltration) and re-operation is not advised lightly.

PARATHYROID GLANDS

Surgical anatomy and function

The development of the parathyroid glands is considered on page 232. The glands receive a rich blood supply from the inferior thyroid artery, the branches of which are a valuable guide to their position. Histologically the glands contain chief cells (classified as dark, light and water clear) which secrete parathormone; after the age of 5–7 years, eosinophil cells appear, the function of which is not known.

Parathormone (PTH) is a polypeptide hormone which maintains serum calcium levels in the range 2.25–2.6 mmol/l. Its secretion is controlled by the level of ionized calcium, the fraction which normally makes up 50% of the total plasma calcium (the remainder is protein-bound and not directly available). There is a dynamic reciprocal relationship between the levels of calcium and phosphate in extracellular fluid (ECF).

Calcium metabolism

Plasma calcium levels are kept constant by regulating the amounts absorbed from the intestine, deposited in or withdrawn from bone, and excreted in the urine. PTH and vitamin D are the main regulators, with an uncertain contribution from calcitonin.

Parathormone

PTH acts on two target organs:

- It mobilizes calcium from *bone* by stimulating osteoclastic activity
- It increases *renal* phosphate excretion and calcium reabsorption, and promotes renal conversion of less active forms of vitamin D to the highly active form, 1,25-dihydroxycholecalciferol. When there is excessive PTH secretion in hyperparathyroidism, hypercalcaemia results in increased excretion of calcium and risk of renal stone formation.

Vitamin D

1,25-dihydroxycholecalciferol promotes calcium absorption from the intestine, and augments the effects of PTH on osteoclasts, perhaps by an action on macrophages.

Calcitonin

Calcitonin inhibits osteoclast activity and may be used to treat conditions such as Paget's disease. However, it is doubtful whether it is involved in calcium homeostasis, and although its production

Table 19.1   Causes of hypercalcaemia
Hyperparathyroidism
Primary hyperparathyroidism
Tertiary hyperparathyroidism
Increased calcium absorption
Vitamin D excess
Sarcoidosis
Drugs (e.g. diuretics, lithium)
Excessive bone breakdown
Metastatic disease (particularly breast cancer)
Myeloma
Immobilization following multiple fractures
Ectopic secretion of PTH-like hormone
Cancer of bronchus
Cancer of breast

Table 19.2   Causes of hypocalcaemia
Hypoparathyroidism
Thyroid surgery
Parathyroid surgery
Hypoproteinaemia
Nephrosis (excessive protein loss)
Malnutrition (inadequate intake)
Cirrhosis (deficient synthesis)
Severe inflammation (e.g. burns, acute pancreatitis)
Vitamin D deficiency
Pseudohypoparathyroidism

increases in medullary carcinoma of the thyroid, there are no consistent changes in plasma calcium levels.

Hypercalcaemia and hypocalcaemia

Hypercalcaemia is a common biochemical abnormality and may be due to many causes other than excess PTH secretion (Table 19.1). Similarly, hypocalcaemia may be due to causes other than parathyroid removal or damage (Table 19.2).

HYPERPARATHYROIDISM

Primary hyperparathyroidism

In 90% of cases, primary hyperparathyroidism is due to an adenoma (Fig. 19.7), in 10% it results from hyperplasia (usually affecting all four glands), and in less than 1% it results from parathyroid carcinoma. Adenomas are normally small spherical brown nodules but can be 10 times larger than the normal gland. Most are single, but one-in-five patients have multiple adenomas. Histologically there is a mixed pattern of cells in which chief cells predominate. Hyperplasia is due to an increase in the number of chief cells, and by definition, the gland must be at least twice the upper limit of normal (i.e. weigh more than 70 mg).

Clinical features

Women are affected twice as often as men, and the disease is usually found in middle age. It is now diagnosed increasingly in asymptomatic patients who are found to have hypercalcaemia on routine biochemical estimations. If clinical manifestations occur, renal and bone effects predominate. Renal effects include nephrocalcinosis (speckled calci-

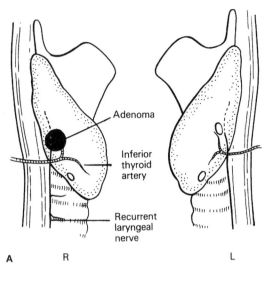

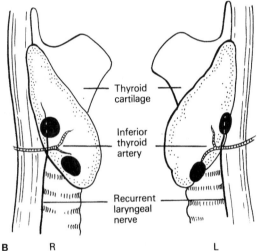

Fig. 19.7 Causes of primary hyperparathyroidism.
A Parathyroid adenoma. **B** Parathyroid hyperplasia.

fication) and formation of urinary calculi due to increased excretion of calcium and phosphate. Polyuria is an early sign of renal failure. Serum calcium levels must be checked repeatedly in all patients with urinary calculi, especially recurrent calculi, if hyperparathyroidism is to be diagnosed in time to avoid renal damage.

Bone damage used to be common but is now rarely seen as the disease is diagnosed earlier. Gross demineralization, subperiosteal bone resorption (seen typically in the middle and distal phalanges of the fingers), cysts in the long bones and jaw, and the moth-eaten appearance of the skull gave rise to the descriptive term, 'osteitis fibrosa cystica' (Fig. 19.8). Multiple fractures were once common.

Other manifestations of hyperparathyroidism include peptic ulceration, acute and chronic pancreatitis, lethargy and muscle weakness, and psychotic symptoms. The clinical picture of florid hyperparathyroidism is often summarized as one of 'bones, stones and groans'.

Diagnosis

If hyperparathyroidism is suspected, serum calcium and PTH levels must be measured on at least three occasions. PTH levels may be normal, but the detection of PTH in a patient with hypercalcaemia supports the diagnosis of primary hyperparathyroidism.

Other supportive findings include a low serum phosphate, hyperchloraemia (and an abnormal Cl/PO_4 ratio), and a raised 24-hour urinary calcium excretion. A *low* urinary calcium excretion should alert the clinician to the possibility of familial hypercalcaemic hypocalciuria, a disease of the renal tubules in which the parathyroids are normal. Alkaline phosphatase (skeletal) levels may be raised even if there is no radiological evidence of bone disease.

Treatment

The aim of treatment is to identify and remove overactive parathyroid tissue. The surgical approach

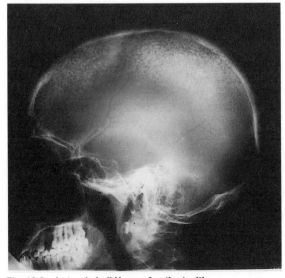

Fig. 19.8 Lateral skull X-ray of patient with hyperparathyroidism showing lytic lesions of osteitis fibrosa cystica.

is similar to that used for thyroidectomy. Each lobe of the thyroid is mobilized and all four glands must be identified and inspected. Normal parathyroids are smooth and brownish, their surface resembling the capsule of the liver. Enlarged glands are nodular. Immediate frozen section examination is used to establish the diagnosis and make certain that parathyroid rather than thyroid, thymus or fat has been identified.

In the majority of cases only one gland is enlarged and this is removed. If two or more glands are enlarged they should be removed, unless all four glands are enlarged and thought to be involved by hyperplasia, in which case all but a portion of one gland should be removed. In all cases the integrity of the recurrent laryngeal nerves must be protected.

If exploration fails to identify an adenoma or hyperplasia, the incision is closed and reoperation considered after thallium scintography (Fig. 19.9) and/or selective venous catheterization with PTH assay (to locate the abnormal source of PTH production). Recurrent hyperparathyroidism is approached in the same way.

Secondary and tertiary hyperparathyroidism

In secondary hyperparathyroidism there is oversecretion of PTH in response to low plasma levels of ionized calcium, usually because of renal disease or malabsorption. This is an increasing problem in patients on long-term dialysis for chronic renal failure, and is managed by giving 1-alpha-hydroxyvitamin D_3 (alfacalcidol) to increase calcium absorption and provide negative feedback on the parathyroids.

Excessive PTH secretion in secondary hyperparathyroidism may become autonomous, and is then termed tertiary hyperparathyroidism. This may occur after renal transplantation. Total parathyroidectomy may be needed with autotransplantation of parathyroid tissue equivalent in size to one normal gland into an arm muscle where it can be located readily if problems persist. Postoperatively, alfacalcidol and calcium are continued to heal bone disease and reduce the risk of recurrent hyperparathyroidism.

Hypoparathyroidism

A fall in ionized calcium levels gives rise to paraesthesiae ('pins and needles') in the hands and feet, and muscle cramps and spasms (tetany) which cause bunching and flexion of the fingers and toes. Respiratory obstruction with stridor due to spasm of the laryngeal muscles can prove fatal. Clinical signs

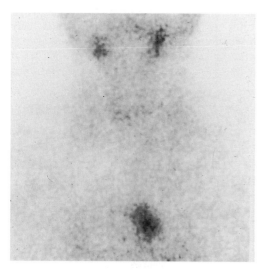

Fig. 19.9 Thallium-technetium subtraction scan showing excess thallium uptake in a mediastinal parathyroid adenoma.

Hyperparathyroidism

- Serum calcium levels are normally controlled by parathormone (mobilizes calcium from bone and increases renal phosphate excretion) and vitamin D (promotes absorption from the intestine and augments effect of PTH on osteoclasts), with an uncertain contribution from calcitonin.

- Hyperparathyroidism may be primary (90% adenoma, 10% hyperplasia, 1% carcinoma), secondary to renal disease/malabsorption (low serum Ca^{++} triggers PTH secretion) or tertiary (development of autonomous secretion in secondary hyperparathyroidism).

- Hyperparathyroidism is now normally diagnosed while asymptomatic but can produce renal effects (nephrocalcinosis, calculi and failure), skeletal effects (demineralization), gastrointestinal upsets (peptic ulcer, pancreatitis), and psychotic symptoms, i.e. 'stones, bones and groans'.

- The diagnosis of primary hyperparathyroidism rests on detection of hypercalcaemia and is supported by detection of circulating PTH in the presence of hypercalcaemia.

- Primary hyperparathyroidism is treated surgically by displaying all four glands and removing a gland enlarged by adenoma formation. If all four glands are involved by hyperplasia, all but a portion of one gland is removed.

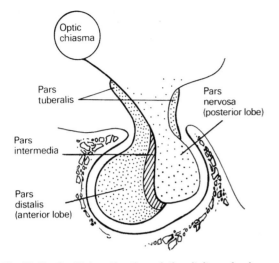

Fig. 19.10 Sagittal section through the pituitary gland.

include Chvostek's sign (twitching of the facial muscles on tapping the facial nerve), Trousseau's sign (spasm of hand and forearm muscles after applying a tourniquet to occlude the pulse), and Erb's sign (hyperexcitability of muscles on electrical stimulation). The patient is lethargic and depressed.

Blood levels of ionized calcium and PTH are low, and the electrocardiogram (ECG) shows a lengthened Q-T interval.

Acute hypoparathyroidism is treated by intravenous calcium gluconate (20 ml of a 10% solution given 4-hourly until calcium levels rise). Oral calcium (effervescent calcium gluconate) and vitamin D (cholecalciferol 20 000 units daily) are prescribed for maintenance. Calcium levels must be monitored regularly.

PITUITARY GLAND

Surgical anatomy

The pituitary gland is small, weighing only 500 mg. It is enclosed within a bony shell, the sella turcica, which is sealed superiorly by a fold of dura mater, the diaphragma sellae. The pituitary stalk connects the pituitary to the hypothalamus. The pituitary has two parts; the anterior pituitary or adenohypophysis, and the posterior pituitary or neurohypophysis (Fig. 19.10).

THE ANTERIOR PITUITARY

The anterior pituitary develops from an epithelial outgrowth from the pharynx (Rathke's pouch). Some cells are thought to be of neural crest origin and belong to the APUD system (p. 442). The anterior pituitary contains solid cords of secreting cells which can be classified as acidophil, basophil or chromophobe on staining with haematoxylin and eosin. On the basis of immunofluorescence and other specific stains these can be subdivided into cell types which secrete the polypeptides growth hormone, prolactin and adrenocorticotropic hormone (ACTH), and the glycoproteins luteinizing hormone (LH), follicle stimulating hormone (FSH) and TSH (Fig. 19.11).

The hypophysial stalk contains a portal venous system which connects capillaries in the median eminence of the hypothalamus with capillaries and sinusoids of the anterior pituitary, and carries neurosecretory hormones which stimulate or inhibit

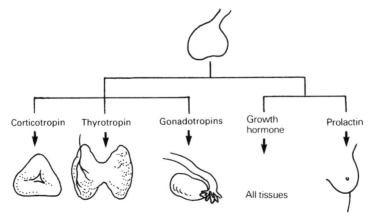

Fig. 19.11 The anterior pituitary hormones and their target organs.

specific endocrine cells in the pituitary. The most important messengers are growth hormone-releasing and -inhibiting factors, corticotropin-releasing factor (CRF), gonadotropin-releasing hormone (Gn-RH), TRH and prolactin-inhibiting factor (PIF). If the portal tract is divided, secretion of all anterior pituitary hormones is suppressed with the exception of prolactin, secretion of which is increased. A number of feedback loops ensure that the secretion of pituitary hormones is adjusted to need.

Functions of anterior pituitary hormones

Growth hormone (GH) has many functions besides growth regulation. It increases uptake of amino acids, promotes protein synthesis and increases the size of muscles and viscera. Lipolysis is increased and utilization of fatty acids is enhanced with production of ketosis. It has an anti-insulin effect (increased gluconeogenesis and decreased peripheral utilization of glucose), and in large amounts it augments milk secretion. Some of the growth-promoting effects are due to increased secretion of somatomedin from the liver and kidney. Growth hormone release is stimulated by stress, fasting and hypoglycaemia, and inhibited by bromocriptine and phenothiazines (e.g. chlorpromazine).

Prolactin is normally secreted in only small amounts and levels are highest at night. Secretion increases greatly in pregnancy, and prolactin is essential for lobulo-alveolar development of the breast and initiation of lactation. Release is increased by stress, oestradiol and phenothiazines, and inhibited by L-dopa and bromocriptine.

Corticotropin (ACTH) is a 39-amino acid polypeptide in man. The 4–10 amino acid sequence is similar to that of melanocyte stimulating hormone (MSH) and this accounts for the pigmentation associated with excess ACTH production. ACTH is secreted as part of a larger molecule with three constituents; pro-gamma ACTH, ACTH and beta-lipoprotein (LPH). Pro-gamma ACTH is thought to sensitize adrenal cells to ACTH, whereas LPH mobilizes fat (and by virtue of amino acid sequences shared with metencephalin and beta-endorphin, it may bind to opiate receptors and have analgesic properties). ACTH itself stimulates secretion of cortisol and adrenal androgens by the adrenal cortex. ACTH secretion is stimulated by CRF, which in turn is secreted in response to stress.

The three *glycoprotein hormones* each have alpha- and beta-subunits. The alpha-subunit is common to all three, while the beta-unit is specific and deter-mines the actions of each hormone. FSH stimulates follicle development towards the end of the menstrual cycle and the secretion of oestrogens by thecal cells. LH triggers ovulation and promotes formation of the corpus luteum and secretion of oestrogens and progesterone. In males, FSH stimulates spermatogenesis and LH (known in males as interstitial cell stimulating hormone) stimulates testosterone secretion by the Leydig cells (Fig. 19.12). TSH promotes thyroid growth and thyroid hormone secretion.

Tumours of the anterior pituitary

Functioning pituitary adenomas may result from overstimulation by hypothalamic factors. Initially small and confined within the gland (microadenomas), they grow slowly and can ultimately expand the sella turcica. Eccentric enlargement is common and asymmetry of the pituitary fossa can often be detected by lateral tomograms. Upward extension of the adenoma may stretch the diaphragm or herniate through it to compress the optic chiasma and cause visual defects. It is important that pituitary adenomas are detected before they enlarge the fossa or extend above it. Computerized tomography (CT) scan with contrast enhancement or a magnetic resonance image (MRI) is used to reveal the tumour and delineate its extent (Fig. 19.13). Three endocrine

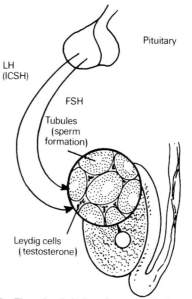

Fig. 19.12 The role of pituitary hormones in the control of male sexual function. ICSH is interstitial cell stimulating hormone.

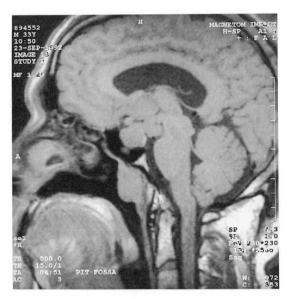

Fig. 19.13 MRI scan showing a pituitary tumour.

syndromes due to anterior pituitary disorders have surgical relevance.

Acromegaly

Excess secretion of GH occurs most often in early adult life and results in overgrowth of the soft tissues of the hands, feet and face, giving the patient 'large extremities' and a characteristically coarse face with bulging supraorbital ridges and protruding jaw. Endochondral ossification and periosteal new bone formation account for some of these changes. All viscera are enlarged and there is muscle hypertrophy, although muscle weakness and cardiac failure develop later. The skin is coarse and greasy and acne is common. Headaches, sweating and the carpal tunnel syndrome often develop. Glucose tolerance is impaired and galactorrhoea can occur in females. GH and somatomedin levels are increased and secretion is not suppressed by glucose or a meal.

Treatment is directed at restoring GH levels to normal. External radiation achieves this in 70% of patients, but only after 10 years, whereas radioactive implants act more quickly (see below). For small adenomas, trans-sphenoidal removal is the treatment of choice.

Although bromocriptine inhibits GH release, it achieves normal levels in only 20% of patients with acromegaly. Somatostatin analogues offer a more effective way of normalizing GH levels, and can be used to reduce the size of macroadenomas and treat recurrent or residual tumour.

Hyperprolactinaemia

Prolactin is the commonest hormone secreted by pituitary tumours. Hypersecretion results in galactorrhoea and amenorrhoea (due to suppression of gonadotropin secretion) in young women, while in males, gynaecomastia and impotence may result. Basal levels of prolactin are high, the nocturnal increase is absent, and the response to TRH and metoclopramide is dimished. It is important to exclude other causes of hyperprolactinaemia, notably administration of drugs such as metoclopramide.

To preserve pituitary function in younger patients, small adenomas are enucleated while larger tumours are treated by bromocriptine with monitoring to ensure that tumour expansion does not threaten visual integrity.

Cushing's disease

This may be due to a functioning adenoma of ACTH-secreting cells. Only 15% of cases show expansion of the pituitary fossa. Removal of the microadenoma or its irradiation will relieve symptoms.

Pituitary surgery and irradiation

Surgical hypophysectomy

The preferred approach for removal of a normal-sized gland or enucleation of a small adenoma is trans-sphenoidal. An operating microscope is used to approach the gland through the sphenoidal or ethmoidal sinuses (Fig. 19.14). The pituitary stalk is divided low so that diabetes insipidus is rare. Cerebrospinal fluid (CSF) rhinorrhoea is prevented by placing a free flap of muscle in the fossa. The transcranial approach is a major neurosurgical procedure and results in loss of sense of smell and diabetes insipidus; it is now used only to remove large tumours with suprasellar extension (often in combination with a trans-sphenoidal approach).

External radiation

The pituitary is radioresistant and at least 100 Gy is needed to affect function of the normal gland. Smaller doses (40–50 Gy) are used to treat acromegaly and Cushing's disease. A rotational

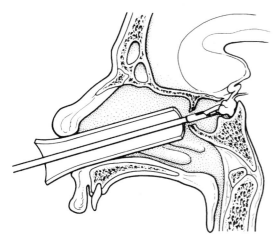

Fig. 19.14   Trans-sphenoidal removal of a pituitary adenoma.

technique avoids excessive irradiation of surrounding nervous tissue. Larger doses of radiation can be delivered by the narrow focused beam of heavy particles which are generated by a cyclotron.

Internal irradiation

Radioactive sources can be implanted by the trans-sphenoidal or transethmoidal route under radiological control (Fig. 19.15), although trans-sphenoidal surgery is now preferred. Yttrium[90] is a beta-particle emitter of high energy and short half-life (64 hours) and was once commonly used. Diabetes insipidus followed only if the hypothalamic nuclei were irradiated; CSF rhinorrhoea was an occasional complication.

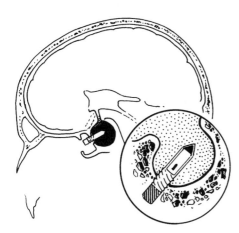

Fig. 19.15   Implantation of radioactive yttrium into the pituitary fossa.

Maintenance therapy

After total hypophysectomy, cortisol or cortisone replacement therapy is required for life (e.g. hydrocortisone 20 mg each morning and 10 mg in the evening), and all episodes of stress or trauma (including hypophysectomy itself) require additional cortisol or cortisone to cover the metabolic response. The patient is advised to wear a band or bracelet advising medical attendants that he is receiving steroid replacement therapy. Aldosterone secretion is unaffected and there is no need for mineralocorticoid replacement. TSH secretion is suppressed and hypothyroidism is avoided by giving thyroxine (0.1–0.2 mg daily). Diabetes insipidus is a common, often transient, complication of pituitary surgery or insertion of radioactive implants; polyuria can be relieved by intramuscular injection or intranasal instillation of the vasopressin analogue, desmopressin (DDAVP).

THE POSTERIOR PITUITARY

The neurohypophysis is part of a secretory and storage unit which includes the nerve cells of the supraoptic and paraventricular hypothalamic nuclei (Fig. 19.16). Fibres pass from these nuclei by the hypothalamo-hypophysial tract to the median eminence of the hypothalamus and posterior pituitary. The nerve cells secrete arginine vasopressin (antidi-

Tumours of the anterior pituitary gland
- The tumour may be detected while still small (microadenoma) or after it has expanded, often with upward extension to compress the optic chiasma.
- The three endocrine syndromes which have surgical importance are acromegaly, hyperprolactinaemia and Cushings disease.
- Acromegaly is due to excessive secretion of growth hormone (GH). Somatostatin analogues (or bromocriptine) can be used to normalize GH levels but small adenomas are treated by trans-sphenoidal removal while radiotherapy (usually by radioactive implants) can be used for larger tumours.
- Hyperprolactinaemia causes galactorrhoea and amenorrhoea in females and impotence and gynaecomastia in men. Small adenomas are usually enucleated while larger tumours are treated by bromocriptine.
- Cushing's disease may result from a functioning adenoma of ACTH secreting cells and is treated by removal or irradiation.

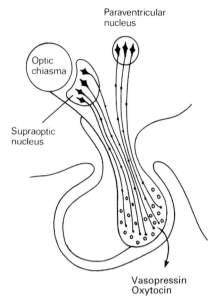

Fig. 19.16   The neurohypophysial system.

uretic hormone, ADH) and oxytocin, both of which pass down the nerve fibres to be stored in vesicles in the pituitary. The close anatomical relationship of the anterior and posterior pituitary has functional significance in that oxytocin release during lactation is paralleled by increased TSH and prolactin production, while the posterior pituitary may influence prolactin secretion by dopamine release.

Vasopressin has surgical importance. It increases permeability in the distal tubule, facilitating water reabsorption and reducing plasma osmolality. Its release is governed by osmoreceptors in the hypothalamus and baroreceptors in the heart and great vessels which react to changes in arterial and venous pressure. Failure of vasopressin secretion results in diabetes insipidus, and may follow trauma, irradiation, inflammation or neoplasia. Surgical hypophysectomy causes diabetes insipidus only if the hypothalamic nuclei are damaged irreparably by traction on the pituitary stalk or its high division. Diabetes insipidus produces thirst and polyuria, with passage of 5–12 litres of dilute urine (osmolality 50–200 mmol/l) in 24 hours. Plasma osmolality is normal (270–290 mmol/l) or slightly increased. Diabetes insipidus is treated by giving DDAVP.

Inappropriate vasopressin secretion can occur in patients with bronchial carcinomas or other para-endocrine tumours, and results in hyponatraemia, increased extra-cellular fluid (ECF) volume, and renal loss of sodium. Inappropriate secretion can also complicate positive pressure ventilation.

ADRENAL GLAND

Surgical anatomy and development

Each adrenal gland weighs approximately 4 g and lies immediately above and medial to the kidneys. The right adrenal lies in close contact with the inferior vena cava into which it drains by a short wide vein that can be difficult to ligate at surgery. The left adrenal vein is joined by the inferior phrenic vein before draining into the left renal vein (Fig. 19.17). The arterial supply of the glands comes from small vessels which arise from the aorta, and renal and phrenic arteries.

Each gland has an outer cortex and inner medulla. The cortex, like the gonads, is derived from mesoderm, whereas the medulla is derived from the chromaffin ectodermal cells of the neural crest. The cortex secretes steroid hormones, and while steroids are also secreted by the ovary, testis and placenta, only those synthesized in the adrenal cortex are called corticosteroids. The medulla is part of the sympathetic nervous system and its APUD cells (see p. 256) secrete catecholamines (adrenaline, noradrenaline and dopamine) and are supplied by preganglionic sympathetic nerves.

ADRENAL CORTEX

Cortical function

Microscopically the adrenal cortex has three zones

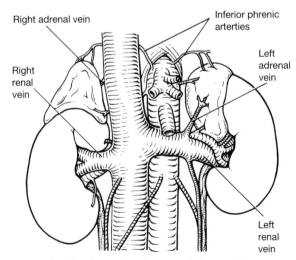

Fig. 19.17   Blood supply and venous drainage of the adrenal glands. IVC = inferior vena cava.

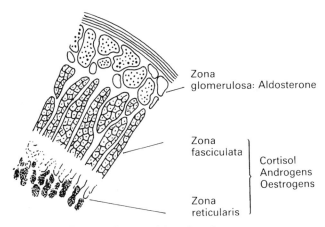

Fig. 19.18   Functional zones of the adrenal cortex.

(Fig. 19.18). The outer *zona glomerulosa* secretes the mineralocorticoid, aldosterone, while the *zona fasciculata* and *zona reticularis* act as a functional unit and secrete glucocorticoids (cortisol and corticosterone), androgenic steroids (androstenedione, 11-hydroxy-androstenedione and testosterone) and the inactive androgen and oestrogen precursor, dehydro-epiandrosterone sulphate (DHA-S). Precursors of aldosterone are also synthesized by the fasciculata-reticularis, as are small amounts of progesterone and oestrogen.

Control of adrenocortical secretion

Only a fraction of the amount of hormone needed daily is stored in the cortex; the hormones are secreted 'to order' and circulate free (5%) or bound to alpha-globulin.

Cortisol secretion (15–20 mg/day) is controlled by pituitary ACTH through a feedback loop (Fig. 19.19). ACTH also stimulates the secretion of androgenic steroids, and if excessive, this can cause virilization. Output of testosterone and androstenedione is normally low while DHA-S output is high.

Aldosterone is secreted in small amounts (100–200 µg/day) and circulating levels are low. Angiotensin is the main determinant of aldosterone production and is controlled in turn by renin liberated from the juxtaglomerular apparatus of the kidney in response to diminished perfusion (Fig. 19.20). Aldosterone secretion is also influenced by the concentration of sodium and potassium in adrenal blood, and can increase in response to high levels of ACTH.

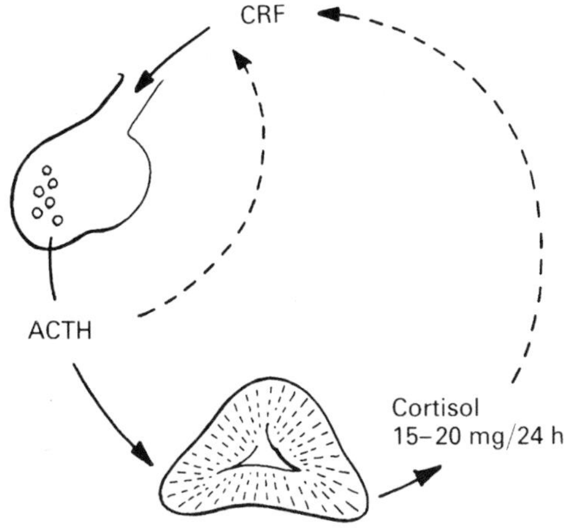

Fig. 19.19   **Feedback loop in the control of cortisol secretion.** CRF = corticotropin releasing factor.

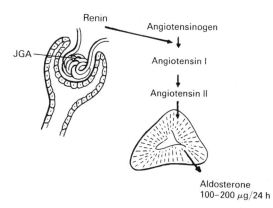

Fig. 19.20   **Control of aldosterone secretion by the adrenal cortex.** JGA = juxtaglomerular apparatus.

Functions of adrenocortical hormones

Cortisol. This is essential for life and has ill-defined but vital intracellular functions which protect the body against stress, maintain blood pressure and aid recovery from injury and shock. Important metabolic activities include protein breakdown (catabolic effect), increased gluconeogenesis and reduced glucose utilization (diabetogenic effect), and mobilization and redistribution of fat stores and water. In excess, cortisol has mineralocorticoid activity (promotes reabsorption of sodium and excretion of potassium) and can cause psychosis and mental instability. It has anti-inflammatory effects and reduces the number of circulating lymphocytes and eosinophils, inhibits fibroblastic activity, and depresses antibody formation (effects employed in the treatment of rejection after organ transplantation).

Aldosterone. It conserves ECF sodium by facilitating its exchange for potassium or hydrogen in the kidney (and to a lesser extent in all cells). In low potassium states the urine may be acid despite extracellular alkalosis because hydrogen ions are more available for exchange. Sodium retention increases plasma volume but this is limited by an exchange mechanism which can override the effect of aldosterone.

DHA-S. This is biologically inactive but is converted in fat, liver and other tissues to testosterone, its 5-alpha-reduced products, and oestrogen. Peripheral aromatization of DHA-S is the main source of oestrogen in postmenopausal women.

Adrenocortical hormones

- Cortisol secretion is controlled by pituitary ACTH. Cortisol protects against stress, maintains blood pressure and aids recovery from injury/shock. Its metabolic activities include protein breakdown, increased gluconeogenesis, reduced glucose utilization and mobilization/redistribution of fat and water.

- In excess, cortisol has mineralocorticoid activity, can cause psychosis and has anti-inflammatory effects (used in transplantation immunosuppression),

- Aldosterone secretion is controlled mainly by angiotensin levels (and thus by renin release from the juxtaglomerular apparatus during decreased perfusion).

- Aldosterone conserves sodium (by facilitating its exchange for potassium and hydrogen ions in the kidney) and is a major determinant of ECF conservation.

- Androgenic steroids and dehydroepiandrosterone sulphate (DHA-S) are also secreted by the adrenal cortex. DHA-S is converted to testosterone and oestrogen by fat and liver and this peripheral aromatization is the main source of oestrogen in postmenopausal women.

Cushing's syndrome

This syndrome was first described by the American neurosurgeon, Harvey Cushing, and results from prolonged inappropriate secretion of cortisol. The syndrome may be due to the following causes.

Tumours of the adrenal cortex (20%). Benign adenoma is the commonest adrenal cause of Cushing's syndrome. It is almost invariably unilateral and is more common in females. Histologically the tumour contains clear cells like those of the zona fasciculata, or compact cells like those of the zona reticularis. Autonomous cortisol secretion inhibits ACTH production so that the contralateral gland becomes atrophic and ceases to function (Fig. 19.21).

Adrenal carcinoma is a rare cause of Cushing's syndrome which occurs in young adults and children. The tumour grows to a large size and frequently metastasizes.

Pituitary disease (80%). Pituitary tumours causing Cushing's syndrome are usually basophil or sometimes chromophobe adenomas of ACTH-secreting cells. They range from tiny 'microadenomas' to large and even invasive tumours. Due to the continued ACTH secretion, both adrenals

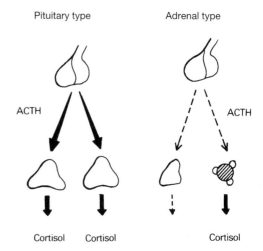

Pituitary type   Adrenal type

ACTH   ACTH

Cortisol   Cortisol   Cortisol

Fig. 19.21   Types of Cushing's syndrome. A Overstimulation of the normal adrenal glands by excess ACTH. **B** Oversecretion of cortisol by a functioning tumour of the left adrenal gland leading to suppression of function in the opposite gland.

become hyperplastic (Fig. 19.21). When Cushing's syndrome is caused by a pituitary tumour, it is referred to as Cushing's disease.

Ectopic ACTH production. Inappropriate secretion of ACTH-like peptide by tumours of non-pituitary origin (e.g. pancreas, bronchus, thymus) is a rare cause.

Clinical features

Cushing's syndrome occurs most frequently in young women. The most striking feature is truncal obesity and a 'buffalo hump' appearance due to redistribution of water and fat, and mooning of the face (in Cushing's original description, a 'tomato head, potato body and four matches as limbs'). As a result of protein loss, the skin becomes thin with purple striae, dusky cyanosis and visible dermal vessels. Proximal muscle weakness is prominent. Other features include increased capillary fragility, purpura, osteoporosis, acne, loss of libido, hirsutism, diabetes, hypertension and amenorrhoea. The clinical signs develop insidiously over years and are best recognized by reviewing old photographs. In some cases, the disease runs a fulminant course, particularly when due to an adrenal carcinoma or ectopic ACTH secretion. Electrolyte disturbances, cachexia, pigmentation, severe diabetes and psychosis are common in these patients.

Investigation

Before proceeding to adrenalectomy, the surgeon must be convinced:

- That cortisol secretion is outwith normal control. In Cushing's syndrome, plasma cortisol levels are high, diurnal variation is lost, and secretion is not suppressed by low-dose dexamethasone or increased by insulin-induced hypoglycaemia.
- That the primary problem is in the adrenal. In patients with a functioning adrenal tumour, ACTH cannot be detected in the plasma and urinary excretion of cortisol is not suppressed by high-dose dexamethasone (Fig. 19.22).
- That pituitary and ectopic sources of excessive ACTH production have been excluded. In Cushing's disease due to a pituitary adenoma, plasma ACTH levels are inappropriately high and urinary cortisol excretion is suppressed by dexamethasone (Fig. 19.22).
- That attempts have been made to localize the

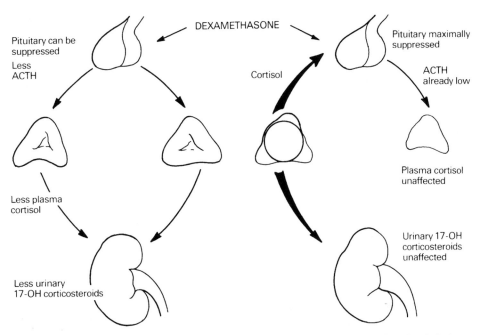

PITUITARY DEPENDENT   AUTONOMOUS ADRENAL TUMOUR

DEXAMETHASONE

Pituitary can be suppressed

Less ACTH

Cortisol

Pituitary maximally suppressed

ACTH already low

Less plasma cortisol

Plasma cortisol unaffected

Less urinary 17-OH corticosteroids

Urinary 17-OH corticosteroids unaffected

Fig. 19.22 **The principle of the dexamethasone test in differentiation between adrenal and pituitary causes of excess cortisol secretion.**

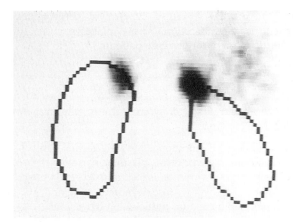

Fig. 19.23 Bilateral uptake of radio-labelled iodocholesterol in a patient with Cushing's disease.

lesion by techniques such as CT scan or isotope scintigraphy using radio-labelled iodocholesterol (Fig. 19.23).

Treatment

Adrenal tumours. Adrenal adenomas are rarely bilateral and unilateral adrenalectomy is indicated. As the other adrenal is suppressed and atrophic, cortisone replacement is needed until the pituitary-adrenal axis recovers. This may take 2 years and steroids must not be reduced or discontinued until a low-dose dexamethasone test shows normal function in the remaining gland.

Carcinomas of the adrenal should be removed whenever possible, and debulking of the tumour may be helpful if chemotherapy is to be used. Patients often present late with large tumours and lung metastases (Fig. 19.24). Even if adrenalectomy appears curative, adjuvant systemic therapy is advisable, and adrenal antagonists such as amino-glutethimide or metyrapone may help to control symptoms.

Pituitary disease. The symptoms of bilateral adrenal hyperplasia due to pituitary hyperfunction can be relieved by bilateral adrenalectomy, but at the expense of life-long steroid therapy. Furthermore, adrenalectomy removes all feedback control so that overproduction of ACTH and MSH produces characteristic skin pigmentation, while continued growth of the adenoma may compress the optic chiasma (Nelson's syndrome). Pituitary irradiation or surgery avoids the side-effects of adrenalectomy, and microsurgical removal of the adenoma is now the treatment of choice after pre-operative preparation with adrenal antagonists.

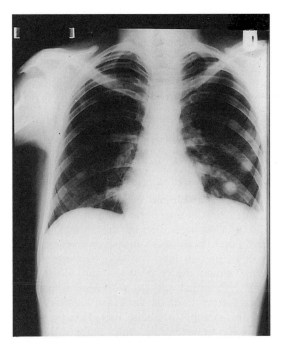
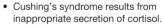

Fig. 19.24 Multiple pulmonary metastases in a patient with Cushing's disease due to an adrenal carcinoma.

Cushing's syndrome
- Cushing's syndrome results from inappropriate secretion of cortisol.

- The syndrome may be caused by tumours of the adrenal cortex (20%), tumours of the anterior pituitary (80%) or ectopic ACTH production (rare).

- The main clinical features are truncal obesity, buffalo hump, mooning of the face ('tomato head, potato body, four matchsticks as limbs'), thinning of the skin, livid striae and proximal muscle weakness.

- Adrenal tumours are usually treated by unilateral adrenalectomy but cortisone replacement is needed until the suppressed contralateral adrenal recovers.

- Before proceeding to adrenalectomy the surgeon should confirm that cortisol secretion is outwith normal control, that the primary problem is not pituitary or ectopic ACTH production, and that attempts have been made to localize the adrenal lesion (CT scan and radio-isotope scan with iodocholesterol).

- Pituitary disease is best treated by pituitary surgery (or irradiation) rather than by bilateral adrenalectomy. This avoids continued growth of the pituitary tumour, problems due to ACTH and MSH production (pigmentation, Nelson's syndrome) and the side-effects of adrenalectomy.

Hyperaldosteronism

Hyperaldosteronism is most commonly *secondary* to excessive renin secretion (and stimulation of the zona glomerulosa by angiotensin) in chronic liver, renal or cardiac disease.

Primary hyperaldosteronism (Conn's syndrome) is usually due to a benign adenoma and is commonest in young or middle-aged women. The adenoma is small, single and canary yellow, and composed of cells of the glomerulosa type; only rarely is the syndrome due to bilateral adrenal hyperplasia or multiple microadenomas. The high circulating levels of aldosterone suppress renin secretion.

Clinical features

Retention of sodium increases plasma volume and produces hypertension, often in association with headaches and visual disturbance (although serious retinopathy is uncommon). Potassium loss leads to worsening hypokalaemia, episodes of muscle weakness, and nocturnal polyuria. Unrecognized, the syndrome progresses to severe hypokalaemic alkalosis, with periodic muscle paralysis, paraesthesia and tetany.

Diagnosis

A low serum potassium in a hypertensive patient should signal the possibility of hyperaldosteronism. Diagnosis then rests on the following:

- *Confirm hypokalaemia.* This may require repeated blood sampling without an occluding cuff; 24-hour urine collection usually shows increased potassium excretion.
- *Demonstrate hypersecretion of aldosterone.* Plasma and/or urinary aldosterone levels are measured at 4-hourly intervals to allow for diurnal variations. Giving the aldosterone antagonist, spironolactone, should reduce blood pressure and reverse hypokalaemia.
- *Exclude secondary hyperaldosteronism.* Measurement of plasma renin is the critical investigation; renin levels are increased in secondary hyperaldosteronism but undetectable in the primary form. Spironolactone causes further increases in renin levels in secondary hyperaldosteronism.
- *Localize the adenoma.* If primary hyperaldosteronism is confirmed, attempts should be made to localize the adenoma by CT scanning (Fig. 19.25) or scanning with radio-labelled

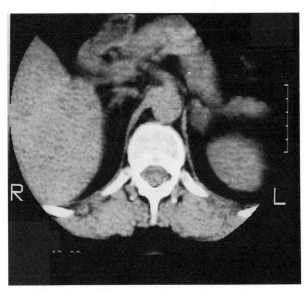

Fig. 19.25   CT scan showing a 1-cm adrenal adenoma immediately anterior to the left kidney.

iodocholesterol. Failure to 'see' an adenoma may mean that there is no discrete tumour and that the patient has bilateral cortical hyperplasia. Plasma cortisol levels should always be measured to exclude Cushing's syndrome.

Treatment

Primary hyperaldosteronism due to an adenoma is treated by removing the affected gland *after* correcting the hypokalaemia (by oral potassium and spironolactone or triamterene). Hyperaldosteronism due to adrenal hyperplasia can be cured by bilateral adrenalectomy but at such a high price that long-term drug treatment with triamterene or amiloride (potassium-retaining diuretics) is preferable.

Adrenogenital syndrome (adrenal virilism)

This syndrome is due to a genetically-determined enzyme defect which impairs cortisol synthesis. The resultant increase in pituitary ACTH production causes adrenal hyperplasia and inappropriate adrenal androgen secretion.

The effects depend on the patient's sex and age. Female infants show enlargement of the clitoris and varying fusion of the labial folds. Later, other signs of virilism appear leading to precocious heterosexual puberty. Young boys have precocious isosexual puberty. In both sexes growth is at first rapid, but the epiphyses fuse early so that the final height is stunted. Excess muscle growth produces an 'infant Hercules' appearance. Milder forms of the disease may affect older girls and cause hirsutism and acne.

The syndrome is treated by giving cortisol to supply the patient's needs and suppress ACTH production. Surgical correction of the genital abnormality may be needed. Rarely, virilism is due to an adrenal tumour, which is usually large and malignant.

Adrenal feminization

Exceptionally, a tumour of the adrenal cortex may secrete oestrogens. Such tumours are usually large and malignant. In the female there is isosexual precocity; in the male there is feminization with gynaecomastia, decreased libido and testicular atrophy. Treatment consists of removing the tumour although recurrence and metastatic spread are invariable.

ADRENAL MEDULLA

The adrenal medulla is not essential for life, and there are other collections of chromaffin cells in paraganglia in the retroperitoneum, mediastinum and neck. The normal adrenal medulla secretes catecholamines in the ratio 80% adrenaline to 20% noradrenaline, and also secretes the noradrenaline precursor, dopamine. Small amounts of catecholamines are excreted in the urine in free and conjugated form. Larger amounts are excreted as metabolites such as the meta-derivatives, metnoradrenaline and 3-methoxy-4-hydroxymandelic acid (VMA).

Adrenaline. This acts on alpha- and beta-adrenergic receptors to redistribute blood flow by constricting skin and splanchnic vessels and dilating those of the heart, skeletal muscles and brain. It causes tachycardia, induces anxiety and has metabolic effects which include hepatic conversion of glycogen to glucose and increased levels of circulating free fatty acids.

Noradrenaline. This acts on alpha-receptors to constrict all blood vessels and raise systolic and diastolic blood pressure.

Phaeochromocytoma

Phaeochromocytomas are tumours of the adrenal medulla (90% of cases) which secrete large amounts of adrenaline and noradrenaline, or tumours arising in extra-adrenal paraganglionic tissue (10% of cases) which secrete only noradrenaline. Virtually all phaeochromocytomas (99%) arise within the abdomen, 10% are multiple and 10% are malignant.

Benign tumours are usually about 5 cm in diameter, chocolate brown and highly vascular. Associated conditions are neurofibromatosis, medullary carcinoma of the thyroid (as part of MEN type II), duodenal ulcer and renal artery stenosis. If it presents in pregnancy, phaeochromocytoma can be mistaken for eclampsia and may cause maternal and fetal mortality.

Clinical features

Phaeochromocytomas usually present before the age of 50 years. Excess noradrenaline secretion causes hypertension, while adrenaline excess has metabolic effects (e.g. diabetes and thyrotoxicosis) and may even give rise to hypotension. Paroxysmal hypertension is the most characteristic symptom and is due to sudden release of catecholamines which may be precipitated by abdominal pressure, exercise or postural change. During an attack, the blood pressure may rise to 200/100 mmHg and there is headache, palpitation, sweating, extreme anxiety, and chest and abdominal pain. Pallor, dilated pupils and tachycardia are prominent features. In some patients, persistent and severe hypertension develops at the age of 30–40 years, often in association with severe retinopathy which can cause optic atrophy and blindness. Glycosuria is common, and the skin may be mottled with tingling of the extremities. Extra-adrenal phaeochromocytomas are always associated with persistent hypertension. On rare occasions, the tumour is in the bladder and micturition may precipitate a syncopal attack.

A few patients present with predominantly metabolic effects such as thyrotoxicosis, and occasionally, a phaeochromocytoma may cause sudden and unexplained death after trauma or surgery.

Investigation

All young hypertensives should be screened for a catecholamine-secreting tumour. The most reliable test is urinary VMA determination following a paroxysm. A CT scan may show the tumour or it can be demonstrated by scintigraphy after giving radio-iodine labelled meta-iodobenzylguanidine (MIBG), a substance which is taken up by catecholamine

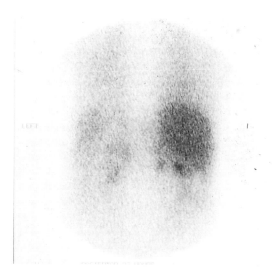

Fig. 19.26   Markedly excessive uptake of MIBG in a huge right-sided phaeochromocytoma.

precursors (Fig. 19.26). Abdominal ultrasonography, intravenous urography with tomography, arteriography and selective venous sampling are now used less frequently. Preliminary blockade (see below) is essential if invasive angiography is used.

Treatment

Surgical removal of the tumour is the treatment of choice. Use of alpha- and beta-blocking drugs has greatly reduced the risk of hypertensive attacks, tachycardia and arrhythmias during induction of anaesthesia or tumour handling. The patient should come to operation with blood pressure and pulse rate controlled. Adrenergic blockade also restores blood volume so that sudden hypotension after removal of the tumour is now unusual. To achieve blockade, the alpha-blocker phenoxybenzamine is started 7–10 days pre-operatively to control hypertension and the beta-blocker propranolol is added if tachycardia develops. Long-acting preparations are preferred. Beta-blockers are never given first as this can precipitate cardiac failure.

Atropine and thiopentone are best avoided, and enflurane is the preferred anaesthetic. Pulse and blood pressure are monitored throughout operation, and blood volume must be maintained. Short-acting alpha- and beta-blocking agents, sodium nitroprusside (which acts directly on vessels independent of adrenergic receptors and gives additional control of hypertension), and blood should be available.

Phaeochromocytoma

- Phaeochromocytomas are usually benign tumours of the adrenal medulla (90% of cases) but 10% arise in extra-adrenal paraganglionic tissue, 10% are multiple and 10% are malignant (the '10% tumour').

- Phaeochromocytoma may be associated with neurofibromatosis, medullary carcinoma of the thyroid (MEN II), duodenal ulcer and renal artery stenosis.

- The tumour presents clinically with hypertension which is often paroxysmal, and with metabolic effects, notably diabetes mellitus and thyrotoxicosis.

- All young hypertensive patients should be screened for phaeochromocytoma, and urinary VMA and catecholamine determination is the most reliable method of diagnosis.

- The location of a phaeochromocytoma is best defined by CT scanning and radiolabelled MIBG scanning.

- Treatment consists of adrenalectomy after careful preparation to control blood pressure and heart rate, and to re-expand blood volume (by alpha-adrenergic blockade with beta-blockade if tachycardia develops).

Non-endocrine adrenal medullary tumours

Ganglioneuromas.   These are benign, firm, well-encapsulated tumours of ganglion cells. They grow slowly, may become large, and can cause diarrhoea. Surgical excision gives excellent results.

Neuroblastomas.   These are highly malignant tumours arising from sympathetic nervous tissue. They are one of the commonest malignant tumours of infancy and childhood, and metastasize widely. About 75% of these tumours secrete catecholamines. Treatment by radical excision, radiotherapy and chemotherapy offers the only hope of benefit, although spontaneous regression has been reported occasionally.

Adrenal 'incidentaloma'

Increasing use of imaging has led to adrenal tumours being discovered as incidental findings in patients being investigated for other reasons. In such patients it is important to determine whether there is cortical or medullary hyperfunction. If there is no hyperfunction, the swelling is less than 5 cm in diameter, and fine-needle aspiration excludes malignancy, further investigation and exploration are unwarranted. Endocrine hyperfunction, a swelling larger than 5 cm, or the suspicion of malignancy are indications for further assessment and exploration.

Adrenalectomy

Indications

Normal adrenal glands were once removed as palliative treatment in postmenopausal women with breast cancer (to remove the source of DHA-S and prevent its peripheral conversion to oestrogen). Aromatase-inhibitors (e.g. aminoglutethimide) have made this approach obsolete.

Indications for adrenalectomy now include adrenal adenomas which may be producing Cushing's syndrome, Conn's syndrome or phaeochromocytoma. Bilateral adrenalectomy may be needed for bilateral tumours, nodular hyperplasia producing Conn's or Cushing's syndrome, and if pituitary surgery fails to eradicate Cushing's syndrome.

The adrenals are inaccessible whether approached from in front, from the side or from behind. The anterior transperitoneal route requires a large incision, inevitably causes ileus, has a high incidence of wound and respiratory complications (especially in patients with Cushing's syndrome), and is now seldom used.

Large tumours may be malignant and are best approached through a flank incision after removing a rib to allow access; if possible the diaphragm, pleura and peritoneum are left intact.

The posterior approach through the bed of the 11th or 12th rib is technically more difficult but has lower morbidity and patients have a quicker return to normal activity. If the pleura is breached in the course of adrenalectomy, it should be drained with a small suction drain for 24–48 hours.

Replacement therapy

Corticosteroid replacement is needed for life after bilateral total adrenalectomy, but may not be needed permanently after unilateral adrenalectomy. Replacement is best achieved by a combination of oral hydrocortisone (30 mg daily in divided doses) and the mineralocorticoid, fludrocortisone acetate (0.1 mg daily). If both adrenals are removed, or the remaining adrenal is non-functional, the operation must be covered by commencing steroid replacement at the time of surgery. Adequacy of replacement is assessed by monitoring blood pressure in the erect and supine position, by serum electrolyte determinations, and by patient well-being.

Hydrocortisone sodium succinate is water soluble and can be given by intravenous infusion during the first 24 hours. Further doses are given intramuscularly until the patient can take oral steroid. It cannot be overemphasized that blood pressure is the best guide to therapy. If hypotension occurs, 100 mg hydrocortisone sodium succinate is given immediately by intravenous injection, followed by 100 mg every 6–8 hours in a saline infusion. All adrenalectomized patients must be warned to increase the dose of steroid if stress or infection occurs. Failure to anticipate the need for added steroid may precipitate an 'adrenal crisis' with acute hypotension and collapse. Such patients should carry a 'steroid card' giving details of dosage and possible complications, and should be able to recognize the symptoms of adrenal insufficiency (i.e. loss of appetite, nausea, cramps, muscle pains and malaise). If such symptoms occur, the patient should take an extra two tablets of hydrocortisone and report urgently to his doctor.

OTHER SURGICAL ENDOCRINE SYNDROMES

APUDOMAS AND MULTIPLE ENDOCRINE NEOPLASIA

The APUD cell series

Distributed throughout the body are cells which have in common the capacity to store amines (e.g. catecholamines), take up their precursors (e.g. dopamine) and possess the decarboxylating enzymes necessary for their synthesis. The term APUD is an acronym denoting *A*mine *P*recursor *U*ptake and *D*ecarboxylation. The cells can be demonstrated by specific histochemical and immunofluorescent techniques.

It is thought that these cells migrate from neural ectoderm to endocrine organs and to the respiratory and gastrointestinal tract. Examples of APUD cells in endocrine organs are the ACTH-secreting cells of the anterior pituitary, catecholamine-secreting cells of the adrenal medulla, and calcitonin-secreting cells of the thyroid. In the gastrointestinal tract, APUD cells are present as single cells (e.g. argentaffin cells of the small intestine) or as large conglomerates, as in the pancreatic islets. The products of gastrointestinal APUD cells include 5-hydroxytryptamine and histamine, and a large number of polypeptide hormones (e.g. secretin, gastrin, cholecystokinin, enteroglucagon, somatostatin, vasoactive intestinal peptide).

Hyperplasia and tumours of any APUD cells can produce specific endocrine syndromes. Occasionally, they give rise to ectopic hormone production, as in the secretion of ACTH by bronchial tumours.

Multiple endocrine neoplasia (MEN) syndromes

In MEN syndromes, patients develop benign or malignant tumours in more than one endocrine gland. The aetiology of the syndromes is uncertain but they are inherited as autosomal dominant traits of variable penetrance and expression. The glands most often affected are the anterior pituitary, adrenal medulla, pancreas and C-cells of the thyroid. Although the cells which make up the parathyroid glands are derived from pharyngeal pouch endoderm, parathyroid hyperplasia and adenomas are also found in these syndromes.

MEN type I

This form of the syndrome is characterized by hyperplasia and/or tumours of the parathyroid, pancreatic islets and anterior pituitary. There may also be non-functioning tumours of the thyroid, pituitary, adrenal cortex, soft tissues (lipomas), and functioning carcinoid tumours of the gut or lungs. The earliest biochemical sign in affected individuals is hypercalcaemia from hyperparathyroidism, or hyperprolactinaemia from an asymptomatic pituitary tumour. Families are often uncovered when the index patient presents dramatically, as for example with small bowel perforation or bleeding due to the Zollinger-Ellison syndrome (see below), or hypoglycaemia due to an insulinoma of the pancreas. Family members should be screened by measurement of fasting serum calcium and other hormonal markers such as prolactin. Once the genetic abnormality responsible has been defined and the gene cloned, screening may be feasible on a blood sample.

Affected individuals may have mixed pancreatic tumours which produce a variety of hormones (e.g. gastrin, insulin and glucagon). Acromegaly is rare and prolactin-secreting tumours are more common. If a person in an affected kindred is shown to have hypercalcaemia, he must be kept under close surveillance for biochemical or clinical signs of other forms of endocrine overactivity. In some cases, familial hyperparathyroidism occurs without involvement of other endocrine glands.

Treatment is directed at the dominant clinical or biochemical feature. For example, pancreatic endocrine tumours are localized by ultrasound or CT scanning and removed as necessary (see Ch. 34). Hypercalcaemia is treated by parathyroid surgery.

Diseased glands are excised, while four-gland hyperplasia may be treated by excising all four glands and implanting small fragments from the most normal gland into an accessible site such as the forearm. This allows easy identification and further removal of parathyroid tissue if hypercalcaemia recurs.

MEN type II

This variant is also inherited as an autosomal dominant condition and is characterized by medullary carcinoma of the thyroid, phaeochromocytoma and parathyroid hyperplasia. Three subtypes are described:

- Familial medullary thyroid carcinoma alone.
- MEN type IIa consisting of medullary thyroid carcinoma (all cases) with phaeochromocytomas and/or parathyroid hyperplasia. The phaeochromocytomas are often bilateral but rarely malignant.
- MEN type IIb consisting of medullary thyroid carcinoma, bilateral phaeochromocytomas (but no parathyroid abnormality), and complex neural abnormalities including mucosal neuromas, thickened nerves (e.g. corneal nerves) and ganglioneuromatosis of the gut. These patients have a typical facies with thick blubbery lips, irregular dentition, and a Marfanoid body habitus.

All of these syndromes are diagnosed by detecting high levels of circulating calcitonin, if necessary after provocation by calcium or pentagastrin. In some cases, diagnosis is achieved when the thyroid abnormality still consists of C-cell hyperplasia, the forerunner of medullary thyroid cancer. The thyroid disorder is treated by total thyroidectomy and dissection of nodes from the central compartment of the neck (modified block dissection).

Phaeochromocytomas are diagnosed by determination of urinary VMA and catecholamine excretion, and localized by CT scanning and met-iodo benzylguanidine (MIBG) scanning (see p. 255). Adrenal medullary hyperplasia is a precursor of phaeochromocytoma, and can also be diagnosed by increased MIBG uptake. Surgical treatment of the adrenal medullary abnormality must take precedence over treatment of thyroid and parathyroid disease, as anaesthesia and surgery in patients with undiagnosed or untreated phaeochromocytoma can be life-threatening.

The genetic abnormality in MEN IIa syndrome has now been localized to the pericentromeric region of chromosome 10. Once the abnormality has been identified with certainty, screening will be possible on the basis of a single blood sample.

Carcinoid tumours and the carcinoid syndrome

Carcinoid tumours can occur in any part of the gastrointestinal tract or respiratory tree. They are found most frequently in the appendix as incidental findings in a patient presenting with acute appendicitis, and account for 85% of all appendiceal tumours. The carcinoid is usually near the tip of the appendix, is usually less than 1 cm in diameter, and is dealt with by appendicectomy as metastases are exceptional. Carcinoid tumours larger than 2 cm in diameter are rare but may have spread to lymph nodes and are best treated by right hemicolectomy. Liver metastases are extremely rare in patients with appendiceal carcinoids, but carcinoids of the small intestine frequently spread to lymph nodes, and in 10% of cases there are liver metastases by the time the patient presents with obstructive symptoms or bleeding.

Carcinoids in any site produce 5-hydroxytryptamine (5-HT) and other biologically active amines and peptides. In the case of gut carcinoids, these products are normally inactivated by the liver. However, liver secondaries secrete these substances directly into the systemic circulation giving rise to a carcinoid syndrome of periodic flushing, diarrhoea, bronchoconstriction, wheezing and distinctive red-purple discolouration of the face. Right-sided heart disease, notably pulmonary stenosis, may result and can prove fatal.

The diagnosis of carcinoid syndrome is confirmed by detecting 5-hydroxy-indoleacetic acid (a breakdown product of 5-HT) in the urine. If the primary tumour is causing symptoms it should be removed surgically if possible (e.g. right hemicolectomy, small bowel resection, lung resection). Hepatic metastases can be dealt with by excising the involved liver lobe or enucleating the deposits in an attempt to gain symptomatic relief. Alternatively, hepatic metastases may be de-arterialized by hepatic artery ligation or angiographic embolization.

Attempts have been made to relieve symptoms by blocking 5-HT synthesis (e.g. alphamethyldopa) or action (e.g. methysergide), but prevention of 5-HT release by somatostatin analogues or alpha-adrenergic antagonists may be more useful. Chemotherapy (e.g. 5-fluorouracil) is sometimes effective.

20
Cardiac surgery

CONTENTS

Surgery has an important role in the management of many types of heart disease, both congenital and acquired. Ischaemic heart disease is a major cause of morbidity and death in which surgery is now used increasingly. Although relatively simple procedures had been developed for the treatment of congenital heart defects, satisfactory correction of intracardiac anomalies only became feasible with the development of safe cardiopulmonary bypass in the 1950s. Replacement or repair of diseased valves followed in the early 1960s, and aortocoronary bypass surgery for ischaemic disease had become widely established by the end of that decade. The majority of cardiac operations now rely on cardiopulmonary bypass with an extracorporeal circuit (see below) which needs supervision by a trained perfusionist. Patients are usually in the operating theatre for 3 or 4 hours and require intensive care for the first 24 hours after surgery.

PRINCIPLES OF SURGICAL TREATMENT

Rational surgical treatment of heart disease requires:

- Accurate assessment of the patient and his cardiac condition
- Knowledge of the natural history of the condition
- An understanding of the potential risks and benefits of the various forms of management (surgical and non-surgical) that are available.

Assessment of the patient

Cardiac assessment

Patients being considered for cardiac surgery are usually first referred to a cardiologist because of symptoms such as chest pain or dyspnoea, or because an abnormality, usually a heart murmur, has been found incidentally on physical examination. The history, physical examination, electrocardiogram (ECG), chest X-ray, and echocardiogram usually enable the cardiologist to make a precise diagnosis of the heart condition. It is then important to assess the severity of the disease and its effects on the heart itself, the lungs and other organs. Cardiac catheterization and angiocardiography are usually undertaken once surgical treatment is contemplated, but are sometimes used as an aid to diagnosis or as a means of assessing the results of operation.

Cardiac catheterization is used to record pressures and measure oxygen saturation in the major vessels and heart chambers. This allows assessment of the severity of obstruction caused by a stenotic valve (Fig. 20.1), and permits calculation of the amount of blood being 'shunted' through abnormal communications such as atrial or ventricular septal defects.

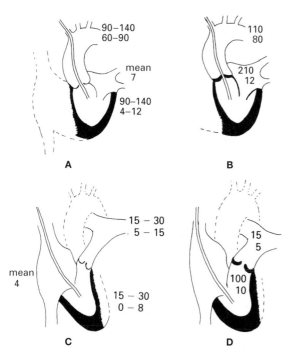

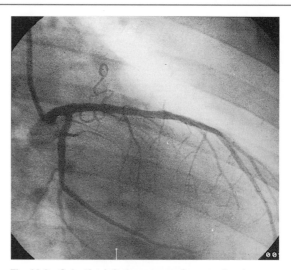

Fig. 20.2   Selective left coronary angiogram showing appearances after balloon dilatation.

Fig. 20.1   Cardiac catheterization. (Top) Catheter inserted via systemic artery showing **A** normal left heart pressures and **B** pressure in aortic stenosis. (Bottom) Catheter inserted via systemic vein showing **C** normal right heart pressures and **D** pressure in pulmonary stenosis.

Angiocardiography (Fig. 20.2) or *selective coronary angiocardiography* (Fig. 20.3) allow clear delineation of abnormalities by injecting radio-opaque contrast medium into a heart chamber or coronary artery during cineradiography.

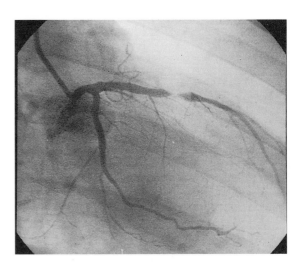

Fig. 20.3   Selective left coronary angiogram, showing stenosis of descending artery.

General assessment

Pulmonary, renal and hepatic function must be assessed. Coagulation status is checked routinely. Lung function is commonly compromised by chronic bronchitis, while liver function is impaired in those with long-standing cardiac failure. Patients with coronary artery disease frequently have evidence of significant vascular disease elsewhere, e.g. a carotid bruit, which merits further investigation. Dental sepsis must be eradicated before cardiac surgery.

Some patients requiring valve replacement may need long-term anticoagulation if a mechanical valve prosthesis is used (see below), so that it is important to make sure that there are no concurrent diseases, e.g. peptic ulcer, which preclude anticoagulation.

With current standards of anaesthesia, surgery and peri-operative care, only very major abnormalities of other systems make surgery inadvisable. The commonest contraindication to cardiac surgery is malignant disease of poor prognosis.

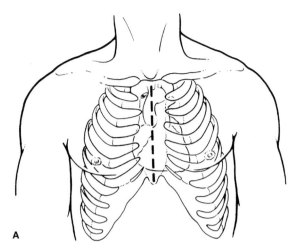

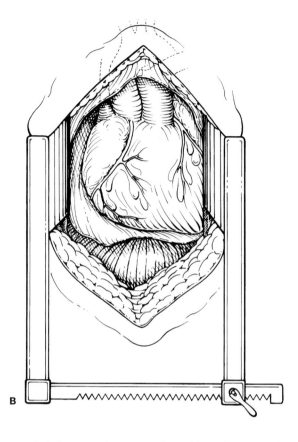

Fig. 20.4 Surgical approach to the heart. A vertical sternotomy incision. **B** Right atrium and ascending aorta exposed.

Natural history of the cardiac condition

Knowledge of the natural history of the heart condition has a major influence on the decision to recommend surgery and on its timing. For example, symptomatic aortic stenosis carries a poor prognosis and early surgery is advisable. On the other hand, ventricular septal defects often close spontaneously in childhood and can be left alone unless there is a large pulmonary blood flow. Atrial septal defects usually cause heart failure in middle life so that elective surgery is advised, even in asymptomatic patients.

Left main coronary artery disease has a poor prognosis without surgery, and triple vessel disease has a worse outlook than single or double vessel disease. On the other hand, the prognosis for patients with single or double vessel disease is generally good and not greatly altered by surgery.

Therapeutic possibilities

The surgeon must be fully familiar with the measures available to the cardiologist and understand the effects of drugs used. The decision to advise surgery is not always easy and knowledge of the natural history of the disease has to be balanced against the hazards of operation, and the long-term results of surgery. For example, closure of atrial

septal defects carries a very low risk and surgery is advised even in symptom-free patients for good long-term results. The low risk of mitral valvotomy makes this operation advisable relatively early in the natural history of mitral stenosis. The greater risk of valve replacement and continuing problems with prosthetic valves means that this operation is less lightly advised.

Surgical treatment of heart disease has two main goals:

1. *Relief of symptoms* by improving cardiac function. Examples are the treatment of exertional dyspnoea due to mixed mitral disease by valve replacement, and relief of angina by coronary artery bypass grafting. Mild symptoms well managed by medical measures usually do not warrant surgery, while severe symptoms or a poor response to conservative treatment usually indicate the need for operation.

2. *Alteration of the natural history of the disease.* Examples are (a) resection of aortic coarctation to avoid hypertension and its complications; (b) treatment of Fallot's tetralogy to avoid the thrombotic

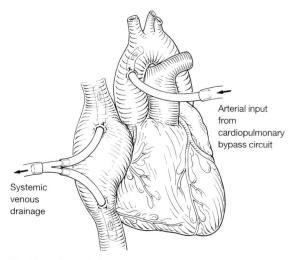

Fig. 20.5 Cannulation for cardiopulmonary bypass.

Arterial input from cardiopulmonary bypass circuit

Systemic venous drainage

complications of polycythaemia or death during a cyanotic spell; and (c) treatment of severe aortic stenosis to prevent life-threatening myocardial damage.

CARDIOPULMONARY BYPASS

Cardiopulmonary bypass is a means of removing systemic venous blood from the body, oxygenating it, and returning it to the systemic arterial system. The blood is returned at reasonably physiological pressure, devoid of gas bubbles or solid particles, at a controlled temperature, and at a rate capable of maintaining normal tissue metabolism.

Surgical approach to the heart

Vertical sternotomy is usually employed. The sternum is split longitudinally in the midline and the pericardium is opened to display the heart and great vessels (Fig. 20.4). Cardiac surgery results in adhesions between the heart and pericardial sac or sternum, increasing the difficulty of further operations.

Cardiopulmonary bypass circuit

Systemic venous blood is removed through two large plastic cannulas inserted into the superior and inferior vena cava respectively through incisions in the right atrium, or through a single large cannula inserted into the right atrium. Oxygenated blood is returned to the systemic circulation through a cannula inserted high in the ascending aorta (Fig. 20.5).

Oxygenators are of two types. *Bubble oxygenators* achieve gas exchange by bubbling a mixture of 95% oxygen and 5% carbon dioxide through a column of blood (Fig. 20.6). Gas bubbles are removed by passing the blood through a defoaming sponge before collecting it in a reservoir and returning it to the patient. *Membrane oxygenators* achieve gas exchange by bringing the blood and gases into close proximity,

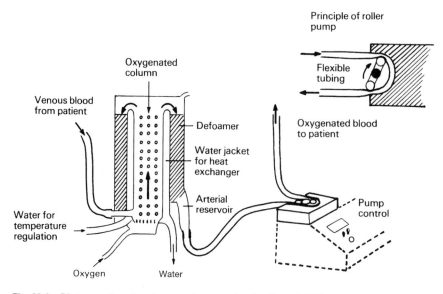

Fig. 20.6 Diagram of cardiopulmonary bypass circuit using a bubble oxygenator.

separating them only by a thin gas-permeable membrane.

The temperature of the returning blood is controlled by a *heat exchanger* (Fig. 20.6) in the oxygenator. This allows the blood to be warmed to 37°C, or to be cooled to induce systemic hypothermia.

A roller pump returns blood to the patient at an even arterial perfusion pressure of between 50 and 100 mmHg. Lack of normal pulsatile pressure does not appear deleterious, although roller pumps are now available which produce pulsatile flow.

Hazards of cardiopulmonary bypass

Before instituting bypass, the extracorporeal circuit is filled with isotonic fluid such as Ringer's lactate. Air embolus is meticulously avoided by excluding air from the arterial side of the circuit and removing all air from the heart chambers at the end of the operation before allowing ejection into the aorta. Intracardiac thrombi and fragments from calcified heart valves can also act as emboli and must be removed.

Clotting in the extracorporeal circuit is avoided by injecting heparin (3 mg/kg) into the patient's circulation before inserting the cannulas. Additional heparin may be needed during long operations, and is neutralized with protamine once the bypass procedure has been completed. Although the extracorporeal circuit is sterile, a broad-spectrum antibiotic is usually given during operation to reduce the risk of bacteraemia.

Myocardial protection

In most cardiac operations the ascending aorta is cross-clamped once cardiopulmonary bypass has been established. This interrupts flow into the coronary arteries and renders the myocardium ischaemic, it allows the aortic root to be opened to give access to the aortic valve, and it helps to provide a bloodless, immobile and relaxed heart. Interruption of coronary flow causes ischaemic cardiac arrest within a few minutes, and increasing myocardial damage after 30–45 minutes. If aortic cross-clamping has to be maintained for more than 30 minutes (as in valve replacement), some form of myocardial protection is required.

Protection is now usually achieved by cooling and arresting the heart (cardioplegia) by infusing either cold (4–10°C) isotonic crystalloid solution with a high potassium content (14–30 mmol/l), or chilled blood with added potassium. The aim is to produce prompt potassium-induced arrest and reduce metabolic requirements by local hypothermia. Cardio-

plegic protection is combined with topical irrigation of the heart and pericardial sac with large volumes of cold (4°C) saline, and by systemic cooling using the heat exchanger within the extracorporeal circuit. Systemic cooling to 28–30°C decreases general metabolic requirements and provides a margin of safety if cardiopulmonary bypass is relatively inadequate. More profound hypothermia (20°C) may be needed to avoid rewarming of the myocardium by non-coronary collateral flow, an important factor in coronary disease where collateral flow may be increased. It is now possible to have safe cardiac arrest for 2 hours or more, sufficient for most cardiac operations.

The myocardium rewarms and regains its activity promptly once coronary flow is restored. Ventricular fibrillation is common during rewarming and is sometimes induced deliberately to prevent ejection of blood until air has been removed. Defibrillating paddles are used to restore an effective beat.

Incisions in ventricular muscle impair contractility and access is obtained through the atria or major vessels whenever possible (Fig. 20.7). Incisions are closed with continuous non-absorbable sutures.

VALVULAR HEART DISEASE

Types of valvular disease

Mitral valve disease. This is usually due to rheumatic fever, although a history of rheumatic fever is not always obtained. The valve may become regurgitant due to annular dilatation during the

---

Open-heart surgery

- Cardiopulmonary bypass removes systemic blood (via cannulas in the inferior and superior venae cavae), oxygenates it, and returns it to the systemic circulation (via an aortic cannula).

- Incorporation of a heat exchanger in the extracorporeal circuit allows blood to be warmed to 37°C or cooled to induce systemic hypothermia.

- Potential hazards of extracorporeal bypass include air embolus, thromboembolism, and introduction of infection.

- During cardiopulmonary bypass, the ischaemic myocardium is protected by potassium-induced cardiac arrest and local cooling (achieved by infusing crystalloid with a high potassium content at 4–10°C).

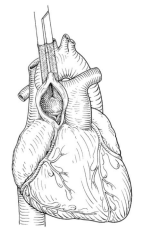

Aortic valve exposed via incision in aorta

A

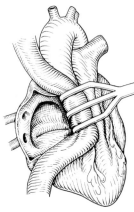

Mitral valve exposed via incision in left atrium Heart retracted

B

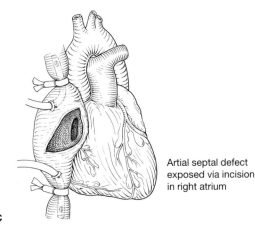

Artial septal defect exposed via incision in right atrium

C

Fig. 20.7 Surgical exploration of intracardiac structures with cardiopulmonary bypass.

acute episode. Surgery is usually required for the late results of chronic inflammation. These may be:

- Predominant *stenosis* due to commissural fusion and leaflet thickening
- Predominant *regurgitation* due to annular dilatation and leaflet retraction
- A *mixed lesion.* Valve calcification is common. Less commonly, mitral regurgitation is due to chordal rupture, leaflet degeneration, infarction or rupture of papillary muscle as a result of ischaemic heart disease, or left ventricular dilatation in severe cardiac failure.

Aortic valve disease. This may also be due to rheumatic fever with predominant stenosis, predominant regurgitation, or a mixed lesion. Calcification occurs in long-standing disease. A congenital bicuspid aortic valve may be stenotic, but stenosis in such cases is more often a late manifestation of calcification. Syphilis and dissecting aortic aneurysm are less common causes of aortic regurgitation.

Tricuspid valve disease. This may be due to rheumatic fever, congenital abnormality, or 'functional' annular dilatation in patients with mitral stenosis and severe pulmonary hypertension.

Pulmonary valve disease. This is usually congenital stenosis with commissural fusion or hypoplasia of the valve annulus.

Infective endocarditis. This may affect any diseased heart valve and cause rapid deterioration in its function.

Conservative surgery for valve disease

Reasonable haemodynamic function of the patient's own valve is preferable to that of any prosthetic valve, so that valves are conserved if at all possible.

A stenosed mitral valve may be opened by *mitral valvotomy* without the need for cardiopulmonary bypass. A finger is inserted through a small incision in the left atrial appendage and used to guide a dilator passed through the left ventricular apex into the mitral orifice; rapid opening of the dilator breaks down commissural fusion.

Pulmonary and *aortic valvotomy* are dealt with by dividing the fused commissures under direct vision using cardiopulmonary bypass.

Regurgitant valves are less easy to conserve although mitral and tricuspid regurgitation due primarily to annular dilatation can be dealt with by annuloplasty (i.e. sewing in a rigid or semi-rigid ring to maintain annular dimensions). Elongated chordae can be shortened, and limited areas of flail leaflets due to chordal rupture can be resected to restore valve competence.

Valve replacement

Using cardiopulmonary bypass the diseased valve is excised, leaving a rim to which the prosthesis is sutured. It is often necessary to remove calcium from the valve annulus. The large choice of available prostheses reflects continuing problems with design and durability; in general there are two types of prosthetic valve.

Mechanical valves are made of non-biological materials (e.g. metal alloys) and do not mimic natural valves. The Starr-Edwards caged ball valve and the Bjork-Shiley tilting disc valve are perhaps the best-known (Fig. 20.8). Mechanical valves are durable but prone to thrombosis, with resulting impairment of valve function and risk of embolism. Indefinite oral anticoagulation (with warfarin) is commenced as soon as operative blood loss ceases.

Bioprosthetic valves are made of porcine aortic valves or bovine pericardium on a supportive frame which can be treated with glutaraldehyde and used to replace aortic or mitral valves. These valves mimic the action of the natural valve, have less tendency to thrombosis, and can often be used without anticoagulants. Unfortunately, their durability is limited and calcification or tissue disruption may develop within 5–10 years. Accelerated calcification is common in young adults and children, the very group in which it is desirable to avoid mechanical valves with their need for anticoagulation.

Valve replacement usually provides marked symptomatic relief and a significant improvement in the natural history of the valve disease. It carries an overall operative mortality of about 5%, the risks being greater in the elderly, and those with coronary disease, impaired liver function or severe pulmonary vascular disease. All prosthetic valves have a small risk of developing infective endocarditis and antibiotics should be taken prophylactically at times of potential bacteraemia, such as dental manipulation and sepsis.

ISCHAEMIC HEART DISEASE

Surgery for coronary artery disease is now increasingly common in most Western countries. In the United States, the number of coronary operations now exceeds 1000 per million of population each year. Angina pectoris is the usual indication, and most agree that surgery should be offered whenever symptoms persist or interfere with activities in spite of adequate medical treatment. It is widely accepted that triple vessel disease and left main coronary artery disease have a better outlook with surgical treatment. This is why detailed investigation, with coronary angiography, is needed before making a decision about management in all patients with angina. Increasingly, younger patients and those with a strong family history are being investigated with a view to surgery whenever a 'coronary event' such as angina or myocardial infarction first occurs.

Coronary artery bypass grafting

The principle of surgery is to insert a conduit which carries high-pressure arterial blood into relatively normal segments of the coronary arterial tree beyond angiographically demonstrated obstruction(s) (Fig. 20.3). In the past, the patient's own saphenous vein was used as the conduit. However, it is now appreciated that about one-half of such grafts become occluded by thrombosis or vein graft atherosclerosis within 10 years, and the patient's own internal mammary arteries are now used in preference.

A bloodless immobile operative field is provided by cardioplegic arrest of the heart and cardiopulmonary bypass. The coronary arteries are opened distal to the known obstructions; typically grafts are needed for the left anterior descending artery, marginal branch of the circumflex artery, and the distal right or posterior descending arteries (Fig. 20.9). Vessels with a lumen diameter greater than 1.5 mm are large enough for grafting. Fine instruments and sutures, and magnification, are

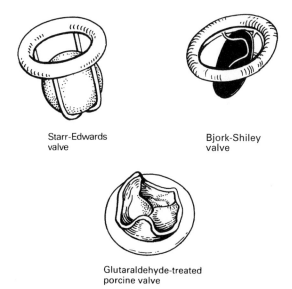

Starr-Edwards valve

Bjork-Shiley valve

Glutaraldehyde-treated porcine valve

Fig. 20.8 Types of artificial heart valve.

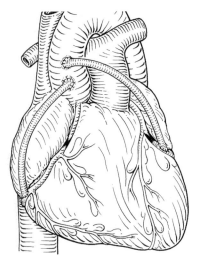

Fig. 20.9   Bypass grafts for right and left anterior descending coronary obstruction.

needed to sew the distal end of the mobilized internal mammary artery (or end of the saphenous vein) to the coronary arteriotomy. When saphenous vein is used, its proximal end is sewn to a small opening in the ascending aorta (Fig. 20.9).

Endarterectomy (i.e. removal of an atheromatous core) will often clear a totally blocked coronary artery and allow graft insertion. Revascularization of a poorly functioning myocardium due to ischaemic fibrosis is unrewarding, but if angina is present (indicating the presence of viable but ischaemic muscle), left ventricular function is rarely so poor as to preclude surgery.

Results of surgery

The operative mortality rate is 1–2% in males under 70 years of age, and is a little higher in females, the elderly and those with widespread arterial disease. Some 60–80% of patients obtain complete relief from angina and the remainder are usually much improved. Angina does gradually return, so that only about 30–50% are free from angina at 10 years. Recurrence is usually due to progression of disease in the coronary arteries or occlusion of vein grafts.

Percutaneous transluminal coronary balloon angioplasty

This technique has become an increasingly popular alternative to surgery since its introduction in the late 1970s. A small balloon is introduced through a peripheral artery and under radiological control it is passed along the aorta to enter the affected coronary artery. The balloon is inflated once it has been positioned across the area of stenosis. The risk of angioplasty is low but its definitive place remains uncertain. Some lesions cannot be dilated while approximately one-third of stenoses recur within 6 months. Balloon dilatation is at present generally reserved for short subtotal stenoses located away from major bifurcations or branching.

Surgery for complications of coronary artery disease

Myocardial infarction. This is the common complication of coronary artery disease. A few centres now undertake prompt coronary angiography followed by immediate bypass grafting, provided that surgery can be undertaken within 4–6 hours of the onset of chest pain. Although low mortality rates have been reported, it is difficult to prove that significant amounts of jeopardized myocardium are salvaged. The same uncertainties apply to thrombolysis using intracoronary infusion of streptokinase or systemic administration of fibrin-targeted lytic agents, although this approach has the attraction of being less invasive and leaves open the possibility of later surgery or balloon angioplasty to deal with stenoses.

Ventricular aneurysm. This is a late complication in which healing of transmural infarction leaves a large fibrous scar which bulges to form an aneurysm. Left ventricular function is compromised and there is breathlessness on exertion. Large symptomatic aneurysms can be resected with improvement in ventricular function, and this may be combined with coronary grafting if appropriate.

Muscle rupture. This may follow infarction involving the interventricular septum or a papillary muscle of the mitral valve. This results in a ventricular septal defect and mitral regurgitation respectively, and places a major and often rapidly fatal haemodynamic load on the already compromised heart. Urgent surgery to close the defect or replace the mitral valve may be life-saving.

CONGENITAL HEART DISEASE

Congenital heart disease occurs in about 6–8 of every 1000 live births. Although symptoms may not appear until later in life (e.g. congenital bicuspid aortic valve), the problem usually presents in childhood. Severe lesions which present in the first few

- Angina pectoris and myocardial infarction are the usual indications to consider coronary arterial surgery.

- Triple-vessel disease and disease affecting the left main coronary artery have the best outlook following surgical treatment, and pre-operative coronary angiography is helpful in defining the extent of disease.

- The patient's own internal mammary arteries are now preferred to saphenous veins as a conduit to bring blood into the distal arterial tree.

- Coronary artery bypass grafting has an operative mortality of 1–2% in good-risk patients. Angina is relieved in 60–80% of cases but often recurs gradually so that only 30–50% of patients remain angina-free at 10 years.

- Percutaneous transluminal coronary angioplasty using balloon catheters offers an alternative to surgical grafting, particularly in patients with short stenoses located away from major bifurcations.

months of life have a high surgical mortality. Although cardiopulmonary bypass is commonly used in neonates for corrective surgery, it is technically more difficult than in older children. For this reason, palliative surgery (e.g. construction of a shunt between systemic and pulmonary circulations in infants with Fallot's tetralogy; see below) may be employed so that definitive repair can be deferred until the child is older and larger.

Patent ductus arteriosus

The ductus arteriosus allows pulmonary artery blood to bypass the airless lungs in utero. Failure of normal closure results in left-to-right shunting of systemic blood into the pulmonary circulation. This can cause cardiac failure in infancy, although it is more common for the shunt to be well tolerated, with the characteristic 'machinery murmur' in the second left interspace being the reason for referral. Surgery carries little risk and is always recommended so as to avoid cardiac failure in later life. The ductus is exposed through a left lateral thoracotomy and is divided and sutured between vascular clamps, or ligated with thick non-absorbable sutures.

Coarctation of the aorta

Narrowing of the aorta most commonly occurs just beyond the origin of the left subclavian artery. The diagnosis is suggested by delayed or absent femoral

pulses, and by rib notching on chest X-ray in older patients. About 50% of patients die within the first year of life from cardiac failure, and complications from proximal hypertension can prove fatal in early adult life. Operation is always advised and is undertaken through a left lateral thoracotomy. The narrowed segment is usually resected with restoration of aortic continuity by end-to-end anastomosis. Long defects may require insertion of a graft, while in infants it may be better to enlarge the narrowed area by patch angioplasty.

Atrial septal defects

Atrial septal defects result in shunting of blood from left to right atrium because the right ventricle and pulmonary arterial tree are more distensible than the left ventricle and systemic arterial system. The typical clinical findings are increased pulmonary blood flow, a delayed pulmonary second sound, and radiological evidence of pulmonary plethora. The defect causes breathlessness on exertion and eventually causes cardiac failure in later life.

Surgical repair is safe and advisable. Using cardiopulmonary bypass, the defect is closed through an incision in the right atrium. A patch of pericardium or Dacron may be needed for large defects. Most atrial septal defects are simple *secundum defects*, but others are more complex. *Sinus venosum defects* lie near the orifice of the superior vena cava while *primum defects* lie close to the mitral and tricuspid valves; greater care is needed during closure to avoid compromising adjacent structures.

Ventricular septal defects

These defects cause left-to-right shunting because left ventricular pressure is higher than right ventricular pressure during systole. The excess pulmonary flow may lead to pulmonary hypertension, with cessation and even reversal of flow through the defect (Eisenmenger's syndrome). Surgery for ventricular septal defects may be needed in infancy because of refractory cardiac failure, and is usually advised before school age if the defect is significant. Spontaneous closure sometimes occurs but raised pulmonary vascular resistance is an indication for early surgery. Surgery is contraindicated once severe pulmonary vascular disease has developed or shunt flow has reversed.

The defect is closed under cardiopulmonary bypass through an incision in the right ventricle or right atrium (if possible). A Dacron patch is usually needed and care must be taken not to damage the tricuspid valve or the conducting system.

Tetralogy of Fallot

This condition consists of:

- Obstruction of right ventricular outflow (due to pulmonary valve stenosis, right ventricular outflow tract muscle hypertrophy, or pulmonary artery hypoplasia)
- A large ventricular septal defect due to malalignment of the aorta and pulmonary artery over the interventricular septum. Both ventricles are at systemic pressure and the right ventricle is hypertrophic. Right-to-left shunting results in cyanosis, compensatory polycythaemia, and spontaneous intravascular thrombosis.

A palliative Blalock-Taussig shunt (i.e. anastomosis of the subclavian artery to the pulmonary artery) may be undertaken in the first year or two of life, and total correction under cardiopulmonary bypass is usually undertaken before school age. The aim of definitive surgery is to remove the palliative shunt, remove outflow obstruction (by patch enlargement if need be), and close the septal defect. The operation has a mortality rate of about 5% but survivors can often return to full activity, with freedom from cyanosis and an improved life expectancy.

PERICARDIAL DISEASE

Chronic constrictive pericarditis has many causes. The commonest is tuberculous pericarditis, which is usually inactive by the time the patient is seen by a surgeon. Systemic venous congestion occurs because the heart cannot expand fully in diastole to accept a normal venous return. The condition is treated by resecting the dense fibrous tissue from around the heart; some surgeons prefer to do so with cover from cardiopulmonary bypass.

CARDIAC TRAUMA

Stab wounds of the heart usually cause rapidly increasing tamponade. Urgent thoracotomy is needed to open the pericardium, relieve tamponade, and buy time for blood transfusion and formal suture of the cardiac injury.

Rapid deceleration injury in road traffic accidents may rupture the first part of the descending aorta. Suspicion is aroused if bruising over the sternum carries an imprint of the hub of a steering wheel. The injury may be rapidly fatal due to intrapleural rupture and exsanguination, or the aortic adventitia and mediastinal tissues may temporarily prevent rupture. The diagnosis is suggested by finding widening of the mediastinum on chest X-ray, and is confirmed by aortography. Using left thoracotomy, the aorta is rapidly clamped above and below the rupture, and aortic continuity is restored by sewing in a short Dacron tube.

CARDIAC TRANSPLANTATION

Transplantation for end-stage cardiac disease is now an established procedure and is discussed in Chapter 15.

POSTOPERATIVE CARE AFTER CARDIAC SURGERY

Before closing the chest after cardiac surgery, tubes are inserted to drain blood and are connected to underwater seal bottles. These tubes allow escape of blood from around the heart and permit measurement of blood loss. If blood loss exceeds 200 ml/hour in an adult, coagulation status is checked and the chest usually has to be reopened. Patients who have undergone cardiopulmonary bypass are usually monitored for 24 hours in an intensive care area and ventilated until spontaneous ventilatory effort has returned and cardiovascular function is stable.

Pulse rate, blood pressure, urine flow and atrial pressure (usually right atrial or central venous pressure) are monitored, and pulmonary arterial wedge pressure may be used as an index of left atrial pressure (see Ch. 3). Low cardiac output is reflected in a fall in skin temperature, tachycardia, hypotension, mental unresponsiveness, oliguria and developing metabolic acidosis. It may be due to the following.

- *Hypovolaemia* is caused by inadequate replacement of blood loss, or vasodilatation in a patient previously vasoconstricted due to hypothermia. Tachycardia, hypotension and low atrial pressure are the typical signs. Rapid blood transfusion is indicated.
- *Heart failure* may be due to surgical trauma, myocardial ischaemia or dysrhythmia. The pulse

rate is variable, and there may be hypotension and high atrial pressure. Treatment consists of administering inotropic drugs and correction of electrolyte and acid–base abnormalities.

• *Cardiac tamponade* is due to accumulation of blood around the heart, usually as a result of clot blocking the drainage tube. Tachycardia, hypotension and high atrial pressure develop rapidly, making tamponade difficult to distinguish from heart failure. Once the diagnosis is suspected, the chest should be opened immediately to evacuate clot and control bleeding.

OTHER COMPLICATIONS OF CARDIAC SURGERY

Cerebral injury. Following cardiac surgery this ranges in severity from minor disturbances of concentration and mood, to severe cerebral lesions resulting in failure to regain consciousness, hemiplegia and other serious disturbances. Minor disturbances may be the result of extracorporeal circulation (e.g. microemboli or inadequate cerebral perfusion). Major cerebral injury complicates 1–5% of cardiac operations and is usually due to air embolism or cerebrovascular accidents during the altered perfusion of cardiopulmonary bypass. Treatment is supportive and the prognosis is variable.

Cardiac arrest. It may be due to ventricular fibrillation (as a result of falling potassium levels) or to asystole. Treatment consists of prompt external cardiac massage, maintenance of ventilation, defibrillation, correction of electrolyte and acid–base imbalance, and inotropic support.

Renal failure. An occasional complication; it may need peritoneal dialysis or haemodialysis.

Repeat cardiac surgery. This has become more common in recent years. For example, it may be needed for definitive correction of congenital abnormalities, replacement of prosthetic heart valves, or further coronary artery surgery in patients with recurrent angina. The increased operative risk is due largely to the hazard of surgical injury to a heart which is adherent to the pericardium or overlying sternum.

Peripheral vascular disease

CONTENTS

Vascular disease is the commonest cause of disability and death in the Western World. Venous disorders are commoner, but arterial diseases are more serious and more likely to require urgent surgical intervention.

ARTERIAL DISEASE

Large vessel disease, affecting the aorta and its branches down to 1–2 mm in diameter, behaves differently from disease affecting small arteries and capillaries. Large vessel disease can threaten life or limb, often presents acutely but can usually be treated successfully by repair or reconstruction. Small vessel disease causes chronic disability and surgery has little to offer. Most arterial disorders are due to atherosclerosis. Morphologically this takes the form of:

• obliterative disease
• ectatic or aneurysmal disease.

ATHEROSCLEROTIC OBLITERATIVE ARTERIAL DISEASE

This disease can affect the circulation to the heart, causing angina or myocardial infarction; to the brain, causing chronic ischaemia or stroke; to the kidneys, causing hypertension or renal infarction; to the gut, causing mesenteric angina or intestinal infarction; or to the limbs, causing claudication, rest pain, gangrene or acute ischaemia. These various manifestations arise from what is essentially the same disease.

Obliterative arterial disease is partly familial. Other important aetiological factors are smoking, hypercholesterolaemia, hypertension and diet. Diabetics are prone not only to atheroma but also to neuropathy which, together with elevated sugar levels in the tissues, makes them vulnerable to sepsis.

Atherosclerosis encompasses a spectrum ranging from pure atheroma, a metabolic lesion affecting large arteries (e.g. aorta, iliac, carotid, renal), to arteriosclerosis, 'hardening of the arteries', which affects the media of the whole arterial tree.

Atheroma has a clear association with smoking and with metabolic disorders, notably hyperlipidaemia and diabetes. It may cause symptoms in young adults. The basic lesion is a subintimal deposit of lipid laid down at points of haemodynamic stress such as vessel bifurcations and branches (Fig. 21.1). In experimental animals and possibly in man these plaques can be made to regress by altering the diet. *Arteriosclerosis* is a disease of older patients. It affects the arterial tree diffusely, including the small arteries, resulting in degeneration of muscle and elastic tissue of the media and their replacement by fibrous tissue and calcification.

Serious complications arise from enlargement or extension of the atheromatous plaque by subendothelial build-up of lipid. Flow may be obstructed or ulceration may lead to thrombosis, embolism or dissection of the vessel wall. Extension of the disease to involve the media and elastic lamina weakens the wall, which may result in aneurysm formation, particularly if the patient is hypertensive.

Thrombosis

The platelet aggregation which starts a thrombus is triggered by several factors, including turbulence and irregularity of the vessel wall. These effects are produced by the developing plaque which, when it obstructs the lumen by about 70%, reduces blood flow. The liability to thrombosis may be further enhanced by ulceration of the plaque to expose thrombogenic subendothelial elements.

Thrombosis of an artery causes infarction only if it is an 'end artery' or when collateral channels are affected by the disease.

Embolism

Before a plaque and/or thrombus completely occludes a vessel, fragments of atheroma or platelet aggregates may pass into the distal arterial tree as emboli. These can be single or multiple and may give rise to pain or necrosis.

An embolus may also arise from an aneurysm but usually comes from the heart. The patient may give a history of recent myocardial infarction (with mural thrombosis) or the thrombus may have formed in a fibrillating atrium. Less often the source is an artificial heart valve, a cusp vegetation or, very rarely, an atrial myxoma. The effects of embolism depend on the site and the adequacy of collateral compensatory flow.

Dissection

Ulceration of the arterial wall allows blood to drive a haemodynamic wedge under the endothelium. A flap may be raised which obstructs flow and exposes subendothelial tissues so that thrombosis is promoted. Dissection may also result from the insertion of an arterial catheter. In the aorta, particularly if there is associated hypertension, the split may extend into

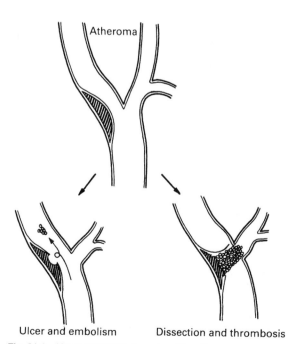

Ulcer and embolism   Dissection and thrombosis

Fig. 21.1 Vascular problems caused by atheroma.

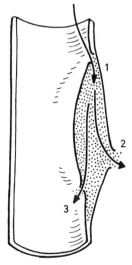

Fig. 21.2 Dissecting aneurysm of aorta. (1) Initial intimal tear. (2) Adventitial rupture. (3) Intimal rupture.

the media and down the wall of the vessel over a distance of many centimetres (Fig. 21.2). Then it may rupture outside the vessel or track back into the lumen to create a false channel carrying blood within the wall of the artery. The process obstructs the orifices of any branches in its path, so that a dissection of the abdominal aorta may cause acute occlusion of the renal, mesenteric or iliac arteries.

Natural history and clinical features

Occlusion of femoro-distal and aorto-iliac segments (Fig. 21.3) causes different clinical features and requires different forms of management.

Femoro-distal obliterative disease

The femoro-distal segment includes the common femoral artery with its superficial and profunda divisions, and the popliteal artery with its three divisions, the anterior and posterior tibial and the peroneal arteries. As a general rule, the older the patient the more the obliterative disease affects the small vessels and therefore the more difficult the surgical repair. The commonest site of occlusion is the superficial femoral artery, but serious effects are limited by the anastomoses between the profunda and the popliteal via the perforating and genicular vessels. Critical ischaemia ensues when there is

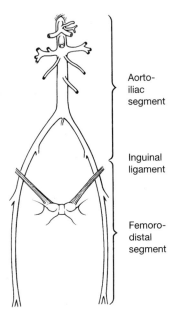

Aorto-iliac segment

Inguinal ligament

Femoro-distal segment

Fig. 21.3 Diagram showing aorto-iliac and femoro-distal segments of the arterial tree.

obstruction of collateral (profunda) channels or of inflow or 'run-off' vessels.

Although obliterative arterial disease is a steadily progressive pathological process, the symptoms follow a pattern of relapse and remission (Fig. 21.4). The earliest lesion to cause symptoms is usually stenosis in the superficial femoral artery in the region of the adductor canal (**A**). The patient reports tightness in the calf muscle (claudication) after walking for about 400 metres. On examination the limb appears normal. Ankle pulses are palpable but diminished and a bruit can be heard at or below the adductor canal.

Over the next few months the collateral vessels of the profunda system enlarge to carry a higher proportion of the blood flow. The symptoms gradually improve or even disappear. With occlusion of the artery by thrombosis there is a sudden deterioration in symptoms. Claudication now comes on after about 200 metres (**B**). The limb still appears relatively healthy but ankle and popliteal pulses can no longer be palpated.

Over the following months, collateral circulation again compensates for the reduced flow and symptoms improve. Stopping smoking greatly facilitates this improvement. The patient may also consciously or subconsciously adapt by relaxing his pace. Thus the inconvenience may be slight, especially if the individual is elderly or relatively inactive.

This phase of moderate claudication may remain apparently stable for several years. However, unless there is a radical change in the patient's life style (notably stopping smoking), the atherosclerosis progresses in inflow, outflow or collateral channels to compromise the blood supply further (**C**). Claudication is now severe, forcing the patient to stop every 50 metres or so and he complains that the foot is cold. On examination the extremity may be cool and capillary refilling slow. Once again there may be a period of relative improvement but the scope for this is steadily diminishing as the disease spreads. In just a few months the occlusions increase and the symptoms worsen (**D**). Severe pain develops in the toes or forefoot at rest, typically arising about an hour after the patient has gone to bed. This 'night pain' is due to the accumulation of metabolites which occurs with the fall in blood flow as the limb rests horizontally. It is severe but is relieved by hanging the limb out of bed, which in turn causes dependent oedema and a risk of infection. There may also be numbness and paraesthesia. Once a patient develops rest pain, gangrene is not far away. This is the stage of 'critical ischaemia'.

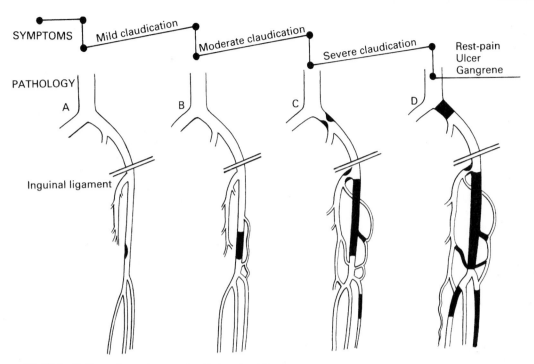

Fig. 21.4 Pattern of symptoms and pathology in obliterative arterial disease (see text for explanation).

By now chronic loss of nutrition will have caused changes in muscles, skin and nails. Necrotic areas (dry gangrene) appear over pressure points such as the knuckles, metatarsal heads and heel (decubitus ulcer), and sepsis supervenes. This is more common if there is dependent oedema or diabetes, when it may lead to a spreading moist gangrene requiring amputation.

An understanding of this cyclical pattern of exacerbation and resolution is important. Medical treatment is usually prescribed when symptoms occur, but improvement is more likely to be due to the natural history than to the medicine. Drug treatment has a very limited place in the treatment of obliterative arterial disease.

Aorto-iliac occlusion

Even when the blockage is above the inguinal ligament, claudication is most commonly felt in the calf. It may also be felt in the buttock and thigh. The commonest sites for occlusion are the lower aorta and the common iliac arteries. If the internal iliac arteries are blocked in a male, the patient may complain of impotence (Leriche syndrome). Relatively young women who are heavy smokers and of small stature, with narrow-calibre vessels, are particularly prone to develop atheroma in the lower aorta.

Femoral pulses are diminished or absent and bruits may be heard. In 'pure' aorto-iliac disease the signs of ischaemia in the lower limb may be minimal, as, at rest, collaterals carry an ample blood supply. When there are blocks in both the aorto-iliac and femoro-distal segments the symptoms are severe.

Assessment of obliterative arterial disease

Particular attention is paid to a history of disease of the cardiorespiratory system, diabetes and smoking, and a family history is obtained. Claudication is the cardinal symptom of early and moderate disease. It is predominantly felt in the calf, occasionally in the thigh and buttock and rarely in the foot. The discomfort, usually described as a 'tightness' rather than a pain, comes on with exercise and goes away within 2–3 minutes of rest. This rapid relief distinguishes it from other causes of exercise-related calf pain, such as spinal cord compression, which takes 5–10 minutes to settle with rest. Pain caused by osteoarthritis of the hip or knee is likely to be present when walking first commences, while that from venous insufficiency obliges the patient to sit down

273

and is associated with leg swelling. Ischaemic rest pain or night pain (see above) is felt in the forefoot or toes and is worse when the leg is elevated. It disturbs sleep and is poorly controlled by analgesics.

In a chronically ischaemic limb the skin is thin and dry. On elevation of the leg there is marked pallor, and on hanging it down the foot becomes bright red; this is known as dependent rubor or 'sunset foot'. In the horizontal position the superficial veins fill sluggishly. The nails are brittle and crumbly and there is muscle wasting. Temperature differences are important. Mottling and extreme pallor are particularly serious signs.

The pulses should be carefully palpated, beginning with the femoral pulses. The strength and regularity of the impulse, the texture of the vessel wall and the presence of any thrill are noted. Auscultation over the common femoral arteries may reveal bruits. To feel the popliteal pulses, the knee should be slightly flexed to relax the muscles and popliteal fascia before palpating deeply between the condyles with the fingers of both hands. The posterior tibial artery is felt midway between the medial malleolus and the tendo-achilles, and the dorsalis pedis just proximal to where it dips down between the bases of the first and second metatarsals. The patient must be carefully examined for other evidence of arterial disease.

Doppler ultrasound is used to measure the systolic blood pressure at the ankle. If there is any doubt about the diagnosis or the severity of claudication, pressures are measured before and after treadmill exercise. Exercise causes a fall in systolic pressure proportional to the severity of the disease. The speed of recovery is quicker with aorto-iliac than with femoro-distal disease. Of the non-invasive radiological or laboratory tests in current use, the most valuable is colour-coded Duplex B-mode ultrasound imaging. This offers the possibility of visualizing the vessel and making a simultaneous blood velocity measurement. Arteriography (Fig. 21.5) is only used if active treatment such as angioplasty or operation is being considered.

Treatment of obliterative arterial disease of the lower limb

Conservative care

Many patients with claudication simply need reassurance and advice. If smoking can be stopped, the prognosis greatly improves. Patients are encouraged to undertake a programme of graded exercise such as walking but pausing momentarily *before*

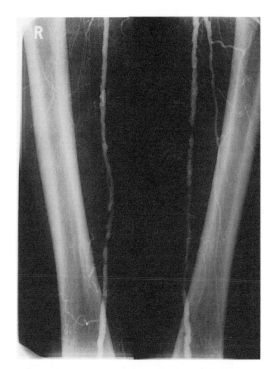

Fig. 21.5 Femoral arteriogram showing irregularity of outline of arteries with stenosis in left superficial femoral artery.

being forced to stop by their claudication, and gradually increasing their walking distance. Patients are advised to take plenty of cereal, fruit and vegetables and to reduce intake of animal fats. Hyperlipidaemia and obesity are corrected as far as possible. Associated diseases such as diabetes, cardiac failure and hypertension should be controlled. Hygiene, care of the skin and chiropody are important to avoid septic complications and gangrene. Extremes of temperature and all forms of trauma should be avoided.

Vasodilator drugs are of no benefit. Drugs with more complex actions such as oxpentifylline (Trental) may be worth a trial in elderly patients with severe claudication for whom no more active intervention is possible. Antiplatelet therapy (one 300 mg aspirin tablet per day) is advised; long-term anticoagulants are not.

When possible, rest pain is controlled with sufficiently strong analgesics to obviate the patient's need to hang the leg out of bed. The head of the bed is elevated. Pressure on the heel must be avoided. Sepsis should be treated promptly with antibiotics. Skin lesions are kept as dry as possible with a spirit-

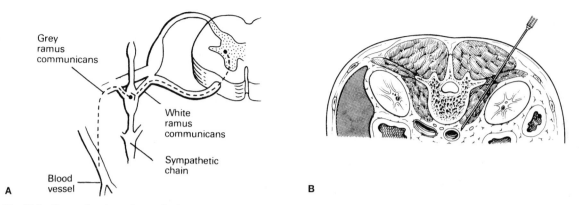

Fig. 21.6 Sympathectomy for occlusive arterial disease. Diagram showing **A** vascular sympathetic supply and **B** direction of insertion of paravertebral needle for phenol block.

based antiseptic. If gangrene occurs, the limb is kept cool and dry. Reflex heating is of no value.

Sympathectomy

Where there is normal autonomic control, sympathectomy results in a warm, dry limb. It does not increase blood flow to muscles.

The principal place for sympathectomy in obliterative arterial disease is in critical ischaemia before any tissue necrosis has developed. In some patients it relieves coldness and rest pain. Chemical sympathectomy avoids operation and is performed by paravertebral injection of phenol in the region of the lumbar sympathetic chain under radiological control (Fig. 21.6).

Percutaneous angioplasty

Balloon angioplasty has added a new dimension to the management of obliterative arterial disease. The technique can be used to dilate stenoses or to re-open short occlusions (i.e. 10 cm). It has been used successfully at a variety of sites, notably the iliac, femoral and renal arteries. The balloon catheter is introduced into the femoral artery over a guide wire (Seldinger technique) under local anaesthesia and advanced through the stenosis (Fig. 21.7). Inflation of the balloon splits the atheromatous plaque, thereby enlarging the lumen. Related percutaneous techniques include the insertion of a metal stent to hold the artery open after balloon angioplasty, and excision of atheroma by atherectomy devices. Various lasers have also been used but, to date, have proved disappointing. Angioplasty can be repeated if necessary. It may avoid the need for a major operation or it can be combined with surgery. It should only be undertaken by a radiologist in collaboration

with a vascular surgeon since complications such as dissection and thrombosis may require emergency surgical repair.

Arterial reconstruction

For the patient with claudication balloon angioplasty may be used, failing which surgery is considered if the occlusion is in the aorto-iliac segment or if the patient's way of life or livelihood is seriously affected. A failed graft not only leaves the patient worse off than before but makes subsequent reconstruction for critical ischaemia more difficult. Thus surgery is usually reserved for a limb whose viability is under threat.

In such patients, most of whom have been lifelong smokers, the risks of operation must always be considered carefully. Impaired respiratory function is very common. Since atherosclerosis is a multifocal disease, there is a much greater risk than average of

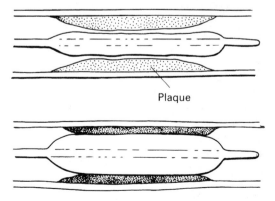

Plaque

Fig. 21.7 Balloon angioplasty used to dilate an atheromatous plaque occluding a vessel.

cardiac complications and of stroke. Indeed, myocardial infarction is the commonest cause of death both in the peri-operative period and during long-term follow-up.

Surgical techniques involve either removal of atherosclerotic plaques and thrombus (thrombo-endarterectomy) or bypass grafting. Synthetic (Dacron) grafts are used to replace large vessels. Vein is preferred for small ones. Fundamental requirements for non-thrombosis of a graft are good cardiac output and patent inflow and run-off vessels.

Aorto-iliac segment. If the occluding lesion is relatively localized, it can be treated by opening the artery and removing it (thrombo-endarterectomy) and then closing the artery with a patch of vein or Dacron to ensure patency (Fig. 21.8). Most aorto-iliac lesions are treated by using an aorto-iliac or aorto-femoral Dacron graft to bypass the diseased sections (Fig. 21.9).

If the iliac artery is blocked only on one side and the patient is unfit for abdominal surgery, a femoro-femoral graft can be brought suprapubically from the patent side to bypass the iliac block. This is an example of 'extra-anatomic' bypass, i.e. one which does not follow a normal anatomical path. Another, which is used in aorto-iliac disease in patients unfit for abdominal surgery, is the axillo-femoral graft. This graft is taken from one axillary artery down the side of the chest and flank to one or both femoral arteries. The results are less satisfactory than direct aorto-iliac reconstruction.

Patency rates are around 80% at 5 years. Graft occlusion may occur for the reasons given above. Other complications such as graft infection or

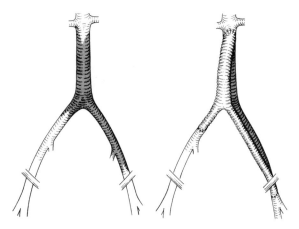

Fig. 21.9 Reconstruction of an occluded aorto-iliac segment by a bifurcation bypass graft.

pseudoaneurysms are rare. Infection in the graft necessitates its removal and an alternative reconstruction. Pseudoaneurysm can usually be repaired locally as long as there is no sepsis.

Femoro-popliteal segment. Saphenous vein is the preferred material for grafts in arteries smaller than the iliacs. Other commonly used materials are polytetrafluorethylene (PTFE) or human umbilical vein (Dardik biograft). The latter is glutaraldehyde-treated to prevent graft–host reaction. These materials are very expensive, patency rates are poor, and sepsis is more likely than with autogenous vein.

An isolated stenosis or a short occlusion can be successfully treated by a vein patch graft with, if necessary, an endarterectomy. For example, the narrowed orifice of the profunda can be widened (profundoplasty). However, since atheroma is never confined to one area and most femoral blocks are many centimetres long, the preferred option is to take a bypass from the common femoral artery to the popliteal, tibial or peroneal artery beyond the block (Fig. 21.10). Using microsurgical techniques femoro-distal bypasses may be taken down to the ankle or even the foot.

Saphenous vein is available in 70% of cases requiring femoro-distal bypass. To eliminate the effect of the valves the vein removed has to be inserted upside down (reversed vein bypass) or it can be left in position and the valves disrupted by a valvulotome. This 'in-situ' technique is preferred in many centres. All the tributaries of the vein have to be individually ligated or clipped. Intravenous heparin is given before arteries are clamped. Grafts are anastomosed to arteries with fine non-absorbable sutures.

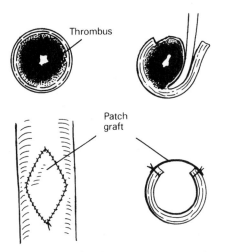

Thrombus

Patch graft

Fig. 21.8 Thrombo-endarterectomy and repair of the vessel by a patch graft.

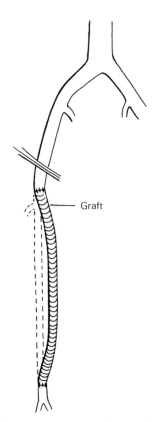

Fig. 21.10 **Femoro-popliteal graft inserted to bypass an occluded femoral artery.**

Graft

Obliterative arterial disease

- Atherosclerosis is the major cause of obliterative arterial disease and aetiological factors include familial predisposition, smoking, hypercholesterolaemia, hypertension, diabetes mellitus and diet.

- Aorto-iliac and femoro-distal disease are the major clinical forms of obliterative arterial disease dealt with in peripheral vascular surgery, and progressively severe intermittent claudication is the major symptom.

- Clinical appearances of ischaemia in a limb include a thin dry skin, pallor with marked reddening on dependency ('sunset foot'), brittle crumbly nails, hair loss, muscle wasting, temperature differences, and mottling.

- Assessment includes palpation of all pulses, Doppler ultrasonography to measure systolic blood pressure at the ankle, and Duplex B-mode ultrasonography to examine flow and velocity. Arteriography is now only used if intervention is being considered.

- Flow can be improved in selected cases by balloon angioplasty or arterial reconstruction. Fundamental requirements for success in arterial reconstruction are a good cardiac output and patent inflow and run-off vessels.

- Patency rates following aorto-iliac reconstruction are 80% at 5 years while after femoro-distal bypass they vary between 30 and 50%.

Patency rates with femoro-distal bypass are not as good as with the large-bore reconstructions, being around 50% at 5 years with vein and 30% with synthetics. The prognosis is better if the patient stops smoking. When a graft blocks, amputation is likely, although some grafts can be cleared or replaced if the patient is referred very promptly.

Diabetes and arterial disease

About 10% of patients with arterial disease are diabetics, while the proportion of patients with critical ischaemia who are diabetic is around 40%. The extent to which microvascular disease plays a part in this is debated. Two other very important factors are the high sugar content of tissues which favours bacterial growth and spread, and the anaesthesia from diabetic neuropathy which leaves the patient unaware of minor traumas that allow ingress of bacteria. Skin care, avoidance of pressure or trauma, hygiene and chiropody are doubly important in the diabetic. Good control of the diabetes and early antibiotic treatment of infections are essen-

tial. Large vessel atherosclerotic disease should be treated in the same way as in non-diabetic patients. Sympathectomy may be tried but usually has little effect. Drainage of pus and debridement of dead tissue are particularly important. Amputations can usually be more conservative than in non-diabetic ischaemia.

Amputation

Vascular disease is responsible for more than 90% of all amputations carried out in Western countries. Amputation is indicated only after arterial reconstruction for 'limb salvage' has failed or is impractical. Fortunately the majority of patients with atherosclerosis do not reach this end-stage and it is important to reassure those with early claudication that if they follow medical advice, especially concerning smoking, amputation can be avoided.

The level of amputation is determined by local blood supply and by the state of the joints, general health and age. The broad principle is to amputate at the lowest level consistent with healing. It is particularly important to conserve the knee joint since the energy required for walking with a below-knee prosthesis is only a fraction of that required for one above the knee. However, if the patient has other disabilities which make walking with a prosthesis impossible, there is no point in attempting to conserve the knee joint at the expense of healing.

Thermography and percutaneous oxygen measurements can be used to assess the local blood supply and determine the correct level for amputation, but clinical judgement and meticulous technique remain the most important factors.

Some 50% or more of major vascular amputations are performed below the knee, the remainder being mostly mid-thigh (Fig. 21.11). A few are performed through the knee or foot (transmetatarsal). Normally the stump is closed by primary suture. In severe septic conditions the stump may be left open with a dressing, to be closed or revised to a higher level when infection has been controlled.

Haemostasis is important. The end of the bone is carefully smoothed, nerves are cut cleanly as high as possible to avoid neuroma formation, muscles and fascia are approximated with fine absorbable sutures, and the skin is closed over a drain. Inadequate blood supply, haematoma, infection and tension on the stitch line are the main causes of failure to heal. Antibiotic cover is routine. A firm but not tight bandage is applied to an above-knee stump. A light plaster is preferred for below-knee stumps. Early return to active exercise helps to avoid contracture at the hip and/or knee. At about one week the patient should begin to bear weight on the other limb between parallel bars, and at 10 days to walk with a pneumatic walking aid. If healing is progressing well, a temporary prosthesis can be fitted at about 3 weeks. Final fitting of the artificial limb must await shaping and firming of the stump. Approximately 70% of below-knee amputees and 30% of above-knee amputees eventually walk independently or with a stick or Zimmer support.

'Phantom limb' pain can be a late and troublesome complication, especially if pain has not been well controlled before and after operation. With analgesia, reassurance and time this usually settles.

Even patients who cannot manage an artificial limb can achieve considerable independence in a wheelchair, especially if they can transfer from chair to toilet or bed and if the appropriate modifications such as ramps, wide doors and bathroom handles are made to the home.

Patients who undergo amputation for critical ischaemia are usually elderly, frail and disabled in other ways. Amputation then presents a huge psychological and physical burden. Such patients need strong support and their care is a matter of team work, with surgeon, nursing staff, physiotherapist, occupational therapist, prosthetist and social worker all playing vital parts. Amputation for vascular disease has high morbidity and mortality and only a few patients remain alive for 5 years.

Occlusive disease of the upper limb

Obliterative arterial disease is much less of a problem in the upper limb. Muscular activity is less, collateral circulation is good, and atheroma does not occur to the same extent. The commonest site of occlusion is the first part of the subclavian artery proximal to the origin of the vertebral artery (Fig. 21.12). Occlusion at this level has two effects:

- Reduced blood pressure in the arm
- Compensatory reversal of flow down the vertebral artery to supply the limb.

This effect, known as 'subclavian steal', can give rise to symptoms of vertebrobasilar ischaemia such as dizziness, classically occurring during muscular activity of the arm. More often the patient presents with weakness, tiredness or claudication in the upper limb, and subclavian steal is a radiological finding on arteriography.

Subclavian occlusion is corrected by inserting a bypass graft between the subclavian and one of the other arteries in the neck, usually the common carotid.

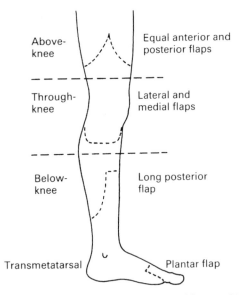

Above-knee

Equal anterior and posterior flaps

Through-knee

Lateral and medial flaps

Below-knee

Long posterior flap

Transmetatarsal

Plantar flap

Fig. 21.11 Levels of amputation and types of flap used to close the residual defect.

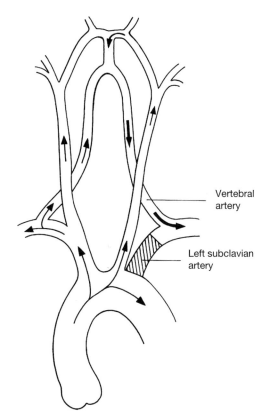

Vertebral artery

Left subclavian artery

Fig. 21.12 Occlusion of the left subclavian artery causing 'subclavian steal'.

Occlusive disease of the carotid and vertebral arteries

Stroke

Stroke is an episode of focal neurological dysfunction whose symptoms last more than 24 hours and which is caused by a vascular disturbance in the brain. When such symptoms last for less than 24 hours, the episode is described as a transient ischaemic attack (TIA). Most TIAs last only a few minutes.

In the United Kingdom about 100 000 people a year suffer their first stroke. As a cause of death, stroke is exceeded only by heart disease and cancer. It is the most important cause of severe disability. Four-fifths of strokes are caused by thrombosis and the majority of these are due to occlusive disease in the *extracranial* vessels, i.e. the carotid and vertebral arteries. Occlusions in these vessels give rise to two distinct syndromes: carotid ischaemia with effects in the related cerebral hemisphere, and vertebrobasilar ischaemia with effects referrable to the hindbrain.

TIAs, especially if clearly in the carotid territory, may be an indication for carotid endarterectomy (see below).

Carotid distribution events

The origin of the internal carotid artery is particularly prone to atheroma. Following the formation of a plaque, emboli of aggregated platelets, fibrin or fragments of atheroma may pass into the carotid territory. If they enter the retinal artery, they cause transient blindness (amaurosis fugax) or sometimes permanent blindness. These emboli can be seen in the retina with an ophthalmoscope. If they enter the territory of the middle cerebral artery, they may cause dysphasia, dysarthria, hemiparesis, hemisensory loss, deviation of the head and eyes towards the side of the lesion, or disorientation. A TIA is a precursor of major stroke, the risk of which is 5–10% per year. Investigation and treatment should not be delayed.

Vertebrobasilar distribution events

These are more varied but frequently produce dizziness, diplopia, cortical blindness, dysarthria, 'drop attacks' and unilateral or bilateral motor and sensory deficits.

Examination and investigation

It is important to exclude other causes of cerebral ischaemia, especially cardiac arrhythmias. The carotid pulse may be diminished or absent and a bruit may be audible over the affected carotid or vertebral artery. However, the absence of a bruit does not rule out significant disease. Cerebral computerized tomography (CT) scanning is an important investigation which can quickly exclude haemorrhage and detect infarcts of more than 0.5 cm in diameter.

Useful screening tests include Duplex B-mode ultrasound imaging and digital subtraction angiography, but perfemoral arch and selective carotid arteriography are the critical investigations on which decisions regarding surgery depend.

Treatment

There is evidence that antiplatelet therapy with aspirin (300 mg per day) reduces arterial thrombotic events. Surgery, since it carries a 1–5% risk of stroke or death, is not justified unless there have been unequivocal transient ischaemic attacks or minor stroke with good recovery. The aim of surgery is to remove the source of embolism and protect the patient from major stroke. To achieve this, carotid disease must be detected before it proceeds to complete occlusion. A completely blocked internal carotid artery cannot be re-opened and operation is not indicated in the presence of a stroke with substantial residual deficit.

At *carotid endarterectomy* heparin is given and the arteries are clamped and opened. Cerebral blood flow is usually quite adequately maintained via collaterals but can be further protected by a shunt (Fig. 21.13). The stenosing plaque is shelled out and the artery repaired with direct suture or patch graft.

Stenosing plaque at the origin of the vertebral artery can be removed through an incision in the subclavian artery, although this operation is rarely performed.

Occlusive disease of the renal artery

Stenoses of the renal arteries can be caused by fibromuscular hyperplasia, particularly in young females, or by congenital lesions, but the great majority are due to atherosclerosis. Such narrowing reduces perfusion of the juxtaglomerular apparatus, which in turn leads to increased release of renin and angiotensin, and hypertension.

Hypertension of renal origin should be suspected if the patient is relatively young or resistant to antihypertensive therapy. There may be an audible bruit on auscultation of the abdomen. Investigations include renin estimations on selective venous catheter samples, renal isotope perfusion scanning and renal angiography.

There are two indications for active intervention in cases of renal artery stenosis:

• Control of hypertension
• Preservation of renal tissue.

Perfemoral balloon angioplasty has proved to be effective in some types of stenosis. Operative reconstruction may be carried out by means of a vein graft. In technically difficult cases, especially where there are multiple renal arteries, the kidney can be removed from the body and preserved by perfusion with cooled electrolyte solution while the arteries are repaired under magnification. The kidney is then returned to its previous position or autotransplanted to the iliac fossa as in renal transplantation.

When the operation is performed for hypertension, about two-thirds of patients are either cured or the hypertension becomes easier to control.

Acute arterial occlusion

The commonest vascular emergency is sudden arterial occlusion. The causes are thrombosis, embolism, trauma or dissecting aneurysm. The effect on distal tissues depends on the level of the block and the adequacy of collateral circulation. Trauma and dissection of aneurysm aside, about

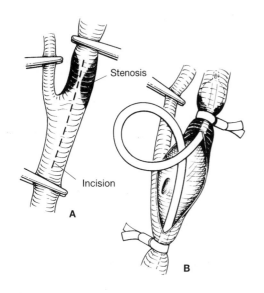
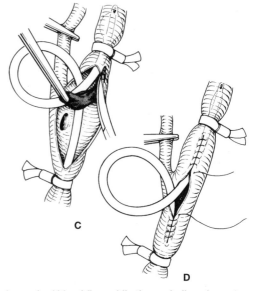

Fig. 21.13 Carotid endarterectomy using an internal shunt to maintain cerebral blood flow while the occluding plaque is removed.

one-third of acute occlusions are due to embolism and one-third to thrombosis. In the remaining third it is not possible to distinguish between the two.

Thrombosis. This usually occurs as the end stage of chronic obliterative disease, so the patient is likely to have a history of previous chronic ischaemia such as claudication. Aneurysms are also prone to thrombosis, especially popliteal aneurysms. The onset may be dramatic with severe pain or, because collaterals have had an opportunity to develop, may simply consist of sudden numbness and coldness. Thrombosis is often precipitated by a fall in blood pressure due to cardiac failure, myocardial infarction or shock from any cause.

Embolism. This is most commonly associated with ischaemic heart disease with atrial fibrillation, cardiac failure or recent myocardial infarction. Sometimes there is a history of previous embolism. Subacute bacterial endocarditis and prosthetic heart valves can produce multiple emboli which may be infected. Emboli may also originate from mural thrombus associated with atherosclerosis in proximal main arteries. Trauma to a vessel during arterial catheterization may dispatch emboli to distal arteries.

A typical embolus consists of partially organized thrombus and lodges at the bifurcation of an artery. Occlusion is aggravated by thrombosis spreading proximally and distally from the embolus, and occluded collaterals can lead to gangrene.

Clinical features

A typical site for acute occlusion is the bifurcation of the common femoral artery. Coldness and pain in the foot and calf are the first symptoms. These are followed by paraesthesia, loss of sensation and loss of power. The loss of sensation is of the 'glove and stocking' variety, i.e. maximal distally and not following any segmental nerve distribution. At first the limb is pale with poor venous filling but later it becomes mottled with cyanotic patches. Muscle tenderness is a sign of ischaemic damage, and is first evident in the anterior tibial compartment. Embolism generally is more dramatic than thrombosis but either can be insidious.

Acute arterial occlusion has to be distinguished from deep venous thrombosis (DVT) and venous gangrene, in which swelling is marked. A careful history and examination, supported by chest X-ray and electrocardiography, will usually define the cause. Arteriography is necessary in most cases, unless loss of power and sensation suggest the need

for urgent surgery. A full blood count, and blood sugar, urea and electrolyte estimations are obtained routinely.

Management

Acute embolic ischaemia can be reversed completely if treated promptly. A main-stem arterial occlusion will cause permanent tissue damage only if more than 6 hours elapse without treatment. Thrombosis is not as easy to correct as embolus because of the underlying disease in the arterial wall but, owing to its more insidious nature, a little more time may be available to investigate and plan treatment.

The first step is to correct any precipitating condition such as hypotension. There is no point in clearing thrombus from an artery if flow cannot be sustained. Volume replacement, digoxin, diuretics, anti-arrhythmics and inotropic agents are used as indicated.

Systemic heparin is started immediately to minimize further spread of thrombus. Acute occlusions with signs of severe ischaemia (loss of sensation, loss of power, muscle tenderness) require urgent operation. For the majority of acute occlusions which have less compelling clinical features, initial medical treatment may be considered. In a few mild cases intravenous systemic heparin will suffice, but most are treated with thrombolytic therapy (streptokinase, urokinase or tissue plasminogen activator) delivered into the thrombus by percutaneous catheter under radiological control. The patient must be very carefully observed for signs of deterioration.

Emergency embolectomy/thrombectomy can be performed under local anaesthesia but an anaesthetist should be available in case of difficulties or in case arterial reconstruction has to be undertaken. Most lower limb thrombi can be removed by passing a Fogarty balloon catheter through an incision in the femoral artery (Fig. 21.14). Embolectomy/thrombectomy is contraindicated in the presence of gangrene, when amputation is the only possible treatment.

Early operation and/or thrombolytic therapy have dramatically improved limb salvage rates but mortality remains around 20%. The degree of ischaemia on presentation gives a good indication of the likely outcome. Lack of motor activity with tender hard muscles suggests that amputation is likely to be necessary. In such cases embolectomy/thrombectomy has to be accompanied by fasciotomy in the compartments of the calf to relieve the tension from swelling which follows restoration of blood

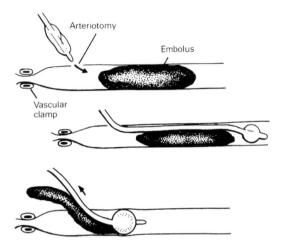

Fig. 21.14 Removal of an embolus with a Fogarty balloon catheter. The balloon is inflated once it is beyond the thrombus and then withdrawn.

flow to ischaemic muscles. Restoration of blood flow, if performed after ischaemic damage has occurred, may cause cardiac or renal complications (arrhythmias, hypotension, oliguria) due to release of breakdown products of myoglobin and haemoglobin.

Femoral embolectomy/thrombectomy. Thrombi in the iliac, femoral, popliteal or more distal arteries can be removed through an opening in the common femoral artery. The artery is incised longitudinally and a Fogarty catheter passed proximally or distally through the thrombus. The balloon is then inflated and the catheter gently withdrawn, extracting the thrombus (see Fig. 21.14). Several passages may be necessary to clear the vessel. The result should be checked by operative angiography. A *saddle embolus of the aorta* is dealt with by removal of the thrombus through bilateral groin incisions.

Acute arterial occlusion of the upper limb. This is less common. Thrombosis may form on an atheromatous area in the subclavian artery, in a subclavian aneurysm, or in an artery mechanically compressed at the thoracic outlet. Thrombosis also occurs in the axillary artery affected by previous radiotherapy for breast carcinoma. Emboli may lodge at any level. Clinical features are similar to those in acute occlusion of the lower limb although, as the collateral supply is better, the symptoms are generally less severe. Exposure of the brachial artery at the elbow gives access to the origins of the radial and ulnar as well as proximal vessels. Arteries of this size or smaller are opened transversely so as to avoid narrowing by the closing suture. Patency should be confirmed by operative angiography.

Postoperative care

The colour, temperature and peripheral pulses of the limb are closely monitored in case re-thrombosis occurs. If fasciotomies were not performed at the initial procedure, the muscles must be carefully checked for swelling or tenderness during the first 12–24 hours. A decompression fasciotomy may be indicated. If the occlusion was due to embolism, heparin is continued for one week and oral anticoagulants for 6 months or more. Patients with atrial fibrillation have to remain on anticoagulants permanently.

Mesenteric embolism

The sudden onset of abdominal pain and diarrhoea in a patient known to be at risk of embolism should suggest the diagnosis of mesenteric embolism. This is based on clinical findings alone as angiography only causes delays which cannot be afforded. Early abdominal signs are non-specific: there may be lower or mid-abdominal tenderness and increased bowel sounds. Urgent laparotomy and balloon embolectomy may prevent intestinal ischaemia, but only 2–4 hours are available before damage

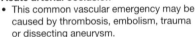

Acute arterial occlusion

- This common vascular emergency may be caused by thrombosis, embolism, trauma or dissecting aneurysm.

- Thrombosis is frequently an end-stage manifestation of chronic obliterative arterial disease, and is often precipitated by a fall in blood pressure due to myocardial infarction, cardiac failure or shock.

- Embolism is most often associated with ischaemic heart disease with atrial fibrillation, cardiac failure or recent myocardial infarction. The embolus usually lodges at the site of bifurcation of an artery.

- The clinical presentation of acute occlusion is one of pain, paraesthesia, pallor and loss of power ('paralysis'). The limb distal to the site of occlusion is pulseless and cold, and may become mottled with cyanotic patches.

- Arteriography is usually advisable unless loss of power and sensation indicate the need for immediate surgery (mainstem arterial occlusion causes permanent tissue damage if unrelieved for more than 6 hours).

- Treatment consists of rectifying any precipitant such as hypotension, prescribing systemic heparin to avoid extension of thrombus, and emergency embolectomy/thrombectomy. Thrombolytic therapy can be used if surgery is not considered mandatory.

becomes irreversible. By the time diarrhoea becomes bloody and there are signs of peritonitis, the bowel has infarcted and the patient's survival is unlikely.

ANEURYSM

An aneurysm is an abnormal dilatation of an artery (or occasionally a vein or a heart chamber). This may be congenital but is more commonly acquired. Aneurysms have three principal complications: rupture, thrombosis or embolism. An arterial aneurysm may be 'true' or 'false' (Fig. 21.15).

True aneurysms

A true aneurysm is enclosed by all three layers of the arterial wall. Acquired aneurysms result from degeneration of the media and elastic lamina due to atheroma or arteritis, with expansion of the affected part of the vessel. Though not strictly an aneurysm, *dissection* of the arterial wall, usually secondary to atherosclerotic destruction of the media, will also be considered here.

In subacute bacterial endocarditis and bacteraemia, septic emboli may lodge within the vasa vasorum and form an intramural abscess. This may give rise to an infective or (as it is often wrongly termed) 'mycotic' aneurysm.

Turbulence of the bloodstream within an aneurysm leads to the laying down of thrombus. As it enlarges, the aneurysm may erode adjacent structures. Since the tension in the wall of a viscus increases with its radius of curvature (Laplace's law), the liability to rupture increases as it expands.

Congenital aneurysms occur in the cerebral arteries and may be saccular or fusiform, depending on whether part or the whole of the circumference of the wall is weakened (see Fig. 21.15).

False aneurysms

If the wall of an artery is pierced, the resulting haematoma sometimes remains in continuity with the lumen. A pulsatile swelling then forms whose wall consists of compacted thrombus. If small (2–3 cm diameter) they usually thrombose and resolve, but if larger they tend to expand and leak.

Abdominal aortic aneurysm

An aneurysm of the abdominal aorta is found in some 5% of autopsies. Such aneurysms appear to be increasingly common in Western countries and they are more common in males. Fortunately 95% occur below the level of the origins of the renal arteries, which simplifies surgical treatment.

Aneurysms are often multiple. An abdominal aneurysm may be in continuity with a thoracic one or there may be associated iliac, femoral or popliteal aneurysms. Most patients are over 70 years of age. Many have hypertension, which increases the risk of rupture. This risk varies with aneurysm size. An aneurysm larger than 6 cm in diameter has at least a 50% risk of rupture within 2 years; however, the risk of dying of myocardial infarction or stroke during that period is almost as great.

Clinical features

An abdominal aortic aneurysm may present in the following ways:

- An asymptomatic pulsatile swelling may be found on routine physical examination, X-ray or abdominal scan.
- Pain may be felt in the central abdomen or more commonly it is referred to the back, loin, iliac fossa or groin; this may simulate renal colic.
- Leakage or rupture may cause severe abdominal or back pain and hypovolaemic shock. An episode of lesser pain (a 'herald bleed') may precede catastrophic rupture by several days or even weeks. Rarely an aneurysm may form a fistula into the bowel or vena cava.

Unless the patient is exceptionally obese, a pulsating mass can be felt. Tenderness is a sign of

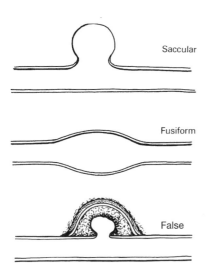

Fig. 21.15 Types of aneurysm.

Saccular

Fusiform

False

impending rupture or of an inflammatory aneurysm. Guarding and distension suggest rupture. Femoral pulses may be diminished.

A plain abdominal X-ray will show a rim of calcification especially on a lateral view. Ultrasound or CT scanning are useful investigations to determine the size and wall thickness and may demonstrate extravascular haematoma. Arteriography is indicated if there is a history of claudication or involvement of the renal arteries is suspected. The diagnosis of a ruptured aneurysm is based on history and physical examination unless the patient remains stable and the diagnosis is in doubt.

Management

The treatment of choice is replacement of the aneurysm with a Dacron graft. The aneurysmal sac is opened between clamps, partly excised and replaced by a straight tube or a 'trouser' bifurcation graft whose legs are anastomosed to the iliac or femoral arteries (Fig. 21.16).

All aneurysms over 5 cm in diameter should be repaired electively unless there are general contraindications to surgery, in which case progress must by monitored by ultrasound.

A leaking or ruptured aneurysm requires immediate operation. Over-enthusiastic resuscitation should be avoided and a systolic blood pressure of 80–90 mmHg is sufficient to sustain renal perfusion. Blood is immediately sent for rapid cross-matching and a urinary catheter and wide-bore venous cannula are inserted. Operative mortality depends on the experience of the surgeon and his team and transfer to a specialist centre is recommended. If the patient is

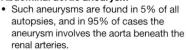

Abdominal aortic aneurysm
- Such aneurysms are found in 5% of all autopsies, and in 95% of cases the aneurysm involves the aorta beneath the renal arteries.

- The risk of rupture depends on size; 50% of aneurysms with a diameter of more than 6 cm will rupture within 2 years. All aneurysms larger than 5 cm should be repaired electively in the absence of contraindications to surgery.

- The aneurysm may be detected as an asymptomatic pulsatile swelling on abdominal examination, ultrasonography or abdominal X-ray, may present with pain in the back, loin, iliac fossa or groin, or may present with rupture (pain ± hypovolaemic shock).

- The treatment of choice is to replace the involved segment of aorta with a synthetic (Dacron) graft. Mortality rates following emergency repair (50%) greatly exceed those of elective repair (5% or less in some centres).

hypotensive, and particularly if he or she has to be transported any distance, a pneumatic 'anti-shock' suit applied to the lower limbs and abdomen will help to maintain blood pressure. Postoperative intensive care is essential. Myocardial infarction and renal failure are the main immediate complications.

Dissection of the aorta

Aortic dissection (see Fig. 21.2) generally begins in the ascending aorta or proximal descending aorta and extends distally. It may cause aortic valve incompetence and/or coronary artery occlusion and has a high mortality. The patients are usually hypertensive but dissection may also occur in pregnancy, as a result of trauma, or in Marfan's syndrome. The onset of dissection is accompanied by excruciating central chest pain which spreads to the back and abdomen. If the ascending aorta is involved, upper limb ischaemia is noted; dissections of the descending aorta affect the lower limbs. Severe chest or back pain with diminution of arm or leg pulses should always raise the suspicion of dissection. Paraplegia, renal failure and mesenteric ischaemia may signal involvement of aortic branches. Pulmonary oedema is often present. External rupture results in hypovolaemic shock.

Management

Pain control, antihypertensive treatment (e.g. with sodium nitroprusside) and stabilization of the circu-

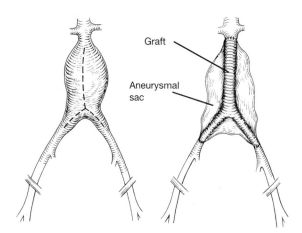

Graft

Aneurysmal sac

Fig. 21.16 Repair of an aortic aneurysm by insertion of a 'trouser' bifurcation graft within the opened aneurysmal sac.

lation are the first steps. The diagnosis is confirmed by aortography or CT scan.

Dissection of the ascending aorta is treated by resection of the affected part and replacement with a Dacron graft, combined if necessary with aortic valve replacement. Uncomplicated dissection of the descending aorta can be treated conservatively with antihypertensive drugs, but grafting is indicated if pain is uncontrolled, if the circulation cannot be stabilized, or if rupture occurs. About 50% of untreated patients die within 48 hours whereas 60% of treated patients survive 5 years.

Peripheral aneurysms

Aneurysms in peripheral vessels form pulsatile swellings in the course of the vessel. The liability to complications varies according to site. For example, in subclavian aneurysm, often associated with mechanical compression at the thoracic outlet (e.g. cervical rib), emboli are carried to the fingers and hand. Popliteal aneurysm frequently presents as acute arterial occlusion. The possibilities for reconstruction are often limited by silting of tibial and peroneal branches by previous small emboli. Aneurysms may also cause symptoms by pressure on adjacent veins or nerves. It is preferable to operate on large aneurysms electively rather than await complications.

Arteriography defines the site and extent of the aneurysm and the state of the distal arteries. Treatment consists of bypassing the affected segment with a vein or synthetic graft, the aneurysm being resected or simply tied off.

ARTERIOVENOUS FISTULA

An arteriovenous (A-V) fistula is an abnormal communication between artery and vein and may be congenital or acquired.

Congenital A-V fistula

Congenital A-V fistulas result from persistence of fetal arteriovenous communications. They are usually multiple and affect small vessels. They usually present in childhood and are commonest in the lower limb or pelvis. There is overgrowth of bone and soft tissues so that the limb is bigger, longer and warmer than normal. Extensive varicose veins cover the posterolateral aspect of the limb and there are areas of purple skin haemangioma. Superficial

venous hypertension may cause skin ulceration. Venous thrombosis is common.

Treatment. Surgery is unrewarding and best avoided. Venous hypertension is controlled with accurately fitted graduated compression stockings. In certain cases, selective catheterization and obliteration of feeding arteries by injected sclerosants is successful, and preferable to surgical ligation. The correction of limb over-growth by bone shortening is deferred until the epiphyses have fused after puberty.

Acquired A-V fistula

Acquired A-V fistulas are generally traumatic in origin and single. A penetrating injury (including surgical mishap) of adjacent artery and vein results in a channel between the two, either directly or with an intervening false aneurysm (Fig. 21.17). Blood is shunted under high pressure into the vein, which becomes thickened and arterialized. Deliberate construction of such a fistula in the forearm is used to provide ready vascular access in patients requiring dialysis for chronic renal failure.

A large communication between an artery and vein gives rise to serious consequences. First, the blood flow to tissues beyond the fistula may be reduced, causing ischaemia in the extremity. Second, the shunt places strain on the heart, leading to valve damage and high-output failure. Fistulas near the heart are more likely to cause cardiac failure, while those situated distally in the extremities tend to cause ischaemia. The clinical features are warmth and venous distension in the region of the fistula, and coldness and signs of atrophy distally. A palpable thrill and a loud to-and-fro 'machinery' murmur at the site of the fistula is characteristic. Occlusion of the fistula by pressure leads to slowing of the heart. Arteriography confirms the diagnosis and outlines the anatomy of the involved vessels.

Treatment. Where access is straightforward,

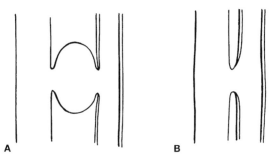

Fig. 21.17 Acquired (traumatic) arteriovenous fistula with A intervening false aneurysm and B direct communication.

the best treatment is operative closure of the fistula and repair or ligation of the vessels. In certain situations a fistula can be blocked by placement of a balloon inserted percutaneously.

ARTERITIS

Buerger's disease (thromboangiitis obliterans)

This obliterative arterial disease is rare in the UK but common in Mediterranean countries. It usually occurs in young males who are heavy smokers and characteristically affects the peripheral arteries, giving rise to claudication in the feet or rest pain in the fingers or toes. There is often a previous history of superficial phlebitis. Wrist and ankle pulses are usually absent, but brachial and popliteal pulses are palpable. Arteriography shows narrowing or occlusion of small peripheral arteries but relatively healthy main vessels. The condition often remits if the patient stops smoking, and sympathectomy is helpful. If amputation is required it can often be limited to the digits.

Giant cell arteritis

Giant cell arteritis is a rare condition involving major limb arteries, particularly the subclavian and axillary. Patients present with claudication and polymyalgia (i.e. pain and weakness) of shoulders and arms. The diagnosis is made by temporal artery biopsy. The condition is treated with steroids; surgery has no place.

Takayasu's arteritis

This rare inflammatory disease affects mainly the aortic arch vessels in young Asian women. Progressive ischaemia of the arms and brain may occur. Steroids may help. Surgical bypass of the affected arteries may be feasible, although further occlusions tend to occur.

Vasospastic disorders

These are very common. Disability is usually relatively minor but in a few patients there is associated thrombosis of small vessels leading to tissue damage.

Raynaud's phenomenon

Exposure to cold causes digital artery constriction so that the fingers become white, numb and painful. Primary and secondary types are recognized.

Primary Raynaud's phenomenon affects 5–10% of young women in temperate climates. It usually appears between the ages of 15 and 30 years; a family history is common. It does not progress to ulceration or infarction. No investigation is necessary and the patient is given reassurance and advised to avoid exposure to cold.

Secondary Raynaud's phenomenon tends to occur in older people as a manifestation of underlying disease such as scleroderma or systemic lupus. It may also be caused by working with vibrating tools or by treatment with beta-blocking drugs. There is thrombosis of small vessels leading to atrophy and necrosis of the finger-tips (Fig. 21.18). Management is often unsatisfactory, particularly when no underlying disease can be found. The fingers must be protected from cold and trauma, and infection treated with antibiotics. Vasoactive drugs have no clear benefit. Sympathectomy helps for a year or two. Prostacyclin infusions are sometimes beneficial. Limited debridement of infected or necrotic digits may be necessary.

Acrocyanosis

Acrocyanosis is characterized by red-blue discoloration of the skin on exposure to cold. When warm

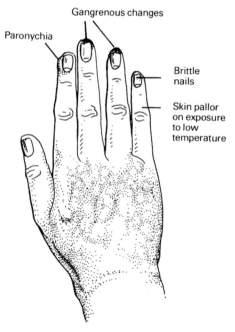

Fig. 21.18 Clinical appearance of long-standing secondary Raynaud's phenomenon.

the extremities become bright pink. It is distinct from, but often coexists with, Raynaud's phenomenon.

Chilblains are a form of this condition. It is also seen in elderly patients with cardiac disease and in limbs affected by neurological disorders such as stroke. Reassurance and protection from cold are usually all that is needed. If symptoms are severe, sympathectomy may be indicated. Vasodilators are ineffective.

Cold injury

Although frostbite is particularly associated with mountaineering, it is also frequently seen in temperate climates in neglected elderly patients or vagrants, particularly alcoholics. At first there is swelling, redness and blistering, followed by infection and superficial gangrene. Treatment consists of reflex heating, analgesics, antibiotics and dextran infusions. Surgical debridement is delayed until the area of dead tissue has become clearly demarcated.

VASCULAR TRAUMA

Arterial damage may occur as a result of blunt or penetrating trauma. Iatrogenic damage during the course of investigations (e.g. cardiac catheterization, arteriography) is relatively common and inadvertent intra-arterial injection of anaesthetic agents or sclerosants can also cause arterial injury. Compression of an artery may follow swelling of tissues within an osteofascial compartment or the application of rigid dressings, or it may be caused by direct pressure from splints or plasters.

Secondary thrombosis at the site of injury occludes the vessel. The degree of ischaemia depends on the state of the collateral circulation. While arterial spasm can occur at or beyond the site of injury, it should never be assumed to be the cause of ischaemia.

Arterial injuries can be divided into three categories:

- Complete severance or transection
- Incomplete or partial severance
- Contusion (Fig. 21.19).

Complete severance (transection)

If the vessel is completely divided, for example by a knife, its ends retract and constrict. Thrombosis occurs rapidly at the cut end and blood loss may be

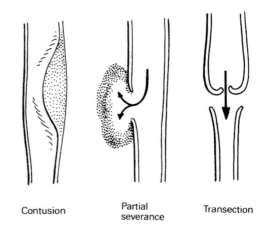

Contusion Partial severance Transection

Fig. 21.19 Types of arterial injury.

surprisingly small. Patients with severe atherosclerosis have less capacity for constriction and retraction so that serious haemorrhage is more likely.

Distal pulses in the limbs are lost immediately, and pallor, paraesthesia, pain, paralysis and poikilothermia (coldness) — the five Ps of acute ischaemia — quickly develop.

Incomplete severance

Partial division of an artery may result from penetrating injuries (including those from surgical knives, drills or needles) or from closed injury, e.g. when the vessel is lacerated by a fragment of fractured bone.

Partial continuity of the vessel prevents retraction, and contraction of the circular muscle at the site of injury tends to hold the laceration open. Haemorrhage is severe. If the overlying tissues are intact, this leads to the formation of a pulsating haematoma (see earlier). Diminution of distal pulses and signs of distal ischaemia are less pronounced than after complete severance. If there is coincident damage to an adjacent vein, an arteriovenous fistula is likely to develop.

Arterial contusion

Contusion results from blunt injury or stretching and is not uncommon in fractures. An intramural haematoma may develop and occlude the vessel. Usually, however, on exploring the vessel the surgeon finds that although the adventitia is intact the intima has been split, often completely circumferentially, with resultant thrombosis.

External bleeding is absent. Pulses disappear and signs of ischaemia develop.

Management

In an open wound, severe haemorrhage indicates the likelihood of arterial damage. In closed injuries, arterial damage should always be considered if limbs and lives are to be saved. Even then, some arterial injuries are not apparent at first but become obvious when complications arise.

Control of haemorrhage is the first concern. The limb is elevated and pressure applied. Tourniquets are seldom required and are potentially dangerous. Blood volume is restored by transfusion. If the peripheral circulation does not improve despite adequate replacement, surgery is indicated. Arteriography may help to define the site and extent of the injury but is often unnecessary and should not delay definitive surgical treatment.

Early reconstruction is advised for injuries of large arteries; small ones may be ligated. Direct closure is sometimes possible but generally a vein patch or tube graft is preferred. Synthetic grafts should be avoided because of their liability to infection, thrombosis and secondary haemorrhage.

Fractures should be stabilized first by external or internal fixation. Antibiotic cover is advisable. Heparin or dextran therapy should be used postoperatively to maintain patency.

Intra-arterial injection of noxious material is treated conservatively in the first instance. The artery is flushed with heparinized saline and irrigated with a vasodilator such as naftidrofuryl, reserpine or prostacyclin. Full systemic doses of heparin, opiates and antibiotics are given.

DISORDERS OF THE VEINS

Venous drainage of the lower limb

The superficial veins of the lower limb are the long and short saphenous veins and their tributaries (Fig. 21.20). The vessels lie outside the deep fascia and carry only 10% of the venous return from the limb. The long saphenous vein begins at the medial end of the dorsal venous arch, crosses in front of the medial malleolus and ascends the medial side of the leg. It penetrates the deep fascia (cribriform fascia) at the saphenous opening 4 cm below and lateral to the pubic tubercle to enter the femoral vein. The short saphenous vein starts at the lateral end of the dorsal venous arch, and passes round posteriorly to

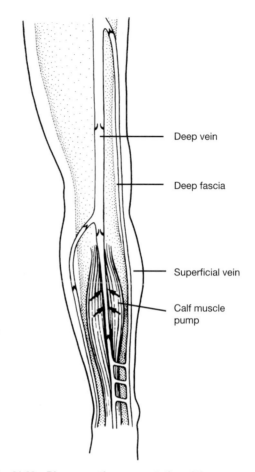

Fig. 21.20 Diagrammatic representation of the venous drainage of the lower limb.

the median line of the calf, in which it ascends to join the popliteal vein behind the knee. Anatomical variations are common.

The deep venous system comprises intramuscular veins and the veins, usually paired in the calf, which accompany the main arteries. There is also liberal venous flow in the medullary cavities of the bones.

The superficial and deep systems are connected by communicating veins which perforate the deep fascia (see Fig. 21.20). The largest perforators are on the medial side of the lower calf, but some occur on the lateral side of the calf and the medial side of the thigh. A point of surgical importance is that in the calf the perforators do not connect directly with the long saphenous vein but join its tributaries.

Venous return is an active process. There is a 'foot pump' as veins of the sole are emptied by weight-bearing and a 'calf pump' comprising veins within the soleus muscle which is activated by muscle contraction within the cylinder of fascia lata. Blood flow is directed inwards and upwards by valves, and during muscle relaxation is sucked in from the superficial veins. Reflux into the superficial system is prevented by valves in the perforators and at the terminations of the saphenous veins. On standing the venous pressure at the ankle is approximately 100 cmH$_2$O (zero in the right atrium) and, provided that valves are intact, falls to 20–30 cmH$_2$O during exercise. It is because of its exposure to this relatively high pressure that the saphenous vein is thick-walled and suitable for arterial grafting.

VARICOSE VEINS

Varicose veins of the leg are particularly common in women (female-to-male ratio 5:1). Incompetence of valves and reflux of blood from the deep system subjects the superficial veins to excessive pressure not only when standing or sitting at rest but also during exercise. The veins become elongated, dilated and tortuous. It is the thin-walled tributaries

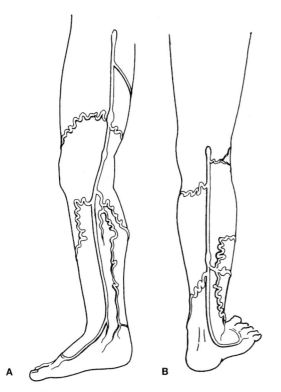

Fig. 21.21 Diagrammatic representation of varicose veins in the lower limb. A Long saphenous system. **B** Short saphenous system.

that undergo these changes; the saphenous veins themselves are relatively little altered (Fig. 21.21).

Primary varicose veins are common and often show a familial tendency. There is debate as to whether the basic fault is in the valves or in the elasticity of the vein wall. The valves at the sapheno-femoral and/or sapheno-popliteal junctions are incompetent and the distension and varicosity spreads progressively through the system. The deep veins are usually normal. Aggravating factors include obesity, pregnancy, constipation and prolonged standing.

Secondary varicose veins develop after valve function has been damaged by disease (thrombosis) or occasionally trauma. The deep veins are either rendered incompetent or are occluded. The high pressure from posture and from the calf muscle pump is transmitted to the superficial veins predominantly via calf perforators, which also become incompetent. Another cause of secondary varicose veins is arteriovenous fistula (see above).

Sustained high pressure in the superficial veins, known as chronic venous insufficiency, results in changes in the skin and subcutaneous tissues of the 'gaiter' area collectively termed lipodermatosclerosis. They consist of oedema, inflammation, fibrosis, pigmentation, eczema and ulceration. Chronic venous insufficiency disturbs the balance between haemodynamic and osmotic pressures (the Starling equation) in the capillaries. The mechanism of the skin changes is not fully understood but it is known that increased capillary permeability permits escape of protein and red cells into the extravascular compartment. Breakdown of the red cells leads to haemosiderin deposition. Fibrin is precipitated outside the vessels and may form a barrier to nutrition. White cell sequestration and activation is also thought to play a part. It is unusual for primary varices to lead to these changes, but they are very common in the secondary variety.

Clinical features

The main anxiety for many patients is that their varices are unsightly, but discomfort in a distended vein and general ache, tiredness and swelling in the limb are common complaints, especially after long periods of standing. The skin changes described above begin with pigmentation or eczema. Minor trauma to such an area often fails to heal and progresses to chronic ulceration.

Rupture of a varix is uncommon but can lead to severe haemorrhage. It is easily controlled by elevation of the limb and local pressure.

Varicose veins are prone to thrombosis (superficial phlebitis), which is discussed later.

Examination

The aim is to identify the sites of incompetent connections between the deep and superficial systems. The patient is examined standing, preferably on a raised platform in a warm room. The experienced examiner will know the likely sites of incompetence from the anatomical pattern of the varices. *Percussion* over a varix while palpating with the other hand at a higher or lower level will help trace the pattern.

The level at which deep-to-superficial reflux is occurring can be checked by the *Trendelenberg test* (Fig. 21.22). The leg is elevated and a rubber tourniquet applied just below the sapheno-femoral junction. The patient is then asked to stand. Veins fill slowly from arterial inflow but quickly from venous reflux. If venous distension below the tourniquet is controlled, the site of reflux must be above it. By moving the tourniquet to different levels in the limb the pattern of incompetence can be mapped out.

A more effective way to demonstrate reflux is to insonate over the site of incompetence and reflux with a portable continuous wave *Doppler ultrasound flowmeter*. This is particularly valuable in obese patients or those with recurrent varicose veins in whom the anatomy may be obscure.

If it is suspected that the varicose veins are secondary to deep vein thrombosis (DVT) (history or the presence of stigmata of chronic venous insufficiency), *ascending phlebography* may be performed. Contrast medium is injected into a foot vein while occluding the superficial system with a tourniquet around the ankle, and taking serial films as the contrast ascends the limb. Before operating on difficult cases of varicose veins, particularly recurrent ones, *varicography* is used, i.e. the direct injection of contrast material into varices to demonstrate deep connections. Duplex ultrasonography is a non-invasive method which can also image veins and study valve incompetence.

Severe varicose veins, especially if in children, of atypical distribution, or associated with cutaneous haemangioma, soft-tissue hypertrophy or limb overgrowth should raise the suspicion of congenital arteriovenous fistulas.

Management

Conservative treatment

Elderly patients or those with mild disease can be treated conservatively. Elastic support hose, weight reduction, regular exercise and avoidance of constricting garments all help to relieve tiredness and reduce swelling.

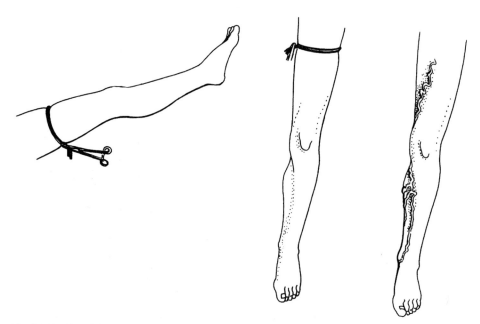

Fig. 21.22   Trendelenberg test to demonstrate sapheno-femoral incompetence.

Sclerotherapy

Injection treatment is used for small varices below the knee which are due to incompetence of local perforators or for recurrent varices after surgery. It is not satisfactory for varices associated with sapheno-femoral or sapheno-popliteal incompetence since recurrence is inevitable. Sclerotherapy also makes subsequent surgery more difficult.

The injection sites are marked with a pen while the patient stands. He or she then sits with the leg hanging over the side of the couch and an elastic self-adhesive bandage is applied, starting at the base of the toes, and wound up to the first injection site. The needle is inserted at the lowest mark and the leg elevated to empty the veins; 0.5 ml of 3% sodium tetradecyl sulphate is then injected while the vein is compressed proximally to keep the segment empty. A cotton wool ball is placed over the injection site and the bandage advanced up to the next point where the injection is repeated – and so on. Compression is maintained for 3 weeks. As the bandage is self-adhesive it stays in place undisturbed. The patient is instructed to walk several miles each day in order to redevelop an efficient muscle pump.

Surgery

When there is sapheno-femoral or sapheno-popliteal incompetence, surgery is the only effective treatment. Varicose vein surgery has three aims:

* To intercept incompetent connections between deep and superficial veins.
* To remove (strip) the main saphenous channels from which pressure is distributed among the superficial veins.
* To eradicate varices.

Sapheno-femoral ligation. The sapheno-femoral junction is displayed and all its tributaries are carefully dissected out, ligated and divided. (Fig. 21.23). The saphenous vein is ligated flush with the femoral vein. In patients with sapheno-popliteal incompetence, the upper end of the incompetent short saphenous vein is dealt with in similar fashion.

Recurrence is less likely if the long saphenous vein is stripped out from knee to groin. However, this part of the operation is omitted if there is any prospect that the patient might later need the saphenous vein as an arterial bypass, e.g. if he or she has arterial symptoms, a strong family history of obliterative disease, is a smoker or has angina or a history of myocardial disease.

Varices are eradicated by dissection and ligation or by the avulsion technique, in which the varices are 'winkled out' through many tiny incisions. Bleeding is controlled by tourniquet or local pressure.

CHRONIC LEG ULCER

Ulceration of the leg is common, especially in the elderly. It affects approximately 4% of individuals over 60 years of age. The female : male ratio is 3 : 1. Some two-thirds are attributable to chronic venous insufficiency. Arterial disease, diabetes and rheumatoid disease are important associated diseases. Added to these causes are many aggravating factors such as old age, obesity, recurrent trauma,

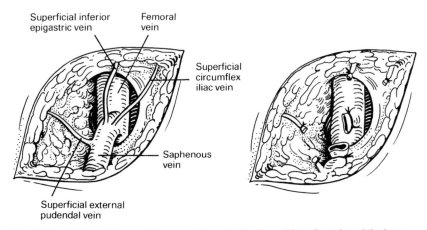

Superficial inferior epigastric vein

Femoral vein

Superficial circumflex iliac vein

Saphenous vein

Superficial external pudendal vein

Fig. 21.23 **Sapheno-femoral disconnection with ligation of the tributaries of the long saphenous vein.**

Varicose veins

- Varicose veins of the lower limb are five times as common in females, and aetiological factors include a familial predisposition, obesity, pregnancy, constipation, prolonged standing, and damage of the deep veins and their valves (usually by deep venous thrombosis).

- The major problem is that the valves guarding the junctions between the superficial and deep venous systems (notably the sapheno-femoral and sapheno-popliteal junctions) are, or become, incompetent.

- Varicose veins may give rise to discomfort, aching and a feeling of tiredness in the leg, particularly after standing, although in many patients the main complaint is that the veins are unsightly.

- Sustained high pressure in the superficial veins may lead to chronic venous insufficiency with oedema, pigmentation, inflammation, eczema and ulceration, these changes being commonest in the 'gaiter' area.

- The Trendelenburg test is used to determine the level at which reflux from the deep to superficial system is occurring.

- Management options include conservative treatment, sclerotherapy with compression, and surgery. The three aims of surgery are to interrupt incompetent perforating veins, eradicate the varices, and (in some cases) strip out the long saphenous vein.

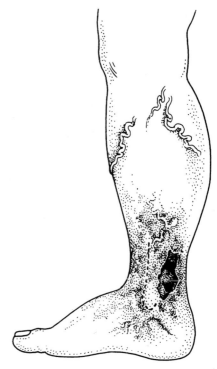

Fig. 21.24   Appearances of a chronic venous ulcer of the leg.

immobility, joint problems (including osteoarthritis and arthrodesis) and neurological deficits following stroke or polio.

Clinical features

Chronic venous ulcer (Fig. 21.24) is the end-stage of lipodermatosclerosis. It is typically situated in the retromalleolar region on the medial side of the gaiter area, just below the calf perforators. Varicose veins are usually obvious. The ulcer is usually single, large and shallow with a base of unhealthy granulation tissue and is surrounded by the signs of chronic venous insufficiency, i.e. pigmentation, induration and eczema. Contact dermatitis is very common because of the chronicity of the condition and the use of injudicious treatments, such as local antibiotics.

If an ulcer does not have these characteristics, an alternative aetiology should be considered. For example, if it is deep and painful and/or extends onto the foot, an arterial element is suspected. If ulcers are multiple and situated higher up on the front or lateral side of the calf, arteritis is the likely cause. An ulcer on the front of the shin or foot may

be traumatic. Some ulcers, for psychological reasons, are self-inflicted.

Management

A careful history should be taken, particularly noting thrombotic episodes, previous vein surgery, arterial symptoms, diabetes, autoimmune disease locomotor problems and allergies. Examination and investigation concentrates on predisposing conditions and should include pedal pulses and Doppler pressures, ankle mobility, gait, full blood count, blood glucose determination and rheumatoid serology. If surgery is contemplated, phlebography is advisable to assess the state of the deep veins. The treatment of chronic leg ulcers depends on the aetiology. Arterial insufficiency is treated by reconstruction or sympathectomy, locomotor disabilities by physiotherapy. Mobility is encouraged, diabetes controlled and obesity, if possible, reduced.

The great majority of ulcers are venous and are treated as follows.

Conservative treatment.   Many venous ulcers can be cured while the patient remains fully active. An absorbent, non-adherent, dressing is applied. Local antibiotics are contraindicated.

Dressing is of secondary importance to careful bandaging designed to counteract the venous hypertension and swelling. This is achieved by *graduated elastic compression* combined with high elevation of the limb at rest. Graduated elastic compression achieves a pressure gradient maximal in the gaiter area and diminishing as it ascends the leg (Fig. 21.25). This has the optimal effect on flow in the deep veins. For a patient of average build a pressure of around 30–40 mmHg at the ankle is appropriate. While the ulcer is still present, compression is achieved by bandaging and after healing, by elastic stocking. Application of effective compression bandages requires skill and experience. It is important to exclude arterial disease before compression is applied.

For inflamed or intractable ulcers bed rest is required with high elevation of the leg to counteract venous hypertension. Once the ulcer is clean, healing can be hastened with skin grafts. When the ulcer has healed, venous hypertension must be controlled by long-term high-quality elastic stockings or surgery. Superficial varices are dealt with as described earlier

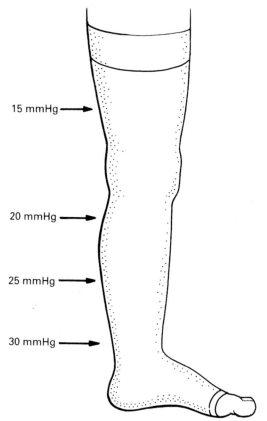

15 mmHg →

20 mmHg →

25 mmHg →

30 mmHg →

Fig. 21.25 Graduated elastic compression for venous ulcer. Compression from the base of the toes to the tibial tuberosity usually suffices.

and incompetent perforators in the lower calf are ligated. This is best done by incising the skin and deep fascia and ligating the perforating vessels under the deep fascia.

VENOUS THROMBOSIS AND PULMONARY EMBOLISM

Superficial thrombophlebitis

Inflammation and thrombosis of a previously normal superficial vein may result from trauma, irritation from an intravenous infusion or from the injection of noxious agents. With the exception of septic puncture sites, it is usually non-bacterial. When superficial phlebitis occurs spontaneously, it almost invariably arises in a varicose vein. Redness and tenderness follow the line of the vein. Thrombosis may spread through communicating channels into the deep veins and give rise to pulmonary embolism. It resolves over 2–3 weeks, leaving a track of pigmentation and fibrosed nodular veins.

Treatment consists of analgesics, support stockings and active exercise. Rapid propagation with deep vein involvement may require heparin therapy and occasionally thrombectomy or vein ligation.

Recurrent, migrating superficial phlebitis is occasionally seen in malignant disease.

Deep vein thrombosis (DVT)

This condition is very common. It is present in some 30% of legs after major operations. It is usually asymptomatic, particularly in the first few days, which is unfortunate because it is the early thrombus which most readily becomes detached and embolizes to the lungs.

The starting point for DVT is usually a valve sinus in the deep veins of the calf (Fig. 21.26). Primary thrombus consists of adherent laminae of platelets and fibrin. When it has accumulated sufficiently to impede flow it is augmented by secondary thrombus which consists of a looser meshwork of red cells and fibrin and which propagates rapidly. It may extend into the popliteal, femoral or iliac veins or vena cava. In a few cases DVT originates in the pelvic veins.

Pulmonary embolism is a serious complication. Life-threatening embolism rarely occurs from calf DVT but the risk is very real when the iliofemoral segment is involved. Since DVT commonly produces no symptoms, the first evidence of its presence may be a fatal pulmonary embolism.

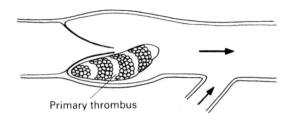

Primary thrombus

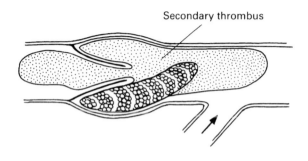

Secondary thrombus

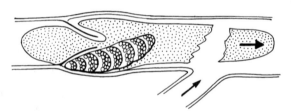

Fig. 21.26   Mechanism of embolus formation from thrombus in a deep vein.

Aetiology

Three factors are traditionally associated with thrombogenesis: venous stasis, intimal damage and hypercoagulability of the blood.

Venous stasis. Many of the factors recognized as increasing the risk of thrombosis, such as immobility, obesity, pregnancy, paralysis, operation and trauma, imply an element of venous obstruction or stasis. However, stasis alone does not cause thrombosis; other factors must be present.

Intimal damage. In most instances of DVT no evidence of intimal damage can be detected, but external trauma to a vein, for example during a hip replacement operation, can provide a starting point for thrombogenesis.

Hypercoagulability. Primary hypercoagulable states include deficiencies of antithrombin III, protein C, protein S and plasminogen activators. One of these should be suspected if there are recur-

rent thrombotic episodes, especially if they occur in a young person or there is a strong family history. Polycythaemia rubra vera is also associated with a tendency to thrombosis.

Secondary hypercoagulable states are conditions associated with thrombosis but the cause is not identified. These include pregnancy and the puerperium, malignancy, Behçet's disease, homocystinuria and paroxysmal nocturnal haemoglobinuria.

It is important to identify patients who are at potential risk of developing venous thromboembolism during or after operation. The most important risk factors are:

- A history of previous DVT or embolism
- Advanced age
- Malignant disease
- Varicose veins
- Obesity
- Thrombophilia.

For reasons which are not clear, smokers have a lower risk of postoperative DVT than non-smokers.

Diagnosis

Early DVT sometimes gives rise to warmth and dilated superficial veins over the affected area. The principal symptoms are pain and swelling, but these may be absent or develop only after the thrombus has begun to organize or has extended to obstruct venous outflow or collaterals. Swelling at the ankle or lower calf indicates that the thrombus is at least at popliteal level; swelling up to the level of the knee means femoral vein thrombosis; thigh swelling indicates iliac vein thrombosis.

Arterial spasm may accompany extensive DVT and cause a swollen white leg (phlegmasia alba dolens). If the limb is both swollen and cyanosed, (phlegmasia caerula dolens) not only are the main stem veins occluded but also the collateral channels. This may go on to venous gangrene and usually indicates a sinister underlying cause such as advanced malignant disease.

The differential diagnosis of DVT includes lymphoedema, dependent oedema, mechanical or tumour obstruction, cellulitis, a ruptured Baker's cyst, haematoma, muscle strain and arterial occlusion.

Because of the inaccuracy of the clinical diagnosis of DVT, anticoagulant treatment (which is potentially dangerous) should not be continued unless the diagnosis has been properly confirmed.

The *radiofibrinogen uptake test* is an excellent perioperative screening test although its use is largely confined to research. The thyroid is first blocked with 100 mg potassium iodide. An intravenous injection of ^{125}I-labelled fibrinogen is then given and the legs are serially scanned on successive days for 'hot spots' with a portable radiation counter. A hot spot which persists on successive readings indicates that fibrinogen has accumulated in a thrombus.

When DVT is suspected clinically, a variety of non-invasive confirmatory tests may be used, including directional Doppler ultrasound, thermography, impedance or strain gauge plethysmography and Duplex B-mode scanning. Each of these improves the accuracy of diagnosis, each has its limitations and none provides as much information as phlebography, which is the 'gold standard'.

Phlebography for DVT is performed by the ascending method unless swelling of the thigh indicates occlusive ilio-femoral thrombus. Ascending phlebography (Fig. 21.27) involves injection of approximately 40 ml of non-ionic (non-irritant) contrast material into a vein on the dorsum of each foot, flow being directed into the deep veins by superficial tourniquets applied above the ankle. For suspected DVT, phlebography should always be bilateral. The aim is to delineate fully any thrombus, especially its upper end since this is the dangerous portion. If ascending phlebography fails to achieve this, perfemoral phlebography with direct injection of contrast into the femoral veins may be necessary. The appearances of the thrombus will indicate how recent it is, how extensive and how likely to embolize. These are the parameters which influence treatment.

An integral part of the investigation of DVT is to find out whether the thrombus is actively embolizing. A lung scan should be obtained at an early stage and provides a baseline for comparison with subsequent scans.

Prevention

Pulmonary embolism is still a common cause of postoperative death. Because of our inability to

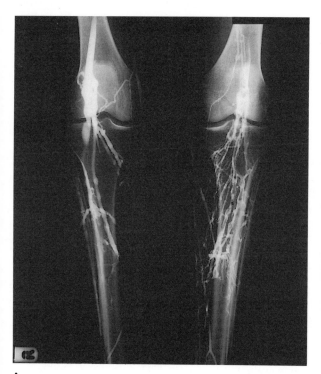

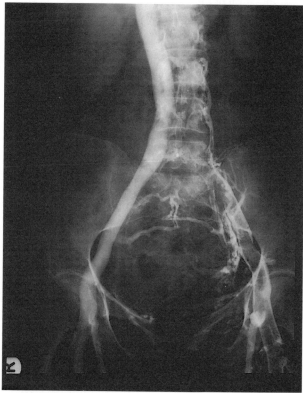

A   B

Fig. 21.27 **Ascending phlebography** showing **A** deep venous thrombosis in the left popliteal vein, and **B** thrombus in left iliac veins.

diagnose DVT in its early and dangerous phase, prophylaxis is very important. Aspects of modern surgical care which help to reduce the likelihood of postoperative venous thromboembolism include regional anaesthesia, accurate fluid replacement, effective pain control and early ambulation. Sometimes these measures are not enough, especially in high-risk patients or high-risk operations. High-risk operations include hip reconstructions, spinal operations, major abdominal or pelvic procedures and others associated with severe illness, malignancy, sepsis or trauma.

Physical methods. Flow in the deep veins can be accelerated and thrombus prevented by graduated compression stockings. These exert a pressure of about 20 mmHg at the ankle. To avoid pressure damage it is vital to check that the patient has readily palpable pedal pulses before applying elastic stockings. If in doubt, the arterial pressure should be measured with a Doppler ultrasonic flowmeter.

Intermittent pneumatic compression can be applied to the legs by means of plastic sleeves connected to a pump during and after operation and is of proven benefit. So is intermittent electrical stimulation of the calf muscles.

Active exercises and early mobilization should be encouraged.

Pharmacological methods. Low-dose subcutaneous calcium or sodium heparin, 5000 units 12-hourly, protects against DVT and pulmonary embolism. The first dose is given with the premedication and treatment is continued until the patient is fully ambulant. There is a slightly increased risk of bleeding and wound haematoma. Low molecular weight heparin is marginally more effective than unfractionated heparin, especially in orthopaedic surgery, but is also more expensive.

Dextran-70 is a starch solution which reduces blood viscosity and coagulability; the protection given is equivalent to that provided by heparin. It is administered by intravenous infusion of 500 ml perioperatively and then daily for 2–3 days. Dextran-70 tends to encourage capillary oozing at operation. Anaphylaxis is a rare but occasionally severe complication.

Oral anticoagulants are effective prophylactic agents but they require laboratory control, react unfavourably with many drugs, and their effects are not easily reversed should bleeding occur. Antiplatelet agents do not provide effective prophylaxis against venous thrombosis.

For patients at particular risk of thromboembolism, physical and pharmacological methods can be combined. The surgeon has to balance the poten-

tial benefit against the inconvenience, side-effects and costs of the methods available.

Treatment of acute DVT

The plan of treatment assumes that the DVT has been reliably diagnosed by an objective method, preferably phlebography. The aims of treatment are:

- To relieve acute symptoms
- To protect against pulmonary embolism
- To facilitate resolution and thereby reduce the likelihood of long-term post-thrombotic damage to the limb.

If thrombus is confined to the calf and the patient is fully mobile, an elastic stocking and physical exercise may be all that is required.

Usually the patient has some underlying cause for the DVT which prevents full activity and there is a risk of thrombus extension. Specific treatment is therefore essential. The foot of the bed is elevated. If there is marked swelling, additional elevation is provided with extra pillows or a foam wedge. Active movement of toes and ankle is encouraged. Elastic compression is not necessary during this phase. Once the patient starts to be mobile, graduated compression stockings are fitted. Mobilization is started as soon as swelling has resolved.

Heparin therapy is started with an intravenous injection of 5000 units and followed by continuous infusion of 1500–3000 units/hour by syringe pump. Calcium heparin can also be given by deep subcutaneous injection in full therapeutic doses of 2500 units per 10 kg body weight 12-hourly, which makes it easier for the patient to become mobile. Subsequent doses of heparin are adjusted to keep the activated partial thromboplastin time at two to three times the normal value. Heparin is continued for 1–2 weeks (depending on the severity of the episode) and overlapped with oral anticoagulants by 3 days. Oral anticoagulants are continued for at least 3 months and patients with a history of recurrent episodes may have to continue treatment indefinitely.

Thrombolytic therapy with streptokinase and urokinase has proved disappointing in DVT of the lower limbs, largely because of the difficulty of making the diagnosis early enough for the thrombus to be readily lysable. New thrombolytic agents such as tissue plasminogen activator and prourokinase are being evaluated.

In some centres venous thrombectomy is practised for ilio-femoral thrombosis but re-occlu-

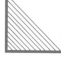

Deep venous thrombosis

- Deep venous thrombosis develops in some 30% of patients after major surgery and commences in the deep veins of the calf (soleal sinuses).

- The three major aetiological factors are venous stasis, intimal damage and hypercoagulability during surgery. Risk factors include previous venous thromboembolism, advanced age, malignancy, varicose veins, obesity and thrombophilia.

- Prophylaxis is recommended and may take the form of low dose subcutaneous heparin (5000 units every 12 hours) and/or physical methods to maintain flow (graduated compression stockings, intermittent pneumatic compression).

- Deep venous thrombosis often produces pain, swelling, local temperature increase and prominence of the superficial veins, but clinical diagnosis is notoriously unreliable and anticoagulation is withheld until the presence of thrombosis has been confirmed (see below).

- Bilateral ascending phlebography remains the 'gold standard' for diagnosis. The key questions are: is thrombus present, is it located in the calf veins or the ilio-femoral segment, and is it occlusive or non-occlusive?

- Thrombus confined to calf veins is treated by supporting (TED) stockings and mobilization. Ilio-femoral thrombus is treated by anticoagulation (heparin with subsequent transfer to warfarin for at least 3 months).

sion may occur and post-thrombotic syndrome is not necessarily prevented.

Pulmonary embolism

Pulmonary embolism is found in approximately 50% of all autopsies. It is the commonest acute lung disorder in hospital patients and an important cause of postoperative death.

Like DVT the majority of pulmonary emboli are silent and many of those which give rise to symptoms are not diagnosed. Approximately 90% of pulmonary emboli arise from the veins of the lower limbs or pelvis. A few come from the right heart. The recent increase in the use of central venous lines for monitoring and parenteral nutrition has caused an increase in emboli from the subclavian veins.

Major embolism

Massive embolism with occlusion of two-thirds or

more of the pulmonary arterial flow causes acute central chest pain, followed by severe dyspnoea, cyanosis, hypotension and collapse.

Early resuscitation is essential and includes cardiac massage, administration of oxygen (at a rate of 6 litre/min) and immediate injection of heparin 15 000 units intravenously to prevent extension of thrombus. Intravenous fluid is given to support right ventricular filling and a pressor agent (i.e. 1 in 1000 noradrenaline made up as 2 mg in 500 ml of isotonic saline) given via a paediatric burette at a rate titrated to maintain blood pressure at a minimum of 80 mmHg systolic.

An urgent pulmonary angiogram is obtained and, if the diagnosis is confirmed and the patient's condition is still serious, thrombolytic therapy is commenced with a loading dose of 250 000 units of streptokinase intravenously, followed by 100 000 units per hour by infusion pump for 24 hours. If life is threatened and pulmonary angiography is not available, thrombolytic therapy should be started on the strength of clinical diagnosis. Hydrocortisone 100 mg intravenously is given before the streptokinase. New thrombolytic agents (tissue plasminogen activator; plasminogen-streptokinase complex; pro-urokinase) may prove to be equally effective but with fewer bleeding complications.

The patient's vital signs are carefully monitored. Thrombolytic therapy is followed by heparin and later by oral anticoagulants.

Rarely pulmonary embolectomy may have to be considered, but few pulmonary emboli occur in circumstances which permit immediate cardiopulmonary bypass.

Minor embolism

This includes any embolism which does not immediately threaten life. Most emboli are multiple and many do not cause infarction. The symptoms may therefore be insidious and a high level of suspicion is essential.

Dyspnoea may be sudden or gradual. Infarction results in pleuritic chest pain, tachycardia and pyrexia. Haemoptysis is relatively uncommon. Auscultation reveals diminished air entry, moist rales and a friction rub. Some pulmonary emboli cause bronchospasm and are mistaken for asthmatic attacks. Others, by reducing cerebral oxygenation, may present as confusion, impaired consciousness or syncopal attacks. Recurrent pulmonary emboli may over months or years lead to pulmonary hypertension.

Blood gas analysis shows a low Pao_2. Electrocardiogram (ECG) may show signs of right heart strain with right axis deviation, a prolonged PR interval, depressed ST segments in leads I and II and an inverted T wave in leads II and III. The chest X-ray may be unremarkable or may show diminished lung markings, a prominent pulmonary artery and enlarged cardiac shadow. Linear atelectasis may be noted. Later there may be pleural effusion, elevation of the diaphragm and wedge-shaped areas of consolidation.

Lung scanning and phlebography are the principal investigations. A perfusion scan is performed with a gamma-camera after intravenous injection of ^{99m}Tc-labelled macroaggregates of albumin. To distinguish perfusion defects from those caused by emphysematous bullae, a ventilation scan may be added. This will reveal areas of increased uptake following the inhalation of xenon-133. If there is doubt about the diagnosis or if thrombolytic therapy is being considered, a pulmonary angiogram is obtained.

At least one-third of the patients who die of pulmonary embolism have had previous episodes of 'herald' embolism. In patients suspected of minor pulmonary embolism, attention must be focused on the lower limbs and residual life-threatening DVT excluded by bilateral phlebography.

The main objective of management is to prevent further embolism. Systemic heparin therapy is started at once, followed by an oral anticoagulant. Antibiotics and analgesics are indicated for pulmonary infarction. If phlebography reveals loose thrombus in femoral or iliac veins or vena cava, embolism can be prevented by insertion of a filter into the inferior vena cava (Fig. 21.28). The filter is introduced percutaneously under radiological control through a femoral or a jugular vein. A further indication for insertion of a caval filter is recurrence of embolism despite anticoagulation. Surgical removal of the thrombus is associated with a high re-thrombosis rate and is seldom indicated. Oral anticoagulants are continued for at least 6 months.

Other forms of venous thrombosis

Inferior vena caval thrombosis

Thrombosis of the inferior vena cava may result from extension of an iliofemoral thrombosis, but more often complicates abdominal malignant disease. The typical signs are bilateral leg and scrotal oedema, distended collateral veins on the abdominal wall and possibly ascites. Management is symptomatic with elevation and anticoagulation (in non-malignant cases followed by mobilization with graduated elastic compression.

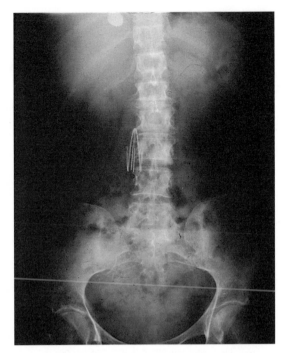

Fig. 21.28 Filter placed in the inferior vena cava to prevent pulmonary embolism.

Superior vena caval thrombosis

Mediastinal tumours or enlarged lymph nodes (e.g. from breast or bronchial carcinoma) may obstruct the superior vena cava and induce thrombosis. Central venous catheters for parenteral nutrition or pressure monitoring may cause thrombosis of the vena cava, or the subclavian or axillary veins. The patient experiences an unpleasant bursting feeling in the head, neck and upper limbs. There is oedema, cyanosis and venous distension.

The obstruction is defined by upper limb phlebography. If the cause is not malignant, gratifying relief may be obtained from thrombolytic therapy followed by heparin and oral anticoagulants. Radiotherapy, chemotherapy or percutaneous stenting may relieve malignant obstruction, but the outlook is poor.

Subclavian and axillary vein thrombosis

Catheter-induced thrombosis has been discussed above. Malignant disease or irradiation of axillary lymph nodes are other causes of axillary thrombosis. Spontaneous axillary thrombosis occasionally occurs in healthy young adults. Sometimes it follows exercise and is then termed 'effort thrombosis'. There may be a previous history of intermittent venous obstruction in the limb due to a mechanical cause at the thoracic outlet. A cervical rib, abnormal muscle or ligamentous bands at the inner border of the first rib, or a narrow interval between the clavicle and the first rib may constrict the vein and lead to thrombosis.

The patient complains of an uncomfortable, heavy, cyanosed arm with venous engorgement. Venous collaterals develop over the shoulder and anterior chest wall.

Upper limb phlebography defines the occlusion. The arm should be elevated, e.g. in a towel suspended from a drip stand. Heparin therapy followed by oral anticoagulants is standard treatment. Thrombolytic therapy can be very effective in early cases. Many surgeons believe that after the axillary thrombosis has been cleared the thoracic outlet should be explored and the first rib or other obstructing element removed.

DISORDERS OF LYMPHATICS

The lymphatic system drains fluid from the interstitial spaces into the venous system. The lymphatics have little if any basement membrane and lack tight junctions between endothelial cells, an arrangement which allows protein molecules to pass through their wall. Flow is directed centrally by endothelial valves and is increased by muscle contraction. The total daily lymph flow is only 2–4 litres.

Solitary lymph nodes occur along the course of the major lymph trunks which then pass to regional nodes. Lymph nodes consist of a supporting framework of reticuloendothelial tissue and contain aggre-

gates of lymphoid tissue (Fig. 21.29). They have filtering, phagocytic and immunological functions.

Lymphangitis

Acute lymphangitis

Inflammation of the dermal lymphatics is most commonly due to streptococcal infection. The primary site of infection is often a minor wound or puncture, and the inflamed lymphatics form red lines in the skin which are often palpable and tender. The regional nodes may also be enlarged and tender (lymphadenitis).

Chronic lymphangitis

Mondor's disease is a rare condition in which there are tense tender strings in the skin and subcutaneous tissues of the breast and cubital fossa.

Lymphoedema

Blockage of lymph flow upsets the normal balance of forces which control the passage of fluid across capillary basement membranes. Accumulation of protein in the tissues increases the osmotic pressure and hence the volume of interstitial fluid (Fig. 21.30). This increase in protein-rich fluid is known as lymphoedema and may be primary or secondary.

Lymphoedema should be differentiated from the accumulation of protein-rich fluid in situations where there is no lymphatic obstruction (e.g. burns, acute pancreatitis), and from the soft pitting oedema of hypoproteinaemia and congestive failure in which the protein content of the fluid is low (1–9 g/l as opposed to 10–50 g/l in lymphoedema).

Primary lymphoedema

This familial condition is caused by developmental failure. The lymphatics may be absent, hypoplastic, or varicose and dilated. Lymphoedema may be present at birth (congenital lymphoedema or Milroy's disease) but commonly develops in adolescence and early adult life (lymphoedema praecox). Lymphoedema praecox affects predominantly females, and may be unilateral or bilateral, and affects the upper or lower limbs. It begins insidiously and is often more noticeable after exercise, exposure to warmth, and in the premenstrual phase. The swelling is at first soft and pitting but becomes permanent and woody. There is a constant threat of

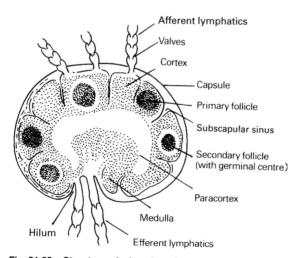

Afferent lymphatics
Valves
Cortex
Capsule
Primary follicle
Subscapular sinus
Secondary follicle (with germinal centre)
Paracortex
Medulla
Hilum
Efferent lymphatics

Fig. 21.29   Structure of a lymph node.

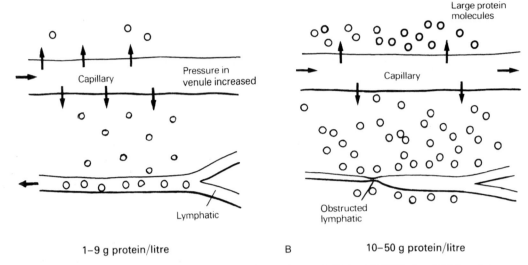

A   1–9 g protein/litre   B   10–50 g protein/litre

Fig. 21.30   Types of oedema. A Low-protein oedema due to abnormally high net fluid filtration. **B** High-protein oedema due to failure of lymphatics to remove interstitial protein.

cellulitis and lymphangitis, and a long-term risk of lymphangiosarcoma.

Lymphangiography can be used to define the extent and severity of the problem. In this technique, the lymphatics on the dorsum of the hand or foot are visualized (by injecting Patent Blue dye into a web space) and then cannulated so that oily contrast medium (lipiodol) can be infused (Fig. 21.31). Treatment consists of elevating the limb at night and intermittent compression from an inflated cuff to drive fluid from the limb. A tailored elastic stocking is worn during the day, and meticulous care is taken to avoid trauma which may cause infection. Minor infections, including athlete's foot, must be treated promptly.

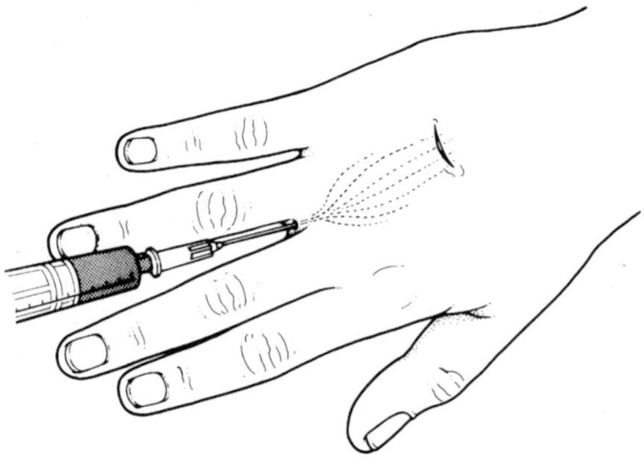

Advanced lymphoedema is unresponsive to these measures. Relief demands complete excision of skin, subcutaneous tissues and deep fascia from the affected limb. Split-skin grafts removed from the excised tissue are then placed directly on the exposed muscle. The limb has a grotesque appearance and the procedure is reserved for patients in whom the swollen limb prevents ambulation or is subject to repeated infection, or when proliferative nodular change affects the skin.

Secondary lymphoedema

Secondary lymphoedema develops if the lymphatic system is obstructed by tumour, recurrent infection, or infestation with filariasis, or obliterated by surgery or radiotherapy. Swelling is accompanied by dragging discomfort, erythema and a high risk of infection. Lymphangiography reveals dilated lymphatics up to the point of obstruction.

Conservative measures such as elevation and compression are of value. Surgery is generally unrewarding although direct anastomosis of dilated lymphatics to the venous system may be of some value. As the upper limb is frequently affected (e.g. after treatment of axillary nodes in breast cancer), the patient is advised to avoid even minor injuries to the hands and to wear protective gloves for activities such as gardening.

Fig. 21.31   Technique of lymphangiography. Patent Blue dye has been injected into a web space to define a lymphatic for cannulation.

22

The chest and mediastinum

CONTENTS

The respiratory system includes the airways, the lungs with their pleural spaces, and the chest wall. Lying between the lungs is the mediastinum.

THE AIRWAYS

Air is conducted into the lungs through the upper (nose, pharynx and larynx) and lower (trachea, bronchi and their subdivisions) respiratory tract.

In the upper respiratory tract air is warmed, humidified and filtered. Food, drink, saliva and other secretions do not normally enter the air passages, but are safely directed down the oesophagus during swallowing. If the upper airway is bypassed, as by an endotracheal tube or after tracheostomy (see below), the epithelium of the lower respiratory tract may be injured by drying, making clearance of secretions ineffective and leading to infection. Similarly, if coordination of swallowing is impaired, e.g. by neuromuscular disease or after anaesthesia, the lower airway may be contaminated by aspiration of food or fluid, again with infection (aspiration pneumonitis).

The trachea has incomplete cartilage rings joined by fibrous tissue where the rings are deficient posteriorly. In the adult the trachea is about 10 cm long and lies half in the neck and half in the chest. The cervical part is easily palpable as a midline structure unless deviated by pressure from a mass or shift of the upper mediastinum.

At the main carina the trachea bifurcates into right and left main bronchi. The right main bronchus is more directly continuous with the trachea than the left and is more commonly entered by inhaled foreign bodies. The lobes of the lungs are supplied by lobar bronchi, which in turn divide into segmental bronchi. The anatomical arrangement is fairly constant (Fig. 22.1). As the bronchi subdivide, the cartilage plates in their walls become less prominent, until after 15–20 divisions the small air passages are devoid of cartilage and are known as terminal bronchioles.

The bronchi and bronchioles are surrounded by smooth muscle which can constrict the lumen (as occurs in asthma). The tracheobronchial tree is lined by ciliated pseudo-stratified epithelium which is three to four cells thick in the upper parts but thins to a single layer in the bronchioles. Goblet cells in the mucosa and discrete submucosal glands produce a film of mucus which is constantly moved up to the larynx to clear inhaled dust particles. Drying of the epithelium interferes with this ciliary clearing action, as does general anaesthesia.

A further protective mechanism is the cough reflex. Stimulation of the sensitive epithelium, especially around the carina, results in forced expiration against a closed glottis. When it opens there is an explosive blast of air which clears secretions or foreign material. Generation of the blast requires adequate muscle strength in the chest wall, which after surgery may be impaired by pain or weakness. Thus general anaesthesia and operations, particu-

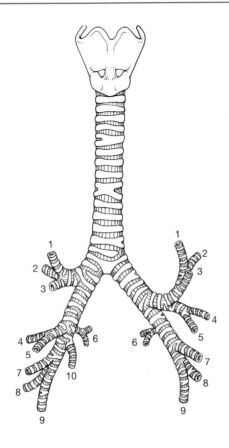

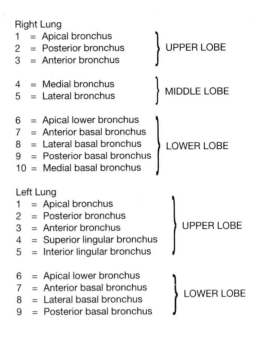

Right Lung
1 = Apical bronchus
2 = Posterior bronchus   } UPPER LOBE
3 = Anterior bronchus

4 = Medial bronchus   } MIDDLE LOBE
5 = Lateral bronchus

6 = Apical lower bronchus
7 = Anterior basal bronchus
8 = Lateral basal bronchus   } LOWER LOBE
9 = Posterior basal bronchus
10 = Medial basal bronchus

Left Lung
1 = Apical bronchus
2 = Posterior bronchus
3 = Anterior bronchus   } UPPER LOBE
4 = Superior lingular bronchus
5 = Interior lingular bronchus

6 = Apical lower bronchus
7 = Anterior basal bronchus } LOWER LOBE
8 = Lateral basal bronchus
9 = Posterior basal bronchus

Fig. 22.1 **Diagram of bronchial tree showing the major bronchi.**

larly on the chest or abdomen, lead to retention of secretions and a risk of infection.

Management of the airways

Maintenance of unobstructed airways and control of ventilation are important in anaesthesia and surgical conditions affecting the chest. The pumping action of the chest wall is interrupted by muscle relaxants, after major chest injury and during thoracotomy. This necessitates mechanical ventilation, with delivery of a humidified mixture of air and oxygen (and anaesthetic gases) directly into the airway. The gas mixture is under intermittent positive pressure, resulting in cyclical expansion of the lungs similar to that which occurs with normal respiration. A cuffed endotracheal tube (Fig. 22.2) is normally used to deliver the gas; the cuff lies in the trachea beyond the vocal cords and is gently inflated until there is an airtight seal.

With modern low-pressure cuffs, the tracheal necrosis is unusual even after many weeks of ventilation, provided overinflation is avoided. For operations on the lungs a 'double-lumen' tube with a separate limb for each main bronchus is available. This allows one lung to be ventilated while the other is collapsed. As the intubated patient cannot cough, bronchial secretions have to be removed from time to time using a sterile suction catheter.

If prolonged ventilation is required, e.g. after head or chest injury, a tracheostomy may be necessary.

Tracheostomy

If possible, tracheostomy is performed only when the airway is already controlled with an endotracheal tube. General anaesthesia, a good light and careful aseptic technique are desirable. Emergency tracheostomy is hardly ever required, except in

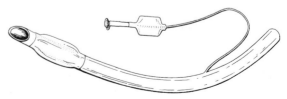

Fig. 22.2 **Cuffed endotracheal tube.**

conditions such as severe facial trauma, when an oral endotracheal tube cannot be inserted. Even then cricothyroidotomy is preferred.

For elective tracheostomy a transverse skin incision is made midway between the cricoid cartilage and the sternal notch. This incision is deepened in the midline, splitting the strap muscles. The isthmus of the thyroid may need to be retracted upwards or even divided. The trachea is opened through the second, third and fourth rings either with a vertical slit or as an inverted U-shaped flap. A short, right-angled cuffed tube is then carefully introduced. This allows easy and reliable access to the airway for ventilation or removal of secretions and is much more comfortable than an oral endotracheal tube, which passes through the sensitive larynx and vocal cords. Complications of tracheostomy include drying of secretions (if the inspired air is not humidified), damage to the tracheal wall from the cuff, and displacement of the tube into the tissues of the neck.

Examination of the airways

Bronchoscopy

Direct viewing of the airways from the larynx down to the beginning of the segmental bronchi is a routine investigation. A rigid or a flexible bronchoscope is used (see Ch. 6, Fig. 6.6, p. 58). The rigid instrument is basically a straight metal tube with a smooth, bevelled end for safer insertion between the vocal cords. It carries a light source near its tip, and a small tube attached to its other end enables a high pressure jet of oxygen to be blown intermittently into the airway. This jet draws in air and ensures satisfactory ventilation of the anaesthetized and paralysed patient. General anaesthesia is preferred, although it is possible to use topical anaesthesia to the larynx. The neck is extended to allow the bronchoscope to be passed gently between the vocal cords and into the trachea. Care must be taken to avoid levering on the teeth. By gently moving the head, each main bronchus can be entered. To examine the smaller bronchi, a right-angled telescope can be used. This is particularly helpful in the upper lobes. If a tumour is identified, it is biopsied with forceps. Tumours beyond direct reach are brushed with a sponge, and these brushings, together with locally collected secretions, are examined cytologically. Compression or distortion of the bronchi by external masses may also be seen on bronchoscopy. An important example is the widening of the usually sharp carina by enlarged subcarinal lymph nodes (a sign of inoperability in lung cancer).

The flexible bronchoscope can be used more readily with topical anaesthesia and can reach further down the bronchi, at least to segmental level. It is less useful for removing foreign bodies and secretions than the rigid instrument. With an experienced operator, a rigid bronchoscope can also be used to assess rigidity or deviation of the distal bronchial tree. Rigid bronchoscopy is frequently used postoperatively to suck out inspissated secretions when the cough mechanism is ineffective.

Removal of foreign bodies. Sudden onset of coughing and dyspnoea, particularly when associated with eating, suggests an inhaled foreign body, especially in children. Stridor is often the only finding. X-ray may reveal no abnormality or may show obstructive emphysema with overexpansion on the affected side. Occasionally the foreign body is radio-opaque. With complete blockage there is collapse or shrinkage of a lobe or lung. Urgent bronchoscopy is essential if there is any suspicion of aspiration. The foreign material is usually found in the right bronchial tree. Skilled anaesthesia is required in children, in whom the airway may be almost completely occluded by the object. A firmly jammed object, particularly if neglected, may require thoracotomy and opening of the bronchus (bronchotomy) for its removal.

Bronchography

Although the trachea and main bronchi can be visualized on a plain film, the distal bronchial tree must first be outlined by coating its walls with a radio-opaque medium (bronchography). This is best done under general anaesthesia. After secretions have been sucked out with a bronchoscope, the medium is injected through an endotracheal tube with the patient positioned so that one side is coated at a time. Bronchography is useful in the investigation of bronchiectasis to outline the extent of dilatation in the distal bronchial tree, but otherwise is seldom now used. As much contrast material as possible is sucked out; once the procedure is completed the remainder is coughed up by the patient, without ill-effect, on awakening.

THE PLEURA

The pleura is a thin sheet of connective tissue with a surface mesothelial cell layer which covers the lungs and lines the inside of the cavities (the hemithoraces) which contain the lungs.

Over the lobes of the lungs it is adherent to the lung tissue and is known as *visceral pleura*. It is insensitive to painful stimuli. This visceral pleura is continuous at the lung hilum with the *parietal pleura*, which lines the inside of the thoracic cage as well as covering the diaphragm and the mediastinum. It is sensitive to pain and has the same blood and nerve supply as underlying structures. The parietal pleura can be fairly readily stripped from the underlying chest wall and mediastinum.

In the normal state the two layers of the pleura are in contact. The slight movement which occurs between them with respiration is permitted by a thin film of fluid. The natural elasticity of the lung, which tends to make it collapse towards the hilum, exerts a negative pressure on this 'potential' space. Collection of air or fluid in this space is abnormal and, if significant, must be dealt with.

Management of the pleural space

Significant amounts of air, blood, effusion or pus in the pleural space compress the lung and interfere with function. Any infection is likely to persist, and the end-result of any inflammatory process in the pleural space is its obliteration by fibrous adhesions or even entrapment of the lung in dense fibrous scar. Techniques of drainage range from simple needle aspiration, through the insertion of intercostal drains, to open operation (thoracotomy). In all cases the aim is to expand the lung fully and obliterate any space. Not only does this allow maximal function of the lung, it also prevents re-accumulation of the collection.

Aspiration. A fine trocar and cannula attached via a two-way tap to a syringe (Fig. 22.3) can be used to aspirate air, remove fluid for diagnostic tests or empty the pleural space completely. The site of aspiration is determined by recent X-rays and by physical examination. Aseptic technique and adequate local anaesthesia of the appropriate intercostal space are important. The needle should pass across the upper border of the rib below so as to avoid the neurovascular bundle.

Intercostal drainage. Large amounts of air or fluid, particularly if they reaccumulate, are best drained continuously through a tube. Ideally this should be inserted laterally, behind the outer border of pectoralis major but in front of the midaxillary line, or anteriorly through the second interspace in the midaxillary line. Prior needle aspiration must always be carried out to confirm the suitability of the selected site. Local anaesthesia is again used and the trocar and cannula are inserted carefully after first

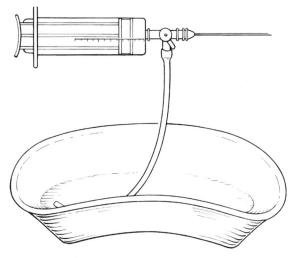

Fig. 22.3 Equipment for aspiration of pleural space.

incising the skin with a scalpel. As with needle aspiration, the cannula should pass just above a rib (Fig. 22.4).

Once the pleural space is entered, the intercostal tube is passed through the cannula, which is then removed. The tube is connected to an underwater seal bottle which acts as a one-way valve, letting out air or fluid but preventing either from re-entering the space.

When drainage is required for long periods (weeks or even months), as in patients with empyema (see

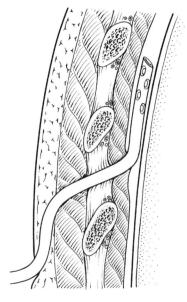

Fig. 22.4 Intercostal drainage.

below), rib resection may allow more efficient drainage. A piece of rib is removed at the site of drainage to permit a large tube to be inserted and the space to be explored by finger or forceps. It is more comfortable for the patient and avoids the risk of the tube eroding into the intercostal vessels (which are ligated when the segment of rib is removed).

As the infection fuses the lung to the chest wall, this type of tube can be converted to 'open drainage', as used for any other chronic abscess cavity in the body, with no risk of producing a pneumothorax.

Pneumothorax

Air in the pleural space is known as pneumothorax. The air usually comes from the lung itself. After penetrating trauma it may come from outside, and occasionally air enters through a perforated oesophagus (e.g. after endoscopy).

Spontaneous pneumothorax

This is the commonest type of pneumothorax. It usually occurs in young adults of either sex who are often tall and thin. It presents with pain and dyspnoea, and on examination there is hyperresonance to percussion and reduced breath sounds over the affected side. On chest X-ray there are no lung markings peripherally, and often an ill-defined line marks the border between lung and air. The lung may be collapsed at the hilum. The cause is usually rupture of a tiny bleb or bulla at the apex of the upper lobe.

If the pneumothorax is small, it may need no action other than observation, or it can be aspirated with a needle. If it is large or under tension (see below) or if there is fluid, a formal intercostal drain should be inserted. As the air comes out of the space, the lung expands and presses against the chest wall, so sealing the site of the leak. Once the drain stops bubbling it can be removed.

Tension pneumothorax

The site of the leak in the lung may act as a flap (one-way) valve, allowing air to enter the pleural space during inspiration and coughing, but preventing it from escaping during expiration, thus raising the pressure within the pleural space. Such pressure, or tension, compresses the lung and then shifts the mediastinum towards the other side (see Fig. 22.5). This in turn compresses the normal lung, impairing its function, and may kink and distort the

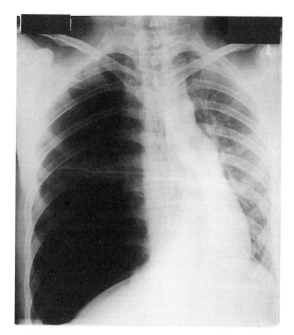

Fig. 22.5   Radiographic appearance of a right-sided tension pneumothorax (note the mediastinal shift to opposite side).

vena cava. The diagnosis should be suspected if there are signs of pneumothorax together with mediastinal shift and perhaps venous obstruction. This is a medical emergency. A large-bore needle plunged into the affected side will, if the diagnosis is correct, be greeted by a hiss of escaping air and relieve the immediate problem. A formal drain should then be inserted.

Recurrent spontaneous pneumothorax

Roughly one-third of spontaneous pneumothoraces will recur. After a second episode the risk doubles. If the same side has been affected twice or more, and particularly if tension has occurred at any time, a *pleurectomy* should be considered. Through a limited thoracotomy the parietal pleura is stripped off the inside of the chest. Any blebs or bullae can be ligated. The anaesthetist then inflates the lung, causing it to adhere to the raw area on the chest wall. A similar effect can be obtained by blowing an irritant such as iodized talc or kaolin into the pleural space. This induces a chemical pleurisy and obliterates the space. Although simpler than pleurectomy, this procedure (*pleurodesis*) carries the risk of introducing foreign (and irritating) material into a body cavity.

Haemothorax

Haemothorax is discussed in detail later in this chapter.

Empyema

Pus in the pleural space is known as empyema. The commonest cause is pneumonia with spread of infection into an associated effusion. A lung abscess can also spread to the pleural space. Infection can be introduced from outside the chest, e.g. by penetrating injury, or contamination of pleural fluid by poor sterile technique during aspiration. Infection can come from the mediastinum, typically after perforation of the oesophagus; the space left after lung resection can become infected (postoperative empyema); or a subphrenic abscess may spread through the diaphragm. The physical signs of empyema are those of a pleural effusion: dullness to percussion, absence of breath sounds, and evidence of infection such as pyrexia and leucocytosis. On X-ray there is a pleural opacity, classically located posteriorly and with a 'D'-shaped outline.

At the earliest stage the pleural space is filled with a thin, watery fluid containing pus cells and known as a 'purulent effusion'. Later, fibrin is laid down on the lung and parietal pleura, and becomes organized as a thick fibrous wall around the cavity. At a very late stage the contained pus may 'point' to the skin surface like any abscess. This is termed 'empyema necessitans'.

The aims of treatment are to drain the infection and obliterate the pleural space by encouraging the lung to expand. At the stage of purulent effusion, needle aspiration alone may be adequate. For thicker pus, a tube drain is required, and for a thick-walled abscess, rib resection (see above) allows much better drainage. The cavity then slowly obliterates by fibrous ingrowth, until eventually just the tube tract is left. Although this may take several months it is safe and effective in the elderly, who now constitute the majority of patients with empyema. In younger patients, open thoracotomy and removal of the walls of the empyema ('decortication') permits full expansion of the lung and more rapid and complete resolution.

THE LUNGS

Each lung is contained within its hemithorax and is attached at the hilum to the mediastinum. The main bronchus, pulmonary artery and veins are the major

---

Pneumothorax
- Pneumothorax is defined as the presence of air in the pleural space, the air coming in most cases from the lung rather than the exterior.

- Spontaneous pneumothorax is the commonest form and usually occurs in young, tall, thin adults.

- Pneumothorax is diagnosed clinically by hyperresonance and absence of breath sounds over the affected side of the chest.

- Tension pneumothorax occurs when a flap of lung acts as a valve allowing air to enter the pleural cavity during inspiration but not leave it on expiration. The increased pressure not only collapses the lung on the affected side but displaces the mediastinum to the opposite side, with potentially fatal compromise of gas exchange. Venous obstruction may also be apparent.

- Tension pneumothorax is a life-threatening emergency which is diagnosed clinically without awaiting radiological confirmation. The condition requires immediate relief by inserting a large-bore needle to allow air to escape, followed by insertion of a cannula with underwater sealed drainage.

---

structures at the hilum; lymphatics and lymph nodes, bronchial arteries and autonomic nerves are also present.

The left lung is divided by an oblique fissure into an upper and a lower lobe. The right lung has an oblique fissure from which a transverse fissure runs forward resulting in an upper, a middle and a lower lobe.

The lobes are divided into bronchopulmonary segments by fibrous septa radiating out from the hilum. Each segment has its own bronchus, always with an accompanying artery. Blockage of a lobar or segmental bronchus results in absorption of air beyond the blockage and collapse or atelectasis (airlessness) of the affected lung. Since areas containing no air appear denser than the surrounding lung on chest X-ray, the collapsed segment or lobe can readily be identified.

Bronchopulmonary segments are further divided into lobules, each with its own bronchiole and accompanying pulmonary arteriole, but without fibrous septa. The terminal bronchioles divide into respiratory bronchioles and then alveolar ducts before reaching the alveoli. These last are surrounded by a web of capillaries. Gas exchange occurs across the very thin alveolar epithelial cells, a basement membrane and the equally thin endothelial cells of the capillaries.

Veins from the smallest respiratory units eventually drain into segmental veins, some of which lie between the fissures. These veins are tributaries of the inferior and superior pulmonary veins, which join the left atrium at the hilum. Because the lobes and segments are discrete anatomical units, they can be removed surgically, leaving the remaining lung intact and viable.

Infective lung conditions

Lung abscess

This term implies infection with localized destruction of lung tissue. A lung abscess may occur within an area of pneumonia, although this is unusual if antibiotics have been given. Inhalation of foreign material, e.g. during a period of impaired consciousness, may be followed by abscess formation in the obstructed and contaminated area. The patient is extremely ill with an elevated temperature. If the abscess communicates with the airway, large quantities of foul sputum may be produced. Chest X-ray characteristically shows an opacity with a fluid level. There may be spillage of pus into healthy areas of the lung, or the pleura may be breached, with empyema or pyopneumothorax.

Postural drainage and physiotherapy, together with appropriate antibiotics, will resolve most abscesses. All such patients must be bronchoscoped—the original opacity may have been a cavitating carcinoma or infection may have developed in a bronchus blocked by tumour.

Bronchiectasis

In bronchiectasis parts of the bronchial tree are abnormally dilated. The bronchial walls are abnormal and there is chronic infection in the bronchi and surrounding lung parenchyma. The condition usually follows childhood infections (particularly tuberculosis, measles and whooping cough) in which transient bronchial obstruction is followed by destruction of the bronchial wall and permanent dilatation. It commonly affects the lower lobes, and sometimes the middle lobe on the right or the lingula on the left. It may also be widespread. The main symptom is persistent cough with production of purulent sputum (up to several cupfuls a day). There may be haemoptysis and recurrent exacerbations of infection. The chest X-ray may be surprisingly normal. Bronchography is required to define the extent and severity of the disease.

Postural drainage and antibiotics given for exacerbations are the mainstay of treatment. If this fails to control symptoms or prevent recurrent severe infection or haemoptysis, surgical resection of the affected segment(s), lobe(s) or even an entire lung may be considered. This can be very successful, but only if the disease is relatively localized. The result of surgery depends on the amount of residual diseased lung.

Benign lung tumours

Benign lung tumours are uncommon. Only bronchial carcinoids and adenoid cystic carcinomas (previously classified as 'bronchial adenomas') are true neoplasms. A number of other non-malignant conditions present as shadows on chest X-ray and must be differentiated from bronchial carcinomas. These include tuberculomas, healed infarcts and hamartomas. Because of the difficulty of proving their benign nature and the importance of not missing a small bronchial carcinoma, many peripheral opacities, or 'coin lesions', are diagnosed only after the suspect area has been surgically removed.

Hamartoma

A hamartoma is a developmental abnormality consisting of a mass of tissue with cartilage, muscle and epithelium. It is firm and mobile within the lung parenchyma, moving around under the surgeon's finger.

Bronchial carcinoid

Bronchial carcinoids account for about 85% of benign lung tumours, and are distantly related to small-cell carcinomas. They typically arise in the major bronchi and cause cough, wheezing or haemoptysis. Unless an airway is blocked, chest X-ray may be normal. Local resection is indicated in all cases. A few may recur and occasionally they develop malignant characteristics and metastasize.

Adenoid cystic carcinoma

This tumour is even rarer. It commonly occurs in the major bronchi or the trachea, and has a striking tendency to recur even years after initial removal. It is only slightly radiosensitive.

Lung cancer

Lung cancer arises from the epithelium of the bronchial tree. Although men are affected more frequently than women (ratio 4:1 in the UK), it is now the commonest cause of death from malignancy in both sexes. It occurs most frequently between the ages of 50 and 60 years but is increasingly seen in younger patients. Cigarette smoking is the major predisposing factor in nearly all cases, but a few are related to exposure to asbestos, radioactive isotopes, arsenic or chromates.

Pathology

Histologically the tumour may be well differentiated or anaplastic. Well-differentiated tumours may be squamous (45–55%) or adenocarcinomatous (20%). Anaplastic tumours are divided into 'large cell' and 'small cell' types. Large cell tumours account for 15% of all types and behave as more malignant forms of the differentiated tumours. Small or 'oat cell' carcinomas account for 20% of all lung cancers and behave as a completely different disease. These cells are believed to be derived from neural crest tissue. They are highly malignant, and many patients have widespread dissemination when first seen.

A lung cancer may be central, i.e. in a major bronchus, and hence visible at bronchoscopy, or peripheral. If it is in a major airway, there may be cough or bleeding (haemoptysis). Airway occlusion leads to silent collapse of the affected area or, more commonly, infection of the distal airways with pneumonia or lung abscess.

The tumour spreads in the lung by local invasion and along lymphatic channels. Once beyond the lung, it may invade adjacent organs such as the pericardium and heart, oesophagus, chest wall or diaphragm. The aorta is curiously resistant to spread.

Lymphatic spread is initially to hilar and mediastinal nodes. Later, supraclavicular nodes may be involved and easily palpable (Fig. 22.6).

Blood-borne metastases occur in most viscera: the commonest sites are the brain, bone, liver, skin and the adrenal glands. Other manifestations of bronchial carcinoma which are not due to metastases are finger clubbing, hypertrophic pulmonary osteoarthropathy, peripheral neuropathy and myopathies, superficial thrombophlebitis and a variety of endocrine disturbances due to inappropriate secretion of hormones.

Presentation

Some tumours are found on routine chest X-rays in asymptomatic patients. A lung shadow in a smoker is presumed to be a bronchial carcinoma until proved

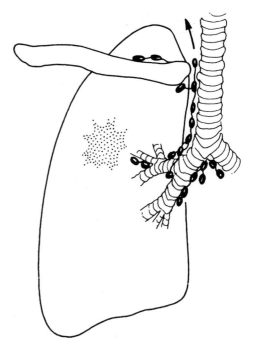

Fig. 22.6 Lymphatic spread of lung cancer.

otherwise. More commonly the patient complains of a cough, perhaps with haemoptysis, and often weight loss. Pneumonia which fails to resolve or which recurs in the same area of lung is another suspicious sign and requires further investigation (i.e. by bronchoscopy). Local spread of tumour may cause pain in the chest wall at the site of invasion. If this occurs at the apex of the lung, the brachial plexus and sympathetic chain may be involved. The combination of severe pain (often down the arm), Horner's syndrome and rib erosion is characteristic of the Pancoast syndrome.

Central invasion may affect the recurrent laryngeal nerve (always the left) and cause hoarseness from vocal cord paralysis. Enlarged lymph nodes in the mediastinum may compress the superior vena cava (SVC) and cause engorgement of the face and arms (SVC syndrome). Occasionally bloodborne metastases are the first manifestation of the disease. For example, bone pain, skin nodules or neurological symptoms (e.g. epilepsy) may all point to metastatic disease.

Investigation

A thorough history and physical examination may suggest the diagnosis and give some idea of the extent of spread. The aim of subsequent investigations is to confirm the diagnosis, define the extent of spread, and determine appropriate treatment. For nearly all types of lung cancer the only hope of cure is by surgery.

Radiological examination. The commonest findings on chest X-ray are a peripheral opacity (Fig. 22.7), enlarged hilar or mediastinal nodes or an area of consolidation in the lung. The examination may also reveal bony erosion or secondary deposits in the ribs, and there may be signs of pleural effusion. Other useful radiological investigations are screening of the diaphragm to detect phrenic nerve paralysis (due to invasion of the mediastinum) and barium swallow or CT scan to determine whether the oesophagus is deviated or indented by enlarged mediastinal lymph nodes.

Bronchoscopy. Central tumours can be biopsied directly. Secretions or brushings from segmental bronchi allow cytological diagnosis of more peripheral lesions. Bronchoscopy can also be used to assess operability. Carinal widening and tracheal invasion are signs of inoperability. Peripheral tumours can be directly biopsied using a percutaneous needle technique under X-ray guidance.

Lymph node sampling. Supraclavicular node metastases indicate inoperability. These nodes can be sampled by direct biopsy or by fine-needle aspira-

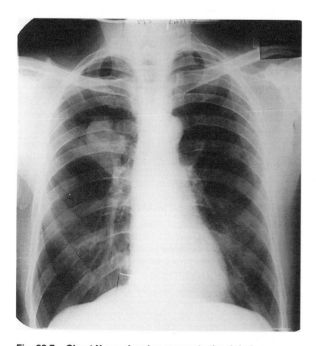

Fig. 22.7 **Chest X-ray showing cancer in the right lung upper lobe.**

tion. Lymph nodes within the mediastinum may be sampled by *mediastinoscopy*. Under general anaesthesia an incision is made in the neck and deepened until a plane beneath the pretracheal fascia is reached. A finger and then an endoscope (similar to a laryngoscope) is introduced as far as the origin of the main bronchi. Involvement of nodes high in the mediastinum or on the opposite side to the tumour denotes inoperability. Routine mediastinoscopy, at least for central tumours, reduces the thoracotomy rate.

Assessment of pulmonary function

When assessing the suitability of a patient for thoracotomy, the surgeon not only has to decide whether the tumour can be resected but also whether the patient has sufficient respiratory reserve to tolerate the operation. As almost all patients will have been smokers, most already have diseased or abnormal lungs. The assessment is based on pre-operative fitness (e.g. ability to climb a flight of stairs), the results of lung function tests and the extent of resection required. Of the large range of pulmonary function tests available, simple spirometry, with measurement of forced expiratory volume in one second (FEV_1) and forced vital capacity (FVC), is the most useful. Postoperative performance obviously depends on the extent of resection, which ranges from a right pneumonectomy, with removal of about 55% of functioning lung tissue, to wedge resection of a slice of lung surrounding a tiny peripheral tumour. Removal of a collapsed lobe is obviously less harmful than removal of one which is fully functional.

Treatment

The principle of surgical treatment is to remove the anatomical unit containing the tumour (segment, lobe or lung) together with its associated lymphatic drainage. Even with apparently curative resection only 35–40% of patients survive for 5 years after the operation. The figure for small peripheral lesions is much better, approaching 90%, and there is worthwhile salvage even if mediastinal lymph nodes have to be removed.

Only a minority of patients with lung cancer are suitable for operation. At presentation, about 50% already have clinical evidence of spread outside the chest or are unfit for thoracotomy. Further investigation usually rules out another quarter or third of the original group, so that only 20–25% are eventually considered for surgery. For the rest, the outlook is hopeless: median survival is 8 months, and only 2–3% are alive after 5 years.

Radiotherapy. Some small tumours can be cured by irradiation, but the resulting damage to the surrounding lung is at least as great as that from surgery. Radiotherapy is useful for pain relief from bony metastases. In the chest it can be used to relieve superior vena cava obstruction and reduce tracheal or bronchial compression.

Chemotherapy. Small cell cancers of the lung are relatively responsive to chemotherapy. Although cure is rare, median survival may be increased from 3 to 18 months. Other types of lung cancer are not responsive, and chemotherapy is rarely indicated.

Principles of operations to the lung

Opening the pleura to gain access to the lungs or other thoracic structures destroys the usual negative intrathoracic pressure. In this situation the lung would collapse. Endotracheal intubation and positive pressure ventilation are therefore necessary. For many operations a standard cuffed endotracheal tube is sufficient. Use of a double-lumen tube allows the lung being operated on to be selectively collapsed ('one-lung anaesthesia'). This is of great help, particularly when a bronchus has to be opened in the course of the operation.

Thoracotomy

The patient is placed on his unaffected side on the operating table. For a standard lateral thoracotomy (such as would be used to gain access to the lung) the skin incision runs from between the medial border of the scapula and the vertebral spines forward to the inframammary crease. It is deepened through the fat and fascia before dividing latissimus dorsi and, anteriorly, serratus anterior. To open the chest the periosteum is stripped off the upper border of a rib (usually the sixth) so that the neurovascular bundle is preserved and the pleura divided. The ribs are gently spread apart using a self-retaining retractor.

Lobectomy

Lobectomy is indicated for tumours or other lesions confined to one lobe. The interlobar fissure is deepened towards the hilum. The lobar vessels are

ligated and divided and the bronchus is divided and closed. Hilar lymph nodes are removed along with the specimen. Small air leaks usually close spontaneously after a few days. Lobectomy has a low mortality and little effect on lung function.

Pneumonectomy

In one-third of cases of tumour, the whole lung must be removed (pneumonectomy). The pulmonary veins and arteries are ligated and divided at the hilum, and the bronchus is divided flush with the carina and closed with non-absorbable sutures or a mechanical stapling device. Breakdown of this closure leads to 'bronchopleural fistula', which is a serious and potentially lethal complication.

It is usual to drain the pleural cavity via a tube connected to an underwater seal bottle after any operation on the chest to deal with continued air leak and oozing of blood from raw surfaces of the lung.

After lobectomy, the remaining lung expands to fill the space left. Crowding of the ribs, elevation of the hemidiaphragm and movement of the mediastinum all reduce the size of the hemithorax on the operated side so that the pleural space is usually obliterated in a week.

Following pneumonectomy there is no lung to fill the space. The drain is removed after 24 hours, and the space allowed to fill slowly with blood and serum over the next few weeks. This undergoes organization and fibrosis.

Lung cancer
- Cancer arising from the epithelium of the bronchial tree is four times commoner in men, but is now the commonest cause of cancer death in both sexes.

- Cigarette smoking is the outstanding cause; other aetiological factors include exposure to asbestos, radioactive drugs and industrial chemicals.

- The tumour may be well differentiated (squamous or adenocarcinoma) or anaplastic (large cell or small cell). Small cell (oat cell) cancers may arise in epithelium derived from the neural crest and have often disseminated widely when first seen.

- The minority (20–25%) of patients with lung cancer are considered for surgery and even after apparently curative resection the 5-year survival rate is only 40%. For the majority with inoperable cancer the median duration of survival is only 8 months.

THE THORACIC CAGE

The main role of the chest wall and diaphragm is to generate the negative intrathoracic pressure required for ventilation. At rest the diaphragm is the principal muscle involved in inspiration; expiration is normally passive. When additional ventilation is required, as during exercise or if there is pulmonary disease, contraction of the intercostal muscles pivots the ribs forwards and outwards, raising the sternum and further increasing the volume of the chest cavity.

Chest wall function may be impaired by damage to the wall itself (e.g. muscle weakness with postoperative pain, fractured ribs) or by pleural disease (e.g. fibrothorax following empyema), both of which restrict lung expansion. Disorders of the lung itself (e.g. pulmonary fibrosis) have similar effects.

Deformities of the chest wall

Pectus excavatum

In this deformity of the thoracic cage the sternum is posteriorly displaced by abnormal development of the costal cartilages. There is a depression in the precordial area, so that the heart is displaced into the left chest. Despite this, the function of the heart is only rarely impaired. Surgery is justified by the cosmetic distress. The operation involves resection of the costal cartilages and elevation of the sternum by a metal bar which passes behind it and rests in front of the ribs on each side. This bar is removed after a few months.

Pectus carinatum

This is the opposite deformity to that described above, in that the sternum is elevated forward as a ridge ('pigeon chest'). Principles of treatment are the same as for pectus excavatum.

Thoracic injury

Blunt injuries to the chest are common in road traffic accidents. There are frequently other injuries, particularly to the head, abdomen and long bones. The thoracic injury is often a cause of early death, which in many cases could be prevented by appropriate and often very simple steps.

Penetrating injury is almost always the result of stab or gunshot wounds.

Airway obstruction

If the cough reflex is suppressed by unconsciousness or the patient cannot cough because of damage to the chest wall, the airway may become obstructed. Gastric contents, pharyngeal secretions or blood may be aspirated. Provision of an open airway is the first priority when dealing with a patient with a chest injury. This may require a pharyngeal airway or sometimes an endotracheal tube. Emergency cricothyroidotomy or tracheostomy is only required if head and neck or upper airway injury precludes insertion of an endotracheal tube.

Fractured ribs

Pain, made worse by coughing and breathing, is the main problem after simple rib fractures. If there is pre-existing lung disease, such as chronic bronchitis, the inability to cough may lead to retention of secretions and pneumonia. Adequate analgesia (e.g. by local intercostal nerve blocks or thoracic epidural anaesthesia) is essential. Immobilization of the ribs by 'strapping' is contraindicated.

Flail chest

Fracture of a number of adjacent ribs in more than one place results in a flail segment of chest wall. Such a 'floating' segment, if large, may show paradoxical movement with respiration, i.e. it moves outwards with expiration and inwards with inspiration, greatly reducing chest wall function (Fig. 19.9). Contusion of the underlying lung is common. The effect of the injury can be limited by good analgesia, physiotherapy and diuretics to prevent local pulmonary oedema. Some patients require artificial ventilation, often for 2–3 weeks, until the injured lung has recovered and the chest wall has become stable.

Traumatic pneumothorax

Pneumothorax (see Ch. 14, Fig. 14.4) implies lung or, very rarely, oesophageal perforation. Damage is usually due to puncture by the sharp ends of fractured ribs. Penetrating injury can have a similar effect. Small pneumothoraces resolve on their own, but if there is a large space, tube drainage is required. The principal aim, as in any pneumothorax, is to fully inflate the lung and obliterate the pleural space. Persistent bubbling of air into the underwater seal bottle with each inspiration denotes bronchial rupture.

If the air in the space is under tension, it may track through the wound into the tissues, where it is palpable as a 'crackling' sensation under the skin. This 'surgical emphysema' may cause massive swelling of the chest, neck and face, producing a 'Michelin man' appearance. It always resolves completely once the air-leak seals and never causes any permanent damage.

Haemothorax

Blood in the pleural space may come from the chest wall, lung or mediastinal structures. Fractured ribs may bleed or lacerate intercostal vessels, which may also be damaged by stab wounds, aspirating needles or chest drains. If the lung itself is injured, bleeding is usually associated with an air leak, leading to a haemopneumothorax. Massive bleeding into the pleura can occur from damage to the heart or the aorta (see below).

The short-term effects are those of blood loss and compression of lung. Blood loss may be insignificant but can be massive and rapidly fatal: the pleural space can contain most of the circulating blood volume. The compressed lung is unavailable for ventilation, so does not contribute to gas exchange. In time, clot in the pleural cavity may organize and permanently compress (or 'trap') the lung in a fibrous case. If contaminated from the outside, the haematoma becomes infected, leading to an empyema.

The principles of management are as for any other fluid in the pleural space, i.e. drainage of the pleural space via a large-bore chest drain connected to an underwater seal bottle, to allow full expansion of the lung and obliteration of the space. If blood loss continues or is excessive, thoracotomy is indicated. The commonest sources of bleeding are the intercostal and internal thoracic vessels. Massive haemorrhage from the heart or great vessels requires immediate repair. It may also be necessary to open the chest to remove large quantities of clot. This should be done early rather than late so that permanent lung compression and empyema are avoided.

Stab injuries to the heart may cause death from tamponade (compression of the heart by blood contained in the pericardium), rather than from exsanguination. Cardiac tamponade rapidly leads to hypotension, tachycardia and elevated jugular venous pressure. Release of tamponade by opening the pericardium through a small anterior thoracotomy often results in dramatic improvement, and allows time for repair.

Aortic rupture

Severe deceleration injuries may disrupt the aorta. In traffic accidents, rupture typically occurs just beyond the subclavian artery at the start of the descending aorta. In falls from a height (or aircraft accidents) rupture more commonly occurs just above the aortic valve.

About 90% of these patients die at the site of the accident from exsanguination. In the remainder, despite a tear of the aortic intima and media, blood is contained within the adventitia for hours or even days. There may be loss of distal pulses or clinical evidence of a left haemothorax. More usually the only clue to the injury is a widened upper mediastinum on chest X-ray, and any patient showing this sign should undergo emergency aortography. Often this reveals no abnormality, but if there is a disruption the injected dye will show an irregularity of the aorta or even leakage into the surrounding tissues.

Operation should be carried out as soon as possible, as the aorta may rupture completely at any time. On opening the chest the surgeon is confronted by an enormous mediastinal haematoma. The damaged vessel is isolated between clamps and a Dacron tube graft inserted between healthy ends of aorta. As the spinal cord is at risk from ischaemia during this part of the operation, bypass to maintain distal circulation is usually advised. This may be a partial bypass (pumping blood from the left atrium to the descending aorta or femoral artery) or, more usually, a temporary bypass of the damaged area by a tube coated on the inside with heparin.

THE MEDIASTINUM

Mediastinal infections

These invariably arise from organs passing through or closely associated with the mediastinum. The commonest cause of mediastinal infection ('mediastinitis') is rupture of the oesophagus. Downward spread of infection from the neck may also occur.

Mediastinal infections spread rapidly through the loosely arranged tissue planes. Clinical features include chest pain radiating to the neck or through to the back, and dysphagia. Pyrexia is invariable. If an air-containing viscus is the source of the infection, surgical emphysema develops. Unless adequately drained, through the pleura or the neck, such infections are often rapidly fatal.

Mediastinal masses

The mediastinum is a relatively silent area. Mediastinal masses are often discovered as an incidental finding on chest X-ray. Sometimes pressure on adjacent structures (oesophagus or trachea, superior vena cava or recurrent laryngeal nerve) may cause suspicious symptoms.

Anterosuperior masses

Retrosternal extension of the thyroid is a common cause of a mass at the thoracic inlet. The trachea may be deviated or compressed (causing stridor) and a goitre is usually palpable in the neck. As sudden bleeding into the thyroid can cause acute tracheal compression, retrosternal goitres are best removed.

Aneurysms of the aorta or vessels arising from the aortic arch can mimic a solid mass in any part of the mediastinum, but are particularly common in the superior part. The wall may be calcified. Aortography or CT scanning with intravenous contrast is indicated to confirm the diagnosis. All aneurysms are at risk of rupture, and if there is evidence of enlargement (pain or erosion of adjacent structures) surgery is advised.

Tumours of the thymus (thymomas) are found in the anterosuperior space. They are usually benign and may be associated with myasthenia gravis. Complete removal of the thymus may result in dramatic improvement, particularly in women with a short history. Surgical removal, which is best done through a median sternotomy, is straightforward, but postoperative ventilation is required.

Lymph node masses may occur at any site in the mediastinum, but most commonly arise at the lung hila, around the lower trachea and in the thymic remnants. They may be the result of benign disease such as sarcoidosis or follow infections, classically tuberculosis. More commonly, however, they are due to malignant disease, either 'primary' disease of lymphoid tissue (as in the lymphomas) or 'secondary' to spread from other tumour (most usually bronchial carcinoma).

Lymphoid masses often have a lobulated appearance on chest X-ray and, if malignant, may show features of local invasion or compression. Obstruction of the SVC causes distension of superficial veins over the trunk, oedema of the arms and head, and a flushed appearance (the SVC syndrome), which is a classical feature of mediastinal invasion from bronchial carcinoma.

Posterior mediastinum

Masses in the posterior mediastinum may originate from abnormalities of the primitive foregut. Oesophageal duplication presents as a fluid-filled mass adjoining the oesophagus, often lined with squamous epithelium. A similar abnormality can arise from the respiratory tract forming a bronchogenic cyst which usually lies around the tracheal bifurcation. The wall may contain cartilage and is lined by ciliated epithelium. A fluid level on X-ray implies communication with the airway, which makes infection inevitable. In children these cysts can rapidly expand and cause respiratory obstruction.

Above the diaphragm, a hiatus hernia may show as a retrocardiac mass containing a fluid level. The gas is in the intrathoracic stomach, and this is the only important situation when a fluid level on chest X-ray does not imply communication with the airway.

Neurogenic tumours are found more posteriorly, in the costovertebral recess. The commonest are tumours of nerve sheath origin (neurofibromas) which are usually benign. They may straddle the intervertebral foramen (dumb-bell tumours) and require a combined thoracic/neurosurgical approach. In children such tumours are nearly always malignant.

General principles of management

Many mediastinal masses are obviously malignant, secondary to bronchogenic carcinoma, and suitable only for palliation. Some forms of malignant disease are readily treated and cured if properly diagnosed and managed. The best examples are the lymphomas, where the disease may be limited to mediastinal lymph nodes. Other masses may be harmless (e.g. benign neural tumours) or non-malignant, but important to detect (e.g. lymph-node enlargement in sarcoidosis). Some benign lesions may enlarge or are at risk of later infection. Aneurysms tend to dilate with time and many eventually rupture, but they often present for the first time relatively late in life.

In some cases, the combination of clinical and radiological features allows precise diagnosis. For example, a patient with myasthenia gravis and an anterior mediastinal mass almost certainly has a thymoma. Most frequently, however, the findings on radiological examination are non-specific and further investigation is needed to confirm the diagnosis. In practice the safest and most efficient way to achieve this is by contrast CT scanning followed by a biopsy. The CT scan accurately localizes the mass and, combined with intravenous contrast, will detect aneurysms and other vascular lesions.

The route of biopsy is determined by the position of a mass. The area around the trachea can be approached by *mediastinoscopy*, while the anterior mediastinum is approached by *anterior mediastinotomy*, through a small incision in the second intercostal space on the appropriate side. Posterior masses require formal thoracotomy.

Large biopsies, ideally of whole lymph nodes, are necessary for accurate diagnosis of lymphomas and thymomas. Fine-needle biopsies are often unsatisfactory.

23
Face, head, and neck

CONTENTS

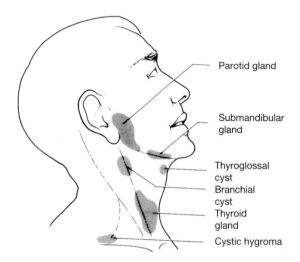

Fig. 23.1   Location of swellings in the head and neck shown relative to the sternocleidomastoid muscle. Thyroglossal swellings are located in the midline.

lymph nodes everywhere in the neck, when pathologically enlarged they usually are in one of the major groupings (Fig. 23.2). As can be seen by comparing Figures 23.1 and 23.2, diagnostic confusion is only likely to arise with swellings in the jugulo-digastric and submandibular region.

The majority of head and neck conditions present as swellings; these are usually in the skin, one of the salivary glands, the thyroid gland or one of the lymph nodes. Thus, from the anatomical position of the swelling it is usually possible to decide which structure is affected (Fig. 23.1). In general, skin lesions can be lifted up in a skinfold; parotid lesions are in front of the ear, over the angle of the mandible or in the upper part of the neck; submandibular gland lesions are in the triangle bounded by the digastric muscle and the jaw; and thyroid lesions are above the suprasternal notch. Though there are

HISTORY TAKING

Once the patient has indicated where they think the swelling is, questions can be directed towards disorders likely to affect structures in that region. In general, the main distinction to be made is between inflammatory and neoplastic conditions. The former are usually painful whereas the latter are not. Lesions considered to have a congenital basis usually present before the age of 25 years, whereas neoplasms tend to present over the age of 45 years, the exception being neoplasms of the reticulo-endothelial system.

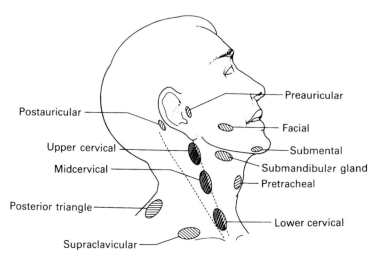

Fig. 23.2   Lymph node groups in the head and neck shown relative to the sternocleidomastoid muscle.

CLINICAL EXAMINATION

Inspection may or may not reveal the swelling, depending on its size. The overlying skin is examined for signs of inflammation or involvement. Operation scars are fairly reliable indications of the organ involved in previous surgery. Palpation will reveal the site of the swelling though sometimes the patient may have to guide the examining hand to it. Under these circumstances, there is a considerable possibility that the patient is concerned about a normal anatomical structure. Tenderness and mobility are assessed though mobility is often limited by the tight fascial sheaths in the neck. All midline swellings including those in the thyroid gland will move up on swallowing because of their investment by the pretracheal fascia. Cysts do not necessarily feel cystic, again because of the fascial sheaths. With lymph node enlargements it is important to examine the oral cavity, including the tongue, the oro-, naso- and hypopharynx and larynx as these are the most likely sites of the primary pathology, be it inflammatory or neoplastic.

RADIOLOGICAL INVESTIGATIONS

Plain X-rays are valuable if a submandibular calculus is suspected. Calcification within a lymph node indicates tuberculosis. The nasopharynx is best examined by lateral views.

Orthopantomograms demonstrate dental and mandibular pathology well.

Ultrasonography can determine whether a mass is cystic.

Contrast can be injected into the parotid and submandibular gland duct to identify obstructive pathology.

Computerized tomography (CT) will delineate most of the important neck structures (Fig. 23.3). It will not only confirm the site and size of the presenting lesion but also reveals non-palpable but pathologically involved lymph nodes.

PATHOLOGICAL INVESTIGATIONS

Fine-needle aspiration cytology can be extremely helpful as an outpatient procedure to diagnose neoplasia, but it must be borne in mind that failure to reveal neoplastic cells *does not* exclude neoplasia.

Endoscopy should be carried out before excision biopsy of a lymph node thought to be secondarily involved by neoplasia. The primary is almost invariably in the head and neck region and though clinical examination of the upper respiratory and alimentary tracts will detect the majority of lesions, sometimes endoscopy is necessary. Biopsy of the primary tumour will give better tissue diagnosis with a minimal risk of tumour spread when compared to node biopsy.

Excision biopsy should only be performed after examination and investigation has excluded a primary pathology in the upper alimentary and respiratory tracts. It is important that the biopsy is total

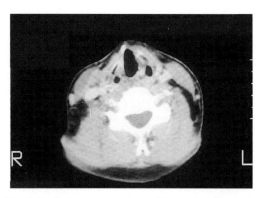

Fig. 23.3 Transverse sections of the neck to illustrate anatomical relationships as seen on CT scanning. Serial scans can be obtained.

excision and not incision. In many instances excision can be curative whereas incision biopsy of a neoplasm increases the risk of tumour spillage and local recurrence even if the tumour is subsequently excised.

SPECIFIC SWELLINGS

Apart from swellings that are thought to be congenital, neck lesions will be considered according to the anatomical structure affected.

CONGENITAL SWELLINGS

Though considered developmental in origin, these swellings present between the ages of 10 to 25 years mainly because they are not evident until they become infected, or enlarged because of accumulation of cystic fluid. The exception is cystic hygroma which presents in the neonatal period.

Thyroglossal cyst

The thyroid gland develops from a midline tubular outgrowth of cells from the foramen caecum at the base of the tongue (Fig. 23.4). This thyroglossal duct tracks through the body of the developing hyoid bone and then bifurcates to give rise to solid masses of cells which form the isthmus and lobes of the thyroid gland. The duct normally disappears in early

fetal life; persistence of any part of it may give rise to midline thyroglossal cysts (Fig. 23.4).

Thyroglossal cysts are the commonest congenital neck swelling. Although they may be present at birth, they more often present in adolescence or early adult life as a painless, smooth, rounded midline swelling. The swelling is usually located between the thyroid isthmus and hyoid bone and is non-tender and rubbery. Characteristically, the cyst moves upwards when the patient protrudes his tongue or swallows. Rarely the patient presents with a discharging sinus if the cyst has become infected.

Thyroglossal cysts are normally excised for cosmetic reasons and to avoid recurrent infection. General anaesthesia is required and the body of the

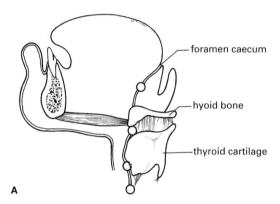

foramen caecum

hyoid bone

thyroid cartilage

A

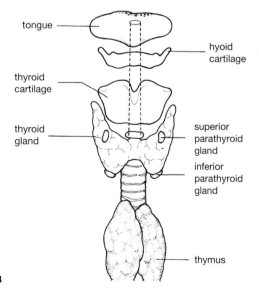

tongue

hyoid cartilage

thyroid cartilage

thyroid gland

superior parathyroid gland

inferior parathyroid gland

thymus

B

Fig. 23.4 Development of the thyroid gland showing A potential sites for the development of thyroglossal cysts and B midline course of descent of the thyroglossal duct.

hyoid may have to be removed so that all of the thyroglossal duct tract can be removed as far as the base of the tongue.

Branchial cyst

Branchial cysts rarely present before adolescence, calling into question the belief that they arise from congenital failure of fusion of the second and third branchial arches. The cyst presents as a deep-seated painless swelling, bulging forwards from the anterior border of the sternomastoid muscle at the level of the hyoid bone (see Fig. 23.1). The cyst has an epithelial lining and contains opaque watery or milky fluid in which cholesterol crystals are suspended. As they contain lymphoid tissue in their walls, branchial cysts are prone to infection, which tends to be recurrent. Rarely, infection is followed by the appearance of a discharging sinus. Even more unusual is the development of a branchial fistula in which there is an internal opening into the tonsillar fossa. Such fistulas are present at birth and are frequently associated with a mucopurulent discharge from the external opening at the anterior border of the lower third of the sternocleidomastoid muscle.

Branchial cysts should be excised for cosmetic reasons and to prevent infective complications. In the case of branchial fistula, complete excision of the tract is essential.

Dermoid cyst

Dermoid cysts result from sequestration of epidermis during fusion of embryonic blocks of tissue. They are lined by stratified squamous epithelium and contain cheesy material produced by desquamation. They present as painless mobile swellings of the forehead, eyebrow region (external angular dermoid), at the base of the nose, and in the midline of the neck (submental dermoid).

Dermoid cysts are excised for cosmetic reasons and to prevent infective complications.

Cystic hygroma

Cystic hygroma is a rare benign lymphangioma which is usually present at birth and can cause problems during delivery. The multilocular cysts contain clear lymphatic fluid and are lined by endothelium. They form a soft and indentable swelling anywhere in the head and neck, but most commonly in the supraclavicular triangle, and may extend into the axilla or mediastinum to cause pressure symptoms.

Surgical removal under general anaesthesia is indicated when the cysts cause problems and may have to be undertaken urgently if there is airway obstruction or infection. Otherwise, the cystic hygroma regresses as the child grows and may be left alone.

SKIN AND SUBCUTANEOUS SWELLINGS

These are the commonest swellings in the head and neck, and the fact that they originate in the skin is relatively easy to determine because they can be picked up in a skinfold.

Sebaceous cysts

These cysts (see Ch. 17) are common in the sebum-producing areas of the skin and are particularly common in the scalp and neck. The presence of a punctum on the swelling is the key to diagnosis. The cyst can be excised under local anaesthesia using an elliptical incision which contains the punctum. Frequently the cysts become infected and then have to be distinguished from furuncles. Incision and drainage allows resolution and if the cyst recurs it can be excised while uninfected.

Furuncles (superficial boils)

These are common on the back of the neck and pinna. Infection begins in a hair follicle and the overlying skin becomes reddened before it turns white and necrotic. Induration, pain and tenderness are common, but lymphadenitis and systemic upset are rare. Most boils discharge spontaneously but incision and drainage may be required. Diabetes must be excluded if the problem is recurrent.

Carbuncles

Carbuncles develop if a hair follicle infection spreads to involve the dermis and subcutaneous tissues. Many of the infected extensions open to the surface as multiple discharging sinuses. There is death of the central portion of the carbuncle and a black necrotic core develops. Carbuncles are usually more extensive than their surface appearance suggests and wide excision is needed to remove all infected sinus tracts. The patient is often febrile and toxic, may prove to be diabetic, and requires antibiotics in addition to surgical drainage.

Lipomas

Lipomas in the head and neck are similar to those found elsewhere in the body and their diagnosis and management are identical (see Ch. 17).

Skin carcinoma

Apart from the hands, the head and neck are the areas most exposed to sunlight and hence are a common site for basal cell carcinomas, squamous carcinomas and malignant melanomas (see Ch. 17). These lesions are all commoner in fair, freckly, non-tanning individuals and should be suspected if any skin lesion increases rapidly in size. Excision biopsy is then indicated from histological diagnosis and is curative in most cases. Excision requires adequate margins and a satisfactory cosmetic result can be achieved by direct closure, local skin flaps or full thickness grafts, depending on the site and size of the lesion. Histological examination will then determine which type of malignancy, if any, was present and whether excision has been complete.

SALIVARY GLAND SWELLINGS AND DISEASE

There are three paired major salivary glands (the parotid, the submandibular and the sublingual) in addition to multiple small unnamed glands scattered throughout the mucosa of the mouth, cheeks, lips

---

Sebaceous cysts
- The cysts occur in sebum-producing areas, notably the scalp and neck.

- They are probably caused by degeneration of a hair follicle (sebaceous glands are normally located within the hair follicles).

- They are epidermal swellings (i.e. located within the skin so that the skin cannot be moved independently over the swelling).

- They have a punctum on close inspection.

- They may become infected, in which case incision and drainage may be needed.

- Uninfected cysts are usually excised under local anaesthesia with an ellipse of overlying skin.

---

and palate. Inflammatory disease and tumours generally involve a single gland, the main exceptions being viral parotitis (mumps) and autoimmune disease.

Surgical anatomy

Parotid gland

The parotid gland lies primarily beneath the subcutaneous tissue anterior to the external auditory canal and overlying the masseter muscle. Its upper pole extends to just below the zygoma, its lower pole into the neck (Fig. 23.5). The gland is enclosed in a sheath of deep cervical fascia so that any acute swelling is extremely painful. Normally the gland is impalpable though sometimes the part overlying the ramus of the mandible can be felt. The parotid duct system combines within the gland to form a common duct which enters the mouth in the cheek opposite the second upper molar tooth. The duct can be readily cannulated to outline the system with contrast medium. The facial nerve runs through the parotid gland after leaving the stylomastoid foramen, and divides within the parotid into its main branches, which emerge to supply the muscles of facial expression. Though the gland is often described as having a superficial and a deep lobe, this division is created surgically when the gland superficial to the facial nerve is removed while preserving the nerve.

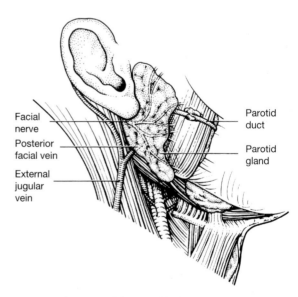

Fig. 23.5 Anatomy of the parotid gland showing its relationship to the facial nerve.

The main diagnostic difficulty with parotid lesions is to distinguish them from enlarged upper cervical lymph nodes when the parotid swelling is in the neck. A small mobile swelling below the angle of the jaw must not be excised without thought that it might arise from the parotid. Otherwise the facial nerve may be imperilled. Less commonly an enlarged preauricular lymph node may be thought to be a parotid swelling. Rarely, retrotonsillar enlargement in the oropharynx may be the result of an infiltrating parotid neoplasm.

Submandibular gland

The larger superficial portion of the submandibular gland fills most of the digastric triangle, extending upwards beneath the body of the mandible (Fig. 23.6). It rests on the mylohyoid muscle, hyoglossus and posterior pharyngeal wall. The smaller deep portion of the gland extends between the mylohyoid and hyoglossus muscles, and from it the submandibular duct runs forward to open on the floor of the mouth at the side of the frenulum of the tongue (Fig. 23.7). In a thin neck the normal gland is sometimes visible and in most it is palpable bimanually with one finger on the floor of the mouth

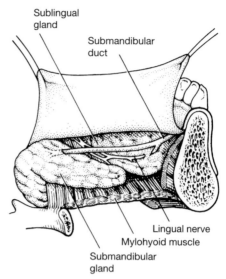

Fig. 23.7 Anatomical relationships of the left submandibular duct as seen from the floor of the mouth.

and the other in the submandibular region. The facial artery and vein and the cervical branch of the facial nerve run over the lateral border of the gland, and the lingual and hypoglossal nerves are deep to it. Damage to these nerves during surgery should be avoided.

Sublingual gland

The sublingual gland is the smallest of the named paired salivary glands. It lies submucosally in the floor of the mouth. It is adjacent to the submandibular duct, into which it secretes, as well as having several other separate openings. It is rarely affected by disease.

Surgical physiology

Saliva has several important functions. It lubricates food to enable swallowing, cleanses the mouth, digests starch, mediates taste and provides an immunological defence system. The composition of saliva secreted by each gland varies, the submandibular gland providing large volumes of high-viscosity calcium-enriched fluid, whereas the parotid gland secretes smaller volumes of serous fluid. Secretion is continuous throughout the day, but is maximal during eating and lowest during sleep.

In diseases where the secretory cells are damaged, such as sialadenitis and autoimmune disease, the volume and composition of saliva changes, although

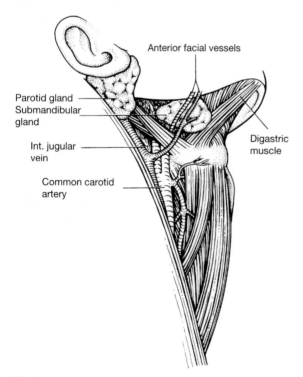

Fig. 23.6 Anatomical relationships of the submandibular gland.

it is not usual to analyse the secretions for diagnostic purposes. The commonest result of altered saliva composition is stone formation—sialolithiasis. This most frequently occurs in the submandibular duct because submandibular secretions are mucinous and high in calcium content. Calculi consist of depositions of concentric lamina of calcareous and organic material.

Examination and investigation of salivary gland disease

Salivary gland disease usually presents as unilateral or bilateral glandular enlargement which may be painful. Distinctions of diagnostic value are given in Table 23.1. The affected gland must be carefully palpated for enlargement and tenderness. Frequently the enlargement is diffuse rather than discrete because the fascia covering the gland is tight. With parotid disease, a change in the contour of the face may be the only sign of enlargement. Bimanual palpation of the submandibular and sublingual glands and ducts (Fig. 23.8) and of the parotid duct should always be carried out. Stones within the ducts can be palpated and the orifices should be inspected to identify any exudate following massage of the gland.

Plain transoral X-ray of the submandibular region is used to detect stones, and sialography can be used to outline any of the duct systems if a secretion abnormality is suspected. In a normal sialogram the arborizations of the duct are fine, regular and symmetrical. Abnormalities include displacement, distortion, stricture, dilatation and sacculation (sialectasis). Radiology is usually of little value in distinguishing benign from malignant tumours, but fine-needle aspiration cytology can be valuable. Antinuclear antibody determinations and lip biopsy to examine the minor salivary glands can provide the diagnosis in autoimmune disease.

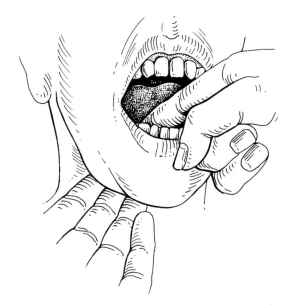

Fig. 23.8   Bimanual palpation of the submandibular gland and duct. Gloves should be worn during examination of the mouth.

Infective conditions

Mumps

After a prodromal period, patients with viral parotitis (mumps) usually develop bilateral, diffusely enlarged and tender parotid glands. These changes subside spontaneously, and symptomatic treatment is all that is needed. Less commonly the condition involves other salivary glands or is associated with sensorineural hearing impairment in children or orchitis in adults. The incidence of mumps should gradually fall in countries with active immunization programmes.

Acute parotitis

The parotid duct is normally flushed continuously by the flow of secretions. Ascending infection is likely if the flow becomes depressed in elderly, debilitated and dehydrated patients with poor oral hygiene. The gland is particularly vulnerable in the postoperative period, and if infection occurs, staphylococcal organisms are usually responsible. With improved standards of peri-operative care the condition has now become extremely uncommon.

Inflammatory conditions

Sialectasis

Sialectasis, or chronic dilatation of the duct system,

Table 23.1 Symptomatology and laterality of parotid gland disease			
	Pain	Swelling	
		Unilateral	Bilateral
Mumps (viral parotitis)	+	+	+
Acute parotitis	+	+	
Sialadenitis	+		+
Autoimmune disease	+		+
Neoplasia	−	+	

usually affects the parotid, and leads to episodes of pain and distension due to stasis and infection. Sialography is diagnostic and shows a dilated, distended duct system. An autoimmune basis should be considered. Management is symptomatic, superficial parotidectomy being reserved for patients with severe problems.

Sjögren's syndrome

This is the commonest form of autoimmune disease affecting both the major and the minor salivary glands. The syndrome comprises the triad of dry mouth, dry eyes (keratoconjunctivitis sicca) and other evidence of collagen disease, most frequently rheumatoid arthritis, or Raynaud's phenomenon. Clinically, there is chronic enlargement of any or all of the major salivary glands and the mouth is dry. If the patient has teeth, there may be gross caries. The diagnosis is best confirmed by biopsy of the minor salivary glands in the lip, and organ-specific and non-organ-specific antibodies can be sought serologically. Management is symptomatic with attention to oral hygiene and eye drops. Rarely, lymphoma develops secondarily.

Sialolithiasis

Salivary calculi are most common in the submandibular gland or duct and the patient usually presents with intermittent painful enlargement of the gland associated with eating. In the chronic condition, the gland becomes fibrosed, enlarged and palpable. If the stone cannot be felt within the duct

---

Salivary calculi
- The calculi are found most commonly in the submandibular gland and its duct.
- They are composed of calcium carbonate and phosphate.
- A salivary calculus initially causes intermittent painful enlargement of the gland, particularly on eating, but in time may cause the gland to become permanently enlarged, fibrosed and palpable.
- The calculus may be felt on bimanual palpation, and its presence can be confirmed by intraoral radiography and sialography.
- If the calculus is within the intra-oral portion of the duct it can be removed through the floor of the mouth; if it is impacted within the gland, removal of the gland is usually required.

---

on bimanual palpation, the duct can be probed, but the final diagnosis is usually made by transoral radiology. The calculi are composed of calcium carbonate and phosphate and are therefore radio-opaque. Sialography may be helpful early in the condition, not only for diagnosis, but also because it flushes out the duct system.

The treatment of a submandibular calculus depends on its site and whether the gland is chronically enlarged. A stone in the intra-oral portion of the duct is removed through the floor of the mouth. However, when the stone is impacted within the gland or when the gland is chronically enlarged, the whole gland must be removed. This is performed through an external approach, taking care to avoid the cervical branch of the facial nerve, and the lingual and hypoglossal nerves.

Salivary gland neoplasia

Neoplasms, benign and malignant, can arise from the secretory tissue, the duct system and from the myoepithelial or lymphoid tissue in the salivary glands. Classification of the many different histological types of tumour is controversial but in the majority of patients the clinical distinction between them does not influence management, although it may have an important bearing on prognosis. Approximately 85% of all neoplasms of the major salivary glands are found in the parotid. The great majority of parotid tumours (roughly 85%) are benign. About half of the tumours arising in the submandibular gland are benign, but the majority of tumours of the minor salivary glands are malignant. The great majority of benign tumours are pleomorphic adenomas. Adenolymphomas are much rarer but are also benign.

Pleomorphic salivary adenoma

A pleomorphic adenoma has a wide variety of histological features. It is composed primarily of epithelial glandular tissue which contains irregular spaces. In the mucoepidermoid type, epidermoid characteristics predominate and there is stratification and prickle cell formation. The epithelial elements form a mucous matrix thought once to be cartilage and responsible for the term 'mixed salivary tumour'. There is a dense collagenous stroma which may enclose tubules of epithelium (the so-called cylindroma) and form a dense capsule. The capsule is incomplete and portions of neoplastic epithelial tissue project into the surrounding salivary tissue.

Pleomorphic adenoma of the parotid gland

Although the superficial portion of the parotid gland is predominantly affected, no salivary tissue is immune. The tumour is found most frequently in middle-aged adults of either sex. Mixed salivary tumours are extraordinarily slow-growing and may reach a large size without causing symptoms. They are not frankly malignant and do not invade or metastasize. However, there is a high incidence of recurrence if the lesion is incompletely excised.

Usually the patient presents with a firm swelling in the lower pole of the parotid gland which often feels surprisingly superficial and may be mistaken for a simple dermoid or sebaceous cyst, or more frequently for a jugulo-digastric lymph gland.

Prior to fine-needle aspiration cytology, all parotid lumps had to be removed by superficial parotidectomy to provide both a tissue diagnosis and cure (as the majority were pleomorphic adenomas). With aspiration cytology, superficial parotidectomy is no longer mandatory as most tumours are slow-growing and surgery is cosmetic. In superficial parotidectomy the tumour is removed together with that portion of the parotid which lies superficial to the facial nerve. The key to success is early identification of the facial nerve where it enters the gland and careful preservation of its branches. In expert hands the operation gives excellent results and is preferable to enucleation with its high recurrence rate.

Post-gustatory sweating (Frey's syndrome) is an unusual complication of surgery in which there is sweating and flushing in the distribution of the auriculotemporal nerve. It is due to aberrant regrowth of parotid parasympathetic secretomotor fibres which innervate sympathetic end-organs of the skin.

Pleomorphic adenomas in other salivary glands

Pleomorphic adenoma affecting the submandibular gland forms a hard nodular swelling. The entire gland should be removed. Tumours of minor salivary glands can occur within the mouth and form lobular firm submucous swellings. They are commonly of cylindromatous type and particularly prone to recur. They should be excised widely and adjuvant radiotherapy may be considered.

Salivary adenolymphomas

This rare benign solid or cystic tumour of the parotid may affect males in later life. It is slow-growing and characteristically soft when cystic. Such tumours contain creamy material and epithelial elements associated with a mixed lymphoid stroma. The tumour feels superficial and is freely mobile. Some believe that it arises from heterotopic salivary tissue in lymph nodes.

Anaplastic carcinoma

Frankly malignant tumours of the parotid occur at a later age than pleomorphic adenomas, grow faster and invade surrounding tissues. They form a stony-hard fixed mass which may be associated with pain in the temple and scalp corresponding to the involvement of the auriculotemporal nerve. Facial palsy due to invasion of the facial nerve is uncommon but diagnostic of malignancy. Complete surgical removal of the entire gland (thus sacrificing the facial nerve) along with radiotherapy, offers the only hope of cure.

THYROID GLAND SWELLINGS AND DISEASE

These are discussed separately in Chapter 19.

LYMPH NODE SWELLINGS AND DISEASE

Several hundred lymph nodes are scattered throughout the head and neck but the majority fall into well-recognized superficial groups (Fig. 23.2). In addition, there is a deep retropharyngeal chain

Pleomorphic salivary adenoma
- Formerly known as 'mixed salivary tumours', these are the commonest histological type to affect salivary gland tissue.

- They can affect any salivary gland tissue in the head and neck but the parotid is the commonest site.

- The superficial portion of the parotid is predominantly affected though this may only be the tail and here there can be confusion with a neck cyst or upper cervical lymph node.

- The tumour is benign and often slow-growing.

- Fine-needle aspiration cytology is often diagnostic. Thereafter removal is for cosmetic reasons, usually by superficial parotidectomy with sparing of the facial nerve.

which cannot be palpated. Drainage to lymph nodes follows a well-defined pattern (Fig. 23.9), so it is often possible to determine the primary site of the disease by knowing which nodes are involved. Unfortunately, nodes along a drainage pathway can be bypassed; for example, dissemination of oral malignancy may skip the submental or submandibular nodes and involve the upper cervical lymph nodes. Nodes have to be at least 1 cm in diameter to be palpable and can be histologically involved by tumour while impalpable. Whether a node is fixed by tumour can be difficult to determine given that the nodes lie adjacent to muscles and within fascial sheaths. Consequently they should not be considered unresectable unless surgery proves them to be so.

Most children have several non-tender palpable nodes in the cervical chain because they are prone to recurrent upper respiratory tract infections. This should not cause concern, but by adolescence and the early twenties, these nodes should have regressed. In contrast, palpable nodes in older patients should always be investigated. In general, tender nodes are inflammatory and non-tender nodes are neoplastic. In all instances, the entire head and neck, and in particular the oral cavity, the nose, the pharynx and the larynx, should be examined endoscopically (under general anaesthesia if necessary) to identify a primary cause. CT is used to assess the extent of lymph node involvement, particularly as it will detect pathologically involved nodes that are impalpable. This is particularly important in neoplasia.

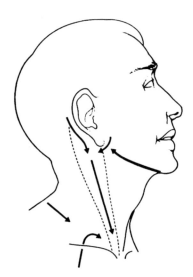

Fig. 23.9   Patterns of spread of infection and neoplasia to involve lymph nodes in the neck.

Disorders affecting the cervical lymph nodes can be classified as follows:

- Infective
    Acute (pyogenic) lymphadenitis
    Chronic (granulomatous) lymphadenitis
- Neoplastic
    Primary lymphoreticular neoplasia
    Secondary carcinoma.

Infective disorders

Acute lymphadenitis

Acutely tender lymph nodes are common in association with infections, particularly of the teeth, tonsils and pharynx. In most instances the cause is evident on examination and management is directed at the primary cause. Rarely the node may suppurate with spread to local tissues so that incision and drainage may be indicated. In some cases the abscess ruptures through the deep fascia so that there are superficial or deep loculi (i.e. 'collar stud' abscess). When draining an abscess, a specimen of pus is sent for bacteriological culture, and a biopsy of the wall is obtained if there is any doubt as to the nature of the condition.

Chronic infective lymphadenitis

In adults, chronically enlarged nodes secondary to infection are relatively uncommon but may be difficult to distinguish from neoplastic nodes as they are often not painful or tender. If no obvious cause can be identified after a thorough examination of the head and neck, including endoscopy, the nodes should be excised and sent for histological examination. This excision should be carried out by an experienced surgeon for two reasons. Firstly, as the node might be neoplastic, it has to be excised without being incised. Secondly, there are many anatomical structures that can be damaged, notably the facial, hypoglossal and accessory nerves.

Histologically the nodes often show non-specific inflammatory changes. In developed countries, diagnoses such as syphilis, actinomycosis, brucellosis, toxoplasmosis and cat scratch fever are exceptionally rare.

Tuberculous lymphadenitis. This is now uncommon in developed countries but should be suspected in any patient with chronically enlarged lymph nodes, particularly when there is an associated sinus, if there are several matted nodes, or when calcification is seen on X-ray. The primary route of infection is through the tonsil. Bovine bacilli in milk are responsible and associated lung tuberculosis is rare. The final diagnosis is made by histological identification of acid-fast bacilli; culture for *Mycobacterium tuberculosis* is more time-consuming. Antituberculous chemotherapy is prescribed.

Infectious mononucleosis (glandular fever). This produces bilateral multiple enlarged lymph nodes in association with a sore throat. This combination of symptoms and signs in adolescents and young adults requires only a mono-spot test to confirm the diagnosis. A skin rash following treatment of a sore throat with ampicillin should raise suspicion of this diagnosis. As this viral infection is spread by mouth, a history of contact with a fellow-sufferer is not unusual. Sometimes the lymph glands remain chronically enlarged for months without oropharyngeal symptoms. The differential diagnosis then includes lymphoma, but a mono-spot test is again diagnostic. Treatment is symptomatic.

Neoplasia

Primary lymphomas

Patients with lymphomas frequently present with bilateral, rubbery, firm, discrete cervical lymph nodes. Nodes elsewhere (e.g. the axilla) may be involved and lymphoid tissue throughout the body can be affected. Hodgkin's disease is the commonest form but non-Hodgkin's lymphoma is an important variant. Extranodal disease is commoner in non-Hodgkin's than in Hodgkin's lymphoma, and the former has a poorer prognosis. Lymphomas are more common in patients with immune deficiency (including those on immunosuppression after organ transplantation). There are few other causes of bilateral, non-tender multiple neck nodes in adolescence and early adult life. Excision biopsy of a node will determine the histological type of lymphoma and after staging the extent of the disease (haematological examination including bone marrow, CT scanning), treatment with chemotherapy and/or radiotherapy is indicated. Laparotomy was once used to stage the disease and perform splenectomy, but is now seldom used.

Burkitt's lymphoma is a poorly differentiated lymphocytic lymphoma which is found in the tropics and has a distribution similar to malaria; it is spread by an insect vector and thought to be virus-induced. Males are predominantly affected, and there is often unsightly swelling due to involvement of tissues around the jaw. Most patients have multiple tumour deposits throughout the body but the disease usually remits with chemotherapy, and remission can often be maintained by further courses of treatment.

Secondary carcinoma

There is virtually only one diagnosis to be entertained when a painless lymph node swelling develops in a patient over the age of 45, namely metastasis from a primary carcinoma which is most frequently, but not always, located in the head or neck. Commonly, there are also symptoms suggestive of a primary tumour but these may be so mild (e.g. hoarseness or the sensation of 'something' at the back of the throat) that the patient does not seek advice until a lymph node appears. Even then he may not mention the other symptoms unless questioned specifically. The primary tumour is often apparent on examination of the mouth, nose, naso-oro-, hypopharynx or larynx, and can then be biopsied. If a primary tumour cannot be identified, endoscopy under general anaesthesia will usually identify a lesion in one of the more difficult areas to examine. If a primary tumour is identified, there is no need to biopsy the cervical node, as the cause for its enlargement is evident. Furthermore, surgery usually consists of excision of the primary tumour and entire lymph node system in a block dissection of the neck. Biopsy of a node prior to thorough head and neck examination is not advisable, as it will not identify the primary site and may compromise subsequent surgery. If a supraclavicular node is involved, potential primary tumours, in addition to those in the head and neck, include a bronchial, breast or gastric neoplasm. If a primary is not found, fine-needle aspiration cytology is indicated.

HEAD AND NECK TRAUMA

Blunt neck injuries

In road traffic accidents, hyperextension of the neck on impact is the rule, hence exposing it to blunt injury. The airway is most at risk from trauma to the laryngeal framework, and the 'ABC' (airway, breathing, circulation) of trauma certainly holds. Stridor may be present from the start or develop due to increasing intralaryngeal oedema. Its management is discussed in Chapter 24.

Cut throat

The majority of such wounds are self-inflicted. The neck is often extended during wounding so that the

> **Lymphadenopathy**
> - Nodes become palpable when their diameter exceeds 1 cm, but impalpable nodes may contain tumour.
>
> - Tender nodes are usually inflammatory whereas non-tender nodes may be malignant.
>
> - The head and neck and, in particular, the oral cavity, nose, pharynx and larynx, must be examined to detect a primary cause for lymphadenopathy.
>
> - Fine-needle aspiration cytology can be diagnostic for secondary head and neck tumours or lymphoma.
>
> - CT scanning helps to find the extent of the lymphadenopathy.
>
> - Painless palpable neck nodes in patients over 45 are almost always due to metastasis from a carcinoma. In most cases the primary is within the head and neck. Such nodes must not be biopsied in the first instance; a thorough search for a primary lesion is the key to diagnosis.
>
> - In lymphoma:
>   - the nodes are often bilaterally enlarged, rubbery, firm and discrete
>   - there is underlying immunosuppression in some cases
>   - extranodal disease is commoner in non-Hodgkin's lymphoma
>   - excision biopsy is diagnostic
>   - bone marrow examination and CT scanning are used in staging.

main blood vessels are protected by the taut sterno-cleidomastoid muscles. However, major vessels within the carotid sheath may be cut and the upper alimentary and respiratory tracts may be opened.

Damage to the airway poses an immediate threat to life. Inhaled blood and secretions should be aspirated urgently and endotracheal intubation or tracheostomy may be needed.

Haemorrhage is the commonest cause of death. The bleeding is frequently venous and usually follows damage to the external jugular vein. Straining and struggling increase venous bleeding and the patient should be nursed in a slightly head-up position to reduce venous pressure. Air embolus may follow the sucking of air into the open vein if the patient is allowed to sit up or stand. Internal bleeding after a stab injury can produce subfascial haematomas, compression of neck structures, and sudden haemorrhage into a pleural space.

Emergency surgical exploration is mandatory if

the airway has been opened, a major vessel continues to bleed, or a haematoma develops. It is also necessary if there is any suspicion that the pharynx or oesophagus has been opened, as leakage of food and fluids into the neck with resultant infection must be prevented. Otherwise it is unnecessary to explore the wound; the risk of infection is low and surgery can damage important structures.

CAROTID BODY TUMOURS

Chemodectoma (carotid body tumour) is a rare cervical tumour which arises from chemoreceptor cells within the carotid body. The tumours are not hormonally active and metastasis is exceptional.

Characteristically, these tumours present as relatively symptomless swellings in the region of the carotid bifurcation. Secondary lymph node involvement from a primary neoplasm in the head and neck is more common and the affected node often appears to pulsate due to pulsations transmitted from the carotid. Carotid angiography is necessary if there is any doubt about the diagnosis before the neck is explored.

Detection of a chemodectoma is not necessarily an indication for surgical removal, particularly in the elderly in whom such surgery can compromise the cerebral circulation. In healthy younger patients the tumour should be excised.

HEAD AND NECK PRESENTATION OF AIDS

As part of the generalized lymphadenopathy associated with positive human immunodeficiency virus (HIV) status, multiple lymph nodes in the neck can be affected, hence the presentation is akin to reticulo-endothelial neoplasia.

At the stage when acquired immune deficiency syndrome (AIDS) has developed, head and neck manifestations are common. The HIV status by this stage will almost certainly be known and the infective conditions are managed as they arise. Oral candidiasis can be particularly troublesome. The pathology that is virtually specific to AIDS is Kaposi's sarcoma which involves the skin or oral/pharyngeal mucosa in 30% of patients.

24
Mouth, nose, throat and ear

CONTENTS

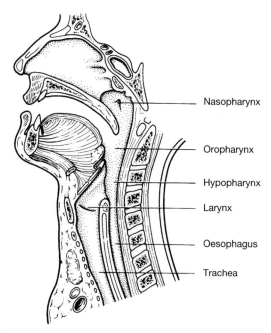

Fig. 24.1 Anatomy of nasopharynx, oropharynx and hypopharynx in relation to larynx and oesophagus.

The upper respiratory tract extends from the nares through the nasal cavities, nasopharynx, oropharynx, hypopharynx and larynx to join the trachea, the first part of the lower respiratory tract (Fig. 24.1). The upper alimentary tract starts at the lips, goes through the oral cavity, past the fauces, over the base of the tongue, into the oro- and hypopharynx and then joins the oesophagus behind the cricoid cartilage of the larynx at the level of the 6th cervical vertebra.

These two tracts might initially appear distinct but the only parts that cannot be used for both eating and breathing are the nose, nasopharynx and larynx.

Because food is relatively abrasive, the upper alimentary tract is lined by a non-keratinized squamous epithelium which is bathed in digestive and lubricative secretions, not only from the named salivary glands but also from multiple small salivary glands scattered throughout the mouth.

Because the primary function of the upper respiratory tract is to filter, warm and humidify the air, it is mainly lined by a mucus-secreting ciliated columnar epithelium. The exceptions are the anterior nares and the glottis, which are lined by squamous epithelium; the nares bear hairs to filter larger particles, while the glottis is subjected to mechanical trauma from vibrations. The Eustachian tube opens on the lateral wall of the nasopharynx and is lined by a

327

ciliated mucus-secreting epithelium in continuity with that of the middle ear. The middle ear can be regarded as an extension of the upper respiratory tract. The Eustachian tube aerates the middle ear space and keeps it at atmospheric pressure while allowing secretions to drain into the nasopharynx.

As potential portals of entry for infection, the two tracts have a well-developed immunological system of lymphoid tissue which is concentrated in a ring (Waldeyer's ring) around the naso- and oropharynx. The tonsils are localized aggregations and therefore excisable (Fig. 24.2). The adenoids are patches of lymphoid tissue scattered within the mucosa of the posterior wall and have to be scraped off to be removed, while the lingual tonsils are spread diffusely within the muscle of the base of the tongue and cannot be removed. Hypertrophy of this lymphoid tissue is normal in childhood, but with ageing there is a variable degree of atrophy. Localized enlargement at any age should be regarded as a possible sign of a reticuloendothelial neoplasm.

DISEASES OF THE UPPER ALIMENTARY AND RESPIRATORY TRACTS

Diseases of the upper respiratory and alimentary tracts can be classified as congenital, inflammatory,

neoplastic and traumatic. Inflammatory and neoplastic conditions are seen more frequently in individuals who smoke or chew tobacco, in alcohol drinkers, those with poor dental hygiene and those in the lower socio-economic groups.

It is not unusual for disease in one part of these tracts to be associated with similar disease in another part. For example, a viral infection may involve the epithelium of the nose, Eustachian tube and larynx causing rhinorrhoea, otitis media with effusion and a hoarse voice. Similarly, it is not uncommon for an individual who has been successfully treated for a tongue tumour, for example, to develop a carcinoma of the larynx some years later.

The commonest histological type of malignant tumour in both tracts is a squamous carcinoma, which is not surprising considering that the tracts are lined mainly by squamous epithelium. Less commonly, reticuloendothelial tumours arise in the lymphoid tissue and very rarely other types of tumours occur, particularly in the nasal passages. The incidence of malignant tumours varies from country to country, depending on culture and habits, but Table 24.1 illustrates what might be expected in a Caucasian country.

Unfortunately, both tracts are relatively capacious so that patients with tumours frequently present late, i.e. when the tumour finally starts to cause obstructive symptoms. The exception to this is the common glottic tumour, which often causes hoarseness early in the course of the disease, prompting the patient to seek medical attention. Another common presentation is with a secondary deposit in a neck node; as might be expected, this usually carries a bad prognosis.

In general, small (T1 and T2) head and neck squamous carcinomas respond well to radiotherapy or excisional surgery, with a 5-year survival rate of over 75%. With larger tumours (T3 and T4) which have spread to adjacent structures or lymph nodes (N1 and N2), the response to either form of therapy

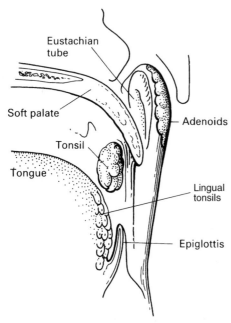

Fig. 24.2 Distribution of lymphoid tissue in pharynx.

Table 24.1	Incidence of head and neck tumours		
	Incidence per 100 000		
	Males	Females	Overall
Larynx	4.3	0.9	2.6
Pharynx	2.1	1.5	1.8
Mouth	2.0	1.2	1.6
Salivary glands	1.4	1.6	1.5
Tongue	1.5	0.9	1.2
Nose/sinuses	0.6	0.4	0.5
Total	11.9	6.5	9.2

is considerably worse. Excisional surgery with or without secondary radiotherapy gives the best survival rates (approximately 35% at 5 years), but there are problems in repairing the defect so that the patient can eat, speak and breathe as normally as possible. Primary radiotherapy is associated with lower cure rates but may be the preferred option for patients such as the very elderly and those with poor support at home. To date, chemotherapy has been reserved mainly for palliation but its benefits are marginal.

THE MOUTH

Infections and swellings

Because the oral cavity is large, lesions tend not to obstruct eating or swallowing unless they are large. Patients often just notice that 'something is there' which can make eating difficult, although the feeling is as frequently relieved by eating. Inflammatory lesions are usually painful whereas malignant ones are not. However, if there is any concern about the nature of a lesion an expert opinion should be sought and biopsy undertaken as a definitive investigation.

Head and neck tumours

- These are mainly squamous carcinomas.

- Tobacco smoke and excessive alcohol ingestion are common aetiological factors to tumours in all sites.

- Non-healing ulcers of the oral cavity raise suspicion of carcinoma.

- Asymmetric tonsil enlargement is suggestive of a tonsillar tumour.

- The sensation of something being there at the back of the throat, but without obstruction to swallowing, requires a pharyngeal or base of tongue tumour to be excluded.

- Individuals with hoarseness of longer than 3 weeks duration must be considered to have a laryngeal carcinoma until shown otherwise.

- Lymph node enlargement due to secondary metastasis is unfortunately the presenting symptom for many head and neck tumours.

- In general, radiotherapy for small tumours and surgery, with or without radiotherapy, for large tumours is the management option for cure.

Mucosal disease

The mouth is the portal of the alimentary tract, and mucosal disease in the ileum or colon, notably Crohn's disease, is occasionally associated with oral ulcers. Deficiences of vitamins (B or C) or minerals (such as iron) can be evident as a general dryness of the lips, cheeks and tongue, with cracking at the angles of the mouth (angular cheilitis).

Aphthous ulcers

These are recurrent painful ulcers which are usually multiple and found on mobile mucosa such as that lining the cheeks, tongue and gingival sulci. The ulcers are small, yellowish-white and punched out with a surrounding halo or erythema. Their aetiology is unknown but they are common in normal individuals and are occasionally seen in patients with Crohn's disease or ulcerative colitis. Treatment may not be necessary but some patients find that topical antiseptics or topical corticosteroid pellets are helpful.

Stomatitis and gingivitis

Inflammation of the oral mucosa (stomatitis) and gums (gingivitis) is particularly common in dehydrated, febrile and ill-nourished patients with faulty oral hygiene. Carious teeth, ill-fitting dentures and heavy smoking favour their development. The mucosa becomes reddened and dry, the tongue is swollen and furred, and halitosis (bad breath) is prominent. Pain on eating may be marked if ulcertion occurs, and fever and malaise are common.

Stomatitis is largely preventable by attention to oral hygiene and adequate hydration. Established stomatitis is treated by removing causal factors, by hydration, regular mouth washes and promoting the flow of saliva. Antibiotics are rarely indicated.

Traumatic ulcers

Trauma from broken teeth or ragged or loose dentures can cause painful ulcers on the lips, cheeks or tongue. Neglecting to remove the dentures to inspect the mouth may mean that the diagnosis is missed. If the ulcer persists after eradication of the dentition problem, it should be biopsied to exclude carcinoma.

Retention cysts

Mucous retention cysts can occur anywhere within the oral cavity or indeed in any part of the upper alimentary and respiratory tracts. Those located under the tongue are *ranulas*. They occur if the drainage of mucous or accessory salivary glands is blocked. Many are discovered incidentally and can be disregarded. Others may have been seen by the patient or given rise to the sensation of 'something being there'. The classical appearance is that of a pearly-white, rounded swelling lying superficially in the mucosa. Excision is curative. Alternatively, the cyst may simply be deroofed. This operation is known as marsupialization.

Candida infections

In otherwise well patients, the commonest site for candida infection is underneath dentures or at the angles of the mouth. In debilitated patients and those on broad-spectrum antibiotic therapy, candidiasis can be a considerable problem anywhere in the mouth but affects particularly the palate, fauces, tongue and oropharynx. The classical appearance is that of a whitish membrane which resembles milk curds and which, when scraped off, reveals a localized area of raw mucosa. The diagnosis is usually obvious but is confirmed by taking scrapings for microscopic examination. Therapy consists of topical nystatin lozenges or suspensions (500 000 units four times a day for 4 days), stopping unnecessary antibiotic therapy, and improving the patient's oral hygiene and general health.

Other forms of specific oral infection

Formerly infective causes of oral ulceration had to be seriously considered but these (e.g. syphilis, tuberculosis, actinomycosis) are now extremely rare.

Leukoplakia

Leukoplakia denotes mucosal hyperkeratosis and is caused by long-standing irritation, notably by tobacco. It appears as white areas located most commonly on the tongue and buccal mucosa. Desquamation may expose sensitive areas resembling raw beef. Hyperkeratosis may proceed to papillomatous proliferation and fissuring, and cancer may supervene. Although premalignant, leukoplakia should regress with attention to oral hygiene and abstinence from tobacco and alcohol. If not, such patients should be observed regularly and any suspicious areas biopsied, particularly if there are red areas associated.

Cancer of the tongue and oral cavity

Cancer arising in the mouth has become less common over the past 50 years but still accounts for some 2% of all malignancies. Tobacco smoking is the major aetiological factor. Other factors include heavy alcohol consumption, poor oral hygiene and betel nut chewing, although it is often difficult to dissociate these factors from the effects of co-existing tobacco consumption. Oral cancer is commoner in males than in females, is uncommon before the age of 45 and the majority of patients are over 70 years of age.

The cancer is usually painless and patients tend to seek advice late. They frequently complain of 'something being there' and the tumour may have become quite large before diagnosis, particularly if located in 'silent' areas such as the gingivo-lingual sulcus or posterior third of the tongue. The diagnosis is usually obvious from the appearance of raised ulcerated areas with overhanging edges which sometimes bleed. The lesions are only painful if there is secondary infection. The diagnosis is confirmed by incision biopsy. The great majority (over 90%) of oral cancers are squamous carcinomas, with pleomorphic salivary adenomas accounting for most of the remainder.

Management depends primarily on the stage of the tumour. Although widespread dissemination is rare, nearly 30% of patients have involved cervical lymph nodes at the time of presentation and in some the mandible is also involved. When the tumour is small, excisional surgery and radiotherapy appear to be equally effective. When it is large and there is mandibular or nodal involvement, the primary method of curative treatment is surgery, with or without radiotherapy. To gain access it may be necessary to temporarily split the mandible. The tumour can then be excised 'en bloc' with any involved bone or cervical lymph nodes. Large defects left after excisional surgery require skilled repair using skin flaps or free grafts with microvascular anastomoses.

Approximately one-third of patients with oral cancer survive for 5 years following diagnosis.

Dental disease

Dental caries is common, and over one-third of the United Kingdom population over the age of 16 years are edentulous. Caries is due to erosion of the dental enamel by the bacterial products associated with plaque formation. In children, the commonest sites are in the cusps and in adults the areas between the teeth and the gum margins. Caries at the gum margin is made worse by chronic gingivitis. The incidence of caries has been dramatically reduced since the introduction of fluoridation of drinking water and toothpaste. Management consists of prevention and avoidance of an oversweet diet along with regular oral hygiene and removal of debris and plaque by a combination of brushing and flossing.

Submandibular abscess

An abscess (Ludwig's angina) can form in the submandibular triangle due to suppuration in a lymph node associated with dental or oral disease. When it spreads to the sublingual space the tongue is swollen and displaced with the potential of obstructing the airway. The patient is ill and toxic with pain, trismus and dysphagia and requires intravenous antibiotics for what is usually a streptococcus or coliform infection.

Congenital abnormalities

Cleft lip and cleft palate

These are the commonest developmental abnormalities of the head and neck, with an incidence of about 1 in 700 live births. Such children pose considerable management problems involving many disciplines for periods which may exceed 20 years. Clefts are due primarily, but not solely, to abnormal fusion of the central premaxillary (nasal) process with the lateral maxillary processes to form the lip, nose, alveolus and its dentition, and the hard and soft palate (Fig. 24.3). They can occur unilaterally or bilaterally and are classified as cleft lip with or without cleft palate, and cleft palate alone (Fig. 24.4). The abnormality is considerably commoner in those

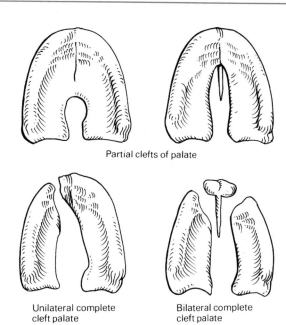

Partial clefts of palate

Unilateral complete cleft palate

Bilateral complete cleft palate

Fig. 24.4 Types of cleft palate.

with a family history, and genetic counselling should be offered.

The diagnosis is usually obvious at birth. Nasal regurgitation during suckling can usually be overcome with special teats. When the child is 3–6 months old, any cleft in the lip is usually repaired, although multiple operations to the lip and nose may be required to achieve a satisfactory cosmetic result. The next objective is to ensure that speech develops as normally as possible by closing any palatal defect surgically at about 18 months of age. Again, many operations may be necessary over the years to lengthen the palate so that the nasopharynx can be closed during phonation and eating. The next problem is to ensure good dentition and encourage maxillary growth by appropriate orthodontic splints and braces. Finally, throughout the growing period, there is the problem of persistent otitis media with effusion (see later) which requires regular observation and management. Needless to say, tonsillectomy and adenoidectomy are contraindicated in children with cleft palates.

THE NOSE

Surgical anatomy

The external nose consists of the nasal bones and the paired upper and lower lateral cartilages (Fig. 24.5).

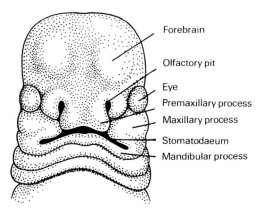

Forebrain

Olfactory pit

Eye
Premaxillary process
Maxillary process

Stomatodaeum
Mandibular process

Fig. 24.3 The development of the lips and mouth.

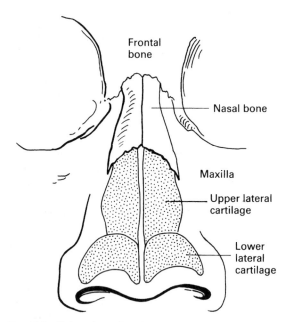

Fig. 24.5   External nasal anatomy.

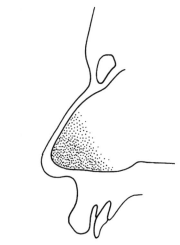

Fig. 24.7   Little's area on septum.

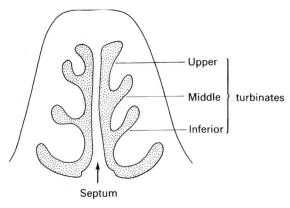

Fig. 24.6   Internal nasal anatomy.

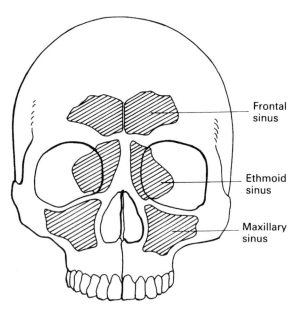

Fig. 24.8   The nasal sinuses.

Internally the nose is divided in two, anteriorly by the cartilaginous septum and posteriorly by the bony septum (Fig. 24.6). The three turbinates on the lateral wall increase the surface area of mucus-secreting mucosa which warms and humidifies the inspired air. The inferior turbinate is readily seen on anterior rhinoscopy and should not be confused with a nasal polyp. Little's area is an area on the anterior septum within reach of a poking finger (Fig. 24.7) from which bleeding is common.

There are four groups of nasal sinuses: the frontal, ethmoid, maxillary and sphenoid sinuses (Fig. 24.8). With the exception of the sphenoid sinus, they drain into the nose below the middle turbinate. Tears from the eye drain into the nose via the nasolacrimal duct, which enters below the inferior turbinate.

Nasal symptoms and diseases

Blockage

The sensation of having a blocked nose may be constant or cyclical, unilateral or bilateral. Constant blockage suggests deviation of the septum or a nasal tumour. Cyclical blockage suggests mucosal problems. Clinical examination will usually reveal the diagnosis.

Deviated nasal septum

Some degree of deviation of the nasal septum is normal and causes no symptoms because of compensatory shrinkage of the turbinates on the narrower side. In a few individuals the deviation is such that the nose feels blocked. Submucosal resection of the deviated part or repositioning the deviated parts (septoplasty; see later) will give relief.

Nasal polyps

Multiple benign polyps are the commonest nasal tumour and most frequently arise bilaterally from the ethmoidal air cells. If small, they may regress with topical steroid application (e.g. beclomethasone) otherwise management consists of surgical removal. Unfortunately, recurrence is common but this may be prevented by prophylactic topical steroids. If this fails, repeat avulsion or ethmoidectomy, in which the air cells are opened to clear them of disease, is indicated.

Nasal cancer

Suspicion that a nasal tumour may not be a simple polyp should be aroused if it is unilateral, does not have the classical glistening pale appearance, and if it bleeds. The many different histological types of nasal tumour can only be distinguished by biopsy. Management almost invariably involves surgery; its extent depends on its histology, on the degree of invasion of neighbouring structures such as the paranasal sinuses and the orbit as assessed by endoscopy and radiology, and on whether there are regional or distant metastases. The tumour is removed together with any involved bone, and any resultant defect in the facial bones is made cosmetically more acceptable by attaching a prosthesis to a dental plate.

Rhinorrhoea

A runny nose is due to an increase in secretions (catarrh) from an inflamed nasal and/or sinus mucosa, and is usually associated with nasal blockage due to mucosal oedema. The secretions are normally clear, but may become yellow, green or brown if secondary bacterial infection occurs.

The common cold

Coryza is the commonest cause of a running nose and the diagnosis is usually obvious.

Allergic rhinitis

Allergic rhinitis is less common than intrinsic rhinitis but, as the latter is diagnosed by excluding the former, allergic rhinitis is considered first. Allergic rhinitis may be seasonal or 'all-year-round' (perennial). Seasonal allergies can be due to pollens and are easy to diagnose from the typical history of a runny nose and watery eyes at a specific time of the year. Perennial rhinitis is less easy to diagnose from the history, and house dust and animal mites are the commonest allergens. The differentiation from non-specific rhinitis rests on the identification of an allergen. Skin tests may be used but false positive reactions are common in asymptomatic individuals and a test battery can be difficult to interpret.

Management consists of avoiding the allergen and prescription of topical steroids (beclomethasone) or sodium cromoglycate. Antihistamines can be given if eye symptoms are dominant. Desensitization is contraindicated because of the dangers of anaphylactic reactions. Surgical trimming or diathermy of enlarged turbinates is an option if medical treatment fails.

Intrinsic non-specific (vasomotor) rhinitis

Intrinsic rhinitis is often attributed (without much evidence) to imbalance in the vasomotor system. The symptoms tend to be perennial but running eyes are infrequent in comparison to allergic rhinitis. The same medications are given as for allergic rhinitis and again turbinate surgery is an option if this fails.

Chronic sinusitis

Chronic sinusitis is akin to chronic bronchitis in that periodically the nasal and sinus mucosa becomes inflamed, resulting in the production of a mucopurulent discharge which is difficult to eradicate. It is like having frequent, mucopurulent colds. Headaches and facial pain are not common. Predisposing factors such as obstruction to the sinus ostia by a deviated nasal septum, dental caries affecting the maxillary sinus, smoking and poor general health should be excluded or dealt with. Conventional X-rays are not helpful in arriving at a diagnosis, because of the poor correlation between radiological mucosal oedema and surgical findings. Computerized tomography (CT) is markedly superior though many would limit its use to only those undergoing surgery, because of cost.

Management consists of encouraging drainage with steam inhalations and topical nasal steroids.

Courses of broad-spectrum antibiotics may be given. In some patients, endoscopic clearance of disease with enlargement of the ostia may be beneficial. Sinus washouts and intranasal antrostomy are less favoured than formerly.

Acute sinusitis

If the ostium of a sinus becomes blocked during an upper respiratory tract infection, an abscess may form. There is acute pain and local tenderness over the affected sinus. Drainage and antibiotics are indicated.

Bleeding (epistaxis)

In younger individuals bleeding occurs most frequently from a small blood vessel in Little's area. In older patients it most frequently arises from a posteriorly located arteriosclerotic blood vessel. Occasionally a nasal tumour presents with bleeding.

In the acute stage the anterior septum should be compressed by pinching the cartilaginous nose. This applies pressure to Little's area (Fig. 24.9) and should stop any bleeding from this site. A pledget of cotton wool soaked in 1 in 1000 adrenaline can be inserted just inside the vestibule to encourage this. The fingernails of children with recurrent epistaxis should be kept short to prevent trauma from picking, and nasal crusts kept soft with vaseline. Prominent blood vessels on Little's area may be cauterized.

If bleeding does not stop with anterior pinching, the epistaxis is arising further back and may be managed by the non-specialist with an epistaxis balloon catheter. Though this may compress the bleeding point it is more likely to work because it closes off the cavity anteriorly and posteriorly. The balloon is kept in for 24 hours after cessation of bleeding. It is usually unnecessary to pack both sides of the nose because, even if blood issues from both sides, it usually originates from only one point. Blood then comes round the septum posteriorly and the side that initially bled is the side to pack. Hospital admission is advisable, because of the dangers associated with any haemorrhage. Sedation and general measures to anticipate and treat shock should be instituted. Coagulation defects should be screened for should the bleeding be troublesome, non-steroidal anti-inflammatory drugs (NSAIDs) such as aspirin being a frequent culprit.

Troublesome epistaxis should be managed by a specialist who may be able to coagulate the bleeding point endoscopically. Nasal packing anteriorly and posteriorly may be required (Fig. 24.10). Surgical ligation of the arterial supply to the bleeding point is sometimes indicated if the problem persists.

Nasal trauma

Nasal fractures

Pugilistic and accidental nasal injuries are common. In the majority there is just bruising and perhaps epistaxis. In some the nasal bones and/or the septal

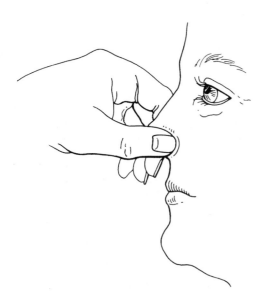

Fig. 24.9 Pressure to control haemorrhage (see text).

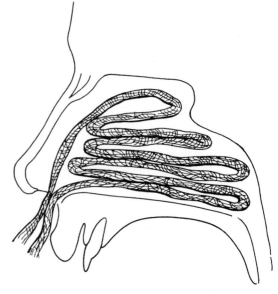

Fig. 24.10 Nasal packing.

cartilage may be fractured (Fig. 24.11). The diagnosis is a clinical one and made by detecting local tenderness over the fracture site(s). Management depends on whether the nose is misaligned. X-rays will not help to make this distinction and even an experienced clinician may find it difficult to differentiate between an old and a newly displaced fracture. Individuals who get their nose bashed tend to do so frequently.

No treatment is necessary for undisplaced fractures apart from dealing with any epistaxis. If the bony or cartilaginous nose is displaced, manipulation under general anaesthesia has to be performed within 10 days of injury because after that time fragments will be difficult to disimpact because of healing.

Chronic deformities

In an age of increasing personal awareness and desire to appear attractive many individuals with previously ignored nasal deformities attend some time after the incident complaining of their appearance and perhaps of increased difficulty in breathing. Other patients may present with an unsatisfactory appearance despite manipulation.

Rhinoplasty with controlled chisel or saw refracturing of the nasal bones via intranasal incisions will improve the appearance. Septoplasty with repositioning of the cartilaginous and bony septum in the midline after partial removal of grossly deviated segments will improve the airway (Fig. 24.12).

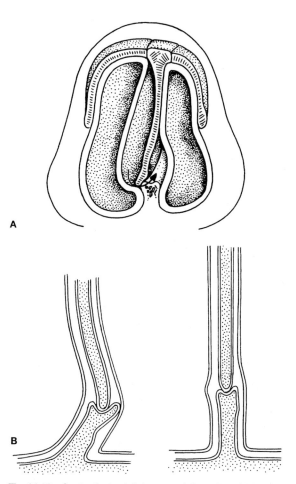

Fig. 24.12   Septoplasty. A Submucosal dissection of inferior part of septum. **B** Before and after repositioning of the cartilaginous and bony septum in the midline.

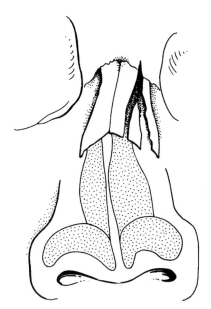

Fig. 24.11   Nasal fracture.

Epistaxis
- Epistaxis in young patients usually arises from a small blood vessel in Little's area; in older individuals it arises from an arteriosclerotic vessel located more posteriorly.

- Pressure on Little's area by compressing the anterior septum usually stops the bleeding, and topical application of 1 in 1000 adrenaline may be helpful.

- Bleeding arising more posteriorly may require balloon compression or packing.

- Coagulation defects should always be excluded in patients with troublesome bleeding. These can be caused by alcohol or non-steroidal analgesics in a high proportion of patients.

- Recurrent or persistent epistaxis may require endoscopic coagulation of the bleeding point (and even surgical ligation of the bleeding point in some cases).

THE PHARYNX

Surgical anatomy

The pharynx is divided into three parts. The nasopharynx extends from the base of the skull to the hard palate and is part of the upper respiratory tract into which the Eustachian tubes open on the posterolateral wall. There are scattered patches of lymphoid (adenoid) tissue on this wall. The oropharynx opens anteriorly to the mouth and is bounded above by the hard palate and below by the tip of the epiglottis. It contains the (palatal) tonsils, the lingual tonsils and the base of the tongue. The hypopharynx is bounded above by the tip of the epiglottis and ends at the cricoid cartilage at the level of the sixth cervical vertebra. The laryngeal inlet is bounded anteriorly on either side by the pyriform fossae, which are the main routes taken by food before it enters the oesophagus at the base of the hypopharynx.

The muscles of the pharynx are under voluntary control via the vagus (X) nerve and mucosal sensation is subserved mainly by the glossopharyngeal (IX) nerve.

The nasopharynx

Adenoid hypertrophy and neoplasia are the two main diseases of the nasopharynx and they usually present with symptoms caused by their size. The nose may become blocked and/or the Eustachian tube may be unable to function, giving rise to otitis media with effusion. Sometimes nasopharyngeal tumours will bleed and, even when small, they may metastasize to the cervical lymph nodes.

Adenoid hypertrophy

Adenoid hypertrophy in childhood is normal and in the majority of cases causes no symptoms. However, large adenoids may be a factor in recurrent nasal infections and otitis media with effusion. The size of the adenoids can be assessed indirectly with a mirror but this is often difficult; lateral X-rays are more reliable. If hypertrophy is considered to be a factor, the adenoids can be removed by curetting. Although a simple operation, it should not be embarked upon lightly because of the dangers of haemorrhage. It is also definitely contraindicated if there is any suggestion of a cleft palate because of the subsequent development of hypernasal speech and nasal regurgitation of food.

Tumours

In children and adolescents the majority of tumours are congenital in origin, and benign. This does not mean that they can be considered trivial. They can erode the base of the skull and cause cranial nerve palsies. The commonest tumour is an angiofibroma which, though not necessarily arising in the nasopharynx, presents with the symptoms of nasopharyngeal obstruction and recurrent bleeding. It is a highly vascular tumour, and blind biopsy is not recommended. CT or magnetic resonance imaging (MRI) with enhancement has replaced angiography as the investigation of choice. Though these tumours are benign and regression with age is likely, it is usual now to surgically remove them, often after arterial embolization.

In adults, particularly those of Chinese extraction who have lived in the Far East, squamous cell carcinoma is the commonest tumour of the nasopharynx. It usually presents late, often with erosion of the base of the skull or with neck metastases. Many patients have otitis media with effusion due to Eustachian tube blockage, hence the importance of considering a nasopharyngeal tumour in adults with this condition. Complete surgical excision of the primary tumour is not possible because of its relationship to important neurological structures, and surgical clearance of the neck can never be complete because of the almost invariable presence of retropharyngeal nodes which cannot be removed. Radiotherapy is therefore the mainstay of management and in the majority of patients is palliative rather than curative, relieving the pain associated with erosion of the skull base.

The oropharynx

As in the mouth, lesions in the oropharynx have to be large before they obstruct swallowing. However, unlike those in the mouth, oropharyngeal lesions frequently cause pain.

Acute pharyngitis

Viral infections of the pharynx are common and present as a sore throat which is exacerbated by tobacco smoke or dust. Usually a runny nose or hoarse voice indicates that other parts of the upper respiratory tracts are involved. Clinically the oropharynx can look surprisingly normal but is hypersensitive to touch. Pain relief pending resolution is obtained in children by paracetamol elixir and in adults by aspirin gargles, which are then swallowed to give both a topical and systemic effect.

Acute tonsillitis

Bacterial tonsillitis due to beta-haemolytic streptococci is a condition of childhood and adolescence. Episodes of sore throat are associated with fever, malaise and cervical lymphadenopathy but without a runny nose, cough or hoarse voice. Both tonsils appear inflamed and enlarged with mucopus in the crypts. Analgesics, as in acute pharyngitis, are the mainstay of management, with prescription of parenteral penicillin for the more severely ill.

In the acute stage, differentiation from acute pharyngitis is easy. Between episodes, it is not possible to make the distinction on the appearance of the tonsils. Some tonsils which are chronically enlarged give no problems while others which are recurrently infected may be small.

If the episodes of tonsillitis are frequent and incapacitating, tonsillectomy is the surgical option. This is done under general anaesthesia with endotracheal intubation to protect the airway from haemorrhage. The tonsils are dissected out and any bleeding points are controlled. Post-tonsillar haemorrhage is the major complication and can be fatal (1 in 10 000 operations). Monitoring, especially of the pulse rate, for 4–8 hours after operation is essential. Fluid replacement, preferably with blood, is vital if bleeding occurs. Once the child is resuscitated, the bleeding point should be ligated. Secondary haemorrhage can occur several days later but is usually minor and does not require surgery.

Because of its dangers and the psychological disturbances associated with admission of children to hospital, tonsillectomy should not be considered a minor operation. The natural history of recurrent tonsillitis is one of spontaneous resolution over a 2-year period so that all tonsillectomy does is hasten this.

Peritonsillar abscess (quinsy)

The most frequent complication of acute tonsillitis is a peritonsillar abscess, which should be suspected when there is asymmetry in the size of the tonsils in a patient with acute tonsillitis. This is due to the abscess displacing the tonsil downwards and medially. Trismus denotes difficulty in opening the mouth due to reflex spasm of the masseter and buccinator muscles and also suggests an abscess.

Drainage of the abscess by needle aspiration, by stab incision under local anaesthesia or by tonsillec-

tomy under general anaesthesia gives quick resolution. In the early stages, parenteral penicillin is an alternative.

Parapharyngeal abscess

The parapharyngeal space is a potential space on both sides of the naso- and oropharynx. Very occasionally infection from the tonsils or teeth may track into this space with gross toxic symptoms of infection, a lateral tender neck swelling and trismus. Treatment consists of systemic antibiotics and internal or external surgical drainage.

Retropharyngeal abscess

The retropharyngeal space is a potential space between the cervical vertebrae and the pharynx which normally contains only lymph nodes. Suppuration in one of these can lead to an abscess but this is uncommon, the usual initial infective cause in children being an upper respiratory tract infection and in adults, tuberculosis of the spine.

Infectious mononucleosis

Infectious mononucleosis (glandular fever) due to the Epstein-Barr virus should be suspected if an adolescent or young adult has grossly enlarged bilateral cervical lymph nodes in association with a sore throat and general malaise. The pharynx may be only mildly infected, there is a mononuclear leucocytosis, and the mono-spot test is positive. Symptoms are often protracted over several months and there is no specific treatment. Interestingly, if ampicillin is given for the sore throat, over 90% of patients will develop a skin rash.

Snoring and sleep apnoea

Snoring, most often, is caused by uncontrolled vibrations of the soft palate and commonly occurs in normal people. It can become particularly annoying to sleeping partners, particularly following an excessive bout of alcohol ingestion and in those that are obese. Advice is initially to lose excess weight, cut down on alcohol ingestion, and sometimes to undergo surgical tightening of the soft palate.

Many normal individuals also have episodes during sleep when respiration slows and temporarily stops. In snorers this can be repeated more than normal and can be associated with hypoxia which becomes evident as daytime somnolence. If sleep apnoea is suspected, overnight monitoring in hospital records the frequency and duration of the episodes along with the degree of hypoxia which on occasion can be life-threatening. Most are considered obstructive in origin due to collapse of a lax oropharynx and tongue musculature, but nasal and oral pathology should be excluded. Once diagnosed, continuous positive airway pressure is provided at home after which weight reduction is encouraged to lessen the risks. Rarely a permanent tracheostomy is required.

The hypopharynx

Pharyngeal problems usually present as a sensation of 'something being there'. There is no difficulty in swallowing or obstruction, indeed swallowing can relieve the symptoms. In many patients, no pathology can be detected despite a thorough clinical examination with a mirror, plain lateral X-rays, and barium swallow.

However, such symptoms should always be treated seriously because of the possibility of an underlying tumour. To exclude this, many patients have to be examined under general anaesthesia to allow evaluation of areas such as the pyriform fossae.

Once pathology has been excluded, the patient can be reassured that symptoms will abate with time. It is likely that in future many of these unexplained symptoms will be diagnosed as due to motility disorders, but in the meantime the term 'globus hystericus', as a label for such idiopathic symptoms, is somewhat inaccurate as there is no hysteria though some patients may be introspective or depressed. The term 'globus syndrome' may be more appropriate.

Gastro-oesophageal reflux

Reflux may produce the sensation of 'something being there' and is not always associated with heartburn. It is easy to understand how refluxed acid and bile can irritate the pharynx. The diagnosis and management of gastro-oesophageal reflux are described in Chapter 27.

Pharyngeal pouch

This is a midline mucosal herniation through the lower pharyngeal muscles (Killian's dehiscence) which gradually enlarges with retained food (Fig. 24.13). The condition is caused by inco-ordination between contraction of the pharynx and relaxation of the upper oesophageal sphincter and usually affects the elderly. It causes progressive

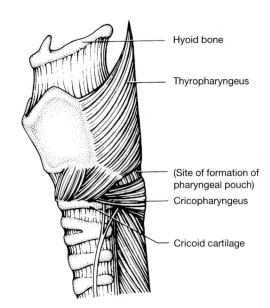

Fig. 24.13 Site of formation of pharyngeal pouch.

Labels: Hyoid bone; Thyropharyngeus; (Site of formation of pharyngeal pouch); Cricopharyngeus; Cricoid cartilage

difficulty in swallowing due to pressure on the hypopharynx and upper oesophagus from the diverticulum. Mirror examination and endoscopy frequently miss the pouch and the diagnosis is best made by barium swallow. It is unusual to palpate a swelling in the neck. Treatment consists of excision of the pouch, repair of the defect and division of the cricopharyngeal muscle (myotomy) below the defect (Fig. 24.14). Endoscopic techniques are also available.

Pharyngeal tumours

These are mainly squamous cell carcinomas and, when small, only cause the sensation of 'something being there'. In some sites, particularly the pyriform fossae, they can grow quite large before causing obstruction to swallowing and, perhaps, hoarseness due to laryngeal involvement. Enlargement of cervical lymph nodes is a common form of presentation.

As these tumours tend to be relatively large by the time they are diagnosed, excision with repair of the pharyngeal defect by a vascularized skin flap such as the myocutaneous deltopectoral flap is the curative method of choice. When the larynx is involved, this has to be removed as well (pharyngolaryngectomy) and repair may involve the use of a free jejunal graft with vascular anastomosis or consist of pulling the mobilized stomach up through the chest to anastomose it with the pharynx. Any involved cervical

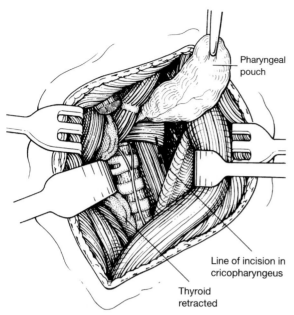

Fig. 24.14 Cricomyotomy and 'suspension' of pharyngeal pouch.

Labels on figure:
- Pharyngeal pouch
- Line of incision in cricopharyngeus
- Thyroid retracted

nodes are excised by block dissection of the neck and radiotherapy can be given as an adjunct.

LARYNX

Applied anatomy

The larynx is the muscular organ of speech and coughing and is enclosed within the cartilaginous framework of the thyroid and cricoid cartilages. It also has the function of preventing food and fluids from entering the lower respiratory tract. This is achieved because the tongue is attached to, and the larynx is suspended from, the hyoid bone. When a bolus of food is propelled by the tongue into the pharynx, the hyoid bone is elevated automatically and this raises and tilts the larynx backwards. Food then goes round the sides of the epiglottis via the pyriform fossae into the hypopharynx and oesophagus. If any material manages to enter the larynx, it is sensed in the supraglottis by virtue of its innervation by the superior laryngeal nerves. The larynx then goes into spasm and coughing subsequently expels the inhaled material.

Sound vibrations produced by the larynx are transformed into articulate speech by movements of the tongue, lips and teeth and by the resonance of the nose. The sound vibrations come from the muscular vocal cords, which are attached to the mobile arytenoid cartilages posteriorly and fixed together anteriorly to the thyroid cartilage. By varying the tension of the vocal cords, vibrations of different pitch can be produced. The motor supply to the vocal cords comes from the recurrent laryngeal branch of the vagus nerve. On the right side of the neck the branch goes directly to the larynx but on the left it first passes intrathoracically below the arch of the aorta.

Coughing is achieved by building up intrathoracic pressure behind a closed glottis, which is then opened, suddenly releasing the air which carries with it any secretions or inhaled particles.

Symptoms of laryngeal disease

As disease most frequently affects the glottis, hoarseness is the commonest laryngeal symptom. It needs only a minor mucosal abnormality to cause hoarseness so that in theory all glottic tumours could be detected early. Stridor or obstruction to breathing is less common but is the way in which supraglottic and subglottic disease most frequently presents. Inhalation of food and loss of the ability to cough it up is the least frequent symptom and when due to loss of sensation in the supraglottis is usually a complication of neck surgery or neurological disease.

Examination of the larynx

The larynx can be visualized indirectly with a mirror or fibreoptic laryngoscope and directly with a rigid laryngoscope. Laryngoscopy is not an investigation for the inexperienced clinician, especially when a tumour has to be excluded. This means referral of all patients with potential laryngeal problems to a specialist. Because of the ability to view the larynx directly, investigations apart from biopsy are usually unnecessary.

Acute laryngeal conditions

Acute laryngitis

Short episodes of hoarseness are common after excessive use of the voice or in association with upper respiratory tract infection. With the avoidance of further trauma, especially from tobacco smoke and voice use, the hoarseness should settle within days and certainly within 3 weeks. Steam inhalations can give symptomatic relief but antibiotics are not indicated.

Acute laryngo-tracheo-bronchitis and epiglottitis

Laryngo-tracheo-bronchitis (croup) and acute epiglottitis are the alternative diagnoses in a child with an upper respiratory infection who develops stridor. Both are life-threatening because of their acute onset and the relatively small size of a child's airway. In laryngo-tracheo-bronchitis the whole mucosa becomes inflamed but particularly in the subglottic region. Acute epiglottitis is a potentially more life-threating infection which is due frequently to *Haemophilus influenzae*. It is almost invariably painful and there is drooling of saliva. Examination of the mouth and throat is contraindicated because it may precipitate obstruction. The child is best managed in hospital, and should be accompanied there by a doctor in case acute obstruction occurs. The majority of patients with laryngo-tracheo-bronchitis will settle with aspiration of secretions, humidification and parenteral antibiotics, usually amoxycillin. Sometimes, however, it will be necessary to intubate the child or perform a tracheostomy as the first step, particularly so in epiglottitis.

Chronic laryngeal conditions

Chronic laryngitis

In chronic laryngitis the whole laryngeal mucosa is inflamed and this is frequently associated with chronic disease elsewhere in the respiratory tract, e.g. bronchitis. Excessive alcohol intake and smoking are often implicated and neoplasia can develop secondarily. Management hinges on the avoidance of predisposing factors, but it is difficult to get patients to comply.

Vocal nodules

Vocal nodules are hyperkeratotic patches which develop in the middle third of the cords, i.e. their main point of contact. They are caused by excessive or inappropriate use of the voice. Voice rest and speech therapy can help. Resolution may be speeded by microsurgical stripping of the cords.

Vocal cord palsy

Vocal cord palsies are commoner on the left because the intrathoracic course of the recurrent laryngeal nerve allows it to be affected by bronchial neoplasms, tuberculosis or arteriosclerosis of the aortic arch. In the neck the commonest cause of palsy is surgical trauma, for example following thyroidectomy. However, many cases are idiopathic, but this should not be assumed until a tumour has been excluded. In addition to a weak or hoarse voice, many patients have difficulty in coughing up sputum and this can be particularly disabling when palsy has been caused by a bronchial neoplasm. The natural history is one of symptomatic recovery either because the palsy recovers or because the other cord compensates. If this does not occur within 6 months, Teflon injection of the cord can be of value. This can be done endoscopically under general anaesthesia or externally under local anaesthesia with fibreoptic vision if the patient is unfit. In individuals whose main problem is coughing up sputum, Teflon injections can give considerable relief and one should not wait to see if spontaneous improvement takes place.

Laryngeal tumours

The larynx is the commonest site in the head and neck for tumours. Thankfully the majority are on the glottis and can be detected early by examining everybody who is hoarse for more than 3 weeks. By comparison, supra- and subglottic tumours present when they are considerably larger, giving rise to occlusion of the airway or hoarseness following extension to the glottis.

The majority of tumours are squamous cell carcinomas and occur in male smokers in the lower socioeconomic groups. Untreated, they spread within the larynx, immobilizing the cord and then spreading outwith the cartilaginous framework to the thyroid gland. Cervical lymph node metastases are frequent with larger tumours but distant metastases are uncommon.

The diagnosis is confirmed by biopsy under direct vision with a rigid laryngoscope. While the patient is under general anaesthesia, the size and extent of the tumour within the larynx are assessed. With small tumours confined to a mobile vocal cord, the 5-year survival rate after radiotherapy is in the region of 80%. However, with larger tumours or cervical lymph node involvement, the survival rate following radiotherapy falls to below 50%. For these patients, laryngectomy with block neck dissection gives superior cure rates but the patient has to develop some other form of speech. Traditionally this is achieved by regurgitation of air from the oesophagus but only about half of all laryngectomy patients manage this successfully; accordingly methods of partial laryngectomy have been developed which are suitable for some patients. Alternatively, a tracheo-oesophageal fistula may be created into which a valved tube is inserted to prevent tracheal aspiration of food or fluids. To speak, the patient closes off the tracheostomy and hence the valved tube with his finger, thus directing air from the trachea into the oesophagus.

MANAGEMENT OF ACUTE AIRWAY OBSTRUCTION (STRIDOR)

Acute difficulty in breathing (stridor) is an alarming problem which requires urgent medical attention. Its cause is usually easy to determine (Table 24.2) and in all cases the first emergency action is to clear secretions from the mouth and pharynx. The next step depends on where the emergency has occurred, its urgency and its cause. If transfer to hospital is deemed advisable, the patient must be accompanied by trained personnel.

Conservative management

Humidified oxygen will rapidly ease symptoms, give confidence, and allow secretions to be more easily aspirated. Hydrocortisone 100–300 mg intravenously will often buy time until a more definitive procedure can be performed.

Heimlich's manoeuvre

Inhaled foreign bodies in children, such as peanuts, are best expelled from the larynx or trachea by a quick bear hug around the chest and abdomen.

Laryngotomy

A large-bore needle inserted through the cricothyroid membrane can give temporary airway relief if necessary. So will the barrel of a ballpoint pen inserted through a stab incision.

Table 24.2 Common causes of acute airway obstruction	
Cause	Distinguishing features
Children	
Inhaled foreign bodies	Sudden stridor in previously well child
Laryngo-tracheo-bronchitis	Increasing illness and fever
Acute epiglottitis	Drooling and painful throat
Adults	
Laryngeal trauma	History of accident
Acute epiglottis	Ill with painful throat
Tumours	Often chronic hoarseness

Intubation

Endotracheal intubation past an obstructing lesion can be difficult but should be attempted if the obstruction persists, and is normally carried out in a hospital environment. If it fails, emergency tracheostomy is necessary.

Emergency tracheostomy

The best site for this is between the second and third tracheal rings, which in adults is two finger-breadths above the suprasternal notch. With the neck extended over a pillow, and under local anaesthesia if the patient cannot be intubated for general anaesthesia, a vertical midline incision is made to expose the tracheal rings; a transverse incision between them at the correct level allows a tracheostomy tube to be inserted. Sometimes the thyroid isthmus has to be divided or retracted to gain access.

THE EAR

Anatomy of the ear

The ear is the organ of hearing and balance. It has three parts: the outer, the middle and the inner ear (Fig. 24.15). These parts have different physiological functions and each has its own diseases.

Acute airway obstruction
- Acute difficulty in breathing (stridor) demands emergency management.

- All secretions, food and blood must be cleared from the mouth and pharynx.

- All patients requiring transfer to hospital must be accompanied by trained personnel.

- Humidified oxygen is invaluable as a means of relieving symptoms and allowing aspiration of secretions.

- Inhaled foreign bodies in children are best expelled by a quick bear hug around the lower chest and abdomen (Heimlich's manoeuvre) if they cannot be held upside down and slapped on the back.

- Temporary access to the airway may be achieved by inserting a large-bore needle through the cricothyroid membrane or by a stab incision.

- If emergency tracheostomy is unavoidable, the trachea is entered through an incision between the second and third tracheal rings.

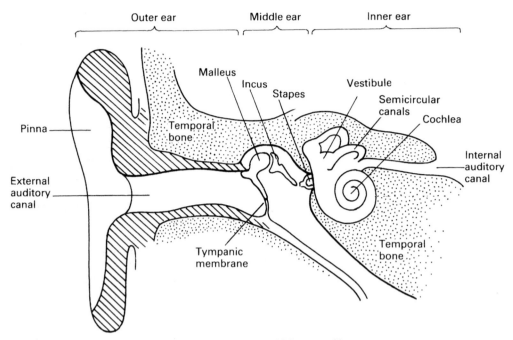

Fig. 24.15   Anatomical relationships of the external ear, middle ear and inner ear.

Outer ear

The outer ear consists of the pinna and the external auditory canal. Both are covered by keratinized squamous epithelium so that skin diseases are common. The substance of the pinna is fibroelastic cartilage and this extends into the outer third of the canal, the remaining two-thirds being bony. In the outer third of the canal there are, in addition, ceruminous glands which secrete wax. The canal terminates at the tympanic membrane (Fig. 24.15), which is part of the middle ear.

Middle ear

The middle ear is an air-containing space in continuity with the nasopharynx via the Eustachian tube and with the mastoid air cells via the mastoid antrum (Fig. 24.16). The Eustachian tube is lined by a mucus-secreting, ciliated respiratory tract epithelium which extends into the middle ear. The remainder of the middle ear and the mastoid spaces are lined by a simple flat mucosa which, when inflamed, undergoes metaplasia to an upper respiratory tract mucosa. The majority of middle ear conditions are due to mucosal disease. The middle ear contains the three ossicles (malleus, incus and stapes) which transmit sounds as vibrations from the external auditory canal to the fluids of the inner ear.

Inner ear

The inner ear is within the temporal bone and consists of the cochlea (the sense organ of hearing) and the vestibular labyrinth (the sense organ of balance). These are supplied by the cochleo-vestibular (VIII) cranial nerve from the brain-stem. The facial (VII) cranial nerve runs alongside the eighth nerve in the internal auditory canal, then progresses through the middle ear and mastoid air cell system to exit via the stylomastoid foramen. In

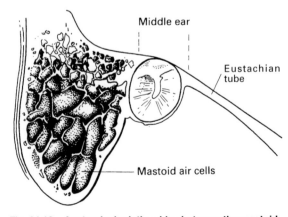

Fig. 24.16   Anatomical relationships between the mastoid air cells and the middle ear.

the inner ear, pathology most frequently affects the neurosensory elements.

Otological symptoms

Otological symptoms are common and their cause is usually easy to ascertain by taking a relevant case history, by examining the ear and by assessing the hearing. Investigations apart from audiology play a minimal role.

Hearing impairment

Hearing impairment may affect one ear, or both ears to an equal or different extent. Although impairments are common they are not always complained of, particularly at the extremes of life. In children, bilateral impairment can seriously hinder education, and screening by health visitors before the age of 1 year (by distraction testing) and again in the first school year (by pure-tone audiometry) is therefore routine in the UK.

Hearing impairments are classified according to whether the defect is in the external or middle ear conduction mechanism or in the sensory or neural parts of the inner ear. The former are called conductive and the latter sensorineural impairments. The distinction has considerable diagnostic and management implications.

Ear discharge (otorrhoea)

Wax is normally shed unnoticed but there are some who consider it to be a discharge. It should not be difficult to distinguish wax from the foul-smelling, watery or mucopurulent discharge that is often associated with inflammation of the external or middle ear. Sometimes there may be blood in the discharge but this is usually due to trauma from attempts to clean out the ear.

Pain (otalgia)

There are two distinct types of otalgia. One is the itchy, uncomfortable pain associated with inflammation of the skin of the external auditory canal which makes the patient want to 'poke' it. The other is a more deep-seated pain due to a difference in pressure across the tympanic membrane. This can be due to a malfunctioning Eustachian tube which is unable to equate pressure in the middle ear with atmospheric pressure. Alternatively, it may be due to pus under positive pressure or fluid under negative pressure.

Otalgia is by no means always otologic in origin; pain from the pharynx, teeth and neck can present as referred otalgia as these areas are supplied by the same nerves (V and IX) as the ear.

Tinnitus

Tinnitus is the intermittent or constant hearing of sounds variously described by terms such as whistling, television interference or rushing water. Tinnitus is usually associated with hearing impairment but this can be of any type or aetiology. Its presence does not make a specific diagnosis more likely, it only determines whether management is required. The vast majority of individuals are able to adjust to their tinnitus.

The pathophysiology of tinnitus is unknown but perhaps the easiest explanation to give a patient is that there has been some damage to the ear which then sends off inappropriate nerve signals which are heard as tinnitus.

Disequilibrium

Balance upset is one of the more difficult symptoms to disentangle. Faulty or absent input from any of the organs that normally help to control balance (Fig. 24.17) can cause disequilibrium. Ophthalmic disease rarely causes disequilibrium and proprioceptor disease is relatively easy to diagnose because of the associated problems of limb control. With time and patience it is usually possible to categorize the patient's symptoms as one of the following.

Vertigo. This is the sensation of rotation, either of the patient or of the environment. Vertigo tends to be episodic, can come at any time, is made worse by

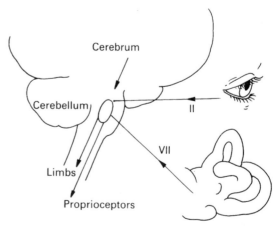

Fig. 24.17 Physiology of balance.

shutting the eyes and is often associated with nausea but not with vomiting. The subject feels off-balance but does not fall, and the episodes last at most for minutes. Vertigo is usually otologic in origin but not all otological balance problems present as vertigo.

Lightheadedness. If this occurs on changing the body's position, the patient can be advised to do this more slowly. The most likely cause is postural hypotension, which occurs when the pressure receptors do not respond quickly enough to a change in posture, notably on getting up from a sitting or lying position. Drugs can cause lightheadedness, including those prescribed for hypertension and for disequilibrium.

Imbalance. This typically occurs only on movement. The patient often staggers to one side and the commonest cause is the general inco-ordination of ageing. Most patients with imbalance have non-otological problems but otological disease can, in the acute stage, cause imbalance. This tends to compensate with time whereas central causes do not.

Blackouts and falls. Patients will usually have no difficulty in deciding whether they temporarily lose consciousness, fall to the ground, or both. A history of loss of consciousness rules out otological conditions as being responsible.

Assessment of the ear

Otoscopy

In most instances, the cause of a conductive hearing impairment will be revealed by otoscopy although this can sometimes be difficult and require a microscope. Otitis media with effusion can be particularly difficult to detect but a pneumatic otoscope, which varies the pressure in the external auditory canal, should help detect an immobile tympanic membrane (see below).

Hearing

Hearing impairment is present if a patient cannot repeat words whispered to him at the quietest level possible from behind and at arm's length while hearing in the non-tested ear is masked by rubbing the tragus. By varying the voice level and distance, the severity of the impairment can be assessed.

Tuning-fork tests, particularly the Rinne test, have been used to identify the presence of a conduction defect. If bone conduction appears louder than air conduction there is conductive impairment, but a high proportion of ears with such impairment do not

give this response. The best way to determine the type of impairment is by pure-tone audiometry.

Audiometry

Pure-tone audiometry determines the thresholds of hearing by both air and bone conduction. The air conduction thresholds reflect the severity of the impairment, while the difference (if any) between air conduction and bone conduction thresholds reflects the magnitude of any conduction defect.

Electric response audiometry measures electrically the neuronal responses to sound stimuli at various levels in the auditory pathway and allows thresholds to be determined in patients who are otherwise difficult to test, notably infants.

Management of hearing impairment

If an individual with a hearing impairment is disabled, the mainstay of management is a hearing aid. However, surgery may be superior if the impairment is of a conductive type.

Hearing aids

These are miniature sound amplifiers whose frequency output and gain can be modified to suit the patient's impairment. The majority are worn behind the ear and are suitable for most types of impairment. In the UK supply and servicing of these aids is free. 'In-the-ear' aids are available commercially but these are mainly suitable for the mildly impaired and are mainly chosen for their presumed cosmetic advantage.

Benefit from a hearing aid is not as simple to achieve as the benefit to vision given by spectacles. Many find the ear mould difficult to insert, and learning to use the aid at different settings in different listening circumstances can be difficult. Follow-up is essential to ensure that the aid can be used. It is unfortunate that extra loudness often does not make speech any clearer for those with poor frequency discrimination due to a sensorineural impairment.

Surgery

Ear surgery (see below) may be necessary to treat ear pathology, but in the majority of patients surgery is undertaken to improve hearing. When successful, the results are superior to those of a hearing aid. Such surgery is usually done with the aid of an operating microscope and under local or general anaesthesia.

General management of tinnitus

The patient should be reassured that tinnitus is common and does not indicate serious brain disease or portend total loss of hearing. Background noise, for example from a radio, can be used to distract the attention when tinnitus is troublesome. The majority require little else. For those more severely troubled, a tinnitus masker, which is worn like a hearing aid but produces a broad band noise, can be a psycho-logical prop. There are no specific anti-tinnitus drugs but sedatives and tranquillizers may be used with caution in selected patients.

General management of vertigo

Thankfully otological vertigo is self-limiting, and long-term medication is seldom indicated. Indeed, drug-induced disequilibrium is common, and many individuals feel better without their medication. The drugs available for treatment are non-specific 'sedatives' and include antihistamines, such as cinnarizine (Stugeron), phenothiazines such as prochlorperazine (Stemetil) or vasodilators such as betahistidine (Serc).

For the rare patient whose vertigo does not subside with time, various destructive surgical procedures, such as labyrinthectomy and vestibular nerve section, may be helpful.

CONDITIONS OF THE PINNA

Bat ears

Bat ears are a common developmental abnormality in which the absence of an antehelix fold causes the ears to stick out. This may cause embarrassment unless covered by long hair. Various methods of surgical correction recreate the absent fold.

Trauma

Because of its position, the pinna is frequently injured. Minor subperichondrial haemorrhage is common and, if repeated, the cartilage will thicken and result in a deformed 'cauliflower' ear (typical of boxers). Any definite haematoma should be surgi-cally drained to prevent cartilage necrosis. If local signs and symptoms of inflammation occur,

secondary bacterial infection has occurred. Such perichondritis should be treated with antibiotics.

CONDITIONS OF THE EXTERNAL AUDITORY CANAL

Wax

Wax is secreted in the outer third of the canal and in this position, even if it obscures the view of the tympanic membrane, will not impair hearing because it does not impede sound vibrations. Only if wax becomes impacted against the tympanic membrane by misguided attempts to remove it with cotton buds will impairment result, and even then the impairment is minor. The mould of a hearing aid can also impact wax.

Wax frequently has to be removed to visualize the tympanic membrane. This is best done by syringing. Impacted wax requires softening with olive oil, almond oil or sodium bicarbonate ear drops. Commercial preparations are not superior and can cause skin irritation.

Otitis externa

Otitis externa is dermatitis of the external auditory canal which sometimes involves the pinna. The ear is uncomfortable and itchy, making the patient want to clean the canal out. There is sometimes a watery discharge and the canal is inflamed, oedematous and weepy. The mainstay of management is to remove the debris initially by syringing and thereafter by mopping. Topical low-strength steroid cream or glycerol and ichthamol ear drops soothe the discom-fort. If the canal is narrow, these medications can be applied daily on a wick. Topical antibiotics are contraindicated, as otitis externa is not normally an infective condition and they can cause allergic skin reactions and fungal overgrowth.

CONDITIONS OF THE MIDDLE EAR

Acute otitis media

Acute otitis media is a bacterial infection of the middle ear which is extremely common in child-hood, especially under the age of 3 years. The typical history is of a child with an upper respiratory tract infection who wakes at night crying with a painful ear. It arises because the products of secondary bacterial infection of the middle ear mucosa are unable to drain down an oedematous Eustachian tube. The differential diagnosis is from transient negative middle ear pressure or from referred pain from the teeth or upper respiratory and alimentary tracts. The distinction is made by the otoscopic finding of an inflamed, bulging tympanic membrane. The natural history is one of spontaneous resolution within 24 hours or drainage after rupture of the tympanic membrane. Such ruptures almost invariably heal spontaneously.

Management consists of analgesics (e.g. paracetamol elixir) and perhaps antibiotics (e.g. amoxycillin to cover upper respiratory bacteria, including *H. influenzae*) if there is gross systemic upset with fever. Drainage of pus by myringotomy is usually unnecessary. Rarely, pus within the mastoid is unable to drain, causing mastoiditis which may spread intracranially to give rise to meningitis or an abscess. Surgical drainage and removal of infected mucosa and bone (mastoidectomy) is then mandatory.

Otitis media with effusion

Otitis media with effusion (secretory/serous otitis media, glue ear) is due to a combination of factors (adenoid enlargement, poor Eustachian tube function, inflammation of the middle ear mucosa) which initially results in negative middle ear pressure and thereafter progresses to non-infected middle ear effusion. This immobilizes the tympanic membrane, causing hearing impairment.

Transient otitis media with effusion will occur in about 50% of children at some time, the incidence peaking around 3 years. The classical history is of a child who previously had normal hearing, as demonstrated by the development of normal speech, becoming dull of hearing. The impairment may or may not be noticed by the parents and is often detected at school screening. Occasionally there is otalgia due to a change in middle ear pressure. The natural history is one of episodes of recurrence and resolution followed by permanent resolution unless there are severe predisposing factors such as poor Eustachian tube function from a cleft palate.

As spontaneous resolution almost invariably occurs, management is expectant unless bilateral hearing impairment (as demonstrated by the inability to repeat a whispered voice at arm's length) persists for 3 months or more. Active management is then indicated because the child may develop speech, language and behavioural problems. Medication is of unproven value, and surgery in any combination

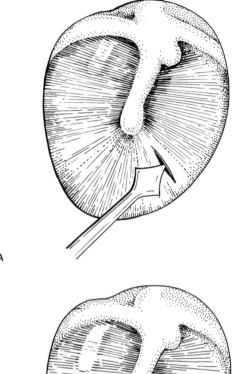

A

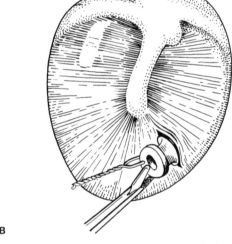

B

Fig. 24.18 Treatment of otitis media with effusion: A myringotomy; **B** insertion of grommet.

of adenoidectomy, myringotomy and aspiration, or insertion of ventilating tubes (grommets) is indicated (Fig. 24.18).

Chronic otitis media

Chronic otitis media is due to chronic inflammation of the middle ear and mastoid mucosa and is associated with permanent perforation of the tympanic membrane. The inflammation may be constant, intermittent or inactive. When active, there is a mucopurulent, foul-smelling discharge which may or may not be noticed by the patient. In all cases there is a conductive hearing impairment the magnitude of which depends on the size of the perforation and on whether the ossicular chain has been eroded. Once mucopus has been removed by mopping with a cotton bud or syringing, the defect in the tympanic membrane should be seen. Sometimes the middle ear mucosa becomes polypoidal and polyps can enlarge through the perforation to fill the external auditory canal. In some ears, in addition to mucosal disease, a cholesteatoma may be identified in the attic. A cholesteatoma is a retraction pocket lined with squamous epithelium in which debris builds up because of its narrow neck.

In inactive ears, surgical closure of the perforation (myringoplasty) will prevent future activity, and if combined with rebuilding any ossicular chain disruption (tympanoplasty) the hearing should improve. Active ears require more aggressive treatment because of the risk (albeit low) of developing meningitis, intracranial abscess or facial nerve palsy due to spread of infection. The discharge is dealt with by regular aural toilet. Instillation of topical antibiotic and steroid drops improves the cyclical resolution rate but permanent cure depends on surgical eradication of the inflammation and repair

> **Otitis media**
> - *Acute otitis media* is extremely common in children under the age of 3, and develops because the products of middle-ear infection cannot drain down an oedematous Eustachian tube.
> - The child typically awakes crying at night with a painful ear and the diagnosis is confirmed by finding a red inflamed bulging tympanic membrane on otoscopy.
> - Spontaneous resolution within 24 hours is common during which time pain relief is important. Antibiotics may be reserved for those particularly ill or not resolving after 24 hours.
> - *Otitis media with effusion* (glue ear) occurs transiently in many children and is manifested by temporary hearing impairment. Most cases settle spontaneously but bilateral hearing impairment may demand surgery (adenoidectomy, myringotomy or insertion of a grommet).
> - *Chronic otitis media* involves the middle ear and mastoid mucosa, and is associated with permanent perforation of the tympanic membrane, hearing impairment and a mucopurulent discharge. Inactive ears require closure of the perforated membrane (myringoplasty) and rebuilding of the ossicular chain. Active ears may require surgical removal of the posterior canal wall to create an open mastoid cavity and so reduce the risk of meningitis, intracranial abscess and facial palsy.

of the tympanic membrane. This may require permanently taking down the posterior canal wall to create an open mastoid cavity.

Otosclerosis

Otosclerosis is new bone growth in the region of the oval window which fixes the stapes. The diagnosis is assumed when a patient with a conductive hearing impairment has a normal tympanic membrane. Surgical alleviation consists of stapedotomy in which a small fenestra is made in the footplate and a piston inserted which is attached to the incus and the stapes superstructure removed.

CONDITIONS OF THE INNER EAR

Sensorineural hearing impairment

Some 20% of adults have a sensorineural hearing impairment, the majority being over the age of 50 years. In most the aetiology is unidentifiable and, in the absence of a history of noise trauma or other cause, the term presbyacusis is often used to describe the syndrome in older patients.

Sensorineural impairments are usually symmetrical. It is important to investigate asymmetrical impairments because of the possibility of an acoustic neuroma, although this is rare (see below).

Noise. Industrial noise from machinery may cause hearing impairment, depending on a combination of genetic predisposition, noise level and duration of exposure. Damage can be mitigated by wearing ear defenders, but cotton wool is useless. Firing guns also causes damage, but occasional 'clubbing' at discotheques will not.

Drugs. Many drugs can cause inner ear damage, particularly in patients with impaired renal function. In this respect the aminoglycosides (e.g. gentamicin) and loop diuretics can be particularly dangerous.

Infection. Mumps and measles can be associated with unilateral sensorineural impairment but the incidence is falling because of increasing immunization of infants. Bacterial meningitis is also fairly frequently associated with deafness.

Head injury. A temporal bone fracture, which is usually evident from the presence of blood in the middle ear and sometimes from the passage of blood or cerebrospinal fluid (CSF) from the ear, may cause sudden unilateral hearing impairment, often associated with vertigo.

Barotrauma. Sometimes, after an aeroplane

flight or underwater diving, unequal pressure between the middle and inner ear ruptures the round window membrane. Sudden unilateral impairment with vertigo results and surgical repair of the rupture may be indicated.

Congenital. Genetic abnormalities, rubella infections, prematurity, birth trauma and haemolytic crises are the main causes of sensorineural impairments in infants. These have to be recognized early so that amplification can be provided to enable speech to develop as normally as possible.

Acoustic neuroma. Acoustic neuromas are benign slow-growing neurofibromas of the eighth cranial nerve which can cause neurological problems and death by pressing on the brainstem. Early diagnosis is vital and is achieved by screening patients with an idiopathic unilateral or asymmetrical impairment by electric response audiometry followed by CT scanning in those failing. The tumours can be excised through the ear (translabyrinthine approach), or the middle or posterior cranial fossa, depending on their size.

Labyrinthine disorders

Acute labyrinthitis

Acute labyrinthitis produces an acute attack of vertigo which lasts for several days, is prostrating, and is associated with a sensorineural hearing impairment and sometimes tinnitus. Temporal bone fracture and ear surgery are readily identifiable causes, while viral infection or transient ischaemia are postulated as more common causes. In the absence of hearing impairment, the pathology is thought to be retrocochlear (as opposed to labyrinthine) and the syndrome is termed vestibular neuronitis. Spontaneous resolution is the rule and medication until this occurs is all that may be required.

Chronic labyrinthitis

Chronic labyrinthitis is diagnosed when there are recurrent episodes of vertigo. Fortunately, most cases resolve spontaneously. The aetiology in most patients is unknown. Chronic otitis media must be excluded because episodic vertigo in this condition implies spread of infection to the inner ear and an increased risk of intracranial complications. Surgical management in such patients is usually mandatory. If the recurrent episodes of disequilibrium are associated with transient deterioration in hearing and perhaps tinnitus or fullness in the ear, the condition is referred to as Ménière's syndrome.

In the rare patient in whom symptoms do not regress with time, destructive operations such as labyrinthectomy (in which the inner ear is totally destroyed) or vestibular nerve section via the middle cranial fossa (which preserves hearing) should be considered. Various other, somewhat controversial surgical procedures have been advocated for Ménière's syndrome but their value is unproven.

Section 7
GASTROENTEROLOGICAL AND ABDOMINAL SURGERY

25

Abdomen, abdominal wall and hernia

THE ABDOMINAL CAVITY AND THE PERITONEUM

Surgical anatomy

The abdominal cavity extends from the level of the
nipples above to the level of the gluteal crease below.
It is lined by the parietal peritoneum, a thin sheet of
smooth glistening mesothelium which also clothes
the abdominal viscera (visceral peritoneum). The
peritoneal cavity has a greater and a lesser sac, the
two being connected by the epiploic foramen. The
omentum (Fig. 25.1) is a double fold of peritoneum
which connects the liver to the stomach (lesser

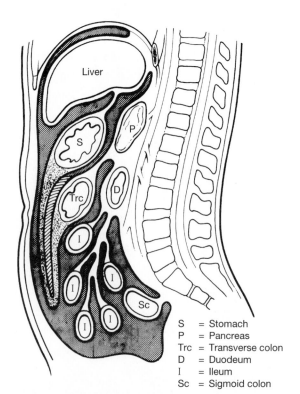

S   = Stomach
P   = Pancreas
Trc = Transverse colon
D   = Duodeum
I   = Ileum
Sc = Sigmoid colon

**Fig. 25.1   Sagittal section through the abdomen showing
the arrangement of peritoneal folds which form the lesser
and greater omentum.**

omentum) and the stomach to the transverse colon (greater omentum). The greater omentum is folded back on itself but the potential extension of the lesser sac is normally obliterated by adhesions. Occasionally, the greater omentum undergoes torsion and produces a tender palpable mass which has to be excised. The peritoneum is relatively resistant to infection but contamination in conditions such as perforation of a hollow viscus, leads readily to peritonitis.

Ascites

Ascites, or the accumulation of free fluid within the peritoneal cavity, can occur in many diseases (Table 25.1). The fluid is frequently clear and straw-coloured as in liver disease; bloodstained fluid suggests malignancy, cloudy fluid suggests infection, and white milky fluid suggests chylous ascites due to blockage of the thoracic duct. Protein concentration is often used to determine whether ascitic fluid is a transudate (<25 g/l) or an exudate (>25 g/l), although this division is of limited value in that protein concentrations show wide variation in different diseases. Particularly high protein concentrations are found in tuberculous peritonitis, hepatic venous congestion, and pancreatic ascites (leakage of pancreatic juice in pancreatitis producing ascitic fluid with a very high amylase content).

Clinical features

Ascites gives rise to dullness to percussion in the flanks when the patient lies supine, but when he lies on one side, fluid gravitates to the dependent part of the peritoneal cavity and the point at which resonance on percussion gives way to dullness

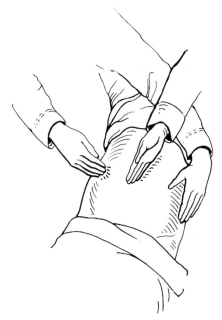

Fig. 25.2   Clinical detection of fluid thrill due to ascites.

changes. A 'fluid thrill' can also be elicited in patients with ascites. One hand is placed flat on the flank while the opposite flank is tapped or flicked with the other hand. If a thrill is felt, transmission through the anterior abdominal wall must be prevented by placing the hand of the patient or assistant on the abdomen (Fig. 25.2).

Investigations

Ultrasonography can detect as little as 100 ml of free fluid and is used when there is doubt clinically. Ascites produces a ground-glass appearance on plain films of the abdomen when there is a large amount of free fluid.

Paracentesis carried out under local anaesthesia (see Ch. 38) can be used to relieve discomfort and obtain samples of ascitic fluid for bacteriology, cytology and biochemistry (protein and amylase concentration). Peritoneal biopsy may also be helpful if tuberculous peritonitis is suspected.

Treatment

Treatment is directed at the cause of ascites where possible. Bed rest, restriction of sodium intake (and in some cases, water intake), and diuretic therapy are the mainstays of treatment of non-malignant ascites. Intractable ascites may be an indication for

Table 25.1   Common causes of ascites
Transudates
Hypoalbuminaemia
Nephrotic syndrome
Malnutrition
Raised central venous pressure
Congestive cardiac failure
Hepatic vein obstruction
Chronic liver disease
Liver malignancy
Portal vein obstruction
Exudates
Inflammatory disease
Malignancy
Chylous ascites
Miscellaneous causes

Ascites
- Free peritoneal fluid may be detected by shifting dullness or eliciting a fluid thrill, while ultrasonography will detect as little as 100 ml of fluid.
- The commonest causes of ascites are liver disease and intraperitoneal malignancy.
- High protein concentrations (> 25 g/l) are found in tuberculous peritonitis, hepatic venous obstruction and pancreatic ascites.
- Pancreatic ascites is due to leakage of fluid from the pancreatic duct system and the amylase content of the peritoneal fluid exceeds that of the serum.
- Bed rest, restriction of salt intake and diuretics (e.g. spironolactone) are the mainstays of treatment if the underlying cause cannot be rectified.
- Intractable ascites may justify insertion of a peritoneo-venous shunt while peritoneal instillation of chemotherapy (e.g. bleomycin) may be worthwhile in malignant ascites.

peritoneo-venous shunting (see p. 481). Instillation of chemotherapeutic drugs (e.g. bleomycin) may be considered for malignant symptomatic ascites.

PERITONITIS

Inflammation of the peritoneum is a common feature of the acute abdomen. Peritonitis can be classified as acute or chronic, septic or aseptic, and primary or secondary. Acute suppurative peritonitis secondary to visceral disease is the commonest form of peritonitis in surgical practice (Table 25.2).

Table 25.2   Causes of peritonitis

Acute suppurative peritonitis
  Primary peritonitis
  Secondary peritonitis
    Inflammatory disease of viscera
    Perforation of bowel or biliary tree
    Infection of the female genital tract
    Penetrating injury of abdominal wall
    Rupture of intra-abdominal abscess
    Strangulation of gut

Tuberculous peritonitis
  Ascitic tuberculous peritonitis
  Plastic tuberculous peritonitis

Aseptic peritonitis
Granulomatous peritonitis
Postoperative peritonitis

whereas primary peritonitis is rare. Chronic peritonitis due to tuberculosis is now rare but can cause abdominal pain, ascites or obstruction due to matting of the bowel by dense adhesions. Granulomatous peritonitis was once seen as an occasional complication after using starch powder with surgical gloves but is now uncommon.

Secondary acute peritonitis

Irritation of the peritoneum by leaking bile, gastric juice, pancreatic enzymes or urine produces an exudate which is initially sterile, but which usually becomes infected within 6–12 hours. In other cases (e.g. perforated diverticular disease), there is infection from the outset. As peritonitis develops, inflammation of the visceral and parietal peritoneum produces a purulent exudate. In some conditions (e.g. acute cholecystitis or acute appendicitis), peritonitis may remain localized for some time, whereas in others (e.g. perforated peptic ulcer) it may rapidly disseminate. Localization depends on adhesions forming between viscera, and the capacity of the omentum to 'wall off' infection. When localization fails, the peritoneal cavity fills with foul-smelling purulent fluid, and the intestine becomes flaccid and dilated, and covered with fibrinous plaques which form adhesions between bowel loops.

Clinical features

The symptoms associated with secondary peritonitis depend on the nature of the primary condition. Inflammation of the parietal peritoneum produces somatic pain which is localized to the site of infection. As infection spreads throughout the peritoneum the pain becomes diffuse. Vomiting is common but is usually not a marked early feature.

The patient usually lies still and is afraid to move. Respiration is shallow, and in the early stages the abdomen is scaphoid. The most important clinical sign is tenderness on palpation, the extent depending on the size of the area involved. There is associated rigidity, guarding and rebound tenderness. The abdomen becomes silent as paralytic ileus supervenes and the pulse rate and temperature rise.

In advanced peritonitis, vomiting becomes more profuse and faeculent, and the patient becomes severely dehydrated, toxic and confused. Pain often abates at this stage, and the abdomen becomes less rigid but more distended. The pulse is rapid and there is often a combination of hypovolaemic and septic shock.

Investigations

Plain abdominal films may point to the cause of the peritonitis, but often merely reveal ileus with dilated flaccid loops of bowel. Biochemical tests are of limited value, but urea, electrolyte and blood gas determinations are essential aids to resuscitation.

Management

The primary objective is to deal promptly and effectively with the underlying cause. For example, perforation of a viscus must be repaired, infarcted bowel must be resected, and infective foci should be removed or drained. Operation is undertaken with minimal delay. The only time which should be spent before operation is that needed to resuscitate an ill patient. Antibiotic cover is indicated in all patients with established secondary peritonitis and is directed against gut flora in the first instance (e.g. an aminoglycoside and metronidazole). Peritoneal lavage is an essential adjunct to operation and many surgeons employ an antibiotic-containing solution (e.g. 1 g of tetracycline in 1 litre of saline).

Primary acute peritonitis

Primary peritonitis is rare, although in childhood it can account for up to 15% of acute abdominal emergencies. The condition used to be common in young girls following ascent of pneumococcal or streptococcal infection from the genital tract. *Escherichia coli* is now the predominant causal organism and probably gains access through the gut wall, or (rarely) by blood-borne spread from a distant focus. Spontaneous bacterial peritonitis in adults is a recognized complication of ascites in cirrhosis or the nephrotic syndrome.

Classically, diffuse peritonitis with generalized abdominal tenderness and rigidity develops within 24 hours. Fever and leucocytosis occur early. Abdominal rigidity is relatively uncommon. Examination of a sample of peritoneal fluid and antibiotic therapy are the mainstays of treatment but laparotomy may be needed to rule out a surgical cause.

Postoperative peritonitis

Peritonitis after abdominal surgery may be a residual effect of the original disease or a direct complication of its operative management (e.g. anastomotic leakage). Diagnosis is difficult as:

1. The patient is usually receiving analgesia and/or sedation and may not complain of pain
2. Any pain and tenderness may be attributed to the wound
3. There is often a 24–48-hour period after abdominal surgery when bowel sounds are absent and the abdomen is distended.

Persisting distension or the development of vomiting and distension after an initial return to normality should raise the suspicion of peritoneal infection. Suspicion is heightened if the patient looks unwell and has fever, tachycardia, and an altered mental state. Plain abdominal films may merely show dilatation of the intestine, but ultrasonography can be used to detect collections, and leakage can be demonstrated by gastrografin.

Fluid and electrolyte replacement, nasogastric suction, and broad-spectrum antibiotic therapy are instituted, and the need for re-operation is considered. If intraperitoneal collections form or abscesses develop, operation can sometimes be avoided by percutaneous drainage under radiological or ultrasound guidance.

INTRA-ABDOMINAL ABSCESS

Intraperitoneal abscess is a common complication of peritonitis and intra-abdominal surgery. The abscess

---

Peritonitis
- Acute suppurative peritonitis secondary to visceral disease is the commonest type of peritonitis seen in surgical practice. Common causes include perforated peptic ulcer, perforated diverticular disease and acute cholecystitis.

- Postoperative peritonitis may represent persistence of the infection which led to surgery or result from a complication, notably anastomotic leakage.

- Intraperitoneal abscesses are a common complication of peritonitis and frequently occur in the subphrenic and subhepatic spaces, the pelvis and between loops of bowel. Ultrasonography and CT scanning allow diagnosis and percutaneous drainage so that surgical drainage can often be avoided.

- Primary acute peritonitis is now rare but was once common in young girls following ascent of the genital tract by pneumococcal or streptococcal infection. Spontaneous bacterial peritonitis in adults may complicate ascites in cirrhosis or the nephrotic syndrome.

- Chronic infective peritonitis (tuberculosis) and granulomatous peritonitis (e.g. following use of starch as surgical glove powder) are now rare.

gives rise to pyrexia, tachycardia and clinical signs of toxicity. Leucocytosis is usual. Common sites for abscess formation are the subphrenic and subhepatic spaces, the pelvis, and between loops of bowel. Complications include rupture with generalized peritonitis, erosion of blood vessels with potentially catastrophic bleeding, and septicaemia. Occasionally, subphrenic abscesses rupture into the pleural cavity, while pelvic abscesses sometimes discharge spontaneously through the rectum.

The site of the abscess may be suspected from the history and clinical examination but localizing signs can be surprisingly lacking (particularly with subphrenic abscess; 'pus somewhere, pus nowhere else, pus under the diaphragm'). Unexplained fever after peritoneal infection or operation should always raise the suspicion of abscess formation. Pain and tenderness over the rib cage, shoulder tip pain and a 'sympathetic' pleural effusion strengthen the suspicion of subphrenic abscess, while diarrhoea and a boggy swelling in the pouch of Douglas on rectal examination are features of a pelvic abscess (Fig. 25.3).

Ultrasound scans and/or computerized tomography (CT) scans are of immense value in diagnosis (Fig. 25.4). Isotope scans following injection of ^{111}In-labelled leucocytes are now used infrequently. Ultrasonography may also be used to guide percutaneous insertion of a needle to obtain material for bacteriological examination and insert a drain. However, surgical drainage may still be needed to ensure effective drainage. Antibiotic therapy is used in conjunction with drainage. Signs usually resolve

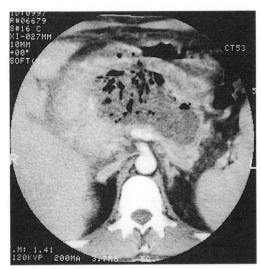

Fig. 25.4 CT scan of upper abdomen showing pancreatic abscess containing streaks of gas.

rapidly following effective drainage, but female patients may be left infertile if the ostia of the Fallopian tubes have been involved in a large pelvic collection.

TUMOURS OF THE PERITONEUM AND RETROPERITONEUM

Primary peritoneal tumours

Such tumours are rare. *Mesotheliomas* in asbestos workers may produce a bulky mass or diffuse peritoneal involvement with ascites. *Pseudomyxoma peritonei* is a low-grade malignant tumour which arises from the ovary or from rupture of a mucocele of the appendix. Lobulated peritoneal deposits give rise to copious secretion of mucus and abdominal distension. Intermittent intestinal obstruction may occur. Repeated operations may be needed to debulk the tumour but can give prolonged survival.

Secondary peritoneal tumours

These tumours are common. Seedlings may stud the peritoneal cavity and produce malignant ascites and a mass in the pouch of Douglas which is palpable rectally.

Retroperitoneal tumours

Arising from connective tissue these occasionally produce an abdominal mass. CT scanning is helpful

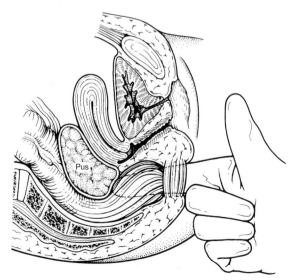

Fig. 25.3 Rectal examination for pelvic abscess.

and a tissue diagnosis must be obtained by radiologically guided sampling or, if need be, by laparotomy. Occasionally such tumours turn out to be lesions with a relatively good prognosis (e.g. lymphomas), provided appropriate treatment is instituted.

THE ABDOMINAL WALL

UMBILICUS

Development abnormalities

Persistent vitello-intestinal duct

The vitello-intestinal duct runs in intrauterine life from the apex of the midgut loop to the yolk sac. It is normally obliterated long before birth but part of it may persist as a Meckel's diverticulum (Fig. 25.5) on the antimesenteric border of the ileum (Ch. 29). Rarer abnormalities include persistence of a band attaching the umbilicus to a Meckel's diverticulum, a patent communication between ileum and umbilicus, an encysted portion of the duct which does not connect with the ileum (enterocystoma), and a persistent umbilical portion of the duct which forms a polypoidal raspberry-like tumour of the umbilicus (enteroteratoma).

Symptomatic remnants may have to be excised, although a broad-based Meckel's diverticulum is usually left alone if found incidentally at laparotomy. Persisting bands can cause intestinal obstruction.

Urachus

The urachus runs from the apex of the bladder to the umbilicus. It is normally obliterated at birth but may give rise to cysts, a urinary fistula, or a discharging umbilical sinus if parts of it remain patent. Symptomatic remnants require excision.

Umbilical sepsis

Umbilical sepsis in neonates may give rise to portal thrombophlebitis, jaundice and portal vein thrombosis. Tetanus can follow application of cow dung to the umbilicus, as once practised in some primitive societies. In adults, sepsis can result from retention of inspissated sebum within the folds of the umbilicus, and from infection of a pilonidal sinus of the umbilicus. Sepsis is treated by removing or excising the causal lesion and prescription of antibiotics.

Umbilical tumours

Umbilical hernias will be discussed later. The umbilicus may be involved by primary neoplasms (e.g. squamous carcinoma or melanoma) and secondary tumour which has tracked along the ligamentum teres from the liver or lymph nodes in the porta hepatis. Neoplasia is an occasional unexpected finding in an umbilicus which has been excised because of persistent discharge.

AFFLICTIONS OF THE RECTUS MUSCLE

Haematoma of the rectus sheath

Spontaneous or traumatic rupture of the inferior epigastric artery occasionally produces a painful swelling of the rectus sheath in association with rigidity. Ultrasonography can be used to confirm the

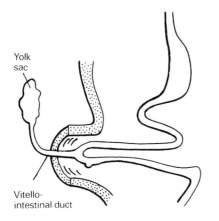
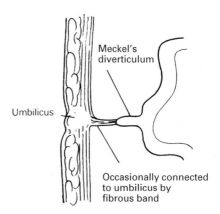

Yolk sac

Vitello-intestinal duct

Meckel's diverticulum

Umbilicus

Occasionally connected to umbilicus by fibrous band

Fig. 25.5   Persistence of the vitello-intestinal duct giving rise to Meckel's diverticulum.

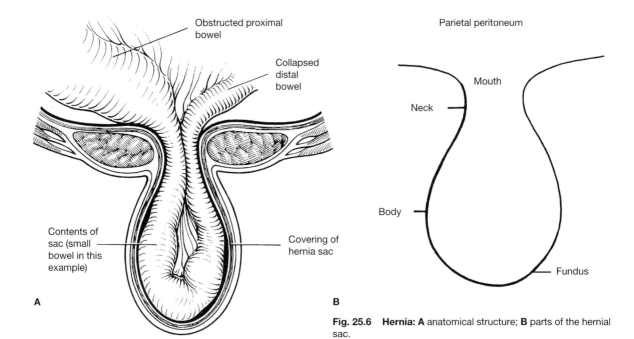

Fig. 25.6 **Hernia: A** anatomical structure; **B** parts of the hernial sac.

diagnosis, and ligature of the bleeding artery with evacuation of clot is indicated.

Desmoid tumour

This rare tumour is thought to arise from fibrous intramuscular septa in the lower rectus abdominis muscle. It is commoner in women of child-bearing age and can be associated with intestinal polyposis in Gardner's syndrome. The lesion must be excised widely as it is prone to recur and can become malignant (fibrosarcoma).

ABDOMINAL HERNIAS

A hernia is an abnormal protrusion of an organ (e.g. intestine, brain, lung) or tissue (e.g. muscle, fat) outwith its normal body cavity or constraining sheath. The hernia may take the name of the organ involved (e.g. cerebral or small bowel hernia), the opening through which herniation occurs (e.g. hiatus hernia), or the region affected (e.g. epigastric or lumbar hernia).

Hernias of the abdominal wall are common. They may exploit natural openings such as the inguinal and femoral canals, umbilicus, obturator canal or oesophageal hiatus, or protrude through areas weakened by stretching (e.g. epigastric hernia) or

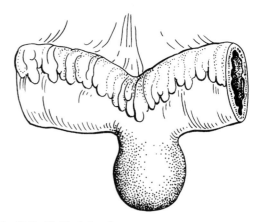

Fig. 25.7 **Richter's hernia.**

surgical incision. The hernia is immediately invested by a peritoneal sac drawn from the lining of the abdominal wall (Fig. 25.6). The sac is covered in turn by those tissues which are stretched in front of it as the hernia enlarges (i.e. the coverings). The neck of the sac is the constriction formed by the orifice in the abdominal wall through which the hernia passes. A hernia may contain any intra-abdominal structure but most commonly contains small bowel and/or omentum. If only part of the circumference of the bowel is involved, the hernia is known as a Richter's hernia (Fig. 25.7).

Hernias

- A hernia is an abnormal protrusion of an organ or tissue outwith its normal body cavity or restraining sheath.

- Hernias of the abdominal wall are common and may exploit natural openings (inguinal, femoral and obturator canals, umbilicus and oesophageal hiatus) or weak areas caused by stretching or surgical incisions.

- Abdominal hernias have a peritoneal sac and the neck of the sac is often unyielding and a potential source of compression of the hernial contents.

- Hernias may be classified as reducible or irreducible, and the contents may become obstructed (e.g. bowel) or strangulated.

- Strangulation denotes compromise of the blood supply of the contents and its development significantly increases morbidity and mortality. The low-pressure venous drainage is occluded first and then the arterial supply becomes occluded with development of gangrene.

A hernia may be reducible, in that its contents can be returned to the abdomen, or irreducible. Bowel within a hernia may become obstructed at the neck of the sac, and can become strangulated if its blood supply is impaired. Omentum may also strangulate.

INGUINAL HERNIAS

Groin hernias account for three-quarters of all abdominal wall hernias. The commonest types of groin hernia are indirect inguinal (60%), direct inguinal (25%) and femoral (15%). Most (85%) groin hernias occur in males. In early life, an indirect inguinal hernia is by far the commonest variety. After middle age, weakness of the abdominal musculature leads to an increasing incidence of direct inguinal hernias. Femoral hernias are relatively more common in females (possibly because of stretching of ligaments and widening of the femoral ring in pregnancy), but indirect inguinal hernia is still the commonest type of groin hernia in women.

Surgical anatomy

The inguinal canal is formed by the descent of the testis through the abdominal wall in fetal life. As it descends, the testis drags with it a tube of peritoneum, the processus vaginalis. The processus is normally obliterated, apart from the tunica vaginalis testis which persists in the scrotum as a covering for the front and sides of the testis (Fig. 25.8).

The testis and processus pass through the layers of the anterior abdominal wall on their way to the scrotum, the track forming the inguinal canal. The canal commences at the internal inguinal ring, an opening in the transversalis fascia which lies 1 cm above the mid-inguinal point. The mid-inguinal point lies midway between the pubic symphysis and the anterior superior iliac spine (*not* at the midpoint of the inguinal ligament), and is the point at which the femoral artery emerges from beneath the inguinal ligament. The internal inguinal ring is bounded medially by the inferior epigastric artery (Fig. 25.9). The inguinal canal ends at the external inguinal ring, an opening in the aponeurosis of the

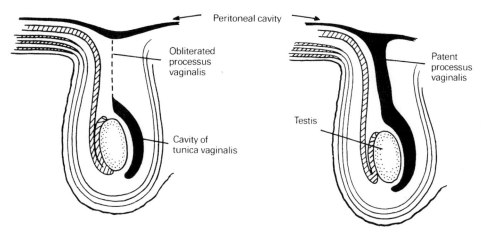

Fig 25.8 Processus vaginalis testis: A normal obliteration of processus vaginalis testis; **B** persistence of patent processus.

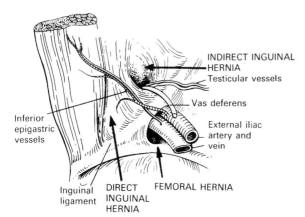

Fig. 25.9 Anatomy of the internal inguinal ring showing sites of herniation from within.

external oblique muscle which lies just above and medial to the pubic tubercle. At birth, the internal and external rings lie on top of each other so that the inguinal canal is short and straight; with growth, the two rings move apart so that the canal becomes longer and oblique.

The testis and spermatic cord receive a covering from each of the layers as they pass through the abdominal wall. The innermost layer is derived from the transversalis fascia (the internal spermatic fascia), the middle layer from the internal oblique muscle (the cremasteric muscle and fascia), and the outer layer from the external oblique aponeurosis (the external spermatic fascia). The spermatic cord consists of the vas deferens, testicular vessels, nerves and lymphatics, and while within the inguinal canal it is covered only by the cremasteric and internal spermatic fascia.

An *indirect inguinal hernia* enters the deep inguinal ring and descends within the coverings of the cord so that it can pass on down into the scrotum. A *direct hernia* bulges into the posterior wall of the inguinal canal; the sac lies behind and outwith the coverings of the cord so that direct hernias do not normally descend into the scrotum. As shown in Figure 25.9, the neck of the sac of an indirect inguinal hernia lies lateral to the inferior epigastric vessels, whereas that of a direct hernia lies medial to them.

Indirect inguinal hernia

Many indirect inguinal hernias are probably the result of failure of obliteration of the processus vaginalis. The hernia may remain within the inguinal canal or extend into the scrotum. Very occasionally it enlarges between the muscle layers of the abdom-

inal wall to form an interstitial hernia. The sac often contains small bowel and/or omentum, but occasionally contains the appendix, ovary, part of the bladder, Meckel's diverticulum or large bowel. When a partly peritonealized organ such as bladder or caecum enters a hernia, it remains only partly covered by peritoneum and forms a 'sliding hernia'.

Clinical features

The moment of herniation (or rupture) may be associated with sudden groin pain, or may pass unnoticed. Thereafter, there may be dragging discomfort in the groin, particularly during lifting or straining, but further pain is unusual in the absence of strangulation.

The hernia forms a swelling in the inguinal canal which may extend into the scrotum. It is often readily visible when the patient stands or is asked to cough. An inguinal hernia which passes into the scrotum passes above and medial to the pubic tubercle, in contrast to a femoral hernia which bulges below and lateral to the tubercle (Fig. 25.10). A cough impulse is normally palpable, and bowel sounds can often be heard within the hernia on auscultation. If there is no visible swelling, a cough impulse is sought while the patient stands with his legs slightly apart, or while the skin of the scrotum is invaginated with the little finger which is then run along the cord to the external inguinal ring.

The hernia often reduces spontaneously when the patient lies down, or it may be reduced by gentle

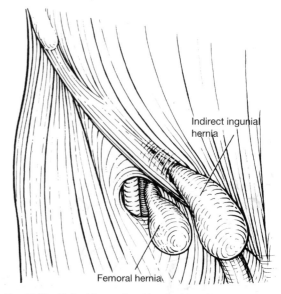

Fig. 25.10 Exit of femoral and inguinal hernias.

pressure applied in an upward and lateral direction. Once reduced, it may be possible to control the hernia by placing a finger or hand over the internal inguinal ring. Clinically, it is frequently impossible to determine whether a hernia confined to the inguinal canal is of the direct or indirect variety.

Direct inguinal hernia

Direct hernias are due to weakness of the abdominal wall and may be precipitated by increases in intra-abdominal tension (e.g. in obstructive airways disease, prostatism or chronic constipation). The hernia protrudes through the transversalis fascia in the posterior wall of the inguinal canal. The defect is bounded above by the conjoint tendon, below by the inguinal ligament, and laterally by the inferior epigastric artery (Fig. 25.9). The hernia occasionally bulges through the external inguinal ring but the transversalis fascia cannot stretch sufficiently to allow it to proceed down to the scrotum. The sac has a wide neck so that the hernia seldom becomes irreducible, obstructs or strangulates.

Clinical features

The hernia forms a diffuse bulge in the region of the medial part of the inguinal canal. It is usually readily reduced by backward pressure and the edges of the defect may then be palpable.

Treatment of uncomplicated inguinal hernia

In infants, an indirect inguinal hernia may disappear spontaneously, and a simple pressure pad inserted in the diaper may be all that is needed to maintain reduction. Infantile hernias seldom strangulate, but operation is indicated if they persist beyond the age of 2 years.

Adult inguinal hernias can be controlled by a truss, but this is uncomfortable and is now seldom indicated, given that the hernia can be repaired under local anaesthesia.

Principles of surgical repair of inguinal hernia

Groin hernias can be repaired by an open surgical approach or by laparascopic insertion of synthetic mesh to occlude the hernial orifice. Laparoscopic repair is used increasingly and may come to supersede the conventional surgical repairs described here.

Indirect inguinal hernia. The first step is to open the inguinal canal, free the hernial sac from the spermatic cord (Fig. 25.11) and remove it after transfixing and ligating its neck. Simple excision of the sac (*herniotomy*) is all that is needed in young children. In older children and adults, the internal ring is often found to be enlarged, and after herniotomy, it is tightened around the cord by non-absorbable sutures placed in the transversalis fascia (Fig. 25.12). In older patients, the posterior wall of the canal is stretched and weakened, and a variety of techniques can be used to tighten the deep ring and strengthen the posterior wall (*herniorrhaphy*). The simplest method is to plicate the transversalis fascia or carry out a Bassini repair in which the conjoint tendon is sutured to the pubic tubercle and inguinal ligament (Fig. 25.13).

Direct hernia. In a direct hernia the sac is not normally excised and it is simply invaginated by sutures placed in the transversalis fascia. Repair of the posterior wall of the canal (as in the Bassini operation) may be difficult if the tissues are stretched and thin. In such cases it may be necessary to use a synthetic mesh (e.g. Marlex) for reinforcement.

Recurrence. The recurrence rate after repair of an inguinal hernia is approximately 10%. The commonest form of recurrence after repair of an indirect hernia is another indirect hernia, usually due to incomplete excision of the sac. After repair of a direct hernia, a recurrent hernia is also likely to be direct.

In all hernia repairs it is important to avoid constricting the spermatic cord by making the deep inguinal ring too tight. This may compromise repair, particularly in large or recurrent hernias, and in

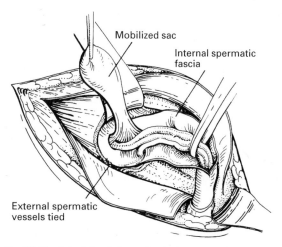

Fig. 25.11   Principle of dissection in the repair of an inguinal hernia.

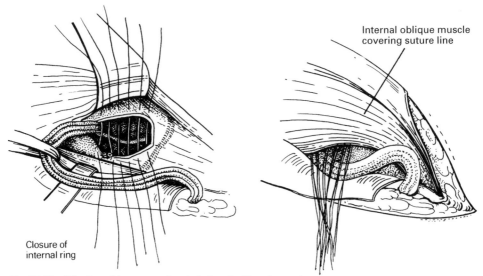

Internal oblique muscle covering suture line

Closure of internal ring

Fig. 25.12 Plication of transverse fascia in inguinal hernia repair.

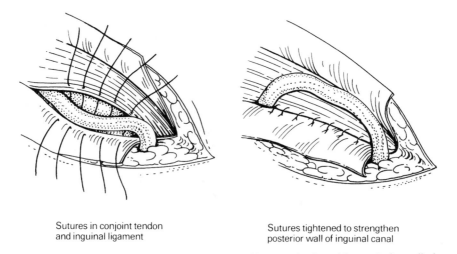

Sutures in conjoint tendon and inguinal ligament

Sutures tightened to strengthen posterior wall of inguinal canal

Fig. 25.13 Bassini-type of inguinal hernia repair with strengthening of the posterior wall of the canal.

older patients removal of the testis may be considered so that the inguinal canal can be completely obliterated.

Femoral hernia

A femoral hernia projects through the femoral ring and passes down the femoral canal. The ring is bounded in front by the inguinal ligament, laterally by the femoral vein, medially by the lacunar ligament, and posteriorly by the superior ramus of the pubis and the reflected part (pectineal ligament) of the inguinal ligament (Fig. 25.14). As the hernia emerges into the groin through the saphenous opening in the deep fascia of the thigh, it turns upwards to lie in front of the inguinal ligament and is often described as retort shaped. The hernia has many coverings and may be deceptively small, sometimes escaping detection. It frequently contains omentum or small bowel, but urinary bladder can 'slide' into the medial wall of the sac.

Clinical features

The hernia forms a bulge in the upper inner aspect of the thigh. It can sometimes be difficult to differen-

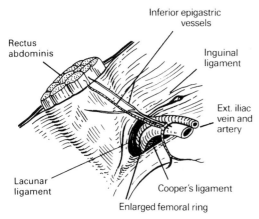

Fig. 25.14 Anatomy of the femoral ring as viewed from within the abdomen. The external iliac vessels become the femoral vessels as they enter the groin.

tiate between an inguinal and femoral hernia, but as indicated earlier, the former passes above and medial to the pubic tubercle as it enters the groin, whereas the latter passes below and lateral to it. Tracing the tendon of adductor longus upwards to its insertion is a useful guide to the position of the pubic tubercle.

A femoral hernia is frequently difficult or impossible to reduce because of its J-shaped course. As well as differentiation from inguinal hernia, it can be confused with inguinal lymph nodes (no cough impulse, irreducible), saphenous varix (positive cough impulse or 'saphenous thrill', prominent on

standing, disappears on elevating the leg) and a lipoma (soft, lobulated, no cough impulse, irreducible).

Surgical repair of femoral hernia

A femoral hernia is particularly likely to obstruct and strangulate, and operation is indicated. As with inguinal hernia, repair can be carried out under local or general anaesthesia.

The aim of operation is to excise the sac and obliterate the femoral ring by suturing the inguinal ligament to the pectineal ligament. The femoral canal can be approached from below the inguinal ligament, through the inguinal canal, or from above by entering the rectus sheath and displacing the rectus abdominis medially (Fig. 25.15). The approach from above (McEvedy approach) gives the best access and is particularly useful if the hernia contains strangulated bowel and intestinal resection is required.

VENTRAL HERNIAS

Ventral hernias occur through areas of weakness in the anterior abdominal wall (Fig. 25.16), namely the linea alba (epigastric hernia), umbilicus (umbilical and paraumbilical hernia), lateral border of the rectus sheath (Spigelian hernia) and the scar tissue of surgical incisions (incisional hernia).

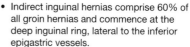

Fig. 25.15 Surgical approach to femoral hernia from above (McEvedy approach). The rectus abdominis muscle is retracted medially to reveal the neck of the hernial sac.

Groin hernias
- Indirect inguinal hernias comprise 60% of all groin hernias and commence at the deep inguinal ring, lateral to the inferior epigastric vessels.
- Direct inguinal hernias account for 25% of all groin hernias and bulge through a weakness in the back wall of the inguinal canal, medial to the inferior epigastric vessels. They rarely obstruct or strangulate.
- Indirect inguinal hernias may pass down within the coverings of the spermatic cord to the scrotum; direct hernias do not descend into the scrotum.
- Femoral hernias account for 15% of all groin hernias and pass through the femoral canal emerging below and lateral to the pubic tubercle (in contrast to inguinal hernias descending to the scotum which pass medial to the tubercle).
- Femoral hernias are often small and easy to miss on clinical examination but are prone to obstruct and strangulate.

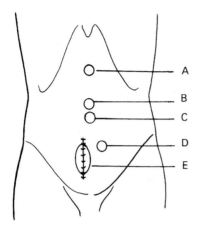

Fig. 25.16 Types of ventral hernias: A = epigastric (through the linea alba); **B** = umbilical (through umbilical scar); **C** = paraumbilical (above or below the umbilicus); **D** = Spigelian (adjacent to rectus sheath); **E** = incisional (anywhere).

Epigastric hernia

Extraperitoneal fat may protrude through small defects in the linea alba to form a soft palpable midline epigastric swelling. The hernia is common in thin individuals and can cause local discomfort. It is repaired by closing the defect with non-absorbable sutures.

Umbilical hernia

A true umbilical hernia occurs in infants. The small sac protrudes through the umbilicus, particularly as the child cries, but is easily reduced. Although these hernias always close spontaneously, persistence beyond the age of 2 years is usually an indication for operation. If the sac has a narrow neck it can be ligated subcutaneously (Fig. 25.17); larger hernias require formal repair.

Paraumbilical hernia

This hernia is caused by gradual weakening of the tissues around the umbilicus. It most often affects obese multiparous women, and passes through the attenuated linea alba above or below the umbilicus. The hernia gradually enlarges, the covering tissues become stretched and thin, and loops of bowel may sometimes be visible under parchment-like skin. The skin may become reddened, excoriated and ulcerated, and a faecal fistula may even develop.

The sac is multilocular and contains adherent omentum and/or loops of bowel. Operation is advised because of the risk of obstruction and strangulation. In the Mayo operation, a horizontal elliptical incision is made around the umbilicus and deepened to define the edges of the defect in the linea alba and rectus sheath (Fig. 25.18). The peritoneum is divided around the neck of the hernia, the omentum and bowel are separated from the sac, and the sac and overlying skin are then removed. The defect is closed by overlapping the layers of the abdominal wall using mattress sutures of non-absorbable material.

Incisional hernia

Midline vertical incisions are most often affected, and poor technique, wound infection, and postoperative distension or chest infection are important factors. The diffuse bulge in the wound is best seen

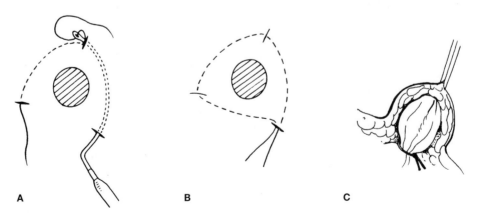

Fig. 25.17 Repair of infantile umbilical hernia. A and **B.** Insertion of subcutaneous suture through three puncture wounds. **C** Suture tied while keeping sac taut and cut short to allow retraction into subcutaneous tissue.

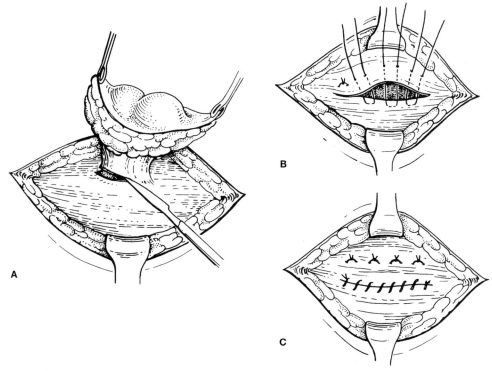

Fig. 25.18 Mayo repair of adult paraumbilical hernia: A excision of sac together with overlying skin; **B** insertion of overlapping sutures into rectus sheath; **C** final appearance.

when the patient coughs or raises his head and shoulders from a pillow, so contracting his abdominal muscles. Strangulation is rare but surgical repair is usually advised. Some patients prefer to wear an abdominal support to control the hernia.

The skin wound is excised and the flaps are elevated to expose the aponeurosis. The sac can be invaginated or excised, and the edges of the defect are then repaired by overlapping sutures or insertion of a synthetic mesh.

RARE EXTERNAL HERNIAS

A *lumbar hernia* forms a diffuse bulge above the iliac crest between the posterior border of the external oblique and latissimus dorsi muscles. It seldom requires treatment.

An *obturator hernia* is a rare hernia which is commoner in women and which passes through the obturator canal. The diagnosis is frequently made only when the hernia has strangulated and is discovered at laparotomy.

INTERNAL HERNIAS

Herniation of the stomach through oesophageal hiatus in the diaphragm is a common cause of internal herniation which is considered in Chapter 27. A variety of cul-de-sacs and peritoneal defects resulting from rotation of the bowel, and other abnormalities of development may be responsible for entrapment of bowel and acute intestinal obstruction. For example, herniation may occur through the foramen of Winslow (opening of the lesser sac), into various fossae around the duodenum, and through various openings in the diaphragm including the oesophageal hiatus (Fig. 25.19).

COMPLICATIONS OF HERNIAS

Irreducibility

An irreducible hernia is one in which the contents cannot be manipulated back into the abdominal cavity. This may be due to narrowing of the neck of

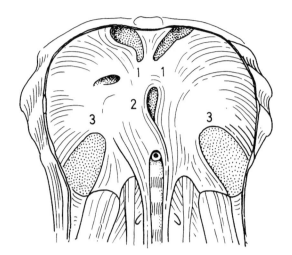

Fig. 25.19 Sites of diaphragmatic herniation.
(1) Parasternal, between the sternal and costal slips of the diaphragm (foramen of Morgagni). (2) Oesophageal hiatus. (3) Pleuroperitoneal canal (foramen of Bochdalek).

the sac by fibrosis, distension of the contained bowel, or adhesions to the walls of the sac.

Obstruction

An irreducible hernia may progress to intestinal obstruction. Abdóminal pain, vomiting and distension signal the need for urgent operation *before* strangulation supervenes.

Strangulation

The vessels supplying the bowel within a hernia may be compressed by the neck of the sac or the constricting ring through which the hernia passes.

The veins are compressed first, and the bowel becomes cyanosed and oedematous with exudation of blood-stained fluid. The arterial supply is then compromised and gangrene follows. Organisms and toxins pass out through the bowel wall causing local peritonitis.

The patient complains of pain in the hernia and usually has features of intestinal obstruction. The hernia is tender, the cough impulse is lost, and there may be increasing evidence of circulatory collapse and sepsis. In a Richter's hernia, only part of the circumference of the bowel is strangulated and there may be no evidence of intestinal obstruction. This type of hernia is relatively common in femoral herniation.

Treatment

If there is no evidence of strangulation, an attempt can be made to reduce an apparently irreducible hernia by giving analgesics, putting the patient to bed with the foot of the bed elevated, and applying gentle pressure. Undue force must never be used for fear of rupturing the bowel or returning the entire hernia to the abdomen with the bowel still trapped within it (reduction en masse). If the hernia does not reduce readily, operation is advised to avoid further complications.

Urgent operation is indicated for all obstructed hernias as one can never be certain that strangulation is not present. The hernial sac is opened and the contents inspected carefully. If they are viable they can be returned to the abdominal cavity and hernia repair undertaken. If there is doubt about the viability of a loop of bowel or omentum, the devitalized tissue must be resected before proceeding to repair.

26

The acute abdomen

Comprehensive coverage of the many conditions which can produce abdominal pain will not be attempted here but the principles of assessment and management will be defined.

Abdominal pain

Visceral pain

Abdominal pain arising from the viscera is mediated by the sympathetic division of the autonomic nervous system. Afferents join the presacral and splanchnic nerves, and pass through rami communicantes to enter thoracic (T6–12) and lumbar (L1–2) segments of the spinal cord. Viscera which develop from the primitive gut (a midline structure) have a bilateral nerve supply, while paired organs (e.g. kidney and testis) have a unilateral supply.

Pain arising from hollow viscera such as the gut, gallbladder or ureter results from distension or excessive contraction. Local ischaemia may contribute, and in conditions such as mesenteric vascular occlusion, can be the dominant factor. Obstruction of a hollow viscus causes accumulation of secretions and gas, and the resulting distension triggers peristaltic contractions in an attempt to overcome the blockage. Such contractions produce bouts of excruciating 'colic' which often last for 1–2 minutes before abating to leave the patient pain-free until the next bout (e.g. intestinal and ureteric colic). In biliary colic the pain characteristically increases to a plateau of intensity, about which it may wax and wane for some hours.

Handling, cutting or clamping the intestine does not cause pain unless the mesentery is put on tension. Pain from solid organs such as the liver and spleen probably arises from congestion and inflammation, while some organs, notably the testis, are exquisitely sensitive to compression. The basis for the pain of peptic ulcer is uncertain, but muscle spasm and irritation of exposed nerve endings by acid may be responsible.

Visceral pain is typically dull and deep-seated. It is localized vaguely to the area occupied by the viscus in embryonic life. Thus, pain arising from the intestine and its outgrowths (liver, biliary system and pancreas) is usually experienced in and around the midline. Pain from the foregut (e.g. peptic ulcer) is usually felt in the epigastrium, midgut colic is felt in the periumbilical area, and hindgut colic is felt in the hypogastrium. Similarly, pain arising from the testis (rather than its somatically innervated coverings) is often felt low in the abdomen rather than in the scrotum.

Somatic pain

The parietal peritoneum is innervated by the somatic nerves (derived from T5–L2) which supply the abdominal wall. The diaphragmatic peritoneum is exceptional in that it is supplied by the phrenic nerve (C3, **4, 5**) (Fig 26.1) which descends with it from the neck during embryological development.

The parietal peritoneum is sensitive to tactile, thermal and chemical stimuli and cannot be cut, cauterized or handled painlessly. Potent chemical irritants include escaped intestinal content, enzyme-rich exudates and pus. Parietal (somatic) pain is often sharp ('knife-like') and localized to the area of its origin. The diaphragmatic peritoneum is again exceptional in that pain is referred to the shoulder tip with which it shares innervation. Painful stimulation of the parietal peritoneum lining the anterior abdominal wall is associated with reflex guarding of overlying muscles, rigidity and hyperaesthesia.

Some acute abdominal conditions have elements of both visceral and parietal pain. For example, acute appendicitis classically commences with periumbilical colic (denoting obstruction of the appendix, a midgut structure) which gradually gives way to more localized (somatic) right iliac fossa pain as the parietal peritoneum becomes inflamed.

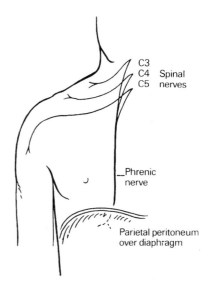

Fig. 26.1   The shared sensory innervation of the shoulder and diaphragm.

ASSESSMENT OF THE ACUTE ABDOMEN

History

Abdominal pain

Explosive *onset* of excruciating pain suggests a vascular catastrophe or perforation of a hollow viscus. Colic can also start suddenly but its onset is rarely explosive. Pain which starts gradually and worsens progressively is typical of peritonitis. Lessening of pain does not necessarily mean that the condition has resolved. The pain of mesenteric vascular occlusion may wane despite the presence of gangrenous bowel, while the pain of perforated peptic ulcer may diminish temporarily despite progressive peritonitis.

The *severity* of pain is difficult to define objectively as patients vary greatly in their reactions. Excruciating pain that is unrelieved by conventional doses of narcotics usually indicates a vascular catastrophe, whereas colic and the severe constant pain of pancreatitis or ulcer perforation are usually more amenable to analgesics.

Parietal pain can usually be *localized* more precisely than visceral pain, but often becomes poorly localized as peritonitis disseminates. *Referral* of pain can confuse if not interpreted correctly. Classic examples are the shoulder-tip pain of

---

Abdominal pain

- *Visceral* abdominal pain is mediated by the sympathetic nervous system and is typically deep-seated and ill-localized to the area originally occupied by the viscus during intrauterine life.

- Colic is a form of visceral pain which arises from a hollow viscus with muscle in its walls (e.g. gut, gallbladder, ureter) and results from excessive muscle contraction (often against an obstructing agent).

- Patients experiencing colic are usually unable to remain still during the bout of pain but are pain-free between attacks. 'Biliary colic' is an exception (and the term colic may be a misnomer) in that pain often waxes and wanes on a plateau and there are no pain-free intervals.

- *Parietal* pain such as that caused by parietal peritonitis is mediated by somatic nerves and is localized to the area of inflammation.

- Reflex guarding and rigidity of overlying muscles is usually present and the patient is reluctant to move for fear of exacerbating the pain.

- Some areas of the peritoneum are 'non-demonstrative' in that parietal peritonitis may be present without tenderness or guarding of overlying muscles (e.g. the pelvis, posterior abdominal wall).

diaphragmatic irritation, the right subscapular pain of biliary pain, and the groin pain of ureteric colic.

Anorexia, nausea and vomiting

These are common but not invariable symptoms in patients with an acute abdomen. Anorexia is usually marked in appendicitis, while nausea, retching and vomiting are prominent in acute pancreatitis, biliary colic and high intestinal obstruction. In gastroenteritis, nausea and vomiting frequently precede the onset of colic and are associated with diarrhoea.

Altered bowel habit

Inability to pass flatus or faeces is a feature of complete intestinal obstruction. Diarrhoea is marked in inflammatory bowel disease and can occur in pelvic sepsis (e.g. acute pelvic appendicitis). Blood is often present in the stool in intestinal ischaemia, but repeated bloody diarrhoea is more likely to be due to ulcerative colitis or dysentery. It must be remembered that upper gastrointestinal bleeding may present with melaena *without* haematemesis.

Menstrual status and gynaecological disease

The frequency of menstruation, date of the last period, and likelihood of pregnancy must be established. Bleeding from rupture of a Graafian follicle, corpus luteum or ectopic pregnancy can cause abdominal pain (see below). Lower abdominal pain and tenderness can also be caused by acute salpingitis, and it is important to establish whether there is a history of purulent vaginal discharge.

Physical examination

Examination of the abdomen

Examination is carried out with the patient lying flat and the abdomen exposed from xiphisternum to groin. Flexing the thighs sometimes helps to relax the anterior abdominal wall. The clinician sits or kneels on the right side of the bed so that his hand and arm extend horizontally across the abdomen. Sedation obscures pain and tenderness, and ideally is withheld until the patient has been examined by the clinician responsible for treatment decisions. In practice, severe pain demands prompt administration of analgesia, and it may be impossible to examine children without appropriate sedation. Bear in mind that physical signs such as tenderness and guarding are often less obvious than might be expected in the elderly, obese, gravely ill, and those on steroid therapy.

Examination follows the standard sequence of inspection, gentle palpation, deep palpation, percussion and auscultation (Table 26.1). Tenderness and guarding on gentle palpation is often the key to diagnosis, and is sought first in areas furthest from the pain. Guarding is due to a reflex increase in tone in the overlying muscles, and in its extreme form the abdominal wall is rigid and board-like (e.g. in perforated peptic ulcer). Some areas of the peritoneal cavity are *non-demonstrative* in that initially there may appear to be no tenderness and muscle guarding despite peritonitis. For example, pelvic peritonitis often produces little abdominal tenderness or guarding, although digital rectal examination reveals marked tenderness. Similarly, inflammation of the peritoneum of the posterior abdominal wall (e.g. acute pancreatitis or retrocaecal appendicitis) may produce surprisingly few signs on abdominal examination. Occasionally in retrocaecal and retroileal appendicitis, irritation of the psoas major causes the patient to lie with the right hip flexed, giving a clue to the correct diagnosis.

In patients with generalized peritonitis, tenderness is often maximal over the site of origin of the inflammation, and there is usually marked muscle rigidity, guarding and rebound tenderness. The abdomen is silent on auscultation. The pulse rate increases and the temperature becomes elevated. The clinical picture deteriorates progressively if the condition remains untreated. Pain becomes less prominent and vomiting more profuse. The vomitus consists initially of gastric contents (which often contain bile), becoming faeculent as small bowel contents are vomited. The bowel dilates as fluid and gas accumulates with the onset of paralytic ileus. Increasing toxicity leads to a lessening of abdominal rigidity and the abdomen distends progressively. The patient becomes increasingly more dehydrated, toxic and confused. The pulse become rapid and thready, and hypovolaemia and sepsis lead to worsening shock.

Guarding and rigidity of the anterior abdominal wall are occasionally found in renal colic, rare neurological disorders, and hysteria or malingering. In renal colic, rigidity is confined to the affected side, while the spasm of hysteria can often be overcome if the examining hand remains on the abdomen while the patient is asked to breathe deeply or is distracted by questioning.

Ascites, abnormal masses and intestinal obstruction are common causes of abdominal distension. In intestinal obstruction, the abdomen is usually

Table 26.1   Checklist for examination of the acute abdomen

Method	Question	Significance
Inspection	What is the abdominal contour?	Distension — intestinal obstruction or ascites
	Does the abdomen move with respiration?	Rigid abdomen — peritonitis
	Can the patient blow out/suck in his abdomen?	Rigid abdomen — peritonitis
	Does the patient lie still or writhe about?	Fear of movement — peritonitis
		Writhe about — colic
	Are there visible abnormalities?	Scars — relevant previous illness, adhesions
		Hernia — intestinal obstruction
		Visible peristalsis — intestinal obstruction
		Visible masses — relevant pathology
Gentle palpation	Is there tenderness, guarding or rigidity?	Tenderness/guarding — inflamed parietal peritoneum
		Rigidity — peritonitis
Deep palpation	Are there abnormal masses/palpable organs?	Palpable organs/masses — relevant pathology
	(Is there rebound tenderness?)	Rebound tenderness — peritonitis
Percussion	Is the percussion note abnormal?	Resonance — intestinal obstruction
		Loss of liver dullness — gastrointestinal perforation
		Dullness — free fluid, full bladder
		Shifting dullness — free fluid
Auscultation	Are bowel sounds present/abnormal?	Absent sounds — paralytic ileus
		Hyperactive sounds — mechanical obstruction — gastroenteritis
	Is there a bruit?	Bruit — vascular disease
Do not forget to: Examine the groin; Do a digital rectal examination; Do a vaginal examination when appropriate; Examine the chest		

resonant or tympanitic to percussion. Ascites gives rise to shifting dullness and in some cases, a fluid thrill (Ch. 25). Shifting dullness is not elicited when fluid is confined within a distended urinary bladder or ovarian cyst, and dullness is restricted to the lower abdomen in these conditions.

Specific clinical signs

Murphy's sign is a reliable sign of acute cholecystitis. The patient is asked to take a deep breath while the examiner palpates the gallbladder region. The breath catches at the zenith of inspiration as the inflamed gallbladder moves down into contact with the examining hand.

Rovsing's sign is an unreliable sign of acute appendicitis in which deep palpation in the left iliac fossa is said to cause pain in the right iliac fossa.

Rebound tenderess denotes resurgence of pain as the examiner's hand is withdrawn sharply after deep palpation. It can also be elicited by heavy percussion. It denotes parietal peritonitis but often adds little to the information gained by gentle palpation and can inflict pain unnecessarily.

Cutaneous hyperaesthesia can sometimes be demonstrated when there is inflammation of the parietal peritoneum, and a triangle of hyperaesthesia to pinprick in the right iliac fossa suggests acute appendicitis. In practice, the test is seldom used.

The *iliopsoas test* detects restriction of the iliacus and psoas major muscles in conditions such as retroileal appendicitis and perinephric abscess. The patient lies on the opposite side and the iliopsoas muscle of the affected side is stretched by hyperextending the thigh. The test is seldom used and is of no value when the abdominal wall is rigid.

Carnett's test helps to determine whether tenderness is due to a problem in the abdominal wall or within the peritoneal cavity. The patient is examined supine and the area of maximal tenderness is defined. He then folds his arms across his chest and sits halfway up while palpation continues. If tenderness abates as the rectus muscles tense, the problem lies within the abdomen; if it does not, the pain is likely to originate in the abdominal wall (e.g. muscle strain, nerve entrapment).

Pitfalls

Failure to conduct a thorough physical examination may lead to serious errors in diagnosis and management. For example, examination of the groin is easily forgotten and a small inguinal or femoral hernia causing intestinal obstruction may be overlooked because all attention is focused on the abdominal signs and symptoms. Failure to perform a digital rectal examination may mean missing important pathology in the anorectum and pelvis, remembering that impaction of faeces is one of the commoner causes of intestinal obstruction. Failure to carry out a vaginal examination may miss the opportunity to diagnose gynaecological and other pelvic disease. Finally, failure to examine the chest may miss causes of referred abdominal pain such as basal pneumonia.

Vital signs and the acute abdomen

Pyrexia and tachycardia are signs of infection and inflammation but are not necessarily *early* features of the acute abdomen. In a shocked patient, the temperature may even be subnormal despite advanced infection. When pain is intermittent, as in renal colic, the pulse rate frequently returns to normal between attacks. Pulse rate, temperature and blood pressure are monitored regularly in all shocked and ill patients, and when the initial diagnosis is in doubt.

Respiration is typically rapid and shallow when abdominal pain is severe. Chest disease can also produce abdominal pain, but high fever, cough, flaring of the alae nasi, and cyanosis point strongly to intrathoracic disease. Hyperventilation may be an early sign in septicaemic shock. Thorough examination of the chest and a chest X-ray are essential in all patients admitted with an acute abdomen.

ESTABLISHING A DIAGNOSIS

The history and physical examination are followed by an attempt to define the nature of the disease and the organ/system involved (Table 26.2). A working

Table 26.2 Common non-traumatic causes of the acute abdomen

Pathological process	Organ commonly involved	Disease
Inflammation	Appendix	Acute appendicitis
	Gallbladder	Acute cholecystitis
	Colon	Diverticulitis
	Fallopian tube	Salpingitis
	Pancreas	Acute pancreatitis
Obstruction	Intestine	Intestinal obstruction
	Gallbladder	Biliary colic
	Ureter	Ureteric colic
	Urethra	Acute retention of urine
Ischaemia	Intestine	Strangulated hernia
		Volvulus
		Mesenteric ischaemia
	Ovary	Torsion of ovarian cyst
Perforation	Duodenum	Perforated peptic ulcer
	Stomach	Perforated ulcer/cancer
	Colon	Perforated diverticulitis
		Perforated cancer
	Gallbladder	Biliary peritonitis
Rupture	Fallopian tube	Ruptured ectopic pregnancy
	Abdominal aorta	Ruptured aneurysm

diagnosis is made, a differential diagnosis constructed, and the need for further investigations is defined.

Laboratory and radiological aids to diagnosis

Haematology

The haemoglobin concentration, haematocrit and white cell count are determined routinely. Leucocytosis is usual in infection but the white count is often normal in the early stages of the acute abdomen.

Clinical chemistry

Urea and electrolyte determinations are essential to assess fluid and electrolyte needs. The results of liver function tests are seldom available in time to influence emergency management, but a baseline must be established as quickly as possible when liver and biliary tract disease is suspected. Serum amylase determinations are diagnostic in acute pancreatitis. Arterial blood gases and hydrogen ion concentration are measured in all shocked patients and those with respiratory problems.

Urinalysis

The urine is tested routinely for sugar, ketones, protein, bile and urobilinogen. Testing for sugar is essential to detect undiagnosed diabetes and assess control in known diabetics. Diabetic patients are just as likely as non-diabetics to develop an acute abdomen, but need special care in the peri-operative period. Diabetic ketoacidosis can produce abdominal pain in the absence of intra-abdominal pathology, and unnecessary laparotomy must be avoided in such cases.

Microscopy reveals pus cells and bacteria in urinary tract infection, and red blood cells in patients with renal colic.

Radiology

A chest X-ray is essential on admission, and may show primary chest pathology, evidence of cardiac failure, or free gas under the diaphragm (e.g. in perforated peptic ulcer). An erect and supine abdominal film may be useful when intestinal obstruction or perforation is suspected. Other radiological signs in patients with an acute abdomen include localized ileus in appendicitis and pancreatitis, radio-opaque stones in the biliary or urinary systems, and vascular calcification in aortic aneurysms (often best seen on a lateral decubitus film).

Gastrointestinal perforation is not always associated with radiological evidence of free gas, and a Gastrografin meal or enema may be indicated. Ultrasonography is frequently useful, as for example when biliary tract disease, acute appendicitis, urinary obstruction, aortic aneurysm or ovarian pathology is suspected. Intravenous urography is also useful in the diagnosis of urinary tract obstruction. Angiography is occasionally indicated to investigate severe gastrointestinal bleeding, mesenteric ischaemia, or genitourinary bleeding.

Peritoneal lavage

Peritoneal lavage is often used to assess the need for surgery in blunt abdominal trauma but is now seldom used to evaluate the acute abdomen.

Laparoscopy

Laparoscopy is used increasingly to diagnose (and in some cases treat) acute abdominal conditions such as acute appendicitis, acute salpingitis, ovarian pathology, and perforated peptic ulcer.

Computer assisted diagnosis

Accuracy of diagnosis of the cause of acute abdominal pain can be improved by using a computer to allow access to a large data base. Part of the success of this approach stems from the use of a standardized approach when recording details of the history and physical examination.

MANAGEMENT

All patients with an acute abdomen are confined to bed and given nothing further by mouth. If the patient has vomited and has upper gastrointestinal disease, obstruction or perforation, a nasogastric tube is passed to keep the stomach empty. Patients requiring urgent laparotomy who have eaten in the past 4–6 hours should also have a tube passed so that the stomach is empty when anaesthesia is induced.

Pulse, temperature and blood pressure are recorded regularly. If there is blood loss, dehydration, shock or electrolyte disturbance (or these are anticipated), an intravenous line is inserted and a fluid balance chart is commenced. In shocked patients, a urinary catheter is inserted to monitor urine output and the need for central venous pressure monitoring is considered.

Antibiotics are prescribed if there are specific indications. For example, they may not be needed in acute pancreatitis, whereas they are prescribed routinely in acute cholecystitis, and are vital when there is colonic perforation. If antibiotic treatment is commenced before surgery in septic patients, blood samples are taken for culture before giving the first dose.

The timing of operation is determined by the nature of the underlying disease, the general condition of the patient, and the need for pre-operative preparation. Considerable delay may have occurred before the patient is first seen by the surgeon, and as a general rule, conditions requiring emergency surgery do deteriorate with time. However, while delay may be disastrous for a patient with ruptured aortic aneurysm, adequate pre-operative resuscitation may prove life-saving for a grossly dehydrated patient with mechanical intestinal obstruction.

In many patients the diagnosis and need for surgery are uncertain at presentation, and re-examination over the next few hours may clarify the position. The risks of undertaking operation needlessly have to be balanced against the dangers of failing to operate promptly. For example, the penalties of not operating early in acute appendicitis outweigh the dangers of needless laparotomy in acute mesenteric adenitis. To await signs which would make the diagnosis of appendicitis certain will inevitably increase morbidity and mortality from gangrene and perforation. For this reason, surgeons accept that the appendix may be normal in 10–20% of emergency appendicectomies.

SURGICAL CAUSES OF THE ACUTE ABDOMEN

The surgical causes of the acute abdomen (see Table 26.2) are considered in detail elsewhere in this volume.

GYNAECOLOGICAL CAUSES OF THE ACUTE ABDOMEN

Mittelschmerz and ruptured corpus luteum

The Graafian follicle normally ruptures 14 days after the start of the last menstrual period, and release of the ovum may be complicated by bleeding. It was thought that this rupture might be the cause of mid-cycle pain in young girls (mittelschmerz translated literally means 'middle pain'), although there is evidence that the pain of mittelschmerz is pre-ovulatory pain. The follicle normally becomes a corpus luteum which degenerates before the start of the next period unless conception occurs. Bleeding from the corpus luteum is an occasional cause of pain in the late stages of the menstrual cycle.

Patients with these causes of pain are usually between 15 and 25 years of age, and experience sudden pain in one or other iliac fossa. Nausea and vomiting may be present but there are no systemic signs and pain usually settles within hours. Tenderness and guarding in the right iliac fossa can simulate acute appendicitis, and a few patients bleed sufficiently to suggest rupture of an ectopic pregnancy. Rectal or vaginal examination may reveal tenderness in the rectovaginal pouch.

The patient is treated conservatively unless appendicitis or ruptured ectopic pregnancy cannot be excluded. Ultrasonography and laparoscopy may help to avoid unnecessary operation.

Ruptured ectopic pregnancy

A fertilized ovum implants at an abnormal site in 1 in 200 pregnancies. The Fallopian tube is by far the commonest site, possibly because of delayed transit of the ovum as a result of previous tubal infection such as gonococcal salpingitis. The erosive trophoblast may penetrate the wall of the tube and often ruptures after about 6 weeks. Alternatively, the conceptus may be extruded from the fimbrial end of the tube.

Bouts of cramping iliac fossa pain may be associated with fainting and vaginal bleeding. Rupture produces sudden severe pain, bleeding, and circulatory collapse. The abdominal pain often becomes generalized and shoulder-tip pain is often elicited by raising the foot of the bed. A missed period is reported by most patients but the menstrual history may be confused by bleeding at the time of implantation or bleeding following death of the embryo.

Signs of pregnancy such as enlargement of breasts and uterus are seldom apparent, but cervical softening and tenderness are detectable on vaginal examination. A haematoma between the layers of the broad ligament may be palpable as a tender mass.

Pregnancy tests are unhelpful in diagnosing an ectopic pregnancy as placental gonadotrophin production is inadequate, but laparoscopy may be helpful if the diagnosis is in doubt. Following rapid resuscitation, laparotomy is indicated urgently and usually involves removal of the involved tube. There is a 10% chance of further ectopic pregnancy.

Torsion of an ovarian cyst

Benign ovarian cysts are a common cause of torsion (Fig. 26.2). Dermoid cysts often have a long pedicle and account for 50% of torsions in young women.

Severe cramping lower abdominal pain is often associated with a smooth round mobile mass which lies higher in the abdomen than might be expected. Tenderness and guarding may be present, particularly if there is leakage, and rupture results in diffuse peritonism. Torsion of a Fallopian tube or fibroid may produce a similar picture.

At laparotomy the twisted pedicle is transfixed and ligated and the cyst is removed. Care must be taken to avoid rupture in case the cyst is malignant. Further radical surgery may be needed if histological examination reveals malignancy.

Acute salpingitis

Acute salpingitis is most often due to gonococcal infection but streptococcal or tuberculous infection can be responsible. Urethritis, cervicitis, and a

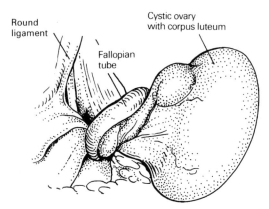

Fig. 26.2 Torsion of an ovarian cyst.

vaginal discharge occur 3–6 days following infection. Tubal involvement is unusual at this stage, but organisms spread to the lining of the uterus and Fallopian tubes after a menstrual period. Both tubes are often involved and adhesions may seal the fimbriated end producing a pyosalpinx.

Bilateral pain is felt just above the pubis and inguinal ligaments. There may be urinary frequency, irregular menstruation, pyrexia and leucocytosis. Vaginal examination reveals unusual warmth, a tender cervix and a vaginal discharge. The cervix appears red and inflamed, and a swab reveals the causative organism. Vaginal findings may be less marked when there is a closed pyosalpinx.

Treatment consists of antibiotic therapy, and laparotomy is only undertaken if conditions such as acute appendicitis cannot be ruled out. Laparoscopy is being used increasingly to avoid unnecessary laparotomy. The inflamed tubes appear inflamed and oedematous, and 'milking' them gently produces a purulent discharge from which a bacteriological swab is taken. The abdomen is normally closed without drainage.

CAUSES OF THE ACUTE ABDOMEN NOT AMENABLE TO SURGERY

Non-specific abdominal pain

Approximately half of the patients sent to hospital with acute abdominal pain have no demonstrable cause or have a minor urinary tract infection of doubtful significance. Such non-specific pain is commonest in young females. Mesenteric adenitis, mild gastroenteritis, irritable bowel syndrome, cyclical ovarian problems, and emotional upset are other possible causes. Tenderness in the right iliac fossa is common, and acute appendicitis is often suspected. Most cases settle on careful observation, but further investigation (e.g. ultrasonography, laparoscopy) and laparotomy may be needed if pain and tenderness persist or worsen.

Acute mesenteric adenitis

Acute mesenteric adenitis is a result of infection with *Yersinia pseudotuberculosis* (and to a lesser extent *Y. enterocolitica*). Most patient are between 5 and 15 years of age and present with central or right-sided abdominal pain, anorexia, nausea and vomiting. There may have been previous attacks and recent upper respiratory tract infection.

The patient is often flushed and pyrexial, and has an inflamed throat and cervical lymphadenopathy. Abdominal tenderness may be slightly higher and more diffuse than is usual in acute appendicitis, and may shift as the patient moves. Guarding and rebound tenderness are unusual. The condition is self-limiting and usually settles in a few days. Serological or stool testing can be diagnostic although these tests are seldom used.

Laparotomy may be unavoidable if appendicitis

cannot be excluded. The mesenteric nodes are fleshy and enlarged, and the terminal ileum is often red and thickened. The appendix is normal but is removed to avoid future confusion.

Diabetes mellitus

Abdominal pain and tenderness occur in 25% of patients with diabetic ketoacidosis. Although hyperamylasaemia is common in such patients, the cause of the pain is uncertain. There is a history of thirst, polyuria, and in some cases, failure to maintain insulin therapy. The patient is dehydrated and looks ill, has acetone on the breath, and may be comatose. Glycosuria, ketonuria, hyperglycaemia, and metabolic acidosis are usually present.

Abdominal pain which is due to diabetic ketoacidosis should disappear rapidly with treatment. Persistence of pain opens the possibility that there is an underlying surgical cause such as acute appendicitis, and that this may have triggered the metabolic problems. If surgery is necessary, ketoacidosis must be treated vigorously beforehand.

Acute intermittent porphyria

This is a rare familial cause of abdominal colic which can be triggered in susceptible individuals by barbiturate ingestion. Vomiting is common but abdominal signs are seldom prominent. The urine reddens on standing or on adding Ehrlich's aldehyde reagent.

Haemochromatosis

Abdominal pain occurs in one-third of patients with haemochromatosis and can simulate acute cholecystitis or appendicitis.

Hereditary spherocytosis

Attacks of abdominal pain and tenderness, nausea and vomiting, and icterus may coincide with episodes of haemolysis, possibly as a result of minor intra-abdominal bleeding. Laparotomy is seldom indicated, although cholelithiasis is common in this condition and acute cholecystitis must be excluded.

Sickle cell disease

This hereditary disease is virtually confined to negroes, particularly those with ethnic roots in West Africa. Abnormal haemoglobin (S) crystallizes when oxygen tension falls, resulting in increased red cell fragility and attacks of haemolysis. This may be associated with abdominal pain, tenderness, guarding and icterus. The abdominal pain is commonly due to splenic infarcts.

The diagnosis is suggested by chronic anaemia, bone and joint pain, and leg ulcers. Blood film examination reveals sickle shaped red cells. Gallstones occur in one-third of patients and cholecystitis must be excluded as a cause of abdominal pain.

Polycythaemia rubra vera

Spontaneous thrombosis in this condition can cause splenic and mesenteric infarcts with acute abdominal pain.

Haemophilia

Abdominal pain in this condition is more often due to bleeding than surgical pathology. The bleeding may be extraperitoneal (e.g. into the psoas sheath) or can occur into the mesentery or gut wall following a large meal. Intussusception can complicate gut wall haematomas. If laparotomy is needed in haemophiliacs, a haematologist must be consulted concerning the availability of factor VIII and other blood products.

Anaphylactoid (Henoch-Schönlein) purpura

This rare cause of abdominal pain in children is usually associated with a streptococcal sore throat. Abdominal colic, vomiting, bloody diarrhoea and intussusception can precede the development of skin purpura.

Polyarteritis nodosa

Nausea, vomiting, abdominal pain and diarrhoea affect 50% of patients with this disease. Severe protracted pain with fever, leucocytosis and abdominal tenderness suggests focal infarction within the abdomen, and pancreatitis, perforation, bleeding and obstruction are recognized complications. Steroid therapy is indicated unless intestinal perforation or infarction is suspected and operation is needed.

Oesophagus

CONTENTS

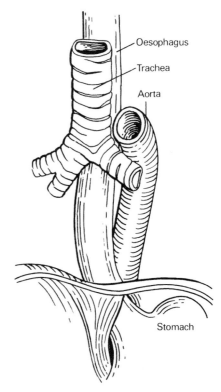

Fig. 27.1   Anatomical relationships of the oesophagus.

Surgical anatomy

The oesophagus extends from the termination of the pharynx (C6) to the oesophagogastric junction (Fig. 27.1). It has cervical, thoracic and abdominal portions and is 25 cm long, the final 2–4 cm lying within the abdomen. It has an inner circular and outer longitudinal muscle layer; the upper third consists of striated muscle and there is a gradual transition to smooth muscle thereafter. The lumen is lined by squamous epithelium with occasional islands of ectopic gastric mucosa, but the distal 1–2 cm are lined by columnar epithelium. The submucosa contains mucous glands, a rich lymphatic network and the neural plexus of Meissner. Auerbach's neural plexus is found between the two muscle layers.

The *upper oesophageal sphincter* is formed by the cricopharyngeus muscle and first few centimetres of oesophagus. It is closed at rest to prevent air entry, but opens on swallowing. The *lower oesophageal sphincter* cannot be defined anatomically but is a 3–5 cm high-pressure zone. It is tonically closed at rest and located in the region of the oesophageal hiatus of the diaphragm. The hiatus consists of an encircling noose of muscle drawn mainly from the right crus of the diaphragm (Fig. 27.2). The oesophagus is held loosely in the hiatus by a condensation of fascia known as the phreno-oesophageal ligament.

The oesophagus receives its arterial blood supply from the inferior thyroid arteries in the neck, bronchial vessels in the chest, and gastric and phrenic vessels in the abdomen. Communication between the left gastric veins (portal system) and

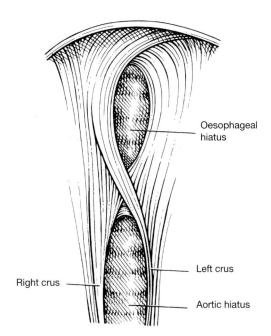

Fig. 27.2 Anatomy of the oesophageal hiatus.

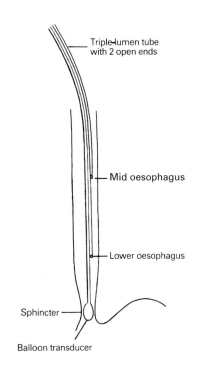

A

thoracic oesophageal veins (azygos and hemiazygos system) are important in the development of oesophageal varices in portal hypertension (see Ch. 33).

The lymphatics run longitudinally in the submucosa before penetrating the muscle coat to drain to regional nodes, and submucosal extension of oesophageal carcinoma is common. Lymph from the upper oesophagus drains first to cervical or thoracic nodes, while that from the lower oesophagus drains to gastric and coeliac nodes.

Surgical physiology

The upper oesophageal sphincter relaxes to allow food to enter from the pharynx. Its subsequent contraction initiates a peristaltic wave which propels food distally. The lower oesophageal sphincter relaxes as the wave approaches and food passes into the stomach. Passage of the peristaltic waves can be monitored by recording luminal pressure at varying levels (Fig. 27.3).

Resting pressure in the thoracic oesophagus reflects intrathoracic pressure and mean values are subatmospheric. Intra-abdominal pressure exceeds atmospheric pressure, but reflux of gastric content is normally prevented by the lower oesophageal sphincter. Additional factors which may prevent

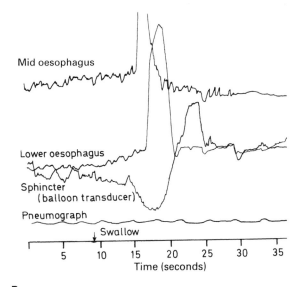

B

Fig. 27.3 Recording of the luminal pressure within the oesophagus: A balloon pressure transducer and open-tipped catheter assembly in place; B pressure recordings of swallowing response in healthy subject. Note that relaxation of the lower oesophageal sphincter precedes arrival of the peristaltic wave.

reflux include the diaphragm, prominent folds of gastric mucosa (mucosal rosette) at the oesophago-gastric junction, and the flap valve created by the oblique entry of the oesophagus to the stomach.

Symptoms of oesophageal disease

Dysphagia

Difficulty in swallowing usually indicates organic disease and requires investigation. Some patients localize the obstruction accurately but many do not. For example, the patient may indicate that food sticks at the level of the sternal angle when the obstruction is actually at the lower end of the oesophagus. It is important to establish length of history, whether dysphagia is intermittent, constant or progressive, and whether solids and liquids are equally affected. Patients with oesophageal obstruction may complain of hiccough on eating, and the symptom may predate dysphagia by several weeks. Some of the major causes of dysphagia are shown in Table 27.1; peptic oesophagitis and carcinoma are particularly common causes. In the Plummer-Vinson syndrome (also known as the Paterson-Kelly syndrome) there is a fibrous web at the entrance to the oesophagus and the patient is typically an edentulous middle-aged woman with atrophic mucosa, iron-deficiency anaemia, and spoon-shaped brittle nails.

Globus hystericus or *globus syndrome* is often confused with dysphagia and is discussed in Chapter 24.

Pain

Heartburn is a retrosternal burning discomfort or pain which is usually associated with gastro-oesophageal reflux. The pain can radiate up to the neck and jaws, through to the back, or down the arms. It is often brought on by recumbency or stooping, occurs soon after meals, and may be precipitated by hot liquids or fruit juice. The pain can usually be reproduced by instillation of 100 mmol/l HCl and is usually relieved by alkali. However, acid is not essential for the production of heartburn, and the symptom can be experienced by achlorhydric patients and after total gastrectomy. Alkaline (bile) reflux may be responsible in such cases. Although conditions which cause reflux oesophagitis usually produce heartburn, there is an inconstant relationship between heartburn and endoscopic and histological evidence of inflammation. Oesophageal motor abnormalities can also produce heartburn.

Oesophageal spasm can produce a diffuse gripping retrosternal pain which may resemble angina pectoris or heartburn. However, the pain of spasm is not related to exercise and in contrast to heartburn, is unaffected by posture or ingestion of alkali.

Regurgitation

Some patients with oesophageal obstruction complain of food regurgitation rather than dysphagia. The patient often states that he vomits, but close questioning reveals that there is no nausea and that

Table 27.1 Causes of dysphagia			
	Intraluminal	Intramural	Extrinsic
Pharynx/upper oesophagus	Foreign body	Pharyngitis/tonsillitis Moniliasis Sideropenic web Corrosives Carcinoma Myasthenia gravis Bulbar palsy	Thyroid enlargement Pharyngeal pouch
Body of oesophagus	Foreign body	Corrosives Peptic oesophagitis Carcinoma	Mediastinal lymph nodes Aortic aneurysm
Lower oesophagus	Foreign body	Corrosives Peptic oesophagitis Carcinoma Diffuse oesophageal spasm Scleroderma Achalasia Postvagotomy	Para-oesophageal hernia

the 'vomiting' is effortless. The patient spits out regurgitated and undigested food that is uncontaminated by gastric juice or bile. Nocturnal reflux and aspiration of food may awaken the patient with coughing fits and can cause aspiration pneumonitis.

Investigation of oesophageal disease

After a careful history and thorough physical examination, the following investigations may be helpful.

Chest X-ray. This may reveal enlarged mediastinal lymph nodes, aspiration pnemonitis or pulmonary metastases. The gastric air bubble may be indented by carcinoma at the cardia, and may be seen in the chest in some patients with hiatus hernia. Air may be seen in the mediastinum and neck after perforation of the oesophagus.

Barium swallow and meal. These are valuable investigations and cineradiography is often helpful in patients with motility disorders.

Fibreoptic endoscopy. This is indicated even when the diagnosis appears certain on radiological grounds. Unsuspected pathology is often revealed (e.g. early carcinoma in a long-standing hiatus hernia), and endoscopy allows biopsy as well as direct inspection. Flexible fibreoptic instruments have eliminated the need to use rigid oesophago-scopes.

Manometry. This is used to assess motility disorders. Pressure readings are obtained from a series of fine tubes perfused with saline and bound together so that their openings are 5 cm apart (Fig. 27.3). The assembly is used to measure pressure in the lower oesophageal sphincter and monitor propulsive activity during swallowing.

Bernstein's test. This entails passing a fine-bore nasogastric tube and infusing 100 mmol/l HCl into the lower oesophagus. Acid reproduces the symptoms if they are due to reflux oesophagitis, but false positive and false negative results are not uncommon.

pH measurement. Measurement by an intraluminal electrode is used to detect gastro-oesophageal reflux and determine the number of swallows needed to clear acid from the lower oesophagus. pH can be monitored over 24-hour periods while the patient goes about his normal activity.

Scintigraphy. Using a gamma counter, this is used to quantitate reflux after taking a meal or a drink labelled with ^{99m}Tc-sulphur colloid.

DISORDERS OF OESOPHAGEAL MOTILITY

Abnormalities of the upper oesophageal sphincter

Lack of co-ordination between pharyngeal contraction and relaxation of the upper oesophageal sphincter is implicated in dysphagia due to conditions such as bulbar palsy and myasthenia gravis, and in the development of pharyngo-oesophageal diverticulum (see Ch. 24).

Achalasia

This common motility disorder affects both sexes equally and can occur at any age, although it is seen most often in middle age. Motility is disordered throughout the oesophagus in that resting pressures are high, propulsive peristalsis is absent, and the lower oesophageal sphincter fails to relax on swallowing. The cause is unknown but degeneration of Auerbach's plexus is the probable explanation, and the denervated oesophagus is hypersensitive to small doses of parasympathomimetic agents. In South America, infection with *Trypanosoma cruzi* (Chagas' disease) causes similar degeneration and produces motor changes indistinguishable from those of achalasia.

Clinical features

Dysphagia is the cardinal symptom and is at first intermittent but gradually worsens. It may be aggravated by anxiety or fatigue, and may be particularly troublesome when taking liquids or cold food. Gravity rather than peristalsis is responsible for food leaving the oesophagus, and the patient may find it helpful to stand when swallowing. Food regurgitation is common, and aspiration during sleep may produce aspiration pneumonitis and pulmonary fibrosis. Retrosternal pain occurs in 25% of cases, and is 'bursting' or 'burning' with radiation to the neck, throat, back or arms.

Minor mucosal erosions of the oesophagus are common but frank peptic ulceration is rare. Carcinoma can develop in long-standing achalasia, even after successful treatment. Its development is insidious and the obstruction may be mistakenly attributed to achalasia, resulting in late diagnosis at an inoperable stage.

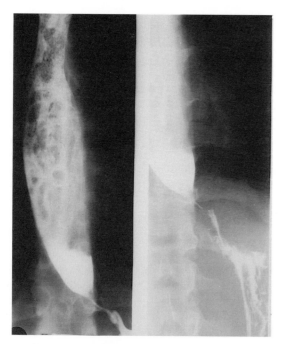

Fig. 27.4 Barium swallow showing gross dilatation of the oesophagus above the lower oesophageal sphincter in achalasia of the oesophagus.

Diagnosis

Barium swallow reveals gross distension and/or tortuosity of the oesophagus, with conical narrowing at the cardia and a 'string-like' passage into the stomach (Fig. 27.4). Cineradiology and manometry confirm that oesophageal contractions are irregular and disorganized, and that the lower oesophageal sphincter fails to relax. The sphincter is not hypertensive, and an endoscope passes easily through it.

Treatment

Medical treatment is ineffective. Hydrostatic balloon dilatation relieves symptoms in 80% of cases, but carries a small risk of oesophageal perforation and may have to be repeated (Fig. 27.5). Cardiomyotomy (Heller's operation) is used if dilatation fails. The oesophagus is approached through the chest, and a 10–12-cm longitudinal incision is made through the musculature but without breaching the mucosa (Fig. 27.6). The incision extends on to the stomach for less than 1 cm and the vagus nerves are carefully preserved. Good results are achieved in 85% of cases, but gastro-oesophageal reflux can be troublesome and some surgeons routinely add an antireflux procedure (see below).

Diffuse oesophageal spasm

This disease differs from achalasia in that the lower oesophageal sphincter is hypertensive as well as failing to relax. The cause is unknown but hypermotility leads to painful spasms which may occur spontaneously or on eating. The pain is retrosternal and ranges from mild discomfort to severe colic or radiating pain which can mimic angina pectoris.

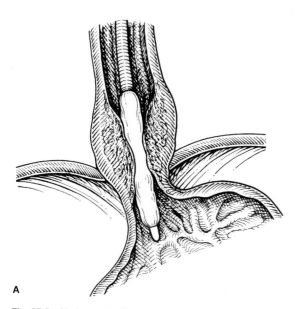
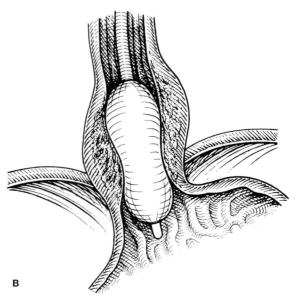

A   B

Fig. 27.5 Hydrostatic dilatation of achalasia.

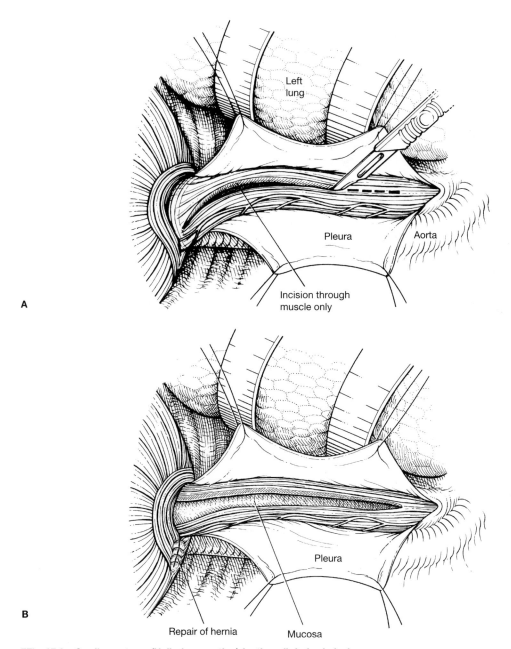

A

B

FFig. 27.6 Cardiomyotomy (Heller's operation) for the relief of achalasia.

Barium swallow reveals a 'corkscrew' oesophagus in 50% of cases, the appearance being due to indentation by contracted muscle (Fig. 27.7). Manometry shows that peristalsis is replaced by simultaneous repetitive contractions ('nutcracker' oesophagus), and confirms that the lower oesophageal sphincter is hypertensive.

Diffuse spasm may be treated in the same way as achalasia, although the results are less satisfactory.

Miscellaneous motility disorders

A number of collagen diseases and neuromuscular diseases can be associated with abnormal oesophageal motility. In scleroderma there is fragmenta-

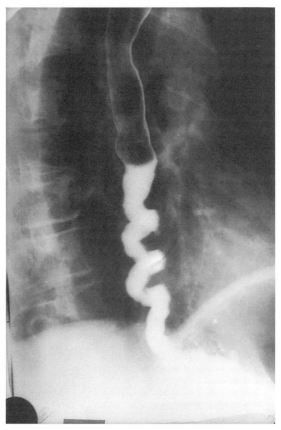

Fig. 27.7 Barium swallow showing appearances of diffuse oesophageal spasm.

tion of the submucosal connective tissue and smooth muscle atrophy. The lower oesophageal sphincter becomes incompetent and reflux oesophagitis leads to stricture formation. Associated fibrosis can produce shortening of the oesophagus and a hiatus hernia. Treatment consists of medical measures to combat reflux oesophagitis, dilatation of strictures and antireflux surgery if these measures fail.

HIATUS HERNIA AND OESOPHAGITIS

Herniation of the stomach through the oesophageal hiatus in the diaphragm is common, particularly in later life. Such herniation is not necessarily associated with symptoms of reflux oesophagitis; conversely, reflux oesophagitis often occurs in the absence of a hiatus hernia. Sliding hiatus hernia is much commoner (95% of cases) than para-oesophageal (or rolling) hernia; mixed hernias in which there is a sliding and a rolling component are exceptional.

Sliding hiatus hernia

The fact that intra-abdominal pressure normally exceeds intrathoracic pressure favours herniation of the stomach through the diaphragm, particularly when intra-abdominal pressure is increased by stooping, straining, coughing and pregnancy. Attenuation of the phreno-oesophageal ligament allows the stomach to herniate increasingly in a concentric fashion, so that the oesophago-gastric junction *slides* upwards into the chest (Fig. 27.8).

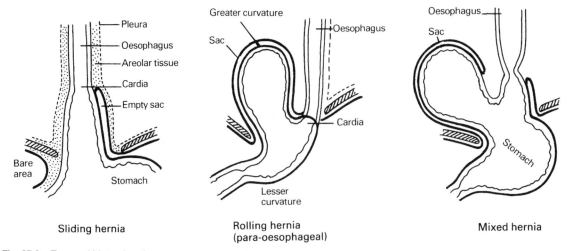

Fig. 27.8 Types of hiatus hernia.

Initially, herniation is intermittent, and provided that the sphincter remains competent, it does not lead to gastric reflux and oesophagitis. If reflux occurs, inflammation and fibrosis may eventually tether the oesophagus and produce a fixed concentric hernia with apparent shortening of the oesophagus.

Clinical features

The majority of individuals with a hiatus hernia have no symptoms, and the condition is only discovered incidentally during barium studies or endoscopy. In others, reflux oesophagitis produces heartburn, particularly after large meals, during recumbency, and when stooping or bending. Patients learn to avoid tight clothing and may sleep with the head of the bed elevated to minimize nocturnal heartburn. Some experience water brash (excessive salivation causing the mouth to fill suddenly with clear taste-less fluid) or the reflux of bitter irritating material into the mouth and pharynx. Aspiration pneumonitis may occur, and dysphagia can be due to spasm or stenosis in the inflamed distal oesophagus. Acute bleeding is uncommon but chronic insidious loss can cause iron deficiency anaemia, particularly in the elderly.

Investigations

The hernia can be demonstrated by barium meal examination, although the patient may have to be placed head-down or have pressure applied to the abdomen (Fig. 27.9). Mucosal irregularity and spasm suggests that reflux oesophagitis is also present. Endoscopy is undertaken to assess the presence and severity of reflux oesophagitis, and the red inflamed mucosa should be biopsied. Endoscopy also allows exclusion of carcinoma in patients with stenotic lesions and excludes more distal problems such as duodenal ulceration. Manometry and the Bernstein test may be helpful in patients with atypical symptoms. Ultrasonography is usually advisable to exclude gallstones.

Treatment

Asymptomatic patients require no treatment. Symptomatic reflux oesophagitis can be managed by non-operative means in 85% of patients. The patient is advised to avoid tight clothing, avoid bending or stooping, sleep with the head elevated (by pillows or bed blocks), stop smoking, and lose weight (if obese). Large meals should be replaced by frequent smaller meals, and foods which induce symptoms

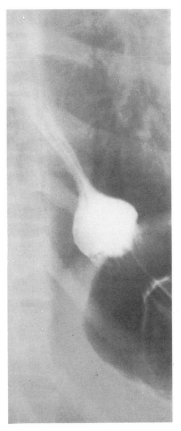

Fig. 27.9 Radiological appearance of sliding hiatus hernia seen on barium meal examination.

are avoided. Agents used to treat reflux oesophagitis include antacid-alginate mixtures such as Gaviscon, antacid-dimethicone mixtures such as Asilone, and antisecretory agents such as ranitidine and omeprazole (see p. 392).

Surgery is indicated if conservative measures fail to control symptoms, gastrointestinal blood loss continues, or dysphagia is due to established stricture. In the past, emphasis was placed on anatomical repair of the hiatus but it has now shifted to prevention of reflux. Many surgeons favour Nissen fundoplication in which the mobilized gastric fundus is wrapped around the lower oesophagus (Fig. 27.10), so that increases in intragastric pressure compress and close the enclosed oesophagus. The margins of the enlarged hiatus are usually approximated behind the oesophagus, although this is not essential. Some 90% of patients are rendered symptom free by this operation, but 10% of patients find difficulty in belching or vomiting ('gas-bloat' syndrome) and it is important not to wrap the gastric fundus too tightly

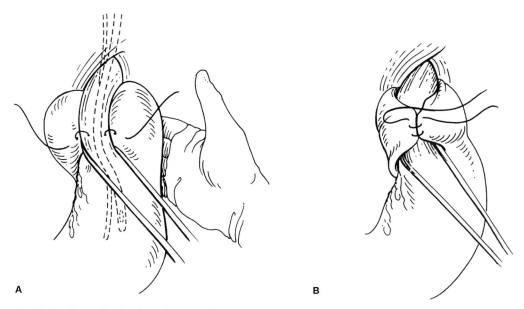

Fig. 27.10 Fundoplication for reflux oesophagitis: A gastric fundus wrapped around lower oesophagus; **B** fundal wrap sutured in position.

around the oesophagus. It is now possible to carry out hiatus hernia surgery laparoscopically.

Para-oesophageal hernia

In this condition there is a wide defect in the hiatus through which the greater curve of the stomach rolls upwards into a well-defined hernial sac lined by peritoneum. In time the entire stomach may roll into the chest so that the cardia and pylorus are approximated and the stomach looks upside down on barium meal examination (Fig. 27.11). In effect, this is a gastric volvulus and can lead to strangulation of the stomach.

Clinical features

The patient is frequently middle-aged or elderly. Reflux symptoms are exceptional and the patient usually complains of deep seated 'crushing' chest pains, often in association with meals. The pain results from distension of the intrathoracic stomach, and can mimic myocardial infarction. Flatulence and belching are common, and reflect attempts to gain pain relief. Weight loss often occurs as the patient tries to avoid trouble by not eating.

Incarceration, pressure necrosis, gangrene, and rupture can complicate para-oesophageal hernia and lead to potentially fatal gastric rupture and mediastinitis.

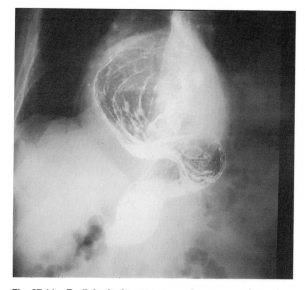

Fig. 27.11 Radiological appearance of para-oesophageal hernia as seen on barium meal examination.

Investigations

Chest X-ray may reveal a gas bubble and fluid level in the entrapped thoracic stomach. Barium meal examination will confirm the diagnosis.

Treatment

Surgery is always advisable in view of the risk of strangulation. The herniated stomach is brought back into the abdomen from below and the margins of the defect are approximated. An antireflux procedure is not needed but many surgeons anchor the stomach to the abdominal wall (gastropexy) to prevent recurrence.

Strangulation of a para-oesophageal hernia may necessitate emergency thoracotomy and gastric resection.

Complications of reflux oesophagitis

Reflux oesophagitis may cause metaplasia of the squamous epithelium so that the lower oesophagus becomes lined by columnar epithelium which is more liable to ulcerate. This situation is known as a Barrett's oesophagus and it was once thought mistakenly that the columnar epithelial lining of the lower oesophagus was a congenital abnormality. Ulceration can be complicated by bleeding, perforation or stricture formation, and adenocarcinoma may develop in 10% of cases. Elective surgery is usually advised to dilate the stricture and perform an antireflux procedure. Bleeding or perforation may necessitate emergency oesophageal resection.

Long-standing reflux can also cause stricture formation in the absence of Barrett's oesophagus. Heartburn is the dominant symptom during episodes of reflux oesophagitis, but gradually gives

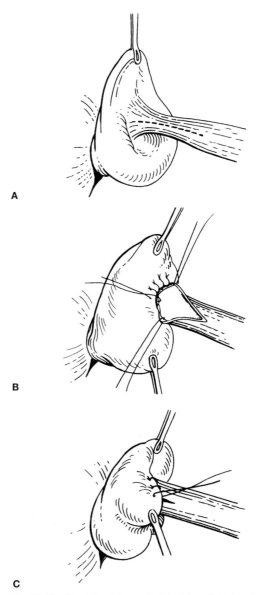

A

B

C

Fig. 27.12   Fundal patch repair: A incision of strictured area; **B** gastric fundus sutured over the defect; **C** completion of fundal patch.

> **Hiatus hernia**
> * Almost 95% of hiatus hernias are of the sliding type. Para-oesophageal (rolling) hernias are rare and mixed hernias are exceptional.
>
> * Sliding hernias are often associated with reflux oesophagitis and heartburn, but reflux can occur in the absence of herniation.
>
> * Symptomatic sliding hiatus hernias can be managed non-operatively in 85% of cases; some form of fundoplication is indicated if symptoms cannot be controlled by conservative measures.
>
> * Longstanding reflux may give rise to ulceration (with risk of bleeding, perforation and stenosis) and metaplasia may produce a Barrett's oesophagus and risk of developing adenocarcinoma
>
> * Para-oesophageal hernias are not normally associated with reflux, but frequently give rise to symptoms and may strangulate so that surgical correction is advisable.

way to dysphagia as the stricture forms. Dilatation with antireflux medication is the first line of treatment. A guide wire is passed through the stricture using a flexible endoscope and a series of bougies of increasing diameter are then passed over the guide wire to dilate the narrowed area. Surgery is indicated if the stricture cannot be dilated or if it recurs. The strictured portion of oesophagus can be resected and the oesophagus anastomosed to the stomach, or the strictured segment can be replaced by a pedicled length of jejunum or colon. Alternatively, the stricture can be opened longitudinally and the defect covered by the mobilized gastric fundus (Fig. 27.12); the serosal surface of the stomach becomes covered by stratified squamous epithelium within a few weeks.

Corrosive oesophagitis

This occurs most often in children who accidentally swallow household caustics but was once a common method of attempting to commit suicide. Necrosis and perforation of the oesophagus can occur, and surviving patients often develop strictures.

Immediate management consists of giving water to dilute the corrosive, providing pain relief, and establishing an intravenous infusion. Early gentle fibreoptic endoscopy will define the extent and severity of injury, and early feeding can be encouraged if there is only mild inflammation. If damage is severe, parenteral feeding will be needed. Urgent surgical resection of the oesophagus and/or stomach may be unavoidable if full thickness necrosis and perforation ensue.

If the patient survives, repeated dilatation is often required to try to maintain a passage through the often extensive and complex stricture. A feeding gastrostomy is often advisable and the stoma can be used for retrograde dilatation of the stricture. If a passage cannot be maintained, the oesophagus is best replaced by a pedicled segment of colon or a segment of jejunum supplied with blood from a microvascular anastomosis to the inferior thyroid artery. Extensive peri-oesophageal inflammation and scarring may make resection so difficult and dangerous that it is better to bypass the oesophagus with a jejunal loop. If the oesophagus is left in place, long-term surveillance is instituted as there is a high risk of oesophageal carcinoma developing.

OESOPHAGEAL PERFORATION

The oesophagus is occasionally perforated at diagnostic endoscopy (incidence less than 1 in 1000 endoscopies) and more commonly during endoscopic intubation or stricture dilatation. The complication was more common when rigid rather than flexible endoscopes were used. Perforation occurs most commonly at the pharyngo-oesophageal junction (due to spasm of the cricopharyngeus muscle), at the site of obstructing lesions, and at the lower end of the oesophagus. It may also be caused by foreign bodies and penetrating trauma, and by operations such as vagotomy. Spontaneous rupture of the lower oesophagus can follow forcible vomiting and retching (Boerhaave's syndrome).

Clinical features

The clinical picture is determined by the size and site of the perforation. Perforation in the neck causes surgical emphysema (so that the tissues become distended with air and there is crepitus on palpation), throat pain and bruising. Perforation of the thoracic oesophagus causes severe substernal pain, inability to swallow, tachycardia and fever. If the perforation is above the diaphragm, mediastinal emphysema may spread upwards to involve the neck, and tearing of the mediastinal pleura results in pneumothorax. Perforation of the abdominal oesophagus produces signs and symptoms resembling those of perforated peptic ulcer.

Investigation

A plain film of the neck and chest usually reveals emphysema and the site of perforation is best defined by a Gastrografin swallow. Endoscopy is indicated if trauma has been caused by a foreign body and may help to rule out intrinsic oesophageal disease.

Treatment

Perforation of the cervical oesophagus can usually be managed conservatively by giving broad-spectrum antibiotics and passing a nasogastric tube. Drainage of the retro-oesophageal space through a neck incision may be required. Perforation of the thoracic oesophagus is a much more dangerous injury. It can sometimes be managed conservatively by antibiotics, nasogastric intubation and insertion of chest drains if there is hydropneumothorax. If perforation has occurred during dilatation of a stricture or cancer, it may be helpful to place a prosthesis through the damaged area. Thoracotomy is needed if there is a large perforation and a clinical picture suggesting mediastinitis. The perforation may be repaired and covered with a patch of gastric fundus (if this is within reach) or the affected segment may have to be resected. The mediastinum and pleural space should be drained. Provided operation is undertaken promptly in such cases, the prognosis is good. A number of series have now been reported in which there was no mortality in patients with benign underlying disease; as might be expected, perforation in patients with cancer carries a worse prognosis.

TUMOURS OF THE OESOPHAGUS

Benign tumours

These account for less than 1% of oesophageal neoplasms. Most are asymptomatic but bleeding and obstruction occasionally occur. Leiomyoma is the commonest benign tumour and is dealt with by local resection.

Carcinoma of the oesophagus

Oesophageal cancer is common in the Far East, Iran, Africa and the West Indies, but in Europe it is relatively uncommon. Men are more often affected although hypopharyngeal cancer is more common in women. The cancer is rare before the age of 40 but its incidence rises progressively thereafter. In Scotland it accounts for just over 1% of all cancers, and has an annual incidence in men of 15 per 100 000 of the population.

Aetiology

The aetiology is unknown but risk factors include chronic irritation, alcohol, smoking and chewing tobacco, betel nut chewing, and hot spicy foods. Dietary deficiency of proteins, vitamins and trace elements (e.g. molybdenum) has also been implicated, ingested nitrosamines may be carcinogenic, and nuts and seeds stored in damp conditions may be affected by moulds such as *Aspergillus flavus* which can produce carcinogens. Local conditions which are premalignant include achalasia, the Plummer-Vinson syndrome, hiatus hernia, Barrett's oesophagus and corrosive strictures. Familial forms of oesophageal cancer have been reported occasionally and there is a recognized association with hyperkeratosis of the palms and soles (tylosis).

Pathology

More than 90% of oesophageal cancers are squamous carcinomas, and most of them occur in the middle third of the oesophagus. Adenocarcinomas can arise in columnar epithelium of the lower third of the oesophagus, although they more often arise from the upper stomach and extend upwards to involve the oesophagus. The cancer may form a polypoidal, ulcerating or hard infiltrating growth and spreads along the mucosa and submucosa. Invasion of adjacent structures and lymph node metastases are common but distant metastases are rare.

Clinical features

Progressive dysphagia and weight loss are typical. Excessive salivation, aspiration pneumonitis, anaemia and lassitude are late effects. The tumour may erode into the bronchus to produce an oesophagobronchial fistula, perforate into the mediastinum, or infiltrate the recurrent laryngeal nerves to cause hoarseness. Clinical examination may reveal involved lymph nodes in the neck, a cervical (or occasionally abdominal) mass, and hepatomegaly.

Investigation

Barium swallow usually reveals an irregular filling defect or stricture (Fig. 27.13) but the oesophagus

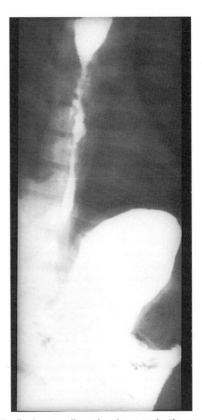

Fig. 27.13 Barium swallow showing neoplastic narrowing of the oesophagus.

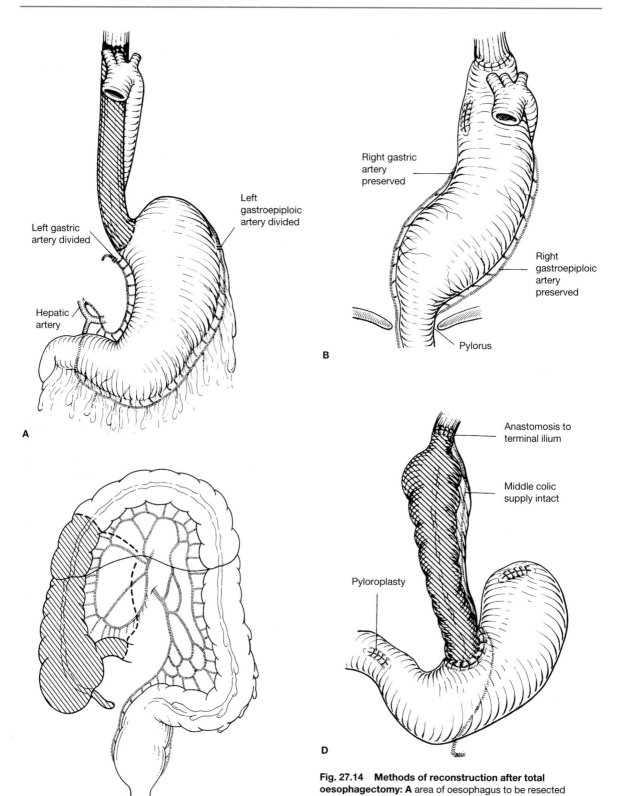

A

Left gastric artery divided

Hepatic artery

Left gastroepiploic artery divided

B

Right gastric artery preserved

Right gastroepiploic artery preserved

Pylorus

C

D

Anastomosis to terminal ilium

Middle colic supply intact

Pyloroplasty

Fig. 27.14 Methods of reconstruction after total oesophagectomy: A area of oesophagus to be resected **B** stomach mobilized to replace resected segment. **C** and **D** use of a pedicled segment of colon for replacement.

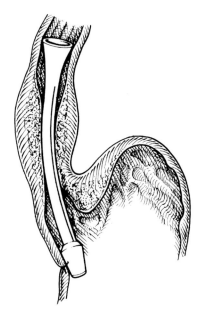

Fig. 27.15   Insertion of a Celestin tube to relieve dysphagia due to an obstructing cancer of the lower oesophagus. When the tube is inserted at laparotomy it is anchored to the stomach by a suture. This is not possible when the tube is inserted endoscopically.

above an obstructing cancer does not dilate to the extent seen in achalasia. Endoscopy reveals an oedematous friable mucosa above the obstruction and it is frequently impossible to advance the instrument into the stomach. The level of the lesion is recorded and biopsies obtained. CT scans are used to assess resectability.

Treatment

Squamous cancer may be radiosensitive whereas adenocarcinomas are not. Cancers of the upper third of the oesophagus are generally treated by radiotherapy, those of the lower third by surgical removal, and those of the mid-oesophagus by either method. Some surgeons prefer to carry out radical total oesophagectomy in all resectable cases, bringing a tube of stomach or colon up to anastomose to the pharynx (Fig. 27.14). The operation may be carried out through a thoracotomy with or without incisions in the neck or abdomen, depending on the position of the lesion and the extent of surgery. Of 100

patients presenting with oesophageal cancer, approximately 60 will undergo surgical exploration and only 40 will prove to have resectable disease. Resection still carries an operative mortality of 10–20%. Fistula formation and hoarseness are signs of unresectable disease, and computerized tomography (CT) scanning may be useful in detecting spread to adjacent structures.

Dysphagia in patients with non-resectable cancer can be relieved by dilating the stricture and inserting a rigid tube to maintain the channel. In the past this was achieved surgically by opening the abdomen and pulling a Celestin tube into position (Fig. 27.15) whereas nowadays tubes such as the Nottingham tube can be inserted endoscopically. Laser photocoagulation is used in some centres to maintain swallowing without intubation. Availability of these techniques now means that surgical bypass of oesophageal cancer is rarely indicated for palliation.

Oesophageal cancer retains a dismal prognosis and the 5-year survival rate is only 5%.

Carcinoma of the oesophagus
- Risk factors include chronic irritation (smoking, alcohol, betel nut, spices), nutritional deficiencies and environmental carcinogens (nitrosamines, *Aspergillus flavus*).

- Premalignant conditions include achalasia, Barrett's oesophagus, Plummer–Vinson syndrome, hiatus hernia and corrosive strictures.

- Histologically 90% of oesophageal cancers are squamous carcinomas while 10% are adenocarcinomas which arise from columnar epithelium in the lower third (or extend upwards from the stomach).

- Late presentation with obstruction (dysphagia and regurgitation), aspiration pneumonitis, local invasion (recurrent laryngeal nerve, bronchus, mediastinum) and metastases is common.

- Approximately 40% of oesophageal cancers are resectable. Squamous carcinomas may be radiosensitive.

- Dysphagia in patients with unresectable cancers can be relieved by endoscopic or surgical intubation, laser treatment or surgical bypass (now rarely used).

- Overall 5-year survival rates are only 5%.

28
Gastroduodenal disorders

CONTENTS

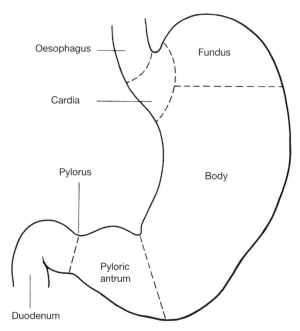

Fig. 28.1   Anatomy of the human stomach.

SURGICAL ANATOMY

The stomach consists of the cardia, fundus, body and pyloric antrum (Fig. 28.1). Its lumen is lined by tall columnar cells which commence abruptly at the cardia at the point of termination of the stratified squamous epithelium of the oesophagus. The gastric epithelium is pitted by the opening of three types of glands.

Cardiac glands secrete mucus and electrolytes and occupy a small ring around the oesophagogastric junction.

Oxyntic glands occupy the fundus and body of the stomach, taking up at least 75% of the gastric mucosal surface area. Undifferentiated mucus neck cells in the narrow neck of the glands divide throughout life to replenish the surface epithelium and oxyntic glandular cells. Parietal cells produce hydrogen ions and intrinsic factor while peptic cells produce pepsinogen. A number of endocrine cells are found between the peptic cells but their function is uncertain.

Pyloric glands in the antrum are lined by cells which secrete mucus and electrolytes, interspersed with G-cells which produce the hormone gastrin.

Nerve supply

The *parasympathetic* nerve supply of the stomach is derived from the anterior and posterior vagal nerve trunks which pass through the diaphragm with the oesophagus. The anterior trunk gives off hepatic branches and then descends along the lesser curvature supplying the front wall of the stomach (Fig. 28.2). The posterior trunk gives off a coeliac branch and then descends along the lesser curve supplying the back wall of the stomach. Almost two-thirds of the vagal fibres entering the abdomen innervate the stomach; the remainder pass in the hepatic branch to innervate the liver and gallbladder, and in the coeliac branch to supply the pancreas, small bowel and large intestine as far as the distal transverse colon.

Postganglionic *sympathetic* fibres from the coeliac ganglion reach the stomach by accompanying the gastric arteries.

SURGICAL PHYSIOLOGY

Gastric motility

Food is stored in the stomach while it is ground,

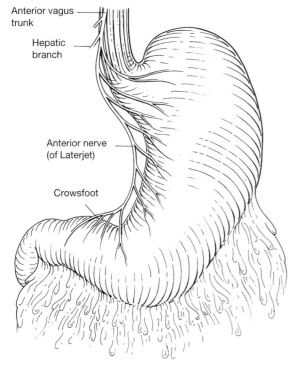

Fig. 28.2 Anatomy of the anterior vagus nerve.

Anterior vagus trunk

Hepatic branch

Anterior nerve (of Laterjet)

Crowsfoot

mixed and prepared for controlled release into the duodenum. The body and fundus act as a *reservoir* and accommodate increasing volumes of food without increases in pressure by a process known as receptive relaxation. The antrum is not concerned with receptive relaxation but serves as a *mill*; its powerful contractions mix and grind the food, and expel it into the duodenum each time the pylorus relaxes. Gastric motility is controlled by intrinsic neural plexuses which are regulated in turn by the extrinsic nerve supply. Truncal vagotomy abolishes receptive relaxation and greatly diminishes the power of antral contraction. The sympathetic nerves inhibit gastric motility.

Gastric secretion

Mucus is secreted in all regions of the stomach. It serves as a lubricant, and protects the surface epithelium against digestion by acid and pepsin by acting as an unstirred layer in which bicarbonate secreted by the surface epithelium is trapped.

Gastric secretion of acid and pepsin is regulated by neurocrine, endocrine and paracrine factors. *Acetylcholine* is the neurocrine regulator released by the vagus, *gastrin* is the endocrine regulator which is carried by the bloodstream from the antrum, while *histamine* is a paracrine regulator released from cells in the immediate vicinity of the parietal and peptic cells. The parietal and peptic cells possess specific receptor sites for each of these three stimulants, and the action of each is potentiated by the other two. This means that surgical vagotomy not only removes stimulation by acetylcholine, but also reduces the efficacy of gastrin and histamine as stimulants. In addition, gastrin and acetylcholine release histamine from mucosal stores (Fig. 28.3), while acetylcholine may also stimulate secretion by inhibiting the local release of another paracrine regulator, somatostatin.

Phases of gastric secretion

Gastric secretion is divisible into three phases.

In the *cephalic (neural) phase*, the vagal centre is activated by the sight, smell, taste, and thought of food. Impulses pass down both vagal nerves to stimulate the peptic and parietal cells *directly* by releasing acetylcholine and *indirectly* by releasing gastrin from the antrum.

In the *gastric phase*, food (notably protein digestion products) in the stomach releases gastrin from the antrum. The release of gastrin is inhibited progressively as the antral lumen becomes more acid. This inhibitory feedback mechanism prevents

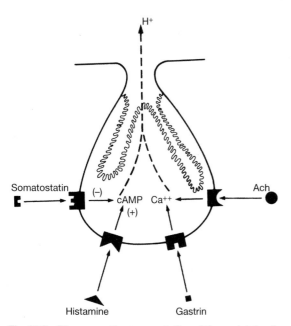

Fig. 28.3 Diagrammatic representation of the parietal cell showing receptor sites for the three major stimulants of acid secretion. Somatostatin inhibits secretion by inhibiting mucosal histamine release and by binding to somatostatin receptors. In addition to liberating acetycholine (Ach), vagal stimulation may also increase mucosal histamine release and inhibit somatostatin release.

is only important in that it provides the environment for peptic activity. Pepsin has maximal activity around pH 2, is inactive above pH 5 and is irreversibly inactivated above pH 7. Excessive acid and pepsin secretion is implicated in *duodenal ulceration* in that the secretory capacity of these patients generally exceeds that of normal subjects. Hypersecretion is not of primary importance in *gastric ulceration* where defective mucosal defences lead to ulceration in individuals with normal or reduced secretory capacity. However, ulceration never occurs in the absence of acid and pepsin and at least some secretion is needed to exploit defective defences. Factors which may damage the gastric mucosa include reflux of bile salts, and the use of NSAIDs is an important aetiological factor in the elderly. The mechanism whereby *H. pylori* causes ulceration is uncertain.

Peptic ulcers may be acute or chronic, may heal spontaneously or may have alternating periods of remission and exacerbation. Complications such as perforation, bleeding and stenosis may arise. The incidence of peptic ulcer has declined for reasons which are not clear; in Scotland the decline since 1975 has been confined to men and may reflect changes in smoking habits.

inappropriate secretion of acid and pepsin. Gastric distension may also stimulate acid and pepsin release through local intramural reflexes involving acetylcholine.

The *intestinal phase* commences as food enters the duodenum and persists for some hours after a meal. Duodenal gastrin, other intestinal hormones, and neural reflexes may all be involved. The marked increase in acid secretion which follows massive small bowel resection suggests that important inhibitory mechanisms are also normally triggered by food in the intestine.

PEPTIC ULCERATION

There are now three known causes of peptic ulceration: *Helicobacter pylori* infection, use of non-steroidal anti-inflammatory drugs (NSAIDs), and pathological hypersecretory states such as the Zollinger–Ellison syndrome (see below). All forms of ulceration result from an imbalance between gastric acid-pepsin secretion and the ability of the gastrointestinal mucosa to withstand autodigestion. The proteolytic enzyme pepsin is the key factor and acid

> **Surgical physiology of gastric secretion**
> - Hydrochloric acid secreted by the parietal cells of the gastric corpus produces an environment in which the proteolytic enzyme, pepsin, is maximally active.
>
> - Acid-pepsin secretion is stimulated by the vagus (acetylcholine), gastrin (hormone secreted by the gastric antrum) and histamine (paracrine regulator).
>
> - Truncal vagotomy reduces acid-pepsin secretion by abolishing the direct vagal drive (and, to a minor degree, by reducing antral gastrin secretion).
>
> - Truncal vagotomy impairs gastric motility by abolishing receptive relaxation of the gastric corpus (reduced reservoir) and diminishing the power of the antral contractions (antral mill) which grind, mix and expel food.
>
> - Because of its effect on gastric motility/emptying, truncal vagotomy is usually combined with a drainage procedure (pyloroplasty or gastroenterostomy).
>
> - Highly selective vagotomy denervates only the body of the stomach. Acid-pepsin secretion is reduced but antral motility is unaffected so that a drainage procedure is not needed and gastric incontinence is avoided.

Special forms of peptic ulceration

Stress ulceration is the development of multiple small superficial ulcers (or erosions) in the stomach or duodenum after major surgery, trauma or severe illness. Altered mucosal resistance is probably a key factor and resistance may be lowered by bile reflux or by a fall in mucosal blood flow during shock. *Curling's ulcer* is a special form of stress ulceration of the duodenum seen in patients with severe burns, while *Cushing's ulcer* may develop in the stomach or duodenum in patients with neurosurgical illness. Cushing's ulcer is associated with increased gastric secretion, possibly because vagal activity is increased as a consequence of raised intracranial pressure. Although normally classified as stress ulceration, Curling's and Cushing's ulcers are usually single and can erode deeply and perforate.

Sites of peptic ulceration

Duodenum

Ulceration of the first part of the duodenum is the commonest form of peptic ulceration. Ulceration of the more distal duodenum is exceptional outwith the rare Zollinger-Ellison syndrome (see p. 405).

Stomach

Gastric ulceration is the second commonest form of peptic ulcer. *Type I* or primary gastric ulcers (Fig. 28.4) are probably due to damage to mucosal defences by agencies such as bile reflux. The ulcer is often on the lesser curve, is usually associated with gastritis, and develops at the junction between acid-secreting and non-acid secreting mucosa. *Type II* gastric ulcers are secondary to duodenal ulceration and usually arise because of stasis due to duodenal deformity. *Type III* ulcers occur in the pyloric channel or prepyloric area, are associated with normal or increased gastric secretion, and have more in common with duodenal than gastric ulceration.

Oesophagus

Oesophageal ulceration is due to reflux of acid and pepsin from the stomach. The ulcers are small and superficial but may be large and penetrating when they occur in columnar mucosa.

Jejunum and ileum

Jejunal ulceration is uncommon but can develop in the Zollinger-Ellison syndrome and when ulceration recurs after gastrojejunal anastomosis (see below). Ectopic acid-secreting mucosa is occasionally found in a Meckel's diverticulum and can ulcerate the adjacent ileum.

Symptoms of peptic ulceration

Pain is the dominant symptom. As the stomach and proximal duodenum develop as midline foregut structures, the pain is usually midline and epigastric. It is usually boring and deep-seated, and may be sharply localized or ill-defined. Days or a few weeks of pain are often separated by weeks or months of remission, although this periodicity may vary considerably. Typically, pain occurs when the stomach is empty (i.e. hunger pains) and is relieved within minutes of taking food, milk or alkali. The patient often awakens with pain in the early hours of the morning. On the other hand, some patients experience pain *after* meals and identify certain foodstuffs (e.g. fatty foods) as responsible.

Other common symptoms of dyspepsia include

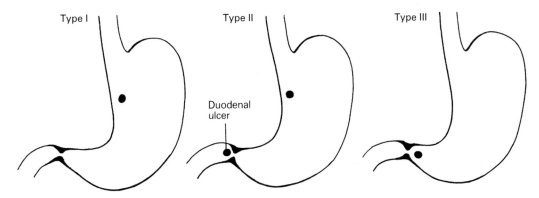

Fig. 28.4 Types of gastric ulcer.

heartburn (burning behind the sternum), waterbrash (sudden flow of saliva), flatulence, and a general feeling of upper abdominal fullness and unease. Vomiting of fluffy secretions mixed with food is common and frequently brings pain relief; some patients actually induce vomiting for this reason.

ELECTIVE PRIMARY SURGERY FOR PEPTIC ULCERATION

The surgeon must make certain that the diagnosis of peptic ulcer is correct, that all necessary investigations have been completed, and that surgery rather than continued medical management is indicated.

Diagnosis of peptic ulcer

Endoscopy. This has now replaced barium meal examination as the mainstay of diagnosis. In addition to confirming the presence of peptic ulceration, endoscopy allows oesophageal disease to be excluded, may reveal unsuspected pathology, and allows gastric ulcers to be biopsied to exclude malignancy (see below). Patients referred to hospital for endoscopy should not be given powerful antisecretory drugs beforehand; normal endoscopy under these circumstances does not exclude the possibility that ulceration has been present.

Acid secretory studies. These are no longer performed routinely. They are of little value in diagnosis, surgeons no longer select the type of operation to be performed on the basis of acid output, and the Zollinger-Ellison syndrome is now diagnosed by measuring serum gastrin levels rather than acid secretion.

Ultrasonography. This is advisable to exclude gallstones as cholelithiasis and peptic ulceration often coexist and share common symptoms.

Indications for surgery in duodenal ulceration

Failure of medical management

The falling incidence of peptic ulceration coupled with the development of effective antisecretory drugs has markedly reduced the amount of elective duodenal ulcer surgery since 1975. Although antisecretory drugs promote healing they do not affect the underlying ulcer diathesis, and long-term treatment is usually required. The drugs most frequently used are the histamine H_2-receptor antagonists (e.g. cimetidine, ranitidine). Proton pump blockers such as omeprazole are very powerful inhibitors of secretion but are usually reserved for patients with intractable ulceration or oesophagitis. The selective antimuscarinic drug, pirenzepine, is as effective as cimetidine, has few peripheral side-effects, and is used occasionally. When *Helicobacter* is present, bismuth preparations and antibiotics (e.g. tetracycline and metronidazole) may be employed. Antacids may still be used for symptom relief.

Some patients require surgery because symptoms break through medical treatment or endoscopy fails to confirm ulcer healing despite symptomatic improvement. Others are reluctant to accept long-term drug treatment. Factors which favour recourse to surgery include onset in adolescence, a strong family history of ulceration, high levels of acid secretion, and previous ulcer complications (see below). Significant loss of time from work may tip the scales in favour of operation. In the Armed Forces, peptic ulceration leads to automatic downgrading with adverse effects on promotion. Patients likely to spend long periods without access to medical care may be better advised to have surgery. If feasible, ulcer patients who require long-term anticoagulants should first have their ulcer treated surgically.

Development of complications

A history of perforation or ulcer bleeding is a strong indication for elective operation in patients with

---

Peptic ulceration

- Peptic ulceration results from an imbalance between acid-pepsin secretion and the ability of the mucosal defences (mucosa, mucus and trapped bicarbonate) of the gastrointestinal tract to withstand peptic digestion.

- Three factors known to cause peptic ulceration are infection with *Helicobacter pylori*, use of non-steroidal anti-inflammatory drugs and the rare Zollinger–Ellison syndrome.

- Duodenal ulceration is commoner than gastric ulceration; other sites which may be affected are the oesophagus, jejunum and Meckel's diverticulum.

- The incidence of peptic ulceration is declining and the need for gastric surgery has fallen dramatically with the availability of potent antisecretory drugs such as the H_2-receptor antagonists and the proton pump blockers.

- Despite the falling incidence, complications of peptic ulceration (bleeding and perforation) are still major causes of death in elderly patients.

recurrent symptoms. Pyloric stenosis is an absolute indication for surgery. Patients with combined gastric and duodenal ulcers are usually advised to have operation because the response to medical management is often poor.

Indications for surgery in gastric ulceration

Patients with gastric ulceration are more likely to require operation than those with duodenal ulceration. The indications for surgery are as follows.

Failure of medical management

Drugs used in the treatment of gastric ulcer include the histamine H_2-receptor antagonists, and combinations of colloidal bismuth and antibiotics (when *Helicobacter* is present). Sucralfate is used occasionally, and prostaglandin analogues such as misoprostol may offer protection against ulceration induced by NSAIDs.

Suspicion of malignancy

When barium meal examination was used extensively, approximately 10% of the gastric ulcers diagnosed radiologically ultimately proved to be malignant. Malignant transformation of benign peptic ulcers is unlikely and in most cases, the ulcer was malignant from the outset. Endoscopy and multiple biopsies to exclude malignancy are essential before commencing medical treatment for gastric ulceration, and endoscopy must be repeated after 6 weeks as a further check. Ulcers at sites other than the lesser curve are regarded with particular suspicion, but ulcers at any site may harbour malignancy.

Development of complications

A history of previous perforation or bleeding, or the development of stenosis (hour-glass stomach) are indications for surgery.

Indications for surgery in endocrine adenopathy

Some 15% of patients with hyperparathyroidism develop peptic ulcer, probably because hypercalcaemia leads to hypergastrinaemia and gastric hypersecretion. The ulcer usually heals once hyperparathyroidism has been corrected. Surgical management of the Zollinger-Ellison syndrome is considered later in this chapter.

Principles of surgery

The aim of surgery is to reduce acid and pepsin secretion to levels no longer associated with ulceration. The ideal operation should achieve this consistently and safely, and should not give rise to significant side-effects. None of the operations available are ideal.

The patient is prepared for surgery as for any elective major abdominal operation. A nasogastric tube is usually passed on the morning of operation to ensure that the stomach is empty, aid the surgeon in mobilization of the oesophagus for vagotomy, and prevent postoperative gastric distension. After conventional operations the patient should expect to stay in hospital for 5–7 days and remain off work for about 6 weeks.

Choice of operation for duodenal ulcer

Truncal vagotomy and drainage

Truncal vagotomy reduces acid and pepsin secretion, but also impairs antral motility and a drainage procedure is needed to facilitate gastric emptying. The drainage procedure may consist of pyloroplasty or gastrojejunostomy (Fig. 28.5). Gastrojejunostomy is preferred if there is marked duodenal inflammation or scarring, but otherwise there is little to choose between the procedures.

Truncal vagotomy and drainage was the operation most commonly performed for duodenal ulcer in the UK over the past 50 years. The operative mortality is less than 1% but 10% of patients develop recurrent ulceration because of failure to identify and divide all vagal trunks. At one time it was considered that side-effects such as diarrhoea and dumping were a consequence of vagal denervation of other abdominal organs, but it is now believed that uncontrolled gastric emptying following the drainage procedure is more important. Bilious vomiting can result from regurgitation of bile through the pyloroplasty or gastrojejunostomy. When the Visick grading system was used to assess the long-term results of surgery (Table 28.1), approximately 75% of patients were classified as having satisfactory results.

Highly selective vagotomy (proximal gastric vagotomy)

This operation has been increasingly preferred to truncal vagotomy and drainage over the past 25 years. Only those vagal fibres passing to the body of the stomach are divided, while those supplying the

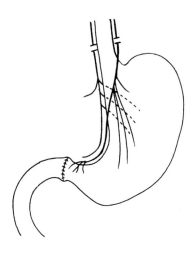

Pyloroplasty

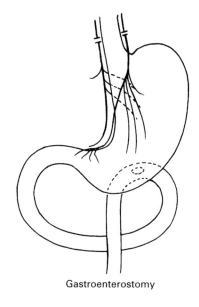

Gastroenterostomy

Fig. 28.5 Truncal vagotomy and drainage.

antrum, pylorus and other abdominal viscera are spared (Fig. 28.6). Acid and pepsin secretion are reduced to the same extent as after truncal vagotomy, but because the antrum and pylorus remain innervated, there is no need to carry out a drainage procedure. The operation is safe, the incidence of side-effects such as diarrhoea, bilious vomiting and dumping is minimal, but recurrent ulceration is somewhat more common than after truncal vagotomy and drainage (Table 28.1). Despite the high recurrence rate, the operation is regarded by many surgeons as the procedure of choice.

A number of modifications of highly selective vagotomy have been described, and the operation has also been carried out laparoscopically with reductions in hospital stay and convalescence. In one modification, the operation is simplified by dividing the branches of the anterior vagus as they pass into the muscle of the body of the stomach

(anterior seromyotomy) and performing a posterior truncal vagotomy.

Truncal vagotomy and antrectomy

This 'two-pronged' approach combines vagal denervation with removal of the major area of gastrin production (Fig. 28.7), and has a recurrent ulcer rate of only 1% (Table 28.1). Gastrointestinal continuity is restored by gastroduodenal (Billroth I) or gastrojejunal (Billroth II) anastomosis. The need for gastric resection means that the operative mortality exceeds that of vagotomy and drainage, but the incidence of side-effects is similar.

Partial gastrectomy

Partial gastrectomy was the standard operation for duodenal ulcer before the introduction of vagotomy. It reduced acid and pepsin secretion by removing the

Table 28.1	Results of surgery for duodenal ulcer			
	Highly selective vagotomy	Truncal vagotomy + drainage	Truncal vagotomy + antrectomy	Partial gastrectomy
Operative mortality	0.3%	0.6–0.8%	1.0–1.5%	2%
Satisfactory long-term results*	86%	75%	85%	75%
Recurrent ulceration	15%	10%	1%	3%

* Visick grades I and II. The Visick grading system has four categories: I and II are often combined as 'satisfactory', while III and IV are 'unsatisfactory'.

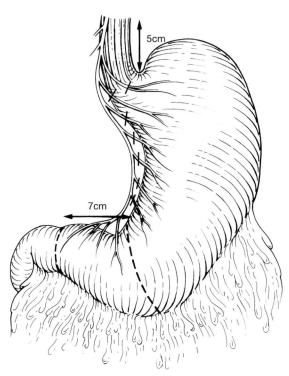

Fig. 28.6   Highly selective vagotomy. The operation divides vagal fibres to the gastric corpus and 5 cm of oesophagus should be cleared.

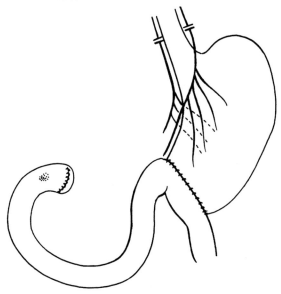

Fig. 28.7   Truncal vagotomy and antrectomy.

antrum and a proportion of the body of the stomach. About one-quarter to one-third of the stomach was left intact; the more extensive the resection, the lower the risk of recurrent ulceration. Gastro-

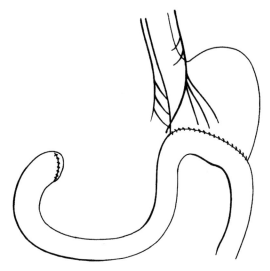

Fig. 28.8   Partial gastrectomy for duodenal ulcer (Polya or Billroth II).

intestinal continuity was usually restored by closing the duodenal stump and anastomosing the gastric remnant to the jejunum (Fig. 28.8) (although this is a Billroth II operation, the commonest variation used is that described by Polya so that the operation is frequently described as a Polya partial gastrectomy). Partial gastrectomy carries an operative mortality of 1–2%, leakage from the duodenal stump being the commonest cause of death. The incidence of long-term side-effects is similar to that following truncal vagotomy and drainage (Table 28.1).

Choice of operation for gastric ulcer

Type I gastric ulcer

The choice rests between partial gastrectomy and truncal vagotomy with drainage. Acid and pepsin secretion can usually be reduced sufficiently by removing 60% of the stomach, including the ulcer, and continuity can usually be restored by Billroth I gastroduodenal anastomosis (see Fig. 28.9). The operation carries a mortality of up to 2% but recurrent ulceration is rare, and the incidence of side-effects is acceptable (Table 28.2). The operation has the advantage that removal of the ulcer allows its complete histological examination and avoids the risk of leaving a malignant ulcer in situ.

Truncal vagotomy and drainage has a lower operative mortality but failure to reduce acid and pepsin secretion means that ulceration recurs in

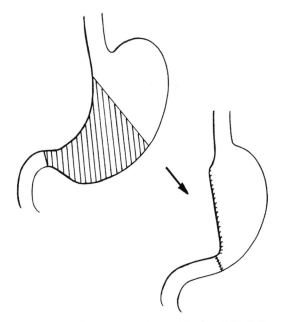

Fig. 28.9   Partial gastrectomy for gastric ulcer (Billroth I).

Table 28.2 Results of surgery for gastric ulcer		
	Truncal vagotomy + drainage	Partial gastrectomy
Operative mortality	1.5%	2%
Satisfactory long-term results*	70%	75%
Recurrent ulceration	10%	3%
Risk of retained cancer	Not known	None
* Visick grades I and II.		

some 10% of patients. There is also the real risk that a malignant ulcer is left behind. If truncal vagotomy and drainage is used, the stomach must be opened and the ulcer biopsied or excised. Truncal vagotomy and drainage is usually reserved for poor-risk patients and those with ulcers so high on the lesser curve that resection would be extensive.

Highly selective vagotomy is not recommended for gastric ulceration.

Type II gastric ulcer

This form of gastric ulcer can be treated by truncal vagotomy and drainage or partial gastrectomy. It is advisable to biopsy the gastric ulcer if it will be left in place, although gastric cancer rarely, if ever, coexists with duodenal ulcer.

Type III gastric ulcer

These ulcers are regarded as variants of duodenal ulcer and are treated accordingly.

Postoperative care

The nasogastric tube is normally removed by the second postoperative day and drinking is then allowed. Some surgeons do not retain the tube once the operation has been completed, particularly in the case of highly selective vagotomy. The patient should be eating normally on discharge, but usually finds it easier to eat small meals at frequent intervals in the early weeks. 'Ulcer diets' are unnecessary. No restrictions are placed on food content, other than instruction to avoid fruits such as oranges with a strong pith which may pass undigested through a wide stoma and obstruct the intestine.

Complications of surgery

Patients can develop the complications of any abdominal operation but the following specific problems deserve mention.

Chest infection.   This is particularly common. Many ulcer patients are smokers and the discomfort of upper abdominal surgery restricts lung expansion and coughing.

Suture line haemorrhage.   During the first 24 hours this is recognized by bright red blood in the nasogastric aspirate. It usually ceases spontaneously but transfusion and reoperation may be needed.

Stomal hold-up.   This is suspected if the patient continues to have large volumes of nasogastric aspirate. Stomal oedema is the usual cause but mechanical factors (e.g. malposition of the stoma, kinks or adhesions) can be responsible. Hypoproteinaemia and electrolyte imbalance should be corrected and a Gastrografin meal is used to confirm obstruction. Most patients settle with conservative management but hold-up which persists beyond 2 weeks usually requires reoperation.

Anastomotic leakage.   This is most likely to occur from the duodenal stump following Billroth II partial gastrectomy (Fig. 28.10). Oedema or kinking at the gastrojejunal anastomosis increases the pressure in the afferent loop, compromising the blood supply of the duodenal stump and its healing. Duodenal stump 'blow-out' usually becomes evident on the 4th or 5th postoperative day. The patient looks and feels unwell, has pyrexia and pain in the right hypochondrium, and discharges bile-stained fluid through the wound or drain track. Local

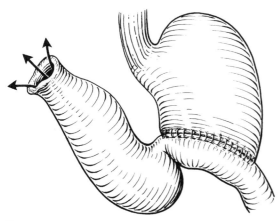

Fig. 28.10 Duodenal leakage following Billroth II partial gastrectomy.

adhesions may prevent generalized peritonitis, but subphrenic and subhepatic abscess formation is common and a persistent fistula forms. Duodenal fistulas rapidly lead to fluid and electrolyte imbalance, and activated pancreatic enzymes cause marked excoriation of the surrounding skin. Urgent treatment is required (see Ch. 29) but most fistulas will heal on conservative management, *provided there is no distal obstruction.* If contrast radiology reveals persisting obstruction, reoperation will be necessary.

TREATMENT OF COMPLICATIONS OF PEPTIC ULCER

Haemorrhage

Bleeding from the upper gastrointestinal tract is common. Peptic ulcer is the commonest cause, bleeding occurring in about 20% of ulcer patients. It may go unnoticed until anaemia raises the suspicion of chronic loss, or it can be acute and sufficiently severe to cause hypovolaemic shock and emergency admission. Vomited blood (haematemesis) may be bright red and fluid, resemble coffee-grounds, or contain clots. If blood passes down the gastrointestinal tract it becomes black (melaena) and treacly.

Some of the other causes of upper gastrointestinal bleeding also involve acid and pepsin secretion. Bleeding from mucosal lesions (gastritis, duodenitis and erosions) is almost as common as bleeding from ulcers, while oesophageal inflammation and ulceration may cause chronic blood loss. Oesophageal varices complicating portal hypertension and mucosal tears at the oesophagogastric junction

(Mallory-Weiss syndrome) are important alternative causes.

Clinical assessment

A history of peptic ulcer, liver disease or previous surgery may point to the likely source of bleeding. Ingestion of NSAIDs, steroids or anticoagulants predisposes to bleeding and is excluded by specific enquiry. A Mallory-Weiss tear is suggested by recent severe vomiting, often in association with excessive alcohol intake. Liver disease and alcohol abuse raise the possibility that oesophageal varices are present. However, it must be stressed that the history may be unhelpful and can mislead; no less than one-third of patients with known upper gastrointestinal lesions such as oesophageal varices will prove to have bled from another cause or site.

A thorough clinical examination is essential to exclude liver disease and portal hypertension, although the presence of such disease does not rule out ulcer bleeding. Pallor, tachycardia and hypotension indicate significant blood loss and the need for transfusion. Blood loss is frequently underestimated when the patient is first seen so that blood replacement often comes too late, is too slow, and involves too little blood.

Principles of management

There are three vital steps in the care of patients with major gastrointestinal bleeding:

- Prompt blood replacement to prevent exsanguination and correct hypovolaemia
- Early investigation to detect the nature and site of the bleeding lesion
- Institution of appropriate treatment to control the bleeding.

Resuscitation. All patients with acute upper gastrointestinal bleeding, even if it appears to be minor, should be referred urgently to hospital for investigation and treatment. A bleed which initially seems trivial may turn out to be major and rapidly cause hypovolaemic shock. Ideally, all such patients should be admitted to the care of an experienced haematemesis team which includes a surgeon. Delay in diagnosis or failure to appreciate the need for urgent resuscitation and/or intervention may compromise survival. Unlike external bleeding, bleeding into the gastrointestinal tract is not directly visible and may not trigger an appropriate sense of urgency.

The aim of resuscitation is to restore the circulation and provide a reserve against further bleeding. An intravenous line is established immediately and 1 litre of crystalloid (saline or Ringer lactate) is infused while blood is grouped and cross-matched. Blood urea, electrolyte concentrations, haemoglobin concentration and haematocrit are measured. A platelet count and prothrombin time (now reported as the International Normalized Ratio or INR) are requested on the first blood sample. Arterial blood gases and hydrogen ion concentration are determined if the patient is shocked.

Pulse rate and blood pressure are monitored, and if the patient is shocked, a central venous line and urinary catheter are inserted to monitor central venous pressure (CVP) and hourly urine output respectively. A large nasogastric tube is passed to prevent aspiration and detect fresh or continuing blood loss.

Whole blood is infused as soon as it is available and replacement needs are assessed by monitoring pulse rate, blood pressure, CVP and urine output. If the patient is elderly or has cardio-respiratory disease, pulmonary wedge venous pressure is monitored by a Swan-Ganz catheter to prevent pulmonary overload. If massive transfusion is needed, the blood must first be warmed.

Impaired haemostasis is expected in patients who need massive transfusion and those with underlying liver disease. Giving stored blood rapidly depletes the labile factors V and VIII, but these defects can be rectified by giving one unit of fresh frozen plasma (FFP) for every 3 litres of blood transfused. Clotting screens to determine thrombin time, INR and kaolin-cephalin coagulation time and platelet count are valuable in patients with massive bleeds. Vitamin K_1 (10–50 mg) is given intravenously to jaundiced patients and those with an abnormal INR.

Early detection of the source of bleeding. *Endoscopy* is now preferred to contrast radiology as the first-line investigation and detects the site of bleeding in 80–90% of patients with upper gastrointestinal bleeding. In general, endoscopy should be carried out as soon as blood volume has been restored in patients with major bleeds, but it can be deferred to the following morning in patients who have had minor bleeds and no signs of hypovolaemia. Patients rarely die from their initial bleed but recurrent haemorrhage is dangerous and the opportunity to define the source of haemorrhage must not be squandered.

Angiography is occasionally indicated when a bleeding site has not been identified by endoscopy. It can show bleeding when loss exceeds 2 ml/min and may reveal that vascular malformation rather than peptic ulcer is the source of haemorrhage. If arteriography does demonstrate a bleeding vessel, selective embolization may avoid the need for emergency surgery.

Treatment to control bleeding. In 90% of cases, bleeding from peptic ulceration ceases spontaneously. The patient is then able to take a light diet within 24–48 hours. Although antisecretory drugs such as H_2-receptor antagonists may not help to stop bleeding, they help ulcers to heal and are prescribed routinely.

If bleeding continues (i.e. need for blood replacement exceeds 4 units) or recurs, intervention is usually needed. Patients with chronic peptic ulcer are more likely to continue bleeding than those with erosive gastritis, and elderly, shocked patients, and those with gastric rather than duodenal ulcers are also at increased risk. The elderly are at particular risk if bleeding continues or recurs, as they are less able to cope with the physical demands of such haemorrhage. Endoscopic appearances denoting increased risk of bleeding include arterial spurting from the ulcer, a visible vessel in the ulcer base, and adherent fresh clot or black slough.

Endoscopic coagulation (by laser, heat or sclerotherapy) or endoscopic injection of alcohol and/or adrenaline solution can control bleeding in 50% of patients who would previously have come to surgery. If a skilled endoscopist is available, this approach should be used initially when bleeding continues or recurs.

If surgery is required, the presence of an ulcer is confirmed on opening the abdomen, although ideally the source of bleeding will already have been determined by endoscopy. If no lesion is apparent the stomach is opened by a longitudinal incision in its front wall (gastrotomy), the clot is evacuated, and the gastric mucosa is inspected and palpated. If a source of bleeding is not found, the gastrotomy is closed and the anterior wall of the pylorus is opened (pylorotomy) to inspect the proximal duodenum.

A bleeding duodenal ulcer is usually treated by under-running the bleeding point with non-absorbable sutures, closing the pylorotomy transversely as a pyloroplasty, and carrying out a truncal vagotomy. A bleeding gastric ulcer can also be treated by under-running the bleeding point and performing a truncal vagotomy and drainage procedure. However, malignancy should always be borne in mind when dealing with gastric ulcers and the ulcer is always biopsied (with frozen section examination if possible) or excised. A bleeding gastric ulcer may also be treated by partial gastrectomy with resection of the distal stomach including the ulcer.

In sick elderly patients, there may be a case for simply under-running the bleeding point, avoiding more extensive surgery, and relying on subsequent medical management to heal the ulcer and prevent recurrence.

If endoscopy reveals that bleeding is coming from gastritis, duodenitis or erosions rather than frank ulceration, antisecretory drugs are used. If bleeding persists, truncal vagotomy with drainage or partial gastrectomy may be needed.

Patients who have had previous ulcer surgery may bleed from recurrent ulceration at the anastomosis. Surgery is frequently needed and the bleeding point is controlled in the first instance by direct suture. If the patient has previously been treated by partial gastrectomy, truncal vagotomy and more extensive resection should be considered. If the patient has previously been treated by vagotomy, any residual vagal trunks must be divided and antrectomy is usually performed to ensure permanent reduction in acid and pepsin secretion.

Anastomotic ulceration should always raise the possibility of the Zollinger-Ellison syndrome. The pancreas, duodenum and liver should be inspected and palpated carefully, and any suspicious lymph nodes biopsied. Serum gastrin levels are determined following operation.

Bleeding from peptic ulceration
- Bleeding affects some 20% of peptic ulcer patients and remains a major source of mortality in patients older than 55 years.

- Bleeding from peptic ulceration is the commonest cause of upper gastrointestinal bleeding, but bleeding from gastritis, duodenitis and erosions is almost as common (each responsible for 30–40% of cases).

- The three priorities are to prevent exsanguination (prompt resuscitation), define the source of bleeding (endoscopy), and institute appropriate therapy.

- Almost 90% of patients stop bleeding on conservative management. Factors associated with further bleeding include old age, shock on admission, endoscopic stigmata (arterial spurting, visible vessel, fresh clot), gastric rather than duodenal ulcer.

- The conventional operation in those who continue to bleed from duodenal ulceration consists of opening the pylorus, under-running the bleeding point, and performing truncal vagotomy and pyloroplasty. Bleeding gastric ulcer can be treated using similar principles or by partial gastrectomy.

- Surgery can now be avoided in many cases by using endoscopic means (injection, laser or heat coagulation) to arrest continued bleeding.

Perforation

Perforation of a duodenal ulcer is 10 times more common than perforation of a gastric ulcer. No age group is immune but the peak incidence is in the fourth and fifth decades of life. A duodenal ulcer which perforates may be 'acute' or 'chronic' depending on whether the history exceeds 3 months. Gastric ulcers which perforate are always regarded as 'chronic'. The overall mortality of perforated peptic ulcer is around 10%. Mortality is greatest in the elderly and those ill from intercurrent disease.

Clinical features

Patients may have no history of significant dyspepsia or a long history of ulceration including complications such as bleeding or perforation. The patient usually presents with sudden severe constant abdominal pain which begins in the epigastrium but soon becomes generalized. The precise time of onset can usually be recalled. Retching may accompany the onset of the pain but vomiting is rare.

The patient is afraid to move for fear of exacerbating the pain. Abdominal tenderness, marked guarding and board-like rigidity are characteristic and denote peritonitis. In some cases, the full clinical picture does not develop because the perforation is sealed rapidly by omentum. In others, fluid leaking down the right paracolic gutter can produce clinical findings resembling those of acute appendicitis. The irritant nature of the leaking fluid causes marked peritoneal exudation and the dilution effect may contribute to a diminution of the abdominal signs after several hours. The peritoneal fluid is initially sterile but bacterial peritonitis develops after an interval of some 6 hours. Leakage of air from the perforation may lead to loss of liver dullness on percussion.

Diagnosis

In two-thirds of patients free air is apparent beneath the diaphragm on chest X-ray or erect abdominal films (Fig. 28.11). Lateral decubitus views in shocked and debilitated patients may also reveal free air. Absence of free air does not exclude perforation, and when the diagnosis remains in doubt, an emergency Gastrografin meal may be helpful. Endoscopy is contraindicated. Acute pancreatitis can be difficult to distinguish from perforated ulcer, particularly as perforation can cause modest hyperamylasaemia.

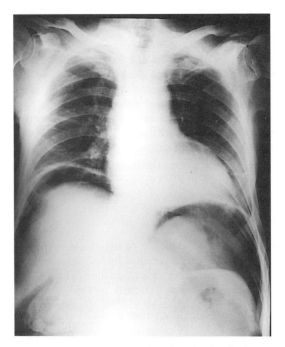

Fig. 28.11 Chest X-ray showing air under the diaphragm.

Initial management

A nasogastric tube is passed to empty the stomach and minimize further peritoneal contamination. Adequate analgesia is provided, blood is withdrawn for haematology and urea and electrolyte measurements, and blood group is determined. An intravenous infusion of crystalloid is commenced. If the patient is severely shocked (uncommon), this must be corrected prior to operation.

Conservative treatment

Perforated peptic ulcer is managed by operation unless:

- The patient is extremely ill on admission and the risks of surgery are greater than those of conservative management
- There has been a long delay between the onset of pain and presentation, and the absence of generalized abdominal signs or leakage on Gastrografin meal suggests that the perforation has sealed
- Facilities for surgery are unavailable.

The patient is then managed conservatively by regular nasogastric aspiration, intravenous fluid therapy, antisecretory drugs, and antibiotic cover if there are signs of peritonitis. Conservative management was once a popular alternative to surgery and had a comparable mortality. However, there was a higher incidence of abscess formation and on occasions, conditions for which surgery was absolutely necessary, e.g. strangulation of bowel, were treated inappropriately.

Operative management

The abdomen is opened through an upper midline incision, all peritoneal fluid is aspirated and the peritoneal cavity is lavaged.

Perforated duodenal ulcer. This may be dealt with by simple closure or by combining closure of the perforation with definitive surgery to prevent ulcer recurrence. Simple closure consists of closing the perforation with three absorbable sutures incorporating a tag of omentum (Fig. 28.12). Definitive surgery usually entails truncal vagotomy and pyloroplasty, the perforation being incorporated into the pyloroplasty. If the duodenum is markedly scarred or friable, it may be safer to close the perforation and employ gastrojejunostomy as the drainage procedure.

Simple closure is usually advocated for *acute* ulcers (i.e those with a history of less than 3 months and no chronic scarring at operation). Following simple closure about one-third of patients have no further dyspepsia, one-third experience mild easily

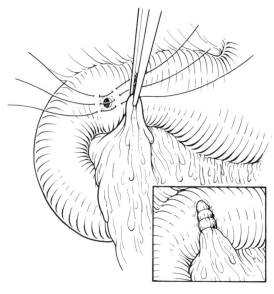

Fig. 28.12 Closure of duodenal perforation.

controlled symptoms, and one-third have significant long-term ulceration that may require definitive surgery. Simple closure of *chronic* duodenal
ulcers carries a much higher risk of recurrent
dyspepsia and definitive surgery is usually advisable.
However, emergency definitive surgery is not
advised:

- In poor-risk patients
- When the perforation is more than 12 hours old
  and heavy bacterial contamination is likely
- When an experienced surgeon and anaesthetist
  are not available. Age in itself is no bar to
  definitive surgery.

Perforated gastric ulcer. This is usually
treated by definitive surgery. Approximately 15% of
perforated gastric ulcers prove to be malignant and
provided that an experienced team is available,
Billroth I gastrectomy is the procedure of choice.
Ulcer excision combined with truncal vagotomy and
drainage may be preferred if the position of the ulcer
would make for extensive or difficult partial gastrectomy. In elderly, poor-risk patients, simple closure
after ulcer excision or biopsy may be the safest
option but careful follow-up for ulcer recurrence is
mandatory.

Perforated peptic ulcer

- Perforated duodenal ulcer is commoner
  than perforated gastric ulcer.

- Ulcer perforation still carries significant mortality
  (10%), particularly in the elderly and those with
  intercurrent disease.

- Free gas beneath the diaphragm on the erect
  abdominal or chest film confirms the diagnosis in two-
  thirds of cases; Gastrografin meal may be helpful if
  free gas is not present.

- Perforated duodenal ulcers can be dealt with by simple
  closure and application of nearby omentum. If the
  ulcer is chronic (i.e. history of more than 3 months and
  scarring at operation) definitive ulcer surgery in the
  form of truncal vagotomy and pyloroplasty can be
  considered.

- Patients who present late or who are deemed too ill for
  operation can be managed by conservative means
  (nasogastric aspiration and intravenous fluids,
  antibiotics and antisecretory drugs).

- Perforated 'gastric ulcers' frequently prove to be
  perforated gastric cancers (15% of cases) and may be
  best treated by partial gastrectomy. Lesser procedures
  (e.g. simple closure or ulcer excision, vagotomy and
  drainage) may be advisable in elderly, poor-risk
  patients.

Pyloric stenosis

The stenosis is usually located in the first part of the
duodenum rather than the pylorus, but the term
pyloric stenosis is time-honoured. Gastric outlet
obstruction can result from oedema during an acute
exacerbation of ulceration, fibrous scarring, or a
combination of the two. The complication is less
common than bleeding or perforation.

A rare form of stenosis in which hypertrophy of
the pyloric musculature is unassociated with peptic
ulceration also occurs in adults. The condition is
similar to the congenital pyloric stenosis of infants,
and may be a mild chronic form of that disease.

Clinical features

The symptoms of pyloric stenosis are frequently
insidious with upper abdominal distension after
meals, eructation, and halitosis. The peptic ulcer
pain may become continuous and intractable
before becoming less intense or even disappearing.
Vomiting eventually supervenes and the patient
brings up copious quantities of bile-free gastric juice
containing partially digested or undigested food
(such as vegetables) that may have been eaten days
earlier.

In some cases the distended stomach is visible and
gentle side-to-side shaking of the patient elicits a
succussion splash. Visible peristalsis is occasionally
present, although gastric atony is usual in long-
standing stenosis.

Investigation

The obstructed fluid-filled stomach is often visible
on plain film and a barium meal will confirm gastric
outlet obstruction. It must be borne in mind that
gastric outlet obstruction can also be caused by
carcinoma and it may not be possible to determine
the true cause of obstruction on barium meal examination. Endoscopy may also be unrewarding in
patients with gastric outlet obstruction, even after
nasogastric lavage, and definition of the cause of
hold-up may have to await laparotomy.

The initial biochemical changes in pyloric stenosis
reflect starvation. Sodium is retained by the kidneys
to preserve salt and water balance, but obligatory
loss of potassium causes hypokalaemia. Lost intracellular potassium is replaced by sodium and
hydrogen ions so that there is intracellular acidosis
and extracellular alkalosis. The onset of vomiting
leads to loss of acid gastric juice with worsening
alkalosis and hypokalaemia. The patient becomes

severely dehydrated. Initially, the urine is alkaline but as body potassium stores become depleted, the kidney begins to excrete hydrogen ions rather than potassium. The resulting *paradoxical aciduria* is a sign of profound biochemical upset. It should be noted that gastric outlet obstruction by carcinoma causes less marked acid–base imbalance as the gastric juice is less acid.

Starvation may also lead to hypoproteinaemia and serum protein levels should be determined.

Treatment

Pyloric stenosis demands surgical relief. This is *not* an emergency procedure and operation is usually undertaken after several days of preparation. Dehydration, electrolyte upsets, and acid–base balance are corrected by intravenous infusion of saline with added potassium chloride. Any anaemia is rectified and gross hypoproteinaemia may necessitate parenteral nutrition. A large-bore (32 Fr) nasogastric tube is used to empty the stomach and allow lavage. Once the aspirate is clear, a smaller tube can be used to avoid distension and encourage the return of stomach muscle tone.

Truncal vagotomy and gastrojejunostomy is the operation of choice but resection is required if malignancy is encountered at operation. Nasogastric aspiration may have to continue for some days if the stomach is slow to regain tone.

LONG-TERM COMPLICATIONS OF ULCER SURGERY

Recurrent ulcer

Gastric ulcer

Recurrence of gastric ulcer is uncommon (Table 28.2). Recurrence after truncal vagotomy and drainage is treated by partial gastrectomy, whereas in the rare event of recurrence after partial gastrectomy, further resection may be needed.

Duodenal ulcer

The incidence and site of ulcer recurrence is influenced by the nature of the previous surgery. Ulceration may recur in the duodenum after pyloroplasty, gastroduodenal anastomosis or highly selective vagotomy, whereas ulceration after gastrojejunostomy usually occurs on the jejunal aspect of the anastomosis. The ulcer recurs because the initial operation failed to reduce acid and pepsin secretion sufficiently. It is signalled by the return of symptoms although the periodicity of the pain may be atypical. The diagnosis is confirmed by endoscopy as barium studies are often difficult to interpret because of the previous surgery.

Although antisecretory drugs usually control symptoms and allow ulcer healing, operation is often advisable. Recurrence after all forms of vagotomy is treated by attempting to complete the vagotomy, usually in association with antrectomy to ensure permanent reduction of acid and pepsin secretion. Recurrence after partial gastrectomy is treated by the addition of truncal vagotomy. Recurrence after truncal vagotomy and antrectomy is rare (Table 28.1) and is dealt with by searching for and dividing any remaining vagal fibres, usually in conjunction with more extensive resection. The Zollinger-Ellison syndrome is a rare cause of recurrent ulceration and is excluded by serum gastrin determinations.

Recurrent ulceration can also cause bleeding, perforation and gastro-jejuno-colic fistula formation. Such fistulas are rare but usually arise because a recurrent ulcer at the site of gastrojejunostomy erodes into the adjacent transverse colon. The communication allows colonization of the stomach and small bowel by faecal organisms resulting in severe diarrhoea, malabsorption and weight loss. The diagnosis is best confirmed by barium enema and early operation is indicated. The fistula is disconnected, the colon is repaired, and an appropriate procedure for recurrent ulceration is undertaken.

Bilious vomiting

Occasional bilious vomiting affects up to one-third of patients after gastric surgery. Frequent and persistent vomiting is much less common and occurs when bile reflux into the stomach causes severe gastritis. Bile lying overnight in an empty stomach gives rise to morning nausea, and vomiting may be precipitated by eating breakfast. Many patients with bilious vomiting are heavy drinkers and/or smokers and abstinence may be the single most effective measure in management.

Afferent loop obstruction after a gastrojejunal anastomosis is a rare cause of bilious vomiting. Pressure builds up in the obstructed loop causing colicky upper abdominal pain; as the obstruction is overcome, bile and pancreatic juice are discharged rapidly into the stomach and vomited.

Persistent bilious vomiting may respond to antisecretory drugs which reduce the amount of acid and pepsin available to exploit damaged mucosal defences. Metoclopramide or cisapride can be used to promote gastric emptying. If medical management fails, bile can be diverted from the stomach by a Roux-en-Y anastomosis (Fig. 28.13). The distance between the gastrojejunal anastomosis and the point of entry of bile should be at least 45 cm to prevent bile from refluxing into the stomach.

Food vomiting

Vomiting of food may be due to fibrotic narrowing of a stoma or faulty siting of a gastrojejunostomy. The problem is evaluated endoscopically or radiologically, and appropriate revisional surgery undertaken.

Occasional patients develop gastric hypotonia despite an adequate anastomosis. Vomiting can be relieved by metoclopramide or domperidone (dopamine antagonists which co-ordinate and improve gastric emptying), or by cisapride (which acts by releasing acetylcholine in the gut wall).

Dumping

The dumping syndrome is characterized by a feeling of epigastric fullness after food associated with flushing, sweating, marked lassitude, increased peristalsis with borborygmi and, in some cases,

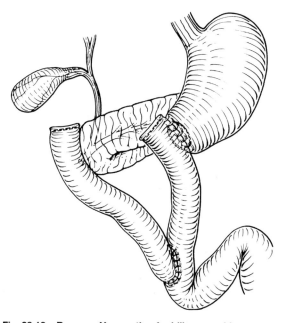

Fig. 28.13   Roux-en-Y operation for bilious vomiting.

diarrhoea. Symptoms commence within 15–30 minutes of eating and usually settle within 30–60 minutes. The patient frequently has to lie down until symptoms pass.

Epigastric fullness occurs in about one-third of patients after gastric surgery, and impaired receptive relaxation following vagotomy is usually responsible. This symptom alone does not constitute dumping; it usually improves spontaneously in a few months and can be avoided by taking smaller meals.

The dumping syndrome proper is due to the uncontrolled rapid emptying of hyperosmolar solutions, particularly carbohydrate solutions, into the small bowel. Large amounts of fluid then move by osmosis into the bowel lumen, and symptoms result from the rapid reduction in extracellular fluid volume and the increased peristalsis produced by jejunal distension. Release of mediators such as 5-hydroxytryptamine and bradykinin may also be implicated.

Dumping symptoms can be ameliorated by taking smaller meals, reducing carbohydrate intake, and avoiding liquids during meals. If troublesome symptoms persist, surgery may have to be considered. However, it must be stressed that it is advisable to wait for at least 1–2 years after the primary operation, as:

• Symptoms often improve spontaneously
• The long-term results of surgery are often disappointing.

If the initial operation included gastrojejunostomy, the stoma should be taken down to restore normal gastrointestinal continuity. If pyloroplasty was undertaken, reconstruction of the pylorus may be attempted. If partial gastrectomy was performed, conversion of a gastrojejunal to a gastroduodenal anastomosis may be worthwhile. If extensive gastric resection has left the patient with a small stomach, it is worth considering interposition of a segment of jejunum between stomach and duodenum (Fig. 28.14).

Reactive hypoglycaemia

This was once known erroneously as 'late dumping'. Symptoms are produced by the rapid absorption of glucose from the upper small bowel, resulting in hyperglycaemia, excessive insulin secretion, and an 'overswing' into reactive hypoglycaemia. Tremor, tachycardia, palpitation and sweating develop 90–120 minutes after a meal and are potentiated by exercise. Approximately 10% of patients develop this symptom at some time after gastric surgery. In

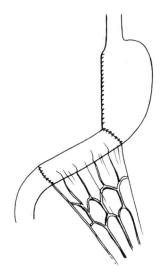

Fig. 28.14 Jejunal interposition to relieve symptoms of dumping.

the great majority of cases the problem is mild, transient and easily controlled. Patients are advised to reduce carbohydrate intake but to carry glucose sweets to take if symptoms arise. Revisional surgery is hardly ever required.

Diarrhoea

Diarrhoea can occur after any form of gastric surgery but is particularly troublesome after vagotomy and drainage. In most cases it is mild and transient, and severe unpredictable episodic diarrhoea affects only 2–4% of patients. Urgency is common, incontinence can occur, and social and professional life can be disrupted. Steatorrhoea and malabsorption are rare.

The cause of diarrhoea is uncertain but loss of gastric continence is a major factor. Avoidance of certain foods may be helpful, and symptoms can often be controlled by kaolin, codeine phosphate or diphenoxylate with atropine (Lomotil). Operation is used as a last resort, the aim being to try to restore continence by taking down a gastrojejunostomy or refashioning a pyloroplasty. Some success has followed reversal of a segment of jejunum to slow transit through the distal small intestine.

Malabsorption

Failure to gain weight or weight loss is a recognized complication of extensive gastric resection. Inadequate intake and fear of dumping may be contributory, and appropriate dietary advice should be given.

True malabsorption with steatorrhoea and weight loss is relatively rare. Causes include lactose intolerance, gastro-jejuno-colic fistula, and the blind loop syndrome. The blind loop syndrome may follow Billroth II gastrectomy or gastrojejunostomy. The diagnosis is confirmed by finding high bacterial counts in the loop and by a good response to antibiotics. Conversion of a gastrojejunal to a gastro-duodenal anastomosis, or replacement of a gastro-jejunostomy by a pyloroplasty eliminates the blind loop and can give permanent relief.

Anaemia

Iron deficiency anaemia is common after all forms of gastric surgery, and particularly after partial gastrectomy. It may be due to a combination of postoperative anaemia, inefficient absorption of dietary iron following reduction of acid secretory capacity, and chronic blood loss from gastritis. Anaemia may take as much as 10 years to become manifest and haemoglobin levels should be monitored regularly. Premenopausal women are particularly susceptible because of menstrual blood loss, and should be advised to take oral iron prophylactically, one month in three.

Anaemia due to vitamin B_{12} deficiency is rare after gastric surgery in the absence of steatorrhoea. Parenteral vitamin B_{12} is required for life.

Calcium malabsorption

This may develop as a consequence of steatorrhoea but can occur 10–15 years after operation in patients without steatorrhoea. Partial gastrectomy favours calcium malabsorption and postmenopausal women (who frequently lack calcium) are particularly prone to develop osteomalacia. For this reason, partial gastrectomy is best avoided in female patients.

Tuberculosis

Patients with a history of tuberculosis are prone to relapse following gastric resection and should be followed carefully.

Gastric cancer

There is increasing evidence that patients who have undergone partial gastrectomy are at increased risk of developing gastric cancer after a latent interval of some 20 years. It has been suggested that reduced acid secretion allows bacterial overgrowth in the stomach with generation of carcinogenic nitrosamines from nitrates in food. However, the risk increase is marginal and as these patients are also at increased risk of cardiorespiratory disease and other forms of cancer (e.g. pancreatic and lung cancer), factors such as smoking habits may be important. The consensus view is that the increase in the risk of developing gastric cancer after partial gastrectomy is not sufficiently strong to justify regular screening by endoscopy. There is little evidence that other forms of gastric surgery might also predispose to gastric cancer.

ZOLLINGER–ELLISON SYNDROME (GASTRINOMA)

The Zollinger–Ellison syndrome is a rare entity in which autonomous secretion of gastrin leads to gastric hypersecretion and fulminant peptic ulceration. The source of gastrin secretion is usually a tumour (gastrinoma) of gastrin-secreting cells (G cells) in the pancreatic islets but tumours can occur in the duodenum or stomach. Two-thirds of gastrinomas are malignant and more than three-quarters of patients have multiple tumours. Men are more commonly affected (sex ratio 3:2) and the peak incidence lies between 20 and 50 years of age.

G-cell hyperplasia is a very rare condition in which hypergastrinaemia is due to hyperplasia of antral G cells rather than tumour formation.

Clinical features

The classical presentation is one of fulminating dyspepsia refractory to routine treatment. However, many patients at first only have mild dyspepsia. Ulceration often occurs at more than one site in the stomach, proximal duodenum or jejunum. Bleeding (33%), perforation (25%) and pyloric obstruction (10%) are common. One-third of patients have diarrhoea due to a combination of jejunitis and steatorrhoea caused by destruction of lipase by acid. Diarrhoea may be the first symptom.

One-quarter of gastrinoma patients have other endocrine abnormalities, including multiple endocrine neoplasia. Parathyroid adenomas are particularly common (see Ch. 19).

Diagnosis

A high index of suspicion is essential. Pointers to the correct diagnosis include:

- Peptic ulceration occurring in childhood or adolescence, particularly in association with a family history of ulceration or endocrinopathy
- Ulceration involving unusual sites such as the distal duodenum or jejunum
- Ulceration with unexplained diarrhoea
- Ulceration associated with endocrine abnormalities such as hyperparathyroidism
- Stomal ulceration which develops rapidly after ulcer surgery, particularly after partial gastrectomy or truncal vagotomy and antrectomy
- Gastric hypersecretion and a ratio of basal to maximal acid output which exceeds 0.6:1.

Serum gastrin determinations are the mainstay of diagnosis. The normal fasting gastrin level for most laboratories is below 150 ng/l. All higher values are regarded with suspicion and a level which exceeds 500 ng/l is strongly suggestive. Provocation tests may be employed; a rapid intravenous bolus injection of secretin causes a marked rise in gastrin levels in most gastrinoma patients. Acid secretory studies are now seldom used in diagnosis unless it is necessary to confirm that hypergastrinaemia is *secondary* to achlorhydria or hypochlorhydria in conditions such as pernicious anaemia and renal insufficiency.

Computerized tomography (CT) scanning and selective angiography are used to try to localize the tumour(s) and detect metastases. Selective venous sampling using a catheter passed through the liver and into the portal and splenic vein may detect high local venous gastrin levels and so localize deposits.

Management

Ideally, an attempt should be made to cure the Zollinger-Ellison syndrome by resecting the gastrinoma and so removing the source of hypergastrinaemia. In practice this is frequently thwarted by the fact that the tumour is malignant or multifocal; in some cases the gastrinoma is so small that it cannot be located.

In the past, *total gastrectomy* was usually employed as the only means of guaranteeing control of acid and pepsin secretion. Modern antisecretory drugs now provide an alternative to such surgery in most patients and although high doses of drug are needed, gastric hypersecretion can usually be controlled. Total gastrectomy is now only used when hypersecretion cannot be controlled medically. Following this operation 60% of patients survived 5 years and 40% 10 years, the pancreatic tumour frequently remaining stable. Similar survival rates should be anticipated with modern medical management. As might be expected, the outlook is worse for patients with metastatic disease and cytotoxic therapy may have to be considered in such cases.

GASTRIC NEOPLASIA

BENIGN GASTRIC NEOPLASMS

Benign tumours of the stomach may arise from epithelial or mesenchymal tissue. Adenomatous polyps are the commonest benign epithelial neoplasm and may be single or multiple. The risk of malignant transformation increases with polyp size. Leiomyomas are the commonest benign mesenchymal neoplasms; neurogenic tumours, fibroma and lipomas are all rare. Benign tumours may be found incidentally during endoscopy or barium meal examination, but they can give rise to bleeding, intermittent pyloric obstruction with vomiting, or intussusception through the pylorus (rare).

The benign nature of the polyp is confirmed by endoscopic biopsy. Some pedunculated polyps can be removed endoscopically using a diathermy snare but large polyps should be resected surgically in view of the risk of malignancy. Multiple polyps may require gastric resection.

MALIGNANT GASTRIC NEOPLASMS

Gastric carcinoma

The stomach is the second commonest site for gastrointestinal cancer and accounts for 10% of all cancer deaths. Unfortunately, gastric cancer has spread through and beyond the confines of the stomach by the time that most patients present with symptoms, and treatment is all too often restricted to palliation. Although there is some evidence that resectability rates are improving and that more extensive lymphadenectomy may improve survival in patients undergoing 'curative' resection, the overall outlook remains gloomy with less than 15% of patients surviving for 5 years. Endoscopic screening offers the possibility of diagnosing gastric cancer while it is still confined to the mucosa. Screening is practised extensively in Japan (where gastric cancer is very common), and 5-year survival rates in excess of 90% have been achieved in patients with screen-detected cancers. In Britain, screening is not practised routinely but there is a strong argument for its use in high-risk individuals such as those with pernicious anaemia.

Aetiological factors

Gastric cancer is more common in Japan, Iceland, Chile and parts of Eastern Europe than it is in the UK or North America where its incidence has declined markedly over the past 50 years. Regional differences may be present within countries, and Scotland, northern England and Wales have a higher incidence than southern England.

Cancer of the stomach is twice as common in men and has its highest incidence in unskilled workers and deprived socio-economic groups. Its incidence increases with age, although 1 in 15 cases occur in patients under 40 years of age. Blood relatives of patients are at increased risk and there is a strong association with blood group A.

Population surveys suggest that a diet rich in carbohydrate but low in fat, fresh fruit and vegetables may have some association with the risk of developing gastric cancer. High intake of nitrates has also been implicated in that carcinogenic nitrosamines can be formed by the bacterial reduction of nitrates to form nitrites which are then nitrosated. Achlorhydria and hypochlorhydria could favour carcinogenesis by allowing growth of bacteria not normally present in the acid-secreting stomach. The presence of carcinogens such as 3,4-benzpyrene in smoked foods has also been implicated in carcinogenesis. Occupational factors include mining and working with rubber or asbestos.

There is a growing belief that H. pylori infection may also be associated with gastric cancer.

The incidence of gastric cancer is increased by three to four times in patients with pernicious anaemia. Atrophic gastritis and achlorhydria, adenomatous polyps, and previous partial gastrectomy are all predisposing factors. Benign gastric ulcer used to be regarded as a potentially malignant condition but this is now discounted.

Pathology

Cancers of the stomach are almost all adenocarcinomas derived from the mucus-secreting epithelial cells. They can occur in any part of the stomach but are most common in the antrum. They are classified as ulcerating, proliferative (or polypoidal), or infiltrating. Diffuse infiltration of the stomach accompanied by a fibrous reaction produces the so-called 'leather bottle stomach' (linitis plastica).

The modes of spread of gastric cancer are:

* Direct extension to neighbouring organs such as liver and pancreas
* Transcoelomic spread to form peritoneal and omental seedlings, and involve the ovaries (Krukenberg tumour) and rectovesical pouch
* Lymphatic spread to regional nodes alongside the stomach, along the hepatic and splenic vessels, and in the porta hepatis. Spread along the thoracic duct may lead to involvement of the left supraclavicular nodes
* Blood-borne spread via the portal vein to the liver, and occasionally to the lung and more distant sites.

The TNM (tumour, nodes, metastases) classification can be applied to gastric cancer. Early gastric cancer (i.e. cancer which has not spread locally beyond the mucosa and submucosa) has a 5-year survival rate following resection of around 90%. When all cases of gastric cancer are considered, lymph node involvement is critical. When there are no involved regional nodes, 5-year survival rates after resection are close to 50% whereas involvement of lymph nodes reduces this figure to about 10%.

Clinical features

The classical symptoms of gastric cancer (anorexia, vomiting, anaemia and weight loss) are all manifestations of advanced disease. Early gastric cancer may produce no symptoms or give rise to vague dyspepsia and epigastric discomfort. A history of recurrent dyspepsia relieved by alkali does not rule out the diagnosis of gastric cancer. Frank haemorrhage is rare but insidious blood loss can produce anaemia, lassitude, pallor and breathlessness. Anaemia should never be treated without full investigation for chronic blood loss.

Rarely, the first symptoms of gastric cancer may arise from pyloric obstruction, perforation or major bleeding. In some cases, the first symptom may be produced by metastatic deposits in the liver, supraclavicular nodes or peritoneal cavity.

Diagnosis

Patients with early disease usually have no physical signs but occult blood may be detected in the faeces. By the time most patients are referred to hospital, weight loss is obvious. An epigastric mass may be palpable (and in some cases, visible), and ascites may be evident. The liver and supraclavicular nodes

are palpated for metastatic disease and a digital rectal examination is essential to detect transcoelomic spread to the pelvis. A full blood count and liver function tests are requested, and endoscopy is arranged.

At endoscopy, any suspicious lesions are biopsied and brushings can be taken for cytological examination. Double contrast barium studies are used less extensively for diagnosis since the advent of endoscopy. Such contrast examinations may reveal a filling defect, ulceration or infiltration (Fig. 28.15). In linitis plastica the stomach is contracted to form a narrow rigid tube which empties rapidly into the duodenum. Radiological differentiation between benign and malignant gastric ulceration may prove difficult. Signs which suggest malignancy include irregularity of the ulcer base, interruption and rigidity of mucosal folds, and an ulcer with raised margins and a raised base. Ulceration at sites not usually affected by peptic ulceration (e.g. the greater curve) is also suggestive of malignancy.

Carcinoma of the stomach must also be differentiated endoscopically from other infiltrative lesions such as lymphoma (see below) which may carry a better prognosis. Giant mucosal hypertrophy may also produce clinical and radiological features similar to those of carcinoma.

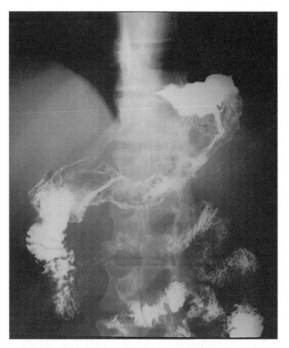

Fig. 28.15 Barium meal examination showing extensive gastric carcinoma causing narrowing of the gastric lumen.

Treatment

Unless there is gross evidence of metastatic disease or general illness severe enough to contraindicate surgery, the abdomen should be explored. CT scanning and laparoscopy may be helpful in tumour staging and in determining whether surgery should be avoided.

On opening the abdomen the extent of the disease is assessed, and biopsies are obtained if the diagnosis of cancer has not already been confirmed by endoscopic biopsy. In some cases, laparotomy does not reveal distant spread but the cancer may be so fixed to adjacent structures that it cannot be resected. If the cancer is not fixed in this way and there is no spread to distant sites, resection may prove to be curative. The standard curative resection for cancer of the distal stomach is a Billroth II partial gastrectomy, removing the distal three-quarters of the stomach in conjunction with the regional lymph nodes. Curative resection for cancer of the body of the stomach necessitates total gastrectomy with removal of regional nodes and the distal 2–3 cm of oesophagus. Following total gastrectomy, a loop of jejunum is brought up to the oesophagus as a Roux-en-Y reconstruction. In recent years there has been considerable emphasis on removing not just the lymph nodes adjacent to the gastric wall (R1 nodes), but also removing common hepatic, splenic, hepato-duodenal and retropancreatic nodes (R2 and R3 nodes). There is some evidence that such extended forms of curative resection may improve long-term survival.

The presence of liver metastases and peritoneal seedlings signifies that treatment will be confined to palliation, but if the patient has symptoms due to blood loss, resection of the involved part of the stomach may still be worthwhile. If the main symptoms are due to obstruction of the distal stomach, gastrojejunostomy can be used to bypass the blockage, accepting that the palliation may be short-lived. In patient with proximal tumours causing obstruction (dysphagia), palliation may be achieved by inserting a tube at operation (Celestin tube) although it is now possible to insert such tubes endoscopically (see Ch. 27).

Radiotherapy has no place in the management of adenocarcinoma of the stomach, but combination chemotherapy has been used to treat recurrence and as a form of adjuvant treatment at the time of surgery.

Gastric carcinoma

- Gastric cancer is the second commonest cause of death from gastrointestinal malignancy (i.e. after colorectal cancer).

- The disease is particularly common in Japan, Chile, Iceland and Eastern Europe, buts its incidence in many Western countries has declined markedly throughout this century for reasons which are not clear.

- Aetiological factors include pernicious anaemia, atrophic gastritis and achlorhydria, and previous partial gastrectomy. Dietary factors (smoked foods, low intake of fresh fruit and vegetables), formation of carcinogenic nitrosamines (from dietary nitrate), and occupational factors (mining, rubber, asbestos) are also implicated.

- Many patients have incurable and unresectable disease at presentation and overall 5-year survival rates in Western countries are less than 15%.

- Lymph node involvement is a major determinant of survival in patients undergoing gastric resection; the 5-year survival rate in patients with uninvolved nodes is 50%, whereas with involved nodes it is only10%.

- 5-year survival rates of 90% have been achieved in Japan following resection of screening-detected cancers confined to mucosa/submucosa.

Gastric lymphoma

About 2% of all malignant gastric tumours are lymphomas. The presentation resembles that of carcinoma but the symptoms may be surprisingly mild despite the presence of a large tumour. The diagnosis is confirmed by endoscopic biopsy. Radical subtotal gastrectomy followed by radiotherapy gives 5-year survival rates of about 50% and tumour size is not a contraindication to surgery. If the tumour is not resectable, radiotherapy can give worthwhile palliation, while systemic disease can respond to chemotherapy.

Gastric leiomyosarcoma

These tumours account for less than 1% of all gastric malignancies. The lesion often bulges into the gastric lumen or into the peritoneal cavity, and its luminal surface may ulcerate and bleed. The tumour grows slowly and metastasizes late, and has a 5-year survival rate of 50% after partial gastrectomy. The tumour is not radiosensitive so that the prognosis is very poor if it cannot be resected.

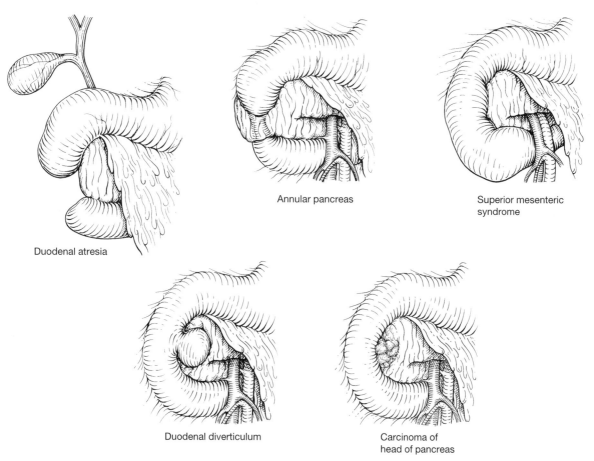

Duodenal atresia

Annular pancreas

Superior mesenteric
syndrome

Duodenal diverticulum

Carcinoma of
head of pancreas

Fig. 28.16   Causes of duodenal obstruction.

MISCELLANEOUS DISORDERS OF THE STOMACH

Gastric diverticula

These rare lesions can be mistaken radiologically for ulcers. Endoscopy provides the correct diagnosis.

Bezoars

A bezoar is a concretion formed in the gastrointestinal tract. Trichobezoars consist of hair and are seen occasionally in young girls or demented patients who chew and swallow their hair. Phytobezoars are less common and consist of vegetable material such as orange pith, fruit skin and seeds. Rare forms of bezoar include the semi-solid bezoars of *Candida albicans* and shellac bezoars in painters or furniture makers.

Bezoars can attain large size and cause obstruction, gastritis and bleeding. The diagnosis is made by barium examination; surgical removal is advisable.

Swallowed foreign bodies

Accidental or deliberate ingestion of foreign bodies is common. Most are radio-opaque and can be followed radiologically as they pass spontaneously through the gut. Surgery may become necessary if the object fails to pass, obstructs the stomach or gives rise to perforation.

Gastric volvulus

Volvulus is usually a sequel to para-oesophageal herniation (see Ch. 27) or eventration of the diaphragm following trauma. The stomach rotates upwards around its long axis. The patient develops epigastric pain, and experiences severe nausea but is unable to vomit. It is impossible to pass a nasogastric tube into the stomach. The diagnosis is confirmed by chest X-ray and Gastrografin meal. Immediate laparotomy is advised to reduce the volvulus, repair any diaphragmatic defect and anchor the stomach in the abdomen so that the twist cannot recur. Untreated, the volvulus readily progresses to strangulation, gastric necrosis and perforation.

MISCELLANEOUS DISORDERS OF THE DUODENUM

Duodenal obstruction

Common causes of duodenal obstruction are pyloric stenosis (see p. 401) and carcinoma of the pancreas. Rarer causes include blockage by mesenteric lymph nodes, duodenal diverticulum, duodenal atresia, annular pancreas and chronic duodenal ileus (Fig. 28.16). If surgical treatment is required, bypass by duodenojejunal or gastrojejunal anastomosis is often appropriate. Symptomatic diverticula may have to be excised. Chronic duodenal ileus is an ill-defined entity which may affect visceroptotic females and rapidly growing thin children. It has been suggested that the duodenum is obstructed by the superior mesenteric vessels as they cross its third part, but most surgeons are sceptical about this explanation. The condition is usually self-limiting in children but in adults surgical bypass may have to be considered.

Duodenal diverticula

The duodenum is the second commonest site for diverticulum formation in the gastrointestinal tract. The diverticula rarely develop before the age of 40 years, and are often found at the point of entry of the common bile duct. They are frequently discovered incidentally at endoscopy or on barium meal examination, but can cause obstruction, bleeding and inflammation (diverticulitis). Symptomatic diverticula should be excised if it is certain that they are the cause of problems.

Duodenal trauma

Duodenal damage may follow severe crush injury of the upper abdomen (see Ch. 14).

29
Intestinal surgery

CONTENTS

The surgery of disorders of the stomach and duodenum is dealt with in Chapter 28. The present chapter deals with surgical conditions of the remainder of the intestine, excluding the appendix (Ch. 30) and anorectal region (Ch. 32).

Surgical anatomy

Development

The gastrointestinal tract develops from a continuous tube which can be divided into the foregut, midgut and hindgut. The bowel derived from the midgut begins at the midpoint of the second part of the duodenum and ends two-thirds of the way along the transverse colon. Each part of the primitive gut has a principal artery of supply; the coeliac axis supplies the foregut, the superior mesenteric artery (SMA) the midgut, and the inferior mesenteric artery (IMA) the hindgut. The ratio of the diameters of the coeliac axis: SMA:IMA is 4:4.5:1. The coeliac axis and SMA anastomose through the pancreaticoduodenal arcade, while the SMA and IMA have a more tenuous anastomosis through the marginal artery (see below).

Structural anatomy

The *small bowel* extends from the pylorus to the ileocaecal valve. There are approximately 500 cm of small bowel beyond the ligament of Treitz, the upper two-fifths constituting the jejunum and the remainder the ileum. The small bowel has an inner mucosa (a single layer of columnar cells interspersed with mucous cells, Paneth cells and APUD (Amine Precursor Uptake and Decarboxylation) cells, a strong fibrous submucosa, an inner layer of circular muscle and an outer longitudinal layer. It is suspended by a mesentery, the root of which runs from the left of L2 to the right sacroiliac joint. Occasionally, embryonic remnants form a mesenteric cyst which presents in later life as a palpable mass which can be moved up and down but not from side to side, and which requires removal.

The SMA runs in the root of the mesentery and supplies the small bowel by a series of straight vessels which originate from arterial arcades (Fig. 29.1). Venous blood drains to the superior mesenteric vein and then to the portal vein. Lymphoid aggregates in the submucosa (Peyer's patches) are more numerous

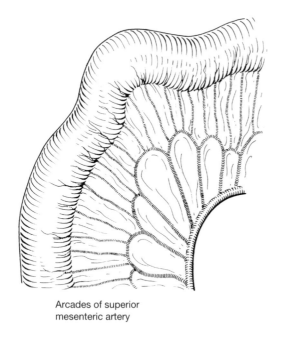

Arcades of superior
mesenteric artery

Fig. 29.1 Blood supply of small intestine showing arterial arcades.

in the ileum. Lymph drains to regional nodes in the root of the mesentery before passing to the cisterna chyli. The mesentery contains parasympathetic and sympathetic nerve fibres which influence motility and blood flow. Intestinal pain is mediated by the sympathetic nervous system.

The principal function of the small bowel is absorption, but its secretory and digestive functions supplement those of the upper digestive tract. The mucosa is thrown into circular folds (plicae semilunares) and is carpeted by finger-like villi, giving an absorptive area of 200–500 m^2. Some 5–8 litres of fluid enter the jejunum each day, of which only 1–2 litres normally pass on to the colon.

The *large bowel* begins at the *ileocaecal valve* (a one-way valve which normally prevents reflux into the ileum). The *caecum* is a blind pouch in the right iliac fossa and the *appendix* opens from its base at the point where the taeniae coli converge. The *ascending colon* passes up to the *hepatic flexure* which overlies the lower pole of the right kidney. The *transverse colon* runs to the *splenic flexure* suspended by the transverse mesocolon. The splenic flexure is higher in the abdomen than the hepatic flexure, a point

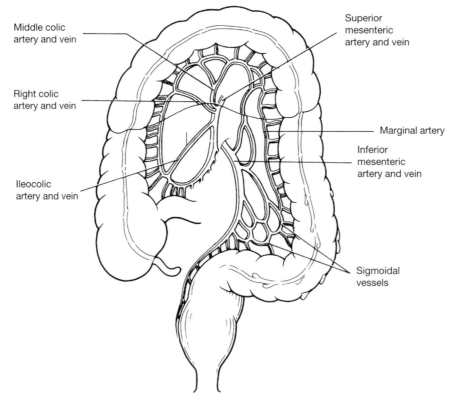

Middle colic
artery and vein

Right colic
artery and vein

Ileocolic
artery and vein

Superior
mesenteric
artery and vein

Marginal artery

Inferior
mesenteric
artery and vein

Sigmoidal
vessels

Fig. 29.2 The blood supply of the large intestine.

which aids orientation of abdominal films. From the splenic flexure, the *descending colon* passes down to become the *sigmoid colon* at the brim of the pelvis. The *sigmoid colon* is suspended by a sigmoid mesocolon which forms an inverted V attached to the pelvic brim at the point where the left ureter crosses the bifurcation of the left common iliac artery. The transverse colon and sigmoid colon have mobility by virtue of their mesentery, whereas the ascending and descending colon are peritonealized on only their front and sides, and are immobile.

The *rectum* commences as the sigmoid colon loses its mesentery, and passes downwards in the hollow of the sacrum to end at the anorectal junction. Its upper third has a peritoneal covering on its front and sides, the middle third is peritonealized only anteriorly, and the lower third lies beneath the peritoneal floor of the pelvis. The pelvic plexus of autonomic nerves lies in the connective tissue behind the rectum. The rectum is attached to the side walls of the pelvis by lateral ligaments which transmit the middle rectal vessels.

The large bowel mucosa consists of columnar epithelium interspersed with mucus-secreting goblet cells. Crypts pass down to the muscularis mucosa, beneath which is a strong fibrous submucosa. An inner circular layer of smooth muscle runs the length of the large bowel, ending as a condensation which forms the internal anal sphincter. The outer longitudinal layer of smooth muscle is condensed in the colon into three bands (taeniae) which coalesce as they approach the rectum to form a continuous investment.

The arteries supplying the colon (Fig. 29.2) anastomose to form a *marginal artery* which allows collateral supply in the event of arterial occlusion. The superior rectal artery is the continuation of the IMA and passes down to supply the rectum and anastomose with the middle and inferior rectal arteries (branches of the internal iliac arteries). The superior mesenteric vein becomes the portal vein as it joins the splenic vein behind the neck of the pancreas, whereas the inferior mesenteric vein drains initially into the splenic vein.

Lymph drains from the colon to epicolic and paracolic nodes close to the bowel wall, and from there to regional nodes at the origin of the superior and inferior mesenteric vessels (Fig. 29.3). Lymph from the rectum drains upwards to superior rectal and inferior mesenteric nodes, whereas anal canal lymph drains to inguinal nodes.

The large bowel actively absorbs sodium and

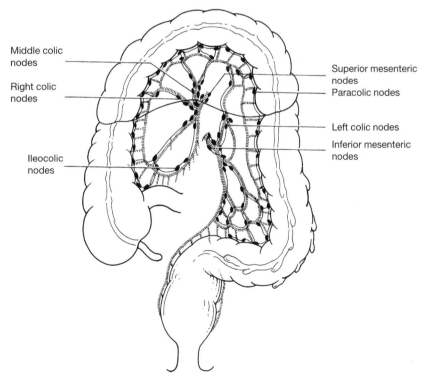

Fig. 29.3 Lymphatic drainage of the colon.

water, particularly on the right side, while the left colon and rectum act as a reservoir until defaecation is appropriate. Mucus is secreted as a lubricant and may become visible as a covering layer or discharge when there is inflammation.

Investigation of bowel disease

History and clinical examination

Diseases of the intestine frequently give rise to abdominal pain, nausea and vomiting, and alteration in bowel habit. The pattern of symptoms is influenced by the location of the problem. For example, obstruction of the small bowel (midgut) produces periumbilical colic, whereas obstruction of the distal large bowel (hindgut) produces colic in the hypogastrium. Nausea and vomiting are early features of high small bowel obstruction, whereas in distal obstruction, vomiting may be a late feature and there may be marked abdominal distension. Diseases of the large bowel are particularly liable to produce alterations in bowel habit with constipation, diarrhoea or alternating bouts of each. It is the *alteration* that is important, as individuals vary greatly in what constitutes a 'normal' bowel habit. Passage of blood or mucus per rectum is a common feature of large bowel disease. Blood originating from the distal bowel is usually bright red whereas blood coming from the upper gastrointestinal tract is often so altered by gut bacteria that it is black (melaena). In some cases, blood is not obvious on inspecting the stool but the faecal occult blood test is positive. Weight loss, malaise and anaemia are common non-specific features of intestinal disease.

A thorough physical examination includes inspection of the oral mucous membrane, hands and finger nails. Examination of the abdomen may reveal distension, a mass or visible peristalsis. The caecum is often palpable in thin subjects, and the descending and sigmoid colon may be palpable when loaded with faeces. Hepatomegaly may be due to metastatic disease in patients with cancer. Abdominal auscultation determines the presence and pitch of bowel sounds, and occasionally reveals an arterial bruit.

Digital rectal examination is essential. Three-quarters of rectal cancers and up to one-third of colon cancers can be felt rectally. An empty rectum in a patient with palpable faecal masses in the colon suggests rectosigmoid obstruction. A cancer in this region can sometimes be felt more easily if the patient turns on to the right side. After digital rectal examination, the withdrawn finger is inspected for blood and mucus, and any faeces are tested for occult blood.

Further investigations

The techniques used to investigate intestinal diseases are outlined in Chapter 6. In general, the small bowel is more difficult to assess than the large bowel, although long fibreoptic enteroscopes are available to inspect and biopsy the proximal small bowel. Small bowel radiology is also more difficult. A barium meal and follow-through is time-consuming, and it is better to instil barium directly through a tube placed in the duodenum (small bowel enema) and so avoid having to await gastric emptying.

PRINCIPLES OF BOWEL SURGERY

Small bowel surgery

Surgery involving the small intestine is usually less problematic than large bowel surgery. The small bowel has a more plentiful blood supply, a stronger wall, and a content which is liquid and has a lower bacterial count. After resection of a segment of small bowel, immediate end-to-end anastomosis can usually be performed with a much lower risk of anastomotic breakdown and leakage than occurs with large bowel anastomoses. The difference is particularly marked in emergency surgery as surgeons often opt to avoid immediate reanastomosis after emergency large bowel resection, exteriorizing one or both ends of the bowel on a temporary basis.

Consequences of small bowel resection

Life can be sustained after loss of the large bowel, but not after loss of the small bowel. The considerable functional reserve of the small bowel may be overcome by massive resection for conditions such as Crohn's disease or mesenteric ischaemia. The consequences of resection are determined by the length and position of the segment(s) resected, the underlying disease, retention or removal of the ileocaecal valve, and the ability of the remaining small bowel to undergo *adaptation*. Loss of absorptive area is compounded by rapid transit, disturbed neurohumoral control of gastric, pancreatic and biliary secretion, continued loss of bile salts, and reflux and overgrowth of bacteria from the colon. Massive gastric hypersecretion is common, due possibly to loss of intestinal inhibitory hormone(s), and the low luminal pH compounds malabsorption by inactivating intestinal lipase and trypsin.

Nutritional consequences are severe when more than 75% of the small bowel is lost. Loss of the jejunum impairs absorption of all nutrients, although the ileum compensates to some degree. Loss of the terminal ileum permanently impairs absorption of bile salts and vitamin B_{12}, whereas iron and folate are absorbed principally from the upper small bowel. Bile salts are cathartic to the colon, and depletion of the bile salt pool results in an increased incidence of gallstones (p. 487).

Severe diarrhoea causes rapid and profound fluid and electrolyte loss, although this usually diminishes within weeks as adaptation takes place. During adaptation the mucosa becomes hypertrophic, the villi increase in length, the crypts of Lieberkuhn deepen, and the bowel wall thickens.

Following massive small bowel resection, fluid and electrolyte loss must be replaced intravenously, parenteral nutrition instituted, and diarrhoea combated with agents such as codeine phosphate. Antisecretory drugs (e.g. ranitidine) are used if there is gastric hypersecretion. Oral isotonic fluids are commenced cautiously as diarrhoea abates, and feeding is resumed thereafter. Elemental diets may be useful initially and are often best given at a controlled rate through a fine-bore nasogastric or nasoenteric tube. Attempts are made to discontinue parenteral nutrition gradually, but long-term total parenteral nutrition is unavoidable in some patients (Ch. 5). It should be borne in mind that adaptation may continue for 12–24 months. The fat-soluble vitamins (A, D and K) are prescribed in those with malabsorption, and parenteral vitamin B_{12} is needed for life after terminal ileal resection.

Large bowel surgery

Pre-operative preparation for elective surgery

Counselling. Large bowel surgery frequently involves the need for a temporary or permanent stoma. This must be discussed fully with the patient and the site chosen before operation by fitting a trial appliance. A stoma-care nurse is invaluable, and a visit from a member of a local Ileostomy or Colostomy Association often provides valuable reassurance and support.

Anaemia and malnutrition. Anaemia must always be corrected, and malnourished patients may benefit from a period of nutritional support if surgery can be deferred.

Consequences of small bowel resection
- Effects are determined principally by length and part of small bowel that is resected, and by the underlying disease process.

- Rapid transit gives rise to diarrhoea with fluid and electrolyte loss, while massive gastric hypersecretion (loss of inhibitory factors) may inactivate pancreatic and intestinal enzymes (lipase and trypsin).

- Loss of the jejunum impairs absorption of all nutrients; iron and folate are absorbed principally from the upper small intestine.

- Loss of the terminal ileum impairs absorption of vitamin B_{12} and bile salts (with depletion of the bile-salt pool and an increased incidence of gallstones).

- Although the remaining small bowel is capable of considerable adaptation, nutritional problems are usually severe if more than 75% of the small bowel is lost.

- Long-term parenteral nutrition may be unavoidable in some patients although adaptation may continue for 12–24 months.

Bowel preparation. The risk of anastomotic leakage and wound sepsis is reduced if the large bowel is empty at the time of resection and if antibiotics are used.

Mechanical bowel preparation may be achieved by purgatives (e.g. picolax) and enemas given over 2–3 days before operation. Alternatively, the bowel can be emptied by whole-gut irrigation on the day before surgery; this involves passing a nasogastric tube and instilling 2–4 litres of crystalloid an hour until the effluent from the anus is clear. Metoclopramide (10 mg) and frusemide (20 mg) are given intramuscularly to accelerate gastric emptying and reduce the risk of pulmonary oedema. Whole gut irrigation and purgation must be avoided in patients with obstructing lesions, and irrigation is contraindicated in frail patients, particularly those with cardiac or renal disease.

Low residue diets can be given for 5 days before operation to ensure an empty colon and rectum, but many units use a 2-day 'no residue, fluids only' regimen.

Antibiotic prophylaxis is combined with mechanical cleansing. The aim of antibiotic therapy is not to 'sterilize' the gut but to provide high blood levels per-operatively. One dose is given at induction of anaesthesia, and another two doses at 8 and 16 hours. The antibiotics are given parenterally and a combination of cefuroxime (750 mg) and metronidazole (500 mg) is popular.

Urinary tract preparation. The ureter(s) can be invaded and obstructed by large bowel cancer, and can be damaged at operation. An excretion urogram is advised before surgery in patients with haematuria, evidence of obstructive uropathy or large rectal cancers.

A urinary catheter is inserted at the start of the operation to ensure that the bladder does not impede access to the pelvis. Postoperatively the catheter is retained to avoid urinary retention and allow hourly urine output to be monitored.

Pre-operative preparation for emergency surgery

Patients presenting with obstruction, perforation, toxic dilatation or bleeding may require emergency surgery. Hypovolaemia and sepsis are common, and adequate resuscitation is essential before anaesthesia. Lost extracellular fluid (ECF) is replaced by crystalloid solutions (e.g. 0.9% saline, usually with added potassium), while colloids and blood may also be needed when there is sepsis and/or blood loss.

Time is often not available for full preparation of the patient for a stoma but the possibility must be discussed before proceeding to surgery.

Operative technique

The extent of resection is governed by the nature of the disease. In malignant disease, the lesion is removed en bloc with an adequate margin of healthy bowel and as much of the regional lymphatic drainage system as possible. In benign disease, only the affected bowel and its immediate mesentery is removed.

If a stoma is not necessary, bowel continuity is restored by an end-to-end anastomosis which can be created by hand suture or stapling. The two ends of bowel must have an adequate blood supply and the anastomosis must be created without tension. This is more often a problem in large bowel anastomoses given the more tenuous blood supply, and adequate mobilization of the bowel is vital. It is also important that the bowel is as empty as possible. 'On table' colonic lavage can be used to empty a loaded colon and permit immediate anastomosis (Ch. 31).

Complications of intestinal surgery

Wound infection

Despite antibiotic prophylaxis, wound infection rates of 10% are not unusual after large bowel surgery. Endogenous gut bacteria are almost always responsible. Infection delays healing, may cause secondary bleeding, and favours wound dehiscence and hernia.

Anastomotic failure

This is more likely when emergency operation is carried out in unprepared bowel, and when operations involve the distal colon and rectum. Some leakage may be detectable radiologically in up to 50% of distal colo-rectal anastomoses, although this is clinically significant in less than 5% of cases. Leakage may lead to peritonitis, abscess and fistula formation (see below), wound infection, and septicaemia.

Treatment consists of resuscitation followed by surgical drainage, and usually requires exteriorization of the ends of bowel used for anastomosis.

Intestinal stomas

Stomas may be temporary or permanent. A permanent intestinal stoma is best sited on a line between the umbilicus and the anterior superior iliac spine, sufficiently far from both to allow easy fixation of an appliance. Temporary stomas may have to be positioned at other sites.

Ileostomy

An ileostomy stoma is fashioned so that a cuff of bowel protrudes from the skin (Fig. 29.4), facilitating delivery of the irritant small bowel content into an appliance and avoiding skin excoriation. The skin is protected further by using a well-fitting appliance and a protective barrier agent such as Karaya

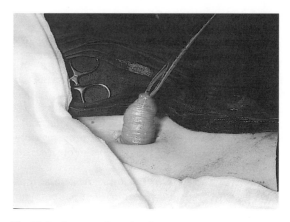

Fig. 29.4 Construction of an ileostomy.

gum. Ileostomy was once common following procto-colectomy for inflammatory bowel disease, but is now needed less frequently (see below).

Colostomy

Two types of colostomy are in common use. *Loop colostomy* (Fig. 29.5) is usually temporary and constructed by bringing a loop of colon to the surface. *End colostomy* may be permanent or temporary, and is created by bringing the divided end of bowel to the surface (Fig. 29.6).

Colostomies can be allowed to move spontaneously, in which case an appliance is worn permanently. These may be one-piece appliances with an adherent fenestrated patch incorporated into the back of a plastic bag, or two-piece appliances where the bag is attached to a moulded flange which adheres to the skin. An air vent can be incorporated into the bag in both cases. An alternative approach is to wash out the colon through the colostomy once a day. This may allow a simple dressing to be worn over the colostomy rather than an appliance. Regardless of the type of colostomy care, patients should avoid foods which cause looseness or excess flatus.

Fistula formation

A fistula is an abnormal communication between two surfaces lined by epithelium (or in the case of arterio-venous fistula, by endothelium). Intestinal fistulas may communicate with the skin (external fistula) or with another loop of bowel or other viscus (e.g. entero-colic and entero-vesical fistulas). Small bowel fistulas are frequently associated with high

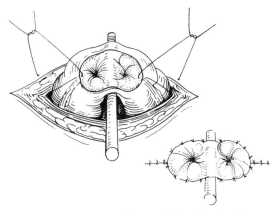

Fig. 29.5 Loop colostomy (the rod is kept in place for approximately 7 days).

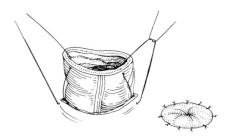

Fig. 29.6 End colostomy.

output of irritant fluid, and are usually more difficult to manage than 'low output' fistulas arising from the large bowel. External fistulas are most often a complication of surgery (over 90% of cases) but can arise spontaneously when the bowel is diseased.

Development of a postoperative fistula is heralded by pyrexia and tachycardia, followed by abdominal pain and tenderness. The clinical picture often suggests wound infection or abscess formation, but surgical incision of the 'abscess' or its spontaneous rupture results in flow of intestinal content. The principles of management of intestinal fistulas are as follows:

Replace fluid and electrolyte losses. Intravenous fluids are commenced and fluid balance is charted with daily measurement of serum urea and electrolytes. High output fistulas can lead to daily losses of 3–4 litres, with rapid dehydration and serious electrolyte deficits.

Ensure adequate external drainage. Material escaping from the bowel must have free egress from the abdomen to avoid abscess formation and disseminated peritonitis. Early surgery may be needed to ensure free drainage; at this stage no attempt is made to repair the site of leakage, but exteriorization of the ends of the anastomosed bowel may be advisable.

Provide nutritional support. Parenteral nutrition is usually required and may be life-saving. Oral intake is discontinued until closure has been achieved, and nasogastric aspiration may be advisable in patients with high fistula.

Protect the skin. Leaking small bowel content contains activated pancreatic enzymes and is very irritant to the skin. Leaking colonic content is less irritant, and leaking pure pancreatic juice (with enzymes which have not been activated by exposure to duodenal enterokinase) causes little or no skin excoriation. The wound margins can be protected by Stomahesive or Karaya gum, and by a snugly fitting ileostomy appliance. If an appliance cannot be attached, suction tubes placed within the fistula may prove useful.

Define whether there is distal obstruction. Most intestinal fistulas will close on conservative management *provided there is no distal obstruction.* Contrast radiology (using water soluble contrast) is used to assess the 'downstream' intestine once the patient is stable. A fistula will not close without surgery if there is distal obstruction or if it originates from bowel involved with Crohn's disease or neoplasia.

Genitourinary problems

Retention of urine is common following intestinal surgery, particularly in males with prostatic disease. The nervi erigentes may be damaged during operations on the rectum as they pass through the pelvis, resulting in loss of bladder motor activity, retention and overflow incontinence. If cystometric studies confirm parasympathetic denervation, the patient is given parasympathomimetic drugs (e.g. bethanecol) and may require bladder neck resection.

The ureters are at risk of damage during mobilization of the colon and rectum, while the prostatic and membranous urethra can be damaged during excision of the anorectum (see Ch. 36).

After rectal excision for cancer, one-third of males become impotent because of division of the nervi erigentes, while a further third are unable to ejaculate because of division of sympathetic nerves in the pelvic plexus. When undertaking rectal surgery for benign disease, particularly in younger males, it is vital to avoid these problems by keeping the plane of dissection close to the bowel.

INTESTINAL DIVERTICULA

Diverticula may be congenital or acquired, protrude from the mesenteric or antimesenteric border of the bowel, and contain some (false diverticula) or all (true diverticula) coats of the bowel wall. Acquired diverticula are most often caused by pulsion from luminal pressure, but can result from traction due to extrinsic disease.

DIVERTICULA OF THE SMALL INTESTINE

Meckel's diverticulum

This is the commonest congenital abnormality of the gastrointestinal tract (see Ch. 25, Fig. 25.5) and results from persistence of part of the vitello-

---

Intestinal fistula
- A fistula is an abnormal communication between two surfaces lined by epithelium (commonly an intestinal fistula involves other loops of bowel, bladder, vagina, or skin).
- Gastrointestinal fistulas may be a complication of surgery (90%) or intestinal disease (Crohn's disease, diverticular disease, carcinoma).
- Small bowel fistulas frequently have a high output (e.g. several litres per day) and irritate the skin (the fluid contains *activated* pancreatic ezymes).
- Large bowel fistulas are usually low output and do not irritate the skin.
- The principles of management are;
  - ensure adequate external drainage
  - maintain fluid and electrolyte balance
  - provide nutritional support (usually by parenteral nutrition)
  - protect the skin
  - ensure that there is no distal obstruction by contrast studies.
- In the absence of distal obstruction or intrinsic bowel disease (Crohn's disease or carcinoma) the great majority of fistulas will close with conservative management.

---

intestinal duct. The diverticulum arises from the antimesenteric border of the ileum some 2 feet from the ileocaecal valve in 2% of people and is on average 2 inches long (the 'rule of twos'). It is a true diverticulum and in 10% of cases its tip is connected to the umbilicus by a fibrous cord. Heterotopic mucosa is found in 50% of symptomatic diverticula and is most often acid-secreting gastric mucosa.

Clinical features

Only 5% of Meckel's diverticula cause symptoms, most frequently in childhood or early adult life. *Bleeding* due to peptic ulceration of the adjacent ileum is the commonest cause of severe gastrointestinal bleeding in childhood. *Intestinal obstruction* may be due to intussusception of the diverticulum, or a loop of bowel may become trapped beneath or twisted around (volvulus) a band extending to the umbilicus. *Acute diverticulitis* produces abdominal pain and tenderness, pyrexia and leucocytosis, and cannot be distinguished clinically from acute appendicitis. Perforation is a common complication.

Management

Symptomatic Meckel's diverticula are excised (Fig. 29.7). Asymptomatic diverticula found inciden-

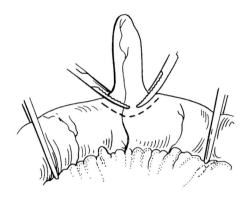

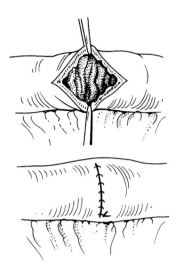

Fig. 29.7 Method of excision of Meckel's diverticulum.

tally at laparotomy need not be excised unless they have a narrow neck or nodularity suggests that they contain abnormal mucosa. In patients with unexplained gastrointestinal bleeding, heterotopic mucosa within a Meckel's diverticulum can be detected by scintiscanning after injection of ^{99m}Tc-labelled sodium pertechnetate (which is taken up by parietal cells).

Jejunal diverticulosis

False diverticula of the jejunum (and less often of the ileum) can develop with age. They are wide-mouthed sacs caused by herniation of mucosa into the mesentery at the site of vessel penetration of the gut wall. The diverticula are often asymptomatic but can cause bleeding, inflammation, malabsorption (due to their contained bacteria), and perforation. They can be demonstrated by barium studies and the affected segment of bowel may have to be resected if the diverticula are causing problems.

DIVERTICULA OF THE LARGE INTESTINE

Diverticulum of the caecum

Solitary diverticulum of the caecum is a rare congenital lesion. The diverticulum arises from the medial wall close to the ileocaecal valve, and can extend upwards retroperitoneally. It may become obstructed by a faecolith and inflamed, producing a clinical picture indistinguishable from appendicitis.

Repeated inflammation and fibrosis may leave a solitary ulcer of the caecum. At laparotomy, it may be impossible to distinguish from carcinoma, and right hemicolectomy is indicated.

Diverticular disease of the colon

Given the rarity of other forms of diverticular disease, the term 'diverticular disease' is usually taken to mean acquired colonic diverticular disease unless otherwise specified. Such diverticula are rare before the age of 35, but by 65, at least one-third of the population are affected. The diverticula are most common in the sigmoid colon and emerge between the mesenteric and antimesenteric taeniae. They result from the herniation of mucosa through the circular muscle at the sites of penetration of blood vessels (Fig. 29.8). Diverticular disease is associated

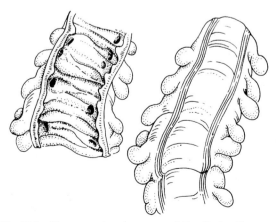

Fig. 29.8 Macroscopic appearance of diverticular disease.

with increased intraluminal pressure in the large bowel and muscular hypertrophy can be detected radiologically before diverticula develop. In general, the disease is uncommon in societies whose staple diet is high in roughage.

Uncomplicated diverticular disease

The disease may be asymptomatic or give rise to intermittent lower abdominal and left iliac fossa pain, altered bowel habit (usually constipation) and occasional minor rectal bleeding. The sigmoid colon is sometimes tender. Barium enema reveals muscle thickening and multiple diverticula (Fig. 29.9).

Most patients improve on a high-fibre diet supplemented if necessary by bran or a bulk laxative such as methylcellulose. Stimulant laxatives and purgatives are best avoided. Antispasmodics such as propantheline or dicyclomine may be useful if there is smooth muscle spasm.

Sigmoid colectomy with end-to-end anastomosis is indicated if there are persistent symptoms or when carcinoma cannot be excluded by radiology or colonoscopy. The need for a temporary 'protective' proximal colostomy has been largely eliminated by pre-operative bowel preparation, or with 'on table' lavage if the bowel is still loaded at surgery.

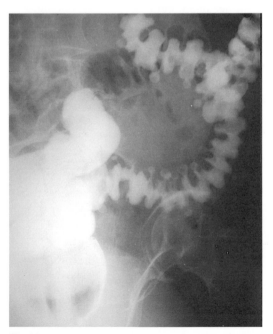

Fig. 29.9 Radiological appearance on barium enema of diverticular disease of the sigmoid colon.

Complications of diverticular disease

Inflammation. Inflammation of a diverticulum may spread to cause peridiverticulitis. There is pyrexia, leucocytosis, nausea and vomiting, and alteration in bowel habit with pain and tenderness in the left iliac fossa. A mass may be palpable despite muscle guarding. The patient is confined to bed, and given nil by mouth, intravenous fluids and antibiotics. Failure to settle suggests that pericolic abscess is developing and that surgical drainage may be needed. Up to one-third of patients admitted with acute diverticular disease undergo surgery during the index admission, half settle and have no further attacks, and 10% eventually require surgery.

Perforation. Rupture of a pericolic abscess gives rise to purulent peritonitis, while free perforation of the bowel produces faecal peritonitis. The patient is usually profoundly ill with septic shock, dehydration, marked abdominal pain, tenderness and distension. Perforation is particularly likely in patients who are immunosuppressed or receiving steroids, and often presents insidiously. The patient is resuscitated vigorously and treated urgently by resection of the affected bowel and peritoneal lavage. Immediate end-to-end anastomosis is not advisable in the face of peritonitis and the bowel ends are both exteriorized (one serving as an end colostomy and the other as a mucous fistula; or the proximal end only is brought to the surface while the rectum is oversewn and left in the abdomen (Hartmann's procedure). Whichever approach is adopted, continuity is restored after bowel preparation some 6–8 weeks later. The mortality of perforated diverticular disease is still about 10–20% and may be as high as 50% in the elderly with faecal peritonitis. In some cases, the patient is so old and frail that a further operation to restore intestinal continuity is not deemed advisable.

Obstruction. Obstruction may be due to oedema or fibrosis in the inflamed segment of colon, or to adherence of small bowel loops. At operation, it may be impossible to distinguish diverticular disease from cancer. Modern management now consists of resection of the involved segment with end-to-end anastomosis (if safe) or a Hartmann's procedure (with later restoration of continuity; see Ch. 31).

Stricture formation. Long-standing diverticular disease may cause stricture formation and subacute intestinal obstruction. Such strictures can be difficult to distinguish from malignant strictures, but are usually longer, show gradual rather than abrupt transition from normal bowel, have associated diverticula and retain an intact mucosa. The presence of diverticula on barium enema does not exclude cancer as the conditions are both common and often coexist. Resection is needed in both cases.

Fistula. Diverticular disease can give rise to fistulas to the skin or other viscera, notably the bladder, small bowel and vagina. It is the commonest cause of *colovesical fistula*, a complication which is less common in women because the uterus is interposed between bladder and sigmoid colon. The patient usually complains of dysuria and passage of a cloudy urine with bubbling on micturition (pneumaturia). The diagnosis is best confirmed by barium enema. Treatment consists of sigmoid colectomy and bladder repair.

Bleeding. Massive rectal bleeding can be caused by sigmoid diverticular disease but in up to two-thirds of cases, bleeding originates from other sources and diverticular disease is incidental. Angiodysplasia (particularly of the right colon), polyps and diverticula elsewhere may all be responsible. Angiography is a valuable (although not foolproof) means of localizing the lesion so that the involved segment of bowel can be resected. If operation has to be undertaken when a source of bleeding has not been localized, total colectomy and ileorectal anastomosis is advised.

INFLAMMATORY BOWEL DISEASE

CROHN'S DISEASE

Crohn's disease was first described in 1932 by Crohn and his associates at the Mount Sinai Hospital, New York as a disease which affected the terminal ileum. It is now clear that any part of the gastrointestinal tract can be involved. Both small and large bowel are affected in one-half of all cases and in one-quarter, the large bowel alone is involved. The incidence appears to have risen to 5–10 cases per 100 000 per year in Western countries. The cause remains unknown but nutritional deficits, increased intestinal permeability and immunological factors have been postulated.

Pathological features (Table. 29.1)

Macroscopically, Crohn's disease produces a cobblestone appearance in which oedematous islands of mucosa are separated by crevices or fissures which can extend through all coats of the bowel wall. Serpiginous ulceration is common, and fibrosis

---

Complications of colonic diverticular disease

Inflammation
- Peridiverticulitis causes pain and tenderness in the left iliac fossa, alteration of bowel habit, fever and leucocytosis, and may produce a palpable mass.
- Surgery may be needed if a pericolic abscess develops.

Intestinal obstruction
- Obstruction may be due to oedema or fibrosis, or to involvement of adherent small bowel loops.
- If emergency surgery is necessary, the Hartmann operation is often performed (resection of the involved segment and temporary end colostomy), although resection with immediate anastomosis is now often feasible.

Perforation
- Perforation of a pericolic abscess gives rise to purulent peritonitis.
- Frank perforation of the colon produces faecal peritonitis (and a greater morbidity and mortality than purulent peritonitis).
- Immediate end-to-end anastomosis is inadvisable in the presence of peritonitis so that the bowel ends are exteriorized after resection of the perforated segment or a Hartmann's procedure is performed.

Fistula formation
- Diverticular disease is the commonest cause of a colovesical fistula (although vagina, other loops of bowel and the skin may be involved).
- Patients with a colovesical fistula frequently present with pneumaturia and complain of a bubbling sensation when passing urine.

Bleeding
- In one-third of patients with major lower GI bleeding, diverticular disease is responsible. Angiodysplasia is another common cause of such bleeding.
- Angiography may be helpful in localizing the site of haemorrhage but it is far from foolproof and total colectomy with ileorectal anastomosis is advisable if surgery becomes necessary

---

produces strictures which can be single or multiple, short or long. Multiple areas of inflammation are common but intervening bowel appears normal (i.e. skip lesions). Penetration of the disease leads to serosal inflammation, adhesion to neighbouring structures, and sinus or fistula formation.

Microscopically, these are deep clefts and fissures (which can be transmural), oedema, and inflammatory cell infiltrates with foci of lymphocytes. In

Table 29.1	Comparison of ulcerative colitis and Crohn's disease	
Criterion	Ulcerative colitis	Crohn's disease
Incidence	5–10 per 100 000 static	5–10 per 100 000 rising
Extent	Large bowel only	May involve entire gastrointestinal tract
Rectal involvement	Almost invariable	Variable
Disease continuity	Continuous	Discontinuous
Depth of inflammation	Mucosal	Transmural
Mucosal appearance	Multiple small ulcers Pseudopolyps	Cobblestone, discrete deep ulcers and fissures
Histological features	Crypt abscesses No granulomas	Transmural inflammation Granulomas (50%)
Presence of anal lesions	25% of cases	75% of cases with large bowel disease 25% of cases with small bowel disease
Frequency of fistula	Uncommon	10–20% of cases
Risk of developing cancer	Significant	Cancer rare

50% of cases there are non-caseating granulomas similar to those found in sarcoid.

One-quarter of patients with small bowel Crohn's disease and three-quarters of those with large bowel disease have anal lesions such as ulceration, abscesses, oedematous skin tags, fissure and fistula.

Clinical features

Crohn's disease is a chronic disorder with exacerbations and remissions and a varied clinical presentation. Continuous or episodic diarrhoea is associated with recurring abdominal pain and tenderness, lassitude and fever. Declining general health, malabsorption, weight loss and retardation of growth (in children) are common.

Examination often reveals malnutrition and a palpable abdominal mass. *Intestinal obstruction* may result from oedematous inflammation, adhesion formation or fibrosis. Typically, there are bouts of subacute intestinal obstruction but complete obstruction may demand surgical intervention. *Fistula formation* occurs in 20% of patients with small and large bowel disease and in 10% of those with large bowel disease only. The fistula may communicate with other loops of bowel, other viscera (e.g. bladder, vagina), or the skin. External fistulas are most often the result of surgical intervention and commonly involve the skin of the anterior abdominal wall or perineum. *Abscesses* can result from sub-

clinical bowel perforation. Free perforation is uncommon because the inflamed segment usually adheres to surrounding structures. Although less common than in ulcerative colitis, *toxic dilatation* can complicate colonic disease, and *carcinoma of the colon* is a rare complication of long-standing disease. *Anal complications* can be particularly troublesome. For example, anal fissures are often multiple and indolent and extend to involve any part of the perineum including the vagina or scrotum.

Systemic manifestations include iritis, ankylosing spondylitis, liver disease (e.g. sclerosing cholangitis) and erythema nodosum. Disease of the terminal ileum or its resection increases the incidence of gallstones (by depleting the bile salt pool).

Investigation

General assessment includes evaluation of nutritional status and search for anaemia. Proliferative changes in the bowel wall produce radiological evidence of thickening, luminal narrowing and separation of loops, and are often associated with ulceration, spike-like fissures and a cobblestone appearance (Fig. 29.10). Fibrosis can produce strictures of variable length, and skip lesions and fistula formation may be apparent.

Proctoscopy, sigmoidoscopy and colonoscopy are used to assess the presence and extent of large bowel disease. Biopsy during sigmoidoscopy and colono-

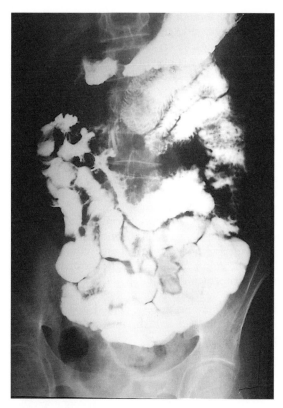

Fig. 29.10 Barium meal and follow-through examination in Crohn's disease showing strictures in the distal ileum.

scopy may reveal disease in macroscopically normal bowel.

Treatment

Medical management

Anaemia is corrected and malnourishment is managed by a high-protein, low-residue diet and provision of vitamins. Hydrophilic colloid preparations and codeine phosphate may help diarrhoea, and cholestyramine can be used to bind bile salts and prevent their cathartic effects on the colon in patients with small bowel disease.

Steroids are used in the acute phase (prednisone 30–60 mg daily by mouth) to reduce inflammatory manifestations, but long-term steroid therapy is avoided. Large bowel disease often responds to sulfasalazine (3–4 g daily by mouth) but small bowel disease is unaffected given that colonic bacteria are required to metabolize the compound to its active principles, sulfapyridine and 5-aminosalicylate. In general, small bowel disease is managed by steroids and large bowel disease by sulfasalazine; combination therapy confers no added benefit. Azathioprine (2 mg/kg daily) can be used in resistant cases.

Surgical management

Almost 90% of patients with Crohn's disease require surgery at some stage. As surgery is not curative in a disease which is often more widespread than it appears, operation is usually reserved for patients who are not thriving on medical management or who have complications (notably obstruction, abscess, perforation and fistula). The aim of surgery is to resect the segment(s) of bowel causing problems, avoid removing uninvolved bowel, and maintain intestinal continuity if at all possible. Extended 'radical' operations are contraindicated as the risk of recurrence is determined more by the natural history of the individual's disease than the extent of surgery. The recurrence rate after resection of small bowel disease is around 33%, as opposed to less than 20% in colonic disease. Bypass of affected segments is no longer recommended. Surgery carries an operative mortality of up to 5%, largely attributable to sepsis, and late deaths bring overall mortality to around 10%.

ULCERATIVE COLITIS

This disease has an annual incidence of 5–10 new cases per 100 000 per year in Western countries. The cause is unknown but most interest centres on an immunological basis. The disease affects all age groups with a peak incidence in young adult life. Whereas the incidence of Crohn's disease appears to be rising, that of ulcerative colitis is static.

Ulcerative colitis is primarily a disease of the large bowel, although systemic manifestations (iritis, arthritis, hepatitis, pyoderma gangrenosum) can occur. In 95% of cases the disease is diffuse, starting in the rectum and extending proximally, often involving the entire colon (see Table 29.1). In 5% of cases, it is segmental and the rectum is occasionally spared.

Pathological features

The characteristic feature of ulcerative colitis is formation of crypt abscesses in the depths of the mucosa. The abscesses have a surrounding inflammatory infiltrate and coalesce to form ulcers which undermine the mucosa. The intervening mucosa becomes oedematous and may form inflammatory pseudopolyps. The bowel loses its haustrations and becomes thick and rigid, although strictures are uncommon. During an exacerbation, the colon may become dilated and paper-thin (toxic dilatation).

Clinical features

Ulcerative colitis characteristically runs an intermittent course of relapse and remission, although a chronic continuous variant is described. In some cases, the initial attack is fulminant, and toxic dilatation with exacerbation of abdominal and systemic symptoms may occur at any time. Diarrhoea with the passage of mucus and blood is typical of relapse. Passage of 10–15 stools a day is not unusual and there is often incapacitating urgency. Abdominal pain and tenderness may be present and intermittent pyrexia is common.

Rectal examination includes careful inspection to detect anal complications such as fissure, fistula and haemorrhoids which are present in 25% of cases. The rectal mucosa often feels thick and boggy.

Sigmoidoscopy (with biopsy) is the key investigation and reveals a red, matt, granular mucosa with contact bleeding.

Complications such as toxic dilatation, bleeding and the development of cancer are considered below.

Investigations

A barium enema is valuable to assess the extent of disease, but is contraindicated in the acute phase for fear of precipitating perforation. Typical changes include loss of haustrations, fluffy granularity of the mucosa, and pseudopolyps (Fig. 29.11A & B). Ultimately, the bowel may become short and featureless so that it resembles a smooth tube. Undermining ulcers can create a double contour to the edge of the colon. Widening of the retrorectal space, due to perirectal inflammation and reduced distensibility of the rectum, is common. So-called 'backwash ileitis' may produce a dilated and featureless terminal ileum, in which the mucosa appears granular.

In an acute attack, plain films of the abdomen

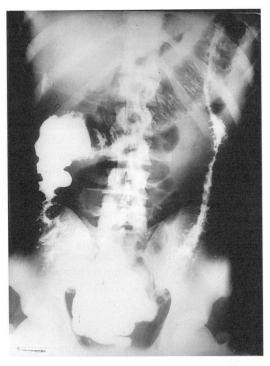

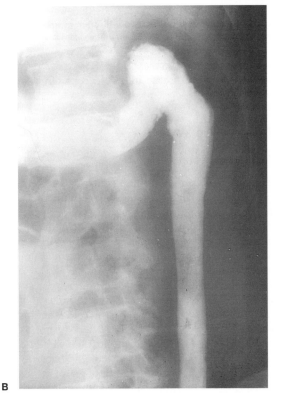

Fig. 29.11 Radiological appearances in ulcerative colitis. A: plain abdominal film showing toxic dilatation of the transverse colon. B: barium enema in long-standing colitis showing a featureless colon with loss of haustrations.

B

may reveal a dilated gas-filled colon in which pseudopolyps are evident. When toxic dilatation is suspected, daily plain films are essential to monitor progress.

Treatment

Medical management

With fluid and electrolyte replacement, correction of anaemia, adequate nutrition and steroid therapy, and timely surgical intervention when appropriate, 97% of patients survive their first attack, although 70% are destined to have further attacks. Systemic steroids (prednisone 10–15 mg orally every 6 hours) are needed during an acute relapse, and topical steroids (prednisone enemas or suppositories) usually control mild attacks. Long-term sulfasalazine (0.5–1 g orally every 6 hours) reduces the risk of relapse when a patient is in remission. Some 15% of patients eventually require surgery. The risk varies from 1 in 50 for those with mild proctitis, to 1 in 20 for those with moderately severe colitis, to 1 in 3 for those with extensive disease.

Elective surgery

Failure to thrive, as reflected in retardation of growth and sexual development in children or malnourishment and anaemia in adults, is a common indication for operation. Local complications which strengthen the decision to operate include stricture, perianal complications and recto-vaginal fistula. Strictures are more common in Crohn's disease than ulcerative colitis, and colonoscopy is indicated to exclude carcinoma. Some complications (e.g. arthritis and eye problems) remit after removal of the diseased bowel, but others (e.g. ankylosing spondylitis and liver disease) do not.

Risk of superimposed large bowel cancer is a major factor in the decision to operate. At least 10% of patients who have had ulcerative colitis for 10 years develop carcinoma, the risk rising to 20% after 20 years. Malignancy is more likely in patients with early-onset and extensive disease, and the mean age for development of cancer in colitics (43 years) is 20 years earlier than in the non-colitic population. It follows that patients with ulcerative colitis should be screened annually by colonoscopy and biopsy of any suspicious areas. However, carcinoma is often difficult to detect in colitis, is usually poorly differentiated, and has a poor prognosis, so that long-standing disease may be an indication for operation in its own right.

The classical operation of pan-proctocolectomy for ulcerative colitis ensured removal of the entire large bowel mucosa but at the expense of a permanent ileostomy. The alternative of colectomy and ileorectal anastomosis was limited by continuing proctitis and diarrhoea and the need to maintain regular surveillance for rectal cancer. Recently there has been an increasing trend to remove the colon and rectum, retain the anal sphincters, and fashion a pouch of ileum which is then anastomosed to the anal canal. A temporary ileostomy is used to protect the ileorectal anastomosis until healing has been assured. This approach removes all 'at risk' mucosa without sacrificing continence, although many patients continue to pass 4–6 motions a day.

Emergency surgery

Perforation (5% of cases), toxic dilatation (5% of cases) and massive bleeding (rare) are all indications for emergency surgery. Acute fulminant colitis which fails to respond promptly to aggressive medical therapy may also mandate urgent operation. Emergency pan-proctocolectomy carries an operative mortality of up to 20% so that it is usual to remove the colon, leave the rectum and form an ileostomy. The rectum is removed subsequently if active disease persists.

OTHER INFLAMMATORY DISEASES OF THE INTESTINE

A large number of infections and infestations of the intestine can cause diarrhoea, abdominal pain and tenderness, and may cause problems in diagnosis. In general, such problems (e.g. shigellosis, salmonellosis, amoebiasis) are more common in tropical medicine and are usually managed by medical rather than surgical means. The remainder of this section will be devoted to inflammatory conditions with surgical implications.

Hypertrophic tuberculous colitis

This condition is rare outside Asia and the tropics. The colon becomes thickened because of granulomatous infiltration, fibrosis and caseation. Strictures may form and the mucosa appears cobblestoned and ulcerated. The patient presents with abdominal pain, alteration in bowel habit and passage of blood and mucus. Differentiation from Crohn's disease and carcinoma may prove difficult, and a number of other infections (e.g. schistosomiasis, amoebiasis and lymphogranuloma venereum) may also cause stricture formation. Resection of strictured bowel may be the only way to exclude cancer. Antituberculous chemotherapy is commenced once the presence of tuberculosis has been confirmed.

Irradiation damage

External and internal irradiation for carcinoma of the bladder or cervix can cause proctocolitis and enteritis. In the acute phase, oedema, inflammation and ulceration produce diarrhoea, lower abdominal pain, tenesmus, mucus discharge and rectal bleeding. Subsequently, the bowel may thicken with fibrosis and stricture. Radiation also damages the vascular endothelium and endarteritis compounds mucosal damage. Topical steroids may give symptomatic relief when there is proctitis. Stricture and fistula formation usually require resection of the affected bowel.

Pseudomembranous colitis

This condition is associated with the use of oral antibiotics, particularly clindamycin, although no antibiotics are free from this side-effect. It was once thought that staphylococcal superinfection was responsible but it is now appreciated that *Clostridium difficile* is usually to blame. Necrosis of the colorectal mucosa causes watery diarrhoea, toxaemia, shock and collapse. The stools are watery-green, foul-smelling and blood-stained, and often contain fragments of mucosal slough (pseudomembrane). The pseudomembrane is often visible on sigmoidoscopy and a biopsy confirms the diagnosis. Detection of *C. difficile* or its cytotoxin in the stool is also used to aid diagnosis. Treatment consists of intravenous fluid replacement and vancomycin (125 mg orally every 6 hours for 10 days).

MEGACOLON

Hirschsprung's disease

This congenital condition affects 1 in 5000 babies and is due to absence of ganglion cells from Auerbach's and Meissner's plexus. A 5–20-cm length of the distal large bowel is usually affected, although longer segments can be involved. Loss of peristalsis in the affected segment leads to large bowel obstruction with gross distension of the proximal intestine. The differential diagnosis in the

---

Inflammatory diseases of the intestines
- Infectious diarrhoeas due to conditions such as shigellosis, salmonellosis and amoebiasis are usually managed by medical means, but strictures can complicate infection with tuberculosis, schistosomiasis and amoebiasis.

- Crohn's disease:
  - often causes diarrhoea, obstruction, fistula, perforation and abscess
  - is frequently complicated by perianal disease
  - is occasionally complicated by the development of carcinoma
  - may be accompanied by systemic effects (iritis, sclerosing cholangitis, erythema nodosum, anaemia, gallstones and malnutrition).

- Ulcerative colitis:
  - causes diarrhoea with loss of fluid, mucus and blood
  - may be complicated by perianal disease, toxic dilatation and carcinoma
  - may be accompanied by systemic effects (arthritis, iritis, ankylosing spondylitis, sclerosing cholangitis).

- Pseudomembranous colitis is a complication of antibiotic use, due to infection with *Clostridium difficile*; it is treated with vancomycin.

- Irradiation damage to the gut may cause inflammation in the acute stage with subsequent development of fibrosis and stricture. Radiation proctitis and enteritis are often the result of irradiation of the cervix or bladder.

---

neonate includes imperforate anus and meconium ileus (a complication of cystic fibrosis in which the gut is plugged by inspissated mucus), and in older children, megacolon acquired from chronic constipation. Ischaemic colitis can develop because of gross distension in all forms of megacolon.

Barium enema reveals dilated bowel above the narrowed aganglionic segment, and lack of ganglia can be confirmed by full thickness biopsy of the abnormal area. In neonates, treatment consists of irrigation of the bowel with saline followed by operation at about 6 weeks to bring ganglionated bowel down to the anal verge. In older children, a preliminary colostomy may be needed to allow the bowel to decompress.

Acquired megacolon

Chronic constipation in childhood can result in megacolon and megarectum. The initial complaint is often faecal soiling. Examination reveals that the colon and the rectum are loaded with faeces. The condition may have a psychological or psychosocial overlay in association with bad toilet training, and can be accompanied by enuresis or anorectal pathology such as an anal fissure. The aim of treatment is to restore muscle tone and function by preventing constipation. This may require faecal disimpaction under general anaesthesia followed by regular colonic washouts.

INTESTINAL ISCHAEMIA

Intestinal ischaemia may result from any of the conditions listed in Table 29.2. Arterial inflow occlusion is commoner than venous outflow occlusion, and is most often due to thrombosis or embolization of the SMA. One-third of patients dying from acute ischaemic necrosis of the midgut have no demonstrable occlusion of a major vessel, and low flow (e.g. due to cardiac failure or arrhythmia) causes non-occlusive infarction. Once ischaemic necrosis has occurred there are three potential outcomes:

1. Progression to necrosis of all bowel layers with gangrene and perforation
2. Full recovery (if flow is restored within 6 hours, the maximum survival time of intestinal muscle deprived of blood flow)
3. Slow resolution of a short segment of ischaemia with fibrosis and formation of a short concentric stricture.

Table 29.2 Causes of intestinal ischaemia	
Arterial inflow occlusion	Atheroma
	Thrombosis
	Superimposed on atheroma
	Polycythaemia
	Sickle cell disease
	Disseminated intravascular
	coagulation
	Oral contraceptive pill
	Embolus
	Aortic disease
	Arteritis
	Polyarteritis nodosa
	Radiation angiitis
	Takayasu's disease
	Neoplasia (rare)
	Iatrogenic injury (operation/ angiography)
Venous outflow occlusion	Associated factors include neoplasia, oral contraceptive pill, infection, portal hypertension
Non-occlusive infarction	Associated factors include ventricular failure, cardiac arrhythmia, heart surgery, shock

Acute intestinal failure

Acute SMA occlusion is predominantly a disease of the elderly and is increasing in frequency. It leads to complete necrosis and gangrene of most of the midgut, and massive resection is inevitable unless flow can be restored within 6 hours. Even if the patient survives, the resulting nutritional problems may prove overwhelming, particularly in the elderly.

Clinical features

Early diagnosis is difficult as the symptoms and signs are so non-specific. A high index of suspicion is essential and a prodrome of chronic or episodic abdominal pain associated with meals, diarrhoea and weight loss, may provide a valuable clue. Cardiac arrhythmias, notably atrial fibrillation, are often present. There is usually abdominal pain, vomiting, and in one-third of cases, watery or bloody diarrhoea. The pain varies in its location (central or epigastric), severity (mild to agonizing), and nature (constant or colicky). Abdominal tenderness, guarding and rigidity are late signs denoting gangrene and perforation, and cardiovascular collapse denotes hypovolaemia and sepsis.

Investigations

Plain abdominal films may reveal atheroma (e.g. calcified aorta) or gas-filled dilated and thickened small bowel loops. Linear streaks of gas in the bowel wall or free gas in the peritoneal cavity are late signs of grave import. Arteriography is confirmatory but time is seldom available because of late presentation. Leucocytosis and hyperamylasaemia are common. In most cases, laparotomy is indicated on clinical grounds.

Treatment

Laparotomy is undertaken promptly after vigorous resuscitation. Gangrenous bowel requires resection but resection of the entire midgut in elderly patients is futile. In some cases of acute SMA occlusion, arterial flow can be restored by embolectomy or thrombectomy. Conservatism is recommended when the mesenteric vessels are pulsating despite evidence of ischaemic bowel. When bowel of doubtful viability is left in the abdomen, 'second look' laparotomy can be undertaken 24 hours later. The prognosis of acute intestinal failure is poor with an overall mortality of 70–90%. Survival is virtually confined to patients in whom a defined vascular occlusion is treated early. Mesenteric venous occlusion has an equally bad prognosis and treatment is usually confined to resection of gangrenous bowel and anticoagulation.

Ischaemic colitis

In addition to its involvement in SMA occlusion, the colon can become ischaemic without small bowel ischaemia. Ligation of the IMA (e.g. during resection of an aortic aneurysm) is occasionally responsible, but in most cases ischaemia arises spontaneously from thrombosis of the IMA or non-occlusive infarction.

Transient ischaemic colitis

In almost 50% of cases, ischaemia is transient and damage is confined to the mucosa and submucosa. The patient presents with lower abdominal pain, nausea, vomiting and bloody diarrhoea, and there may be a history of previous attacks or 'abdominal angina' after meals. Examination reveals tenderness and guarding, often maximal in the lower left abdomen. Sigmoidoscopy is usually normal but plain films and barium enemas reveal mucosal

sloughing and 'thumbprinting' due to oedema and bleeding into the bowel wall (Fig. 29.12A & B). Varying lengths of the colon are involved but the splenic flexure and sigmoid colon are most often affected.

The condition is treated conservatively unless abdominal signs suggest that peritonitis is developing. Symptoms normally resolve within days and resolution can be checked by repeat barium enema.

Gangrenous ischaemic colitis

Some 10% of patients with ischaemic colitis present with gangrene. The presentation and management are as described for acute intestinal failure.

Ischaemic stricture

In almost 50% of cases, ischaemic colitis does not produce gangrene but progresses to stricture formation. Serial barium enemas reveal a narrowed area of bowel with a funnelled appearance at either end. Persistent bleeding and pain suggest that a stricture is forming. The splenic flexure and left colon are the common sites affected. Most patients ultimately require resection but a minority improve spontaneously.

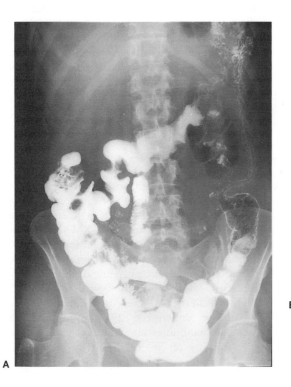

A

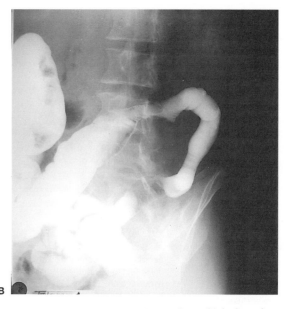

B

Fig. 29.12 A: barium enema in a patient with ischaemic colitis showing oedema and appearance of thumbprinting in transverse colon. B: barium enema showing resolving ischaemic stricture at the splenic flexure.

Chronic intestinal ischaemia

Chronic midgut ischaemia is a rare and controversial condition in which severe epigastric pain is experienced 15–20 minutes after meals (abdominal angina). There may be other evidence of vascular disease, malabsorption and weight loss, and a bruit in the epigastrium. If selective angiography reveals occlusion of one or more of the three visceral arteries, surgical revascularization may be considered. The *coeliac axis compression syndrome* is a variant in which surgery may be contemplated to relieve compression from the median arcuate ligament of the diaphragm.

Focal ischaemia of the small bowel

This rare focal stricture follows strangulation by bands and hernia, traumatic mesenteric haematoma, radiation enteritis and ischaemia induced by drugs such as enteric-coated potassium tablets. Subacute small bowel obstruction may necessitate resection of the stricture.

SMALL BOWEL NEOPLASMS

Small bowel tumours account for less than 5% of all gastrointestinal neoplasms.

Benign tumours

Solitary neoplasms include adenomatous or villous polyps, hamartomas, lipomas, haemangiomas and leiomyomas. Multiple hamartomas are found in the Peutz-Jeghers syndrome in association with brown or blue spots on the lips, buccal mucosa and digits, and diffuse gastrointestinal polyps. The hamartomatous polyps are not true neoplasms so have no malignant potential. Operation is indicated if there are symptoms (e.g. obstruction from intussusception or bleeding).

Malignant tumours

Adenocarcinomas

These are the commonest malignant tumours of the small bowel but are still rare. The periampullary area and duodenum are most often involved. Periampullary tumours frequently present with biliary obstruction (Ch. 33), while other small bowel tumours usually present with obstruction. Resection

of the affected segment is carried out where possible, but palliative bypass may be all that is possible.

Lymphomas

Lymphomas of the small bowel can cause obstruction, bleeding or perforation. Resection may be needed if complications develop, and the disease is staged before planning further systemic or local treatment.

Carcinoid tumours

Carcinoid tumours of the small bowel (the second commonest site for carcinoids after the appendix) have often metastasized to lymph nodes by the time of presentation. Obstruction and bleeding are not uncommon. The primary tumour should be resected where possible (see Ch. 19).

LARGE BOWEL NEOPLASMS

Benign tumours such as lipoma are rare in the large bowel. Polyps and carcinoma are the major problems and will be discussed in detail.

POLYPS

Non-neoplastic polyps

Hamartomas may be found as solitary *juvenile polyps* in young children or as multiple polyps in the *Peutz-Jeghers syndrome*.

Neoplastic polyps

Adenomatous polyps

These account for 90% of all colonic neoplastic polyps. They vary from small seed-like excrescences to large pedunculated masses which can be several centimetres in diameter. They are frequently multiple and their distribution is similar to that of large bowel cancer (see below). Histologically they consist of a mass of glandular tubules fed by a central fibrovascular core and covered by a mucous membrane of varying degrees of differentiation.

At least 5% of the population have adenomatous polyps. Most polyps are symptomless but they can bleed, intussuscept and even prolapse through the anus. They can be seen on colonoscopy or air-contrast barium enema, and be removed colonoscopically using a diathermy snare.

Adenomatous polyps are premalignant lesions and once they exceed 1 cm in diameter, the risk of malignancy rises to 5%. Histological examination must include a search for malignancy and invasion of the stalk. Once a polyp has been diagnosed the large bowel mucosa should be regarded as 'at risk' and the patient followed by regular colonoscopy (or barium examination).

Villous adenomas

These tumours account for 10% of all large bowel neoplasms, and are most often found in the rectum or sigmoid colon. They form soft shaggy sessile growths which spread to involve a considerable area of mucosa. A villous adenoma is also a premalignant lesion and invasive cancer is found in at least one-third of cases. Excessive mucus discharge is the common presenting symptom and may give rise to hypokalaemia, weakness, oliguria and alkalosis. The lesion is often palpable rectally and visible on sigmoidoscopy. Bleeding or areas of induration suggest malignancy. Biopsy will confirm the diagnosis, but given the focal nature of malignancy, a benign biopsy does not exclude malignant transformation. For this reason, all villous adenomas are excised. Transanal excision may be feasible but larger tumours require formal resection of the affected portion of bowel.

Familial adenomatous polyposis

This rare autosomal dominant syndrome is caused by an inherited defect in the adenomatous polyposis coli (APC) gene on chromosome 5. As expected, males and females are affected equally and the chances are that half the children in a given family will be affected. The genetic abnormality is always expressed so that the disease is transmitted only by those who suffer from it. Sessile and pedunculated adenomas develop during childhood and the large bowel is carpeted by hundreds of adenomas. Symptoms often develop between the ages of 10 and 15 years and consist of bleeding, diarrhoea and mucous discharge. Malignant change is inevitable in individuals who have familial polyposis but is virtually unknown before the age of 20 years.

Treatment consists of removing all of the mucosa at risk. At one time this meant proctocolectomy with permanent ileostomy, but it is now possible to remove all of the large bowel and anastomose the anal canal to an ileal pouch. The ideal time for surgery is at about school-leaving age. Individuals affected by polyposis also have a high risk of devel-

oping adenomatous polyps in the duodenum which may progress to periampullary cancer.

Although rare, familial polyposis has important implications. All family members must be screened to see whether they have polyps if malignancy is to be avoided. Polyposis registers are being introduced to facilitate such screening programmes.

Gardner's syndrome. This is an even rarer but related condition in which sebaceous cysts, dermoid cysts, bony exostoses and connective tissue tumours are found in association with multiple adenomas.

LARGE BOWEL CARCINOMA

Carcinoma of the colon and rectum is second only to lung cancer as a cause of cancer death in Western countries (p. 307). Scotland has one of the highest incidences and its population of just over 5 million has 3 200 new cases a year and 1 860 deaths annually. In Scotland the lifetime risk of colorectal cancer is 1 in 22 for men and 1 in 33 for women. Rectal cancer is commoner in men while colon cancer is commoner in women, suggesting that cancer in these sites may have different aetiologies. Two-thirds of large bowel cancers occur in the rectum and sigmoid colon (Fig. 29.13). In 3% of cases there is more than one cancer at presentation and 1% of patients develop cancer of the remaining large bowel with each 10 years of follow-up. The

---

Neoplastic polyps of the large bowel
- Adenomatous polyps:
  - account for 90% of large bowel polyps
  - may bleed, prolapse or intussuscept
  - carry a 5% risk of malignancy when over 1 cm in diameter

- Villous adenomas:
  - account for 10% of all large bowel polyps
  - are most common in the rectosigmoid region
  - may produce a profuse mucus discharge (causing hypokalaemia)
  - in one-third of cases are associated with carcinoma.

- Familial adenomatous polyposis:
  - is transmitted as an autosomal dominant trait in which the inherited defect is located in the APC gene on chromosome 5
  - gives rise to polyps of the colon and rectum in childhood
  - is associated with a 100% risk of malignant transformation (although this is exceptional before the age of 20).

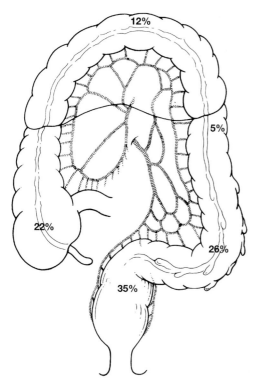

Fig. 29.13 Large bowel cancer: Tumour distribution within the colon and rectum.

disease is uncommon before the age of 40; two-thirds of cases occur in patients over 65.

Aetiology

Large bowel cancer is rare in Africa and the Orient, and in general, its incidence parallels that of coron-

ary heart disease and breast cancer. Dietary factors implicated include a high-fat, low-fruit and vegetable fibre diet and it seems likely that slow intestinal transit prolongs mucosal contact with luminal carcinogens. These factors may also help to explain the frequency with which the rectum and sigmoid colon are affected. Bile salts may also be implicated and clostridia and coliforms with dehydrogenating activity can convert bile acids to carcinogenic sterols.

About one-quarter of patients with colorectal cancer have a family history of the disease. The risk of developing colorectal cancer rises to 1 in 10 if a first-degree relative is affected. It is likely that multiple genetic events are involved and recent interest has centred on a defective gene on chromosome 2 which may be implicated in some 15% of all cases. Although rare, familial adenomatous polyposis accounts for 1–2% of all cases of colorectal cancer. Hereditary non-polyposis colorectal cancer is another autosomal dominant disorder with a high degree of penetrance in which colorectal cancer develops in gene carriers, but without the myriad of adenomas seen in familial adenomatous polyposis; the syndrome accounts for 5% of all cases of colorectal cancer and there may be associated breast, uterine and ovarian malignancies.

Most colorectal cancers arise in pre-existing adenomatous polyps, with a transition interval of 10 to 35 years. Other factors implicated include ulcerative colitis, Crohn's disease and villous adenoma.

Pathology

Three gross types of tumour are described: polypoidal, ulcerating and stenosing (Fig. 29.14). Infil-

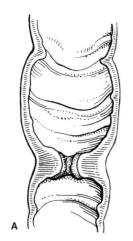 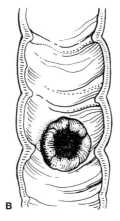 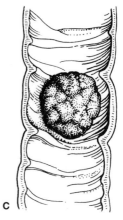

Fig. 29.14 Pathological types of large bowel cancer: A stenosing; **B** ulcerating; **C** polypoidal.

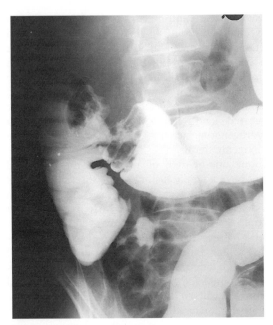

Fig. 29.15   Barium enema showing carcinoma of the proximal transverse colon.

trating tumours frequently spread circumferentially and produce 'apple core' appearance on barium enema (Fig. 29.15). The tumours are adenocarcinomas which arise from the columnar epithelium and show a wide spectrum of differentiation. Tumours with a colloidal or gelatinous structure occasionally arise (particularly in young people) and are associated with a bad prognosis.

The cancer may spread locally and can penetrate and perforate the bowel; spread to the serosa allows transperitoneal dissemination. Lymphatic spread leads to nodal involvement in about half of all cases coming to operation, while spread via the bloodstream gives rise to liver metastases in 20–30% of such patients. The Duke's classification used by pathologists (Table 29.3) has major prognostic implications. It should be noted that the original classification did not have a stage D and that patients are assigned to this category by their surgeon rather than

the pathologist (who only has access to the resection specimen). Resectability is also an important prognostic indicator and is determined by the degree of local extension and fixation.

Clinical features

The key clinical features of large bowel cancer are alteration in bowel habit and rectal bleeding. The patient often feels unwell and may have lost weight, and the presenting signs and symptoms are also influenced by the location of the tumour.

Right colon.   The contents of the caecum and ascending colon are fluid so that altered bowel habit and obstruction are late features. The tumour may be palpable by the time the patient presents and a hypochromic microcytic anaemia is common due to chronic occult blood loss. Right iliac fossa discomfort or pain may be present.

Left colon.   The left colon is narrower and has a more solid content so that obstruction and alteration of bowel habit are common. Blood and mucus are frequently passed per rectum.

Rectum.   Bleeding is often the main symptom and the patient may believe that he has piles. A feeling of incomplete evacuation of the rectum is common after defaecation and the patient may experience urgency and the frequent passage of slime and blood. As the rectum is capacious, obstruction is unusual.

Examination may also reveal hepatomegaly or ascites in patients with advanced disease. Up to one-third of patients with colorectal cancer present on an emergency basis with obstruction (20%), perforation (10%), fistula formation or bleeding (rare).

Investigations

Almost half the patients have a palpable abdominal or rectal mass. Digital rectal examination and sigmoidoscopy are essential in patients with rectal bleeding, even if piles are present, and all suspicious lesions must be biopsied. Barium enema or colonoscopy are needed to exclude colonic neoplasia

Table 29.3 Duke's classification and its impact on outcome in colorectal cancer			
Duke's stage	Definition	Proportion of patients	5-year survival (%)
A	No spread of growth beyond muscularis mucosa	10%	80–100%
B	Spread through bowel wall to serosa	33%	66%
C	Spread to involve lymph nodes	33%	33%
'D'*	Distant metastases (particularly liver metastases)	33%	0–5%
*Duke's original classification did not include a stage D (see text)			

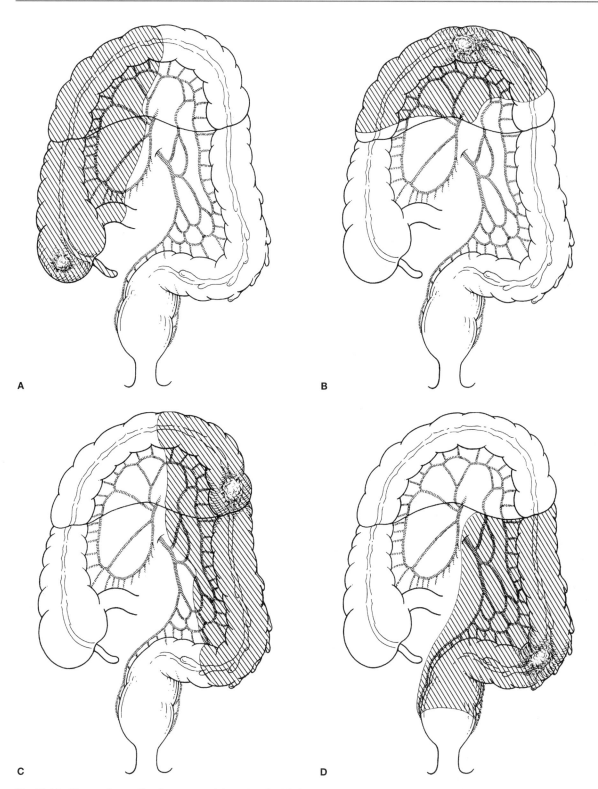

Fig. 29.16   Types of resection for cancer of the colon A: right hemicolectomy. **B**: transverse colectomy. **C**: left hemicolectomy. **D**: sigmoidcolectomy.

when sigmoidoscopy is negative, and to detect a second primary when it is positive.

Liver function tests, liver scans (ultrasound or computerized tomography; CT), and a chest X-ray are obtained to exclude metastatic disease, and an intravenous urogram (IVU) may be advisable (p. 526).

Treatment (Fig. 29.16)

Laparotomy is necessary to assess resectability of the tumour and any fixation to neighbouring structures. Intra-abdominal spread is determined and intra-operative ultrasonography can be used to supplement inspection and palpation of the liver.

Tumours in the right colon and transverse colon are removed by right hemicolectomy with ileocolic anastomosis, while tumours of the descending and sigmoid colon are dealt with by left hemicolectomy or sigmoid colectomy respectively. In all cases, the associated mesentery and regional nodes are removed en bloc with the affected bowel. When operating under emergency circumstances and with unprepared bowel, it may be inadvisable to restore intestinal continuity as part of the primary operation.

Carcinoma of the upper third or middle third of the rectum is dealt with by anterior resection (with restoration of continuity), while cancers of the lower rectum usually require abdominoperineal excision of the rectum (using a combined abdominal and perineal approach) with formation of a permanent colostomy in the left iliac fossa. At one time, almost all cancers within 12 cm of the anus were treated by abdominoperineal excision. However, it is now recognized that a resection margin of only 2 cm is necessary distal to the cancer, and the advent of stapling techniques has allowed easier performance of low colorectal anastomoses. This means that cancers more than 7 cm from the anal verge can now usually be treated by anterior restorative resection. In females, part of the vagina may be excised with the specimen, while in men great care must be taken not to damage the urethra.

'Curative' resection of colon and rectal cancers means that there is no obvious residual cancer once resection has been completed). In many cases it is apparent from the outset that resection will only be palliative, but it may nevertheless be worthwhile in that it avoids complications such as bleeding, perforation and obstruction. When resection is impossible or inadvisable, consideration may be given to palliative bypass (e.g. ileotransverse anastomosis in patients with unresectable caecal cancer).

There is evidence that pre-operative radiotherapy may improve long-term survival rates in patients with rectal cancer. In some centres, local radiotherapy is used as an alternative to surgery in patients with well-differentiated rectal cancers.

Chemotherapy alone has no role in the primary management of colorectal cancer, but intraportal 5-fluorouracil and systemic levamisole may each prove to have a role as adjuvant therapy.

Prognosis

The operative mortality of elective large bowel resection for cancer has fallen to beneath 5%, although emergency resection still carries a mortality of some 10%. The overall 5-year survival rate for patients with colorectal cancer is almost 40% but much depends on the Duke's staging (Table 29.3). If liver metastases are present, survival beyond 1–2 years is exceptional. Occasional patients with isolated liver metastases may be considered for hepatic resection.

Presymptomatic diagnosis

Colorectal cancer can now be diagnosed at a presymptomatic stage (i.e. when curative treatment is often possible) by testing of the stool for the presence

---

Large bowel cancer

- It is the second commonest cause of cancer death in Western countries and has a particularly high incidence in Scotland.

- Aetiological factors include diet, bile salts and a positive family history, while recognized premalignant conditions are ulcerative colitis, pre-existing, adenomatous and villous polyps, and Crohn's disease.

- Two-thirds of all large bowel cancers occurs in the rectum and sigmoid colon and the commonest clinical features are alteration in bowel habit and passage of blood per rectum.

- Presymptomatic diagnosis may be achieved by testing the stool for occult blood and by regular colonoscopy. With the indentification of the genetic abnormalities associated with a high risk of colorectal cancer, genetic screening is becoming feasible.

- The overall 5-year survival rate is 40% and the Duke's staging system is a useful prognostic index. If liver metastases are present, survival beyond 2 years is exceptional.

of blood (haemoccult testing) and so identify patients who require colonoscopy. This allows detection of polyps and presymptomatic cancers, many of which are found to be in Duke's stage A. In some centres, screening colonoscopy is carried out regularly (i.e. every 2–3 years) without haemoccult testing, particularly in high-risk individuals. With advances in molecular genetics, high-risk individuals are now being identified in whom screening may pay particular dividends.

30

The appendix

CONTENTS

Surgical anatomy

The appendix develops as a conical diverticulum which projects from the dependent pole of the caecum. As a result of differential caecal growth, the appendix eventually projects from the medial wall of the caecum some 2 cm below the ileocaecal junction (Fig. 30.1). The taeniae coli converge on the root of the appendix and so aid in its localization at laparotomy.

In most individuals the appendix lies behind the caecum or hangs down over the pelvic brim (Fig. 30.2). In up to 5% of subjects, the appendix lies behind or in front of the terminal ileum. In rare congenital anomalies, such as malrotation of the colon or situs inversus, the caecum and appendix may be outwith the right iliac fossa. The position of the appendix influences the clinical picture in acute appendicitis.

The appendix has no known function in man. Its lumen is lined by colonic epithelium and the submucosa contains lymphoid follicles which are prominent in childhood but regress in adolescence. The appendix lumen may eventually be obliterated by fibrosis in older patients.

ACUTE APPENDICITIS

Incidence

Acute appendicitis is predominantly a disease of Western civilization although its incidence in the United Kingdom has fallen significantly over the past 30 years. It is uncommon in developing countries but its incidence may be increasing with adoption of low-residue Western-style diets.

Acute appendicitis remains the commonest acute abdominal emergency in childhood, adolescence

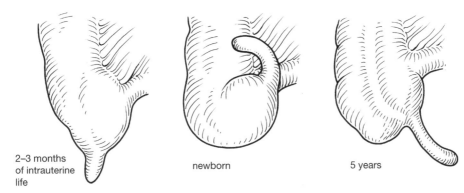

2–3 months
of intrauterine
life

newborn

5 years

Fig. 30.1   The stages in the development of the appendix.

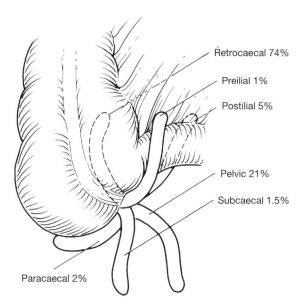

Retrocaecal 74%

Preilial 1%

Postilial 5%

Pelvic 21%

Subcaecal 1.5%

Paracaecal 2%

Fig. 30.2 Variations in the position of the appendix.

and early adult life. It is uncommon before the age of 2 and less than 5% of cases occur in patients above the age of 60 years.

Aetiology and pathophysiology

The fact that acute appendicitis typically commences with central abdominal colic suggests that obstruction of the lumen is an important factor. Accumulation of secretions in the obstructed appendix then leads to distension, necrosis of the mucosa, and invasion of the wall by gut bacteria. The peak-age incidence of appendicitis overlaps the period of maximal development of lymphoid tissue, and lymphoid hyperplasia within the wall could predispose to obstruction. In older patients, inspissated faeces (faecoliths), fibrosis, adhesions and neoplasia are all potential causes of obstruction. Threadworms can cause signs and symptoms resembling mild acute appendicitis but are incriminated in few cases.

Although the acute inflammation occasionally resolves spontaneously, it is far more common for it to progress to gangrene and perforation if the appendix is not removed. Continuing obstruction leads to impairment of blood supply, and even before frank perforation occurs, bacteria migrate through the damaged wall to infect the peritoneal cavity and inflame the parietal peritoneum. Once perforation has occurred, the outcome depends on the ability of the omentum and neighbouring organs

to contain the infection. If it can be contained, an appendix abscess or appendix mass results; if not, generalized peritonitis ensues. The omentum is not fully developed in infants and they may localize infection less effectively. In all age groups, *delay* in diagnosis and treatment is the key determinant of outcome.

Clinical features

It is vital to appreciate that in some patients, the 'typical' signs and symptoms of acute appendicitis are not present or may appear late. As indicated earlier, the clinical picture is also influenced by the position of the appendix.

Symptoms

Pain is usually the first and most impressive symptom. In 'typical' cases, it begins as periumbilical colic which ranges in severity from mild discomfort to severe pain. The colic represents *visceral pain* due to appendiceal obstruction; its periumbilical location reflects the embryonic origin of the appendix as a midline midgut structure. Classically, the pain remains periumbilical for several hours before shifting to the right iliac fossa. This denotes the development of *somatic pain* as parietal peritonitis ensues. Whereas the periumbilical colic is ill-localized, the somatic pain is sharply localized and is exacerbated by moving or coughing. In around one-third of cases, pain commences in and remains in the right iliac fossa without preceding visceral pain. When the appendix is retrocaecal, somatic pain is perceived in the flank and loin. A pelvic appendix may not be associated with somatic pain when inflamed (see below).

Anorexia is almost invariable, to the extent that hunger usually means that the patient does not have acute appendicitis. Nausea is common but vomiting is rarely a prominent feature. Some patients experience fullness and may misguidedly take aperients in an attempt to gain relief; others give a history of constipation. Diarrhoea may occur, particularly when pelvic appendicitis irritates the neighbouring rectum.

Signs

Fever and tachycardia are *not* early signs of appendicitis, and may not develop until perforation has occurred. Foetor is often present but is non-specific.

Tenderness and muscle guarding are the cardinal

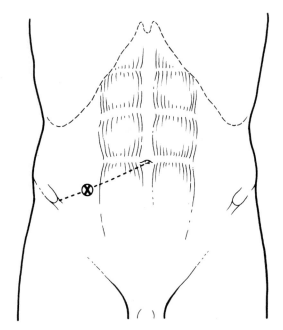

Fig. 30.3   McBurney's point.

signs of acute appendicitis. Tenderness is often maximal over McBurney's point (Fig. 30.3), which lies one-third of the way along a line drawn from the right anterior superior iliac spine to the umbilicus, and is often associated with rebound tenderness and hyperaesthesia of the skin. Less reliable signs include Rovsing's sign (pressure on the left iliac fossa producing pain in the right iliac fossa) and the psoas sign (pain during passive extension of the right hip). In the early stages, bowel sounds are normal or slightly reduced in frequency.

Retrocaecal appendicitis is often difficult to diagnose early in that there may be no signs in the right iliac fossa; tenderness, if present, is maximal in the right flank or loin. Pelvic appendicitis often produces little tenderness or guarding on examination of the abdomen, but tenderness is usually present on digital rectal examination. Digital rectal examination must *always* be performed in patients with acute abdominal pain. It will elicit tenderness in one-third of patients with appendicitis and is a valuable means of excluding gynaecological and other causes of pain.

Perforation of the appendix with diffuse peritonitis leads to generalized tenderness, guarding and rigidity, although even at this stage, tenderness is often still maximal in the right iliac fossa. If infection remains localized, a mass may become palpable on abdominal or rectal examination. This mass consists

of omentum and neighbouring viscera which have adhered to the inflamed appendix.

Diagnosis

The diagnosis of acute appendicitis is essentially clinical and rests heavily on the findings of pain, tenderness and guarding in the right iliac fossa. Polymorphonuclear leucocytosis may be present after some hours but it occurs in many acute abdominal conditions and is not diagnostic. Urinalysis is usually normal in appendicitis, although the urine may contain a few pus cells or red cells if the inflamed appendix lies next to the ureter. Gross pyuria indicates primary urinary tract infection rather than appendicitis, while significant haematuria is more likely to be associated with passage of a urinary calculus.

There are no pathognomic signs of early acute appendicitis on abdominal plain films, although radio-opaque faecoliths are sometimes seen. Fluid levels in the right iliac fossa, obliteration of the psoas border, and free gas in the right iliac fossa are occasional signs of *late* appendicitis. Ultrasonography is not used routinely to diagnose appendicitis but can detect free fluid and exclude other causes of pain such as gynaecological conditions.

Differential diagnosis

Acute appendicitis is seldom absent from the differential diagnosis of acute abdominal pain. The list of conditions included in the differential diagnosis of appendicitis is longer in women, and removal of a normal appendix is more likely in young adult or adolescent females. The following should be noted:

- Most conditions which can be confused with acute appendicitis also require laparotomy. However, 'medical' causes of abdominal pain such as basal pneumonia and diabetic ketoacidosis, for which laparotomy is positively contraindicated, must be excluded.
- The periumbilical colic of early acute appendicitis can suggest gastroenteritis or intestinal obstruction. In gastroenteritis, nausea, vomiting and diarrhoea are prominent and usually precede or accompany the pain; tenderness is seldom localized to the right iliac fossa. The picture in intestinal obstruction depends on the level of obstruction. For example, high obstruction produces marked vomiting but little or no abdominal distension, while low obstruction causes marked distension and constipation and late onset of vomiting. The colic of intestinal

obstruction usually persists for much longer than that of appendicitis, and tenderness is seldom localized to the right iliac fossa.

- Conditions which can produce right iliac fossa pain and tenderness include acute mesenteric adenitis, acute terminal ileitis, inflammation of Meckel's diverticulum and mittelschmertz (see Ch. 26). Although the correct diagnosis may be suspected clinically, laparotomy (or possibly laparoscopy) is indicated if pain and tenderness persist and appendicitis cannot be excluded.
- Acute salpingitis can produce right iliac fossa pain and tenderness but is often bilateral and gives rise to diffuse lower abdominal tenderness. Vaginal examination reveals a hot tender cervix and vaginal discharge in most cases of salpingitis.
- Rupture of an ectopic pregnancy can simulate all stages of acute appendicitis, beginning with cramping abdominal pain and progressing to spreading pain and tenderness as blood diffuses through the peritoneal cavity. The true diagnosis is suggested by a history of menstrual irregularity, vaginal bleeding, and shoulder-tip pain on elevating the foot of the bed.
- Ureteric colic can be associated with tenderness on deep palpation over the ureter, but the severity and radiation of the colic in the presence of haematuria usually indicates the true diagnosis. Abdominal plain films and an intravenous urogram are likely to show the calculus.
- Pelvic appendicitis may be simulated by salpingitis, diverticular disease or perforation of a colonic carcinoma. As a general rule, these colonic diseases cause more diffuse tenderness and may produce a palpable abdominal mass.
- Retrocaecal appendicitis can be mimicked by perinephric abscess, acute pyelonephritis, perforated colon cancer and acute cholecystitis. The renal diseases usually produce a higher fever, pyuria and tenderness in the costovertebral angle, while acute cholecystitis gives rise to a positive Murphy's sign and can produce a palpable mass and mild icterus.
- A mass in the right iliac fossa raises the suspicion of intussusception (in young children), acute terminal ileitis, Crohn's disease, ovarian cyst and bowel neoplasia.
- Perforated peptic ulcer can simulate acute appendicitis when leaking gastroduodenal contents run down the paracolic gutter and produce pain and tenderness in the right iliac fossa. Although perforation of the appendix can give rise to free gas beneath the liver or

diaphragm, it does so much less often and less impressively than perforation of a peptic ulcer or diverticular disease.

Problem areas in diagnosis

Appendicitis in infancy

Although acute appendicitis is rare before the age of 2 years, *it can occur.* The diagnosis can be difficult in that tenderness is often not localized. Anorexia, fever, looseness of the bowels and irritability may be misinterpreted as features of gastroenteritis. The average delay between onset and diagnosis is 4 days in these infants and in the vast majority, the appendix has perforated (often with abscess formation or generalized peritonitis) by the time surgery is undertaken. Fever and abdominal tenderness in infancy should always raise the suspicion of acute appendicitis.

Appendicitis in pregnancy

Acute appendicitis is just as common in pregnant women as in non-pregnant women. Early diagnosis is vital but difficult. The appendix is displaced upwards by the gravid uterus (especially during the third trimester) so that pain and tenderness may be higher than expected. Rectal and vaginal examination are less helpful than normally, the white cell count is normally elevated in pregnancy, and the use of X-rays is contraindicated.

Delay is harmful to both mother and unborn child, and the threshold for diagnosis and surgery must be no different to that applied in non-pregnant women. Maternal and fetal deaths do not result from laparotomy; they are a consequence of delayed diagnosis, reluctance to operate until the diagnosis is certain, and the development of peritonitis. Fetal mortality in uncomplicated appendicitis is 3%, that following perforated appendicitis is 30%.

Appendicitis in the elderly

Appendicitis progresses more rapidly in the elderly, possibly because of the earlier loss of blood supply. Gangrene and perforation are five times commoner in patients over the age of 60 years. Delay in diagnosis is undoubtedly contributory as the 'classical' features of appendicitis may be lacking, and pain and tenderness less marked than normal. Willingness to consider the diagnosis, despite atypical presentation, and prompt surgery are the keys to successful management.

Treatment of appendicitis

The aim is to remove the appendix before gangrene and perforation occur. Pre-operative resuscitation is not normally required in the absence of generalized peritonitis.

Under general anaesthesia, the abdomen is entered through a small skin crease incision which passes through McBurney's point (Fig. 30.3). The muscles of the abdominal wall are split in the line of their fibres as each layer is encountered. The caecum is delivered and the root of the appendix found by following the taeniae coli. The mesoappendix is divided with ligation of the appendicular artery, the appendix is ligated at its base and removed, and the appendix stump is invaginated into the caecum with a purse-string suture. The appendix is sent for histological examination (to confirm the diagnosis and exclude malignancy) and a swab for bacteriological culture is taken from the peritoneal cavity.

The wound is closed in layers. Local antiseptic agents such as povidone iodine reduce the incidence of wound infection and most surgeons also cover the operation by giving metronidazole (1 g suppository) at the time of premedication. A drain is not left into the peritoneal cavity, although some employ drainage if there has been gangrene and perforation. If there has been gross contamination of the wound with purulent material it may be prudent to close only the deeper layers, leaving the skin and subcutaneous tissues open for some 4–5 days. Once it is clear that the wound is uninfected, it can be sutured (delayed primary closure), although in most instances the skin will heal perfectly without the need for suture.

Problems during appendicectomy

The normal appendix

A normal appendix is removed in approximately 20% of emergency appendicectomies. While every effort should be made to avoid unnecessary laparotomy, delaying operation until the diagnosis is certain can lead to an unacceptable incidence of gangrene and perforation, and an increased morbidity and mortality.

If a normal appendix is found at operation, other pathology must be excluded. If peritoneal fluid is present, it may give a clue to the correct diagnosis. For example, mesenteric adenitis may be associated with clear yellow fluid, perforated peptic ulcer with bile-stained fluid, colonic perforation with faecal fluid, and gut infarction with blood-stained fluid.

Free blood suggests rupture of a vessel or ectopic pregnancy.

The distal ileum is withdrawn to exclude a Meckel's diverticulum, terminal ileitis or Crohn's disease. Both ovaries and Fallopian tubes should be inspected and an attempt made to visualize the sigmoid colon. Even if other pathology is present, a normal appendix should be removed when operating through a gridiron incision; this avoids confusion if appendicitis develops in a patient bearing an appendicectomy scar.

Lumps in the appendix

Faecoliths are the commonest cause of a palpable mass within the appendix. They are frequently mobile but can be mistaken for neoplasms (see below) if they become immobile in obstructed appendicitis.

Mucocele of the appendix

This rare condition results from chronic obstruction of the appendix with accumulation of mucin resulting in cystic dilatation (Fig. 30.4). The obstruction is usually due to fibrosis but sometimes a malignant mucus-secreting papillary adenocarcinoma is responsible. Simple mucoceles are cured by appendicectomy. Pseudomyxoma peritonei is a rare complication of rupture of a mucocele.

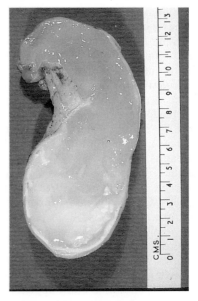

Fig. 30.4 Mucocele of the appendix.

Acute terminal ileitis

This condition was once wrongly regarded as a manifestation of Crohn's disease. It is a self-limiting infection with *Yersinia enterocolitica* or *Y. pseudotuberculosis* and may mimic acute appendicitis. At operation, the terminal ileum is red and thickened, mesenteric adenitis is obvious, and the caecum and appendix are normal. Examination of the lymph nodes reveals non-specific changes and the diagnosis is best confirmed serologically (or by node culture).

When acute terminal ileitis was confused with Crohn's disease, it was thought that appendicectomy was contraindicated because of the risk of fistula formation. It is now accepted that the correct course of action is to remove the appendix and leave the bowel alone. Even in true Crohn's disease, it is now recognized that the appendix can safely be removed as long as it is not itself involved.

Meckel's diverticulitis

Inflammation of a Meckel's diverticulum cannot be distinguished clinically from acute appendicitis but laparotomy is indicated in both conditions. If an acutely inflamed diverticulum is found, it should be resected; if an inflamed appendix is found, it should be removed without looking for a Meckel's diverticulum. Meckel's diverticula which are discovered as incidental findings at laparotomy need not be removed as routine.

Problems after appendicectomy

Complications are uncommon if an inflamed appendix is removed before the onset of gangrene and perforation. Uncomplicated appendicitis has an overall mortality of less than 0.1% whereas mortality rates may be as high as 5% following perforation.

Postoperative complications following appendicectomy include bleeding (rare), wound infection, intraperitoneal abscess formation, leakage from the appendix stump (rare), and urinary tract infection.

Complications of acute appendicitis

Perforation

The appendix rarely perforates within 12 hours of the onset of inflammation, unless the patient is elderly or has been taking aperients. Pain sometimes eases temporarily after perforation, but diffusion of pain and tenderness, increasing fever and tachycardia, and clinical deterioration then follow.

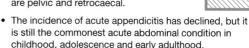

The appendix
- The common positions for the appendix are pelvic and retrocaecal.

- The incidence of acute appendicitis has declined, but it is still the commonest acute abdominal condition in childhood, adolescence and early adulthood.

- The typical history of periumbilical colic (visceral midgut pain) followed within several hours by right iliac fossa pain (somatic pain from parietal peritonitis) is not always present.

- Tenderness and muscle guarding in the right iliac fossa are the most reliable signs of acute appendicitis. Leucocytosis, high temperature and radiological signs are late manifestations which may denote gangrene and perforation.

- The objective is to carry out appendicectomy before gangrene and perforation supervene (with associated increase in morbidity and mortality).

- Gangrene and perforation are common and/or particularly dangerous in infants (diagnosis not considered in children under 2 years), pregnant women (desire to avoid negative laparotomy) and the elderly (more rapid progression of disease).

Prompt appendicectomy is essential but a period of vigorous resuscitation is sometimes needed. Systemic antibiotics (gentamicin and metronidazole) are administered, all portions of the necrotic appendix must be removed, and after taking a bacteriological swab, the peritoneal cavity is lavaged prior to closure. Precautions are taken to minimize wound infection (see above).

Appendix abscess and appendix mass

Development of an appendix abscess is associated with increasing pyrexia, pain and the presence of a mass. The mass is tender and is often palpable in the right iliac fossa. Pelvic abscesses are palpable on digital rectal examination and may produce few abdominal signs. Abscesses behind the caecum or terminal ileum are often difficult to detect but associated psoas spasm may mean that the patient prefers to lie with the right hip flexed. Ultrasonography is often helpful in diagnosis.

Appendix abscesses are treated by surgical drainage, taking care not to disseminate infection throughout the peritoneal cavity. If the appendix cannot be removed readily, it is safer to leave it and perform an interval appendicectomy some weeks later.

If the presentation is delayed and the patient has a

well-defined mass but no toxaemia and an otherwise soft, non-tender abdomen, conservative treatment can be instituted. The aim is to allow the inflammation to settle so that interval appendicectomy can be undertaken easily and safely. The patient is confined to bed, given intravenous fluids and nil by mouth. Vital signs are monitored and the mass is palpated and delineated twice daily. Conservative treatment is abandoned in favour of surgical drainage if the mass increases in size, the general condition deteriorates, or there are signs of dissemination of infection. In general, conservative treatment is inadvisable in the very young, the elderly, and pregnant women.

Portal pyaemia

Suppurative thrombophlebitis of the portal vein with hepatic abscess formation is now an extremely rare complication of appendicitis. There is high swinging pyrexia and icterus, and gas may be seen radiologically in the portal system. Vigorous antibiotic treatment offers the only hope of survival. Patients who do survive are often left with portal hypertension due to portal vein occlusion.

CHRONIC APPENDICITIS

It is debatable whether recurring bouts of low-grade appendicitis can give rise to intermittent 'grumbling' pain in the right iliac fossa. The 'grumbling' appendix is something of a diagnostic scapegoat and appendicectomy should be advised only when all other investigations have proved negative.

TUMOURS OF THE APPENDIX

Carcinoid tumour

The appendix is the commonest site for carcinoid tumours of the gastrointestinal tract. The tumour arises from argentaffin cells of the Amine Precursor Uptake and Decarboxylation (APUD) system and is usually a distinct yellow submucosal lesion located near the tip of the appendix. Carcinoid tumours account for 85% of all appendiceal tumours and are found in 0.5% of all appendices removed surgically. The vast majority are benign but tumours larger than 2 cm can infiltrate the wall of the appendix, and spread to the mesoappendix and regional lymph nodes. It is most unusual for appendiceal carcinoids to give rise to liver metastases and the carcinoid syndrome.

Appendicectomy is all that is required for most appendiceal carcinoid tumours. If the tumour is large, involves the caecum, or involves lymph nodes, right hemicolectomy is necessary.

Adenocarcinoma

Adenocarcinoma of the appendix is a highly malignant neoplasm which spreads rapidly to regional nodes. It may present as acute appendicitis or as an appendix mass. Right hemicolectomy is indicated.

Tumours of the appendix
- The appendix is the commonest site of carcinoid tumour in the gastrointestinal tract, and 85% of all appendiceal tumours are carcinoids.

- Carcinoid tumours are found in 0.5% of all appendices removed surgically.

- The tumour usually takes the form of a small firm yellowish nodule near the tip of the appendix.

- Although carcinoid tumours frequently show spread to the serosa, lymph node involvement is rare and distant metastases are extremely rare.

- Appendicectomy is usually adequate treatment although subsequent right hemicolectomy may be considered in patients who prove to have involved lymph nodes.

31

Intestinal obstruction

CONTENTS

Classification of intestinal obstruction

Intestinal obstruction can be classified according to:

- The level of obstruction of the gut (high or low small bowel, colonic)
- The rate of progression of obstruction (acute, subacute, chronic or acute-on-chronic)
- The location of the pathological process responsible (intraluminal, mural, extramural)
- The nature of the pathological process responsible (simple mechanical obstruction, strangulation, paralytic ileus).

Although all of these methods of classification are of value, the last has critical significance in clinical practice. If an obstructed segment of bowel is allowed to strangulate (i.e. become so congested by constriction that its circulation is arrested), urgent surgical intervention becomes mandatory and prognosis worsens appreciably. For example, prompt operation on an inguinal hernia causing simple mechanical occlusion of the intestine carries little hazard to life, whereas if operation is delayed and strangulation supervenes, significant mortality results.

It is important to appreciate that obstruction may progress to perforation in the absence of devascularization from strangulation. This can be due to penetration of the gut wall by the causal lesion, a situation encountered when obstruction of the colon by carcinoma is complicated by perforation at the site of the tumour.

While in most instances the gut is obstructed at only one point, a segment of bowel may become occluded at both ends. Examples of such 'closed-loop' obstruction are volvulus of the sigmoid colon (Fig. 31.1), obstructed external hernia, and colonic obstruction in the presence of a competent ileocaecal valve which prevents reflux into the small bowel. The contents of the closed loop are unable to escape in either direction, the blood supply rapidly becomes compromised, and there is a much higher risk of strangulation than in simple obstruction.

Causes of intestinal obstruction

The frequency of the various causes of intestinal obstruction changes with age (Table 31.1). Intussus-

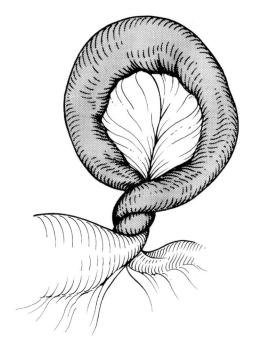

Fig. 31.1   Volvulus – an example of closed-loop obstruction.

Table 31.1 Common causes of intestinal obstruction in various age groups

Neonates	Children	Adults
Meconium ileus	External hernia	Adhesions
Atresia/stenosis	Intussusception	Large bowel cancer
Malrotation of the gut	Adhesions	External hernia
Hirschsprung disease		Diverticular disease
		Crohn's disease

ception, hernia and congenital anomalies are the common causes in infancy, whereas neoplastic obstruction is the major problem in the elderly. In the UK, 35% of adult intestinal obstructions are due to external hernias, 30% to large bowel cancer, and 25% to bands and adhesions. Volvulus is a rare cause in this country whereas sigmoid volvulus is so common in some parts of Africa that it is second only to hernia as a cause of obstruction.

Pathophysiology of intestinal obstruction

Simple mechanical obstruction

The bowel above the obstructing lesion becomes distended with fluid and gas, and this stimulates excessive peristalsis, producing colic. The gas is mainly swallowed air; luminal putrefaction makes only a small contribution. As distension increases, the blood vessels in the bowel wall become stretched and narrowed, so that blood flow is impaired. The mucosa is the first layer of the bowel wall to show the effects of ischaemia. Absorption from the lumen is diminished and there is net loss of water and electrolytes into the lumen, resulting in depletion of extracellular fluid (ECF) and hypovolaemia. The fluid lost is isotonic with ECF but has a higher potassium content. Some of the ECF passing into the gut lumen is lost overtly by vomiting, but there are also substantial occult losses as fluid accumulates in the obstructed bowel. As a very rough guide, 2 litres of ECF are lost in the lumen before vomiting begins; with vomiting and dehydration this increases to 4 litres, and the onset of hypovolaemic shock suggests a loss of the order of 6 litres.

In simple mechanical obstruction, shock occurs relatively late and is due to ECF depletion (i.e. hypovolaemic shock). The patient becomes increasingly dehydrated and has tachycardia, falling central venous pressure and hypotension. Hypoxia is exacerbated by the abdominal distension and reduced excursion of the diaphragm. Bacteraemia is not an important factor in pathogenesis; although the luminal bacterial count rises in mechanical obstruction, bacteria do not migrate through the gut wall unless ischaemia supervenes.

Strangulation obstruction

The initial stage of strangulation is occlusion of the low-pressure venous system by constricting agencies such as the tight neck of a hernial sac or the twist of a volvulus. This results in oedema of the bowel wall. Arterial blood continues to enter until prevented from doing so by increasing back pressure. The bowel becomes ischaemic and infarcted. Losses of blood and plasma in the infarcted segment of gut are often substantial and overshadow the losses of ECF due to preceding simple mechanical obstruction. For example, in strangulated sigmoid volvulus up to two-thirds of the total blood volume may be sequestered in the twisted colon. Shock is in part hypovolaemic, but as bacteria and their toxins begin to migrate through the ischaemic gut into the peritoneum, septic shock supervenes.

Clinical features of intestinal obstruction

Symptoms

Abdominal colic is the cardinal symptom (Table 31.2). Its distribution reflects the region of

---

Causes of intestinal obstruction

- The most important classification of intestinal obstruction is based on the nature of the pathological process; simple mechanical obstruction, strangulation and paralytic ileus.

- In mechanical obstruction, distension of the proximal bowel produces marked peristalsis and colic, while impairment of mucosal function causes net loss of water and electrolytes into the lumen (with ECF depletion).

- In high intestinal obstruction, vomiting is an early feature. In distal obstruction, vomiting may be a late manifestation but fluid sequestration within the gut still leads to ECF depletion.

- Strangulation denotes loss of blood supply and may complicate simple mechanical obstruction. Venous drainage is usually occluded first, followed by arterial occlusion.

- Strangulation increases the morbidity and mortality of intestinal obstruction. Blood and plasma are sequestered in the strangulated intestine and bacteria and their toxins migrate through the devitalized gut wall.

Table 31.2 Clinical and radiological presentation of patients according to the level of mechanical intestinal obstruction

Level of obstruction	Mode of onset	Nature of pain	Clinical findings	Radiological findings
High small bowel	Sudden	Epigastric colic, occasionally continuous	No distension; dehydration often marked.	Abdomen may appear gasless or show distended proximal small bowel
Low small bowel	Gradual	Periumbilical colic	Distension	Gaseous distension of small bowel; fluid levels on erect film
Large bowel	Insidious	Central or lower abdominal colic; may have generalized discomfort	Gross distension	Gaseous distension of large bowel proximal to obstruction. Small bowel may also show distension

the bowel which is distended and undergoing excessive peristalsis. With small bowel (midgut) obstruction, the colic is periumbilical, whereas obstruction of the distal colon produces a combination of midgut and hindgut obstruction resulting in periumbilical and hypogastric colic. In contrast to patients with peritonitis, who are afraid to move during an attack, patients with colic are restless and change position in an attempt to find relief. Development of more constant and more localized pain with tenderness strongly suggests the onset of strangulation. Suspicion is heightened if the patient appears more ill than might be expected from the length of history, pallor is present and there is circulatory collapse. It must be stressed that strangulation is notoriously difficult to detect in its early stages, and can never be excluded with confidence without laparotomy. It is for this reason that with few specific exceptions (see below), early surgical intervention is advised in all patients with simple mechanical obstruction.

Vomiting occurs early in high small bowel obstruction but may be absent or develop late in low small bowel or colonic obstruction. At first, the vomitus may contain altered food but later becomes bile stained and then faeculent and foul smelling. The faeculent material is small bowel content contaminated with faecal organisms and not faeces from the colon. In obstruction due to pyloric stenosis, the vomitus does not become bile stained or faeculent.

Constipation and *failure to pass flatus* are features of complete obstruction but flatus and some faeces may continue to pass in incomplete obstruction and for a time following the onset of high small bowel obstruction.

Physical examination

Abdominal distension is a common feature of intestinal obstruction, although it may be absent in high obstruction. In low small bowel or colonic obstruction, visible loops of small intestine may form a 'ladder' pattern across the abdomen. Peristalsis is occasionally visible. The distended bowel produces a resonant note on percussion, allowing obstruction to be distinguished from obesity or ascites.

Auscultation during an attack of colic reveals runs of exaggerated bowel sounds. When the bowel becomes distended with fluid and gas, bowel sounds become high-pitched and tinkling.

Examination of the abdomen may reveal the cause of obstruction. An abdominal scar raises the possibility of adhesion obstruction or previous surgery for a condition which can cause recurrent obstruction (e.g. Crohn's disease). The hernial orifices must be examined carefully and the danger of overlooking a small groin hernia, particularly a femoral hernia, cannot be overemphasized. The hernia may produce little local pain or tenderness and central abdominal colic tends to focus attention away from the causal lesion.

Digital rectal examination is essential. Faecal impaction is a frequent cause of obstruction in the elderly, while an obstructing colorectal cancer may be palpable. A mass in the rectovesical pouch suggests widespread abdominal neoplasia.

Proctoscopy and sigmoidoscopy can reveal the cause of distal large bowel obstruction; in the case of sigmoid volvulus, sigmoidoscopy may allow a flatus tube to be passed into the obstructed loop with relief of obstruction.

Radiological investigation

Plain films of the abdomen usually reveal gaseous distension of the obstructed bowel with fluid levels in the erect (or lateral decubitus) views. In high obstruction, such as that due to pyloric stenosis, little or no gas is seen in the intestine although a fluid level may be present in the stomach.

The site of obstruction can often be deduced from the plain film. Obstructed small bowel occupies the centre of the abdomen, has markings (valvulae conniventes) which extend across the whole diameter of the bowel, and seldom becomes as grossly distended as the colon. Obstructed large bowel occupies a peripheral position, has haustral indentations, and may become grossly distended, particularly when there is closed loop obstruction such as that caused by sigmoid volvulus.

Contrast radiology, using dilute barium or the water-soluble contrast medium, Gastrografin, may be helpful when the diagnosis is in doubt. Undiluted barium can compound obstruction, and barium must not be used if perforation is suspected.

MANAGEMENT OF MECHANICAL INTESTINAL OBSTRUCTION

Prompt diagnosis and operation are essential to reduce the risk of strangulation. Whenever possible, hypovolaemia and electrolyte deficits should be rectified by vigorous resuscitation prior to surgery. In the presence of strangulation, the benefits of delaying surgery to allow resuscitation have to be balanced against the risk of progressive impairment of the blood supply of the obstructed bowel.

Principles of surgery

Small bowel obstruction

Extrinsic lesions such as hernias, bands and adhesions are the commonest cause of small bowel obstruction. Hernias are reduced and repaired, while adhesions and bands are divided. Lesions within the bowel wall are less common and require resection of the involved segment with end-to-end anastomosis. Obstruction due to an intraluminal mass, such as a gallstone or food bolus, is rare. It is managed by milking the offending agent into the colon; if this is not possible, enterotomy is needed to extract the obstructing material.

Strangulated bowel is blue or black in colour, lacks sheen, is often papery in consistency, and does not show peristalsis when squeezed or flicked. It may be obvious that there is no arterial pulsation in the adjacent mesentery. If the bowel is gangrenous or its viability is in doubt, the involved segment must be resected with end-to-end anastomosis of the remaining bowel.

Large bowel obstruction

Obstruction of the right colon. Obstructing lesions of the right side of the colon are usually managed by right hemicolectomy with immediate ileocolic anastomosis. If the patient has an unresectable carcinoma, the obstruction may be bypassed by carrying out a palliative side-to-side anastomosis between the ileum and the transverse colon (Fig. 31.2).

Obstruction of the left colon. The management of obstructing lesions of the left side of the large bowel is more controversial, given that there is a significant risk of leakage from an end-to-end anastomosis involving obstructed, distended and loaded bowel. The left colon has a poorer blood supply than the right colon and its luminal content is more solid. At one time, a three-stage approach was employed routinely (Fig. 31.3). The first stage consisted of an emergency transverse colostomy to relieve obstruction. After adequate preparation, the affected segment of the bowel was resected at a second operation performed some weeks later, an end-to-end anastomosis being performed between the two bowel ends. The transverse colostomy was retained to divert the faecal stream. Finally, the transverse colostomy was closed at a third operation some 4–6 weeks later after anastomotic healing had been confirmed by barium instilled through the transverse colostomy and into the distal loop.

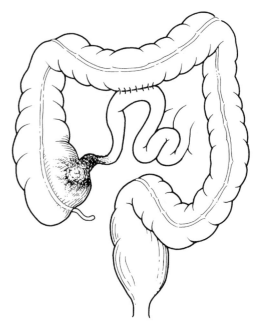

Fig. 31.2   Ileo-transverse anastomosis to bypass an irresectable lesion at the ileocaecal valve.

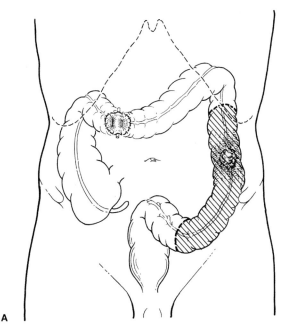

A

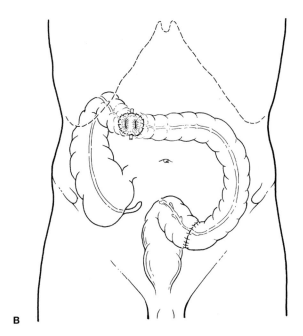

B

Fig. 31.3 Three-stage resection of large bowel:
A emergency transverse colostomy (the site of subsequent resection is also shown); **B** elective resection of large bowel segment, retaining the colostomy to protect the anastomosis; **C** closure of colostomy.

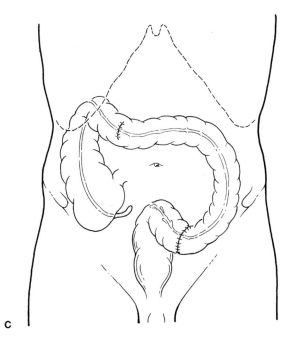

C

This three-stage approach has been superseded by a one-stage or two-stage procedure. The alternatives available are as follows:

1. The segment of bowel containing the obstructing lesion is resected at the emergency operation (Fig. 31.4A). The two ends of bowel are then exteriorized, the proximal end serving as a temporary end-colostomy while the distal end acts as a mucus fistula (Fig. 31.4B). Alternatively, the distal end of bowel can be oversewn and allowed to drop back into the abdomen; this is the Hartmann procedure and it is particularly useful with obstructing tumours of the distal sigmoid colon or rectum. Whichever method is employed, continuity is restored at a second operation carried out electively some weeks later and after appropriate bowel preparation.

2. The segment of bowel containing the obstructed lesion is resected and intestinal continuity restored by immediate end-to-end anastomosis. This approach has been used increasingly by experienced surgeons in recent years. Two techniques have evolved to overcome the dangers of immediate anastomosis in patients with unprepared loaded bowel:

On-table lavage can be employed to empty the obstructed proximal colon. A Foley catheter (24 Fr) is inserted into the caecum (through the base of the removed appendix) and secured by a purse-string suture. The catheter is connected to an irrigation system containing isotonic saline solution (Fig. 31.5). A wide-bore collecting tube is tied into

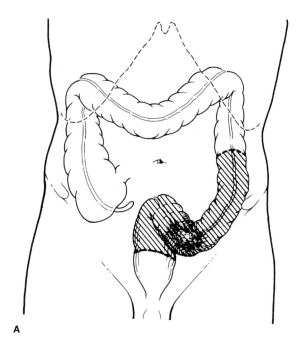

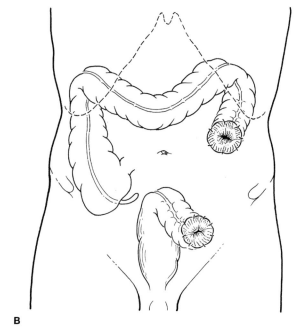

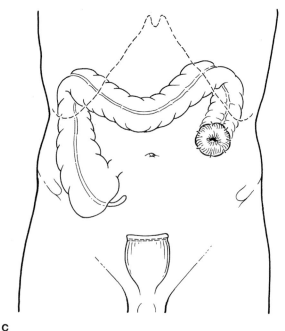

Fig. 31.4 Emergency management of distal colorectal cancer. A tumour of sigmoid colon showing area of bowel to be resected; **B** exteriorization of both ends of bowel; **C** the Hartmann procedure

the proximal cut end of colon and led to a collecting receptacle. The irrigation washes faeces from the obstructed bowel into the collecting system, although harder scybala may have to be broken down manually and massaged along the colon. Irrigation continues until the effluent is clear. As much as 10–12 litres of saline may be needed. The catheter is brought out through a stab incision in the right iliac fossa and can be left in place for a few days as a temporary caecostomy (although the catheter is now rarely retained).

The *Coloshield technique* employs an inner 'stocking' to protect the anastomosis (Fig. 31.6). After resection of the affected segment of bowel, a soft rubber ring, to which the stocking of fine latex rubber is attached, is sewn into the proximal bowel just above the site of the proposed anastomosis. Absorbable sutures are used for this purpose. The posterior layer of the anastomosis is then completed, and using a 'retriever' passed up through the anus and rectum, the stocking is pulled through the distal bowel until it emerges from the anus. The anterior layer of the anastomosis is then completed. If the anastomosis lies below the level of the mid-rectum, the stocking is left protruding from the anus. If the anastomosis is at a higher level, the stocking is cut

at the anus and allowed to retract into the rectum (Fig. 31.6). The stocking protects the anastomosis as it heals and is passed spontaneously some 2–3 weeks later.

3. The proximal bowel is decompressed by a loop colostomy placed close enough to the obstructing lesion that it can be included in the resection

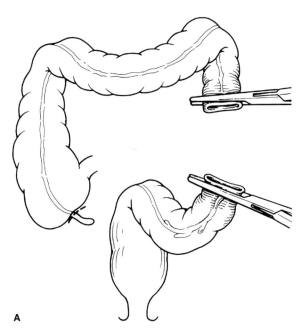

A

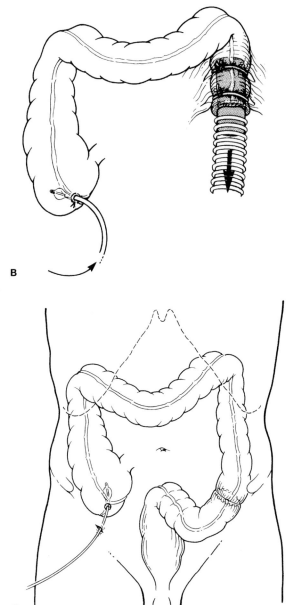

B

C

Fig. 31.5   Principles of one-stage resection and anastomosis using 'on-table' colonic lavage. A The obstructing lesion has been resected. (If present, the appendix is also removed.) **B** A Foley catheter is inserted through the appendix stump, secured by a purse-string suture and connected to the irrigating system. Faecal content is washed from the colon into the collecting system. **C** The anastomosis has been made, the Foley catheter led out from the caecum to form a temporary caecostomy, and the abdomen closed.

specimen at the second operation. Intestinal continuity is restored at this second elective operation.

Strangulation of the colon. Resection is always necessary if strangulation is present. Intestinal continuity can be restored immediately following resection of strangulated right colon, but if there is any doubt about the viability of the remaining bowel or peritonitis is present, it is advisable to exteriorize the two ends as an ileostomy and colostomy respectively.

Immediate anastomosis is not normally recommended following resection of strangulated segments of left colon and rectum. The two ends of bowel are exteriorized or a Hartmann's procedure is performed (see above).

Caecostomy. If a patient with large bowel obstruction is unfit for laparotomy, a 'blind' caecostomy is occasionally considered. The term 'blind' caecostomy refers to the fact that laparotomy is not carried out. A large-bore tube can be inserted into the caecum under local anaesthesia with the object

of decompressing the obstructed colon. The tube has to be irrigated regularly to prevent its blockage.

Role of conservative treatment

Non-operative treatment of mechanical intestinal obstruction is indicated, at least initially, under the following circumstances.

Adhesion obstruction. If a patient has already undergone multiple operations for obstruction due

449

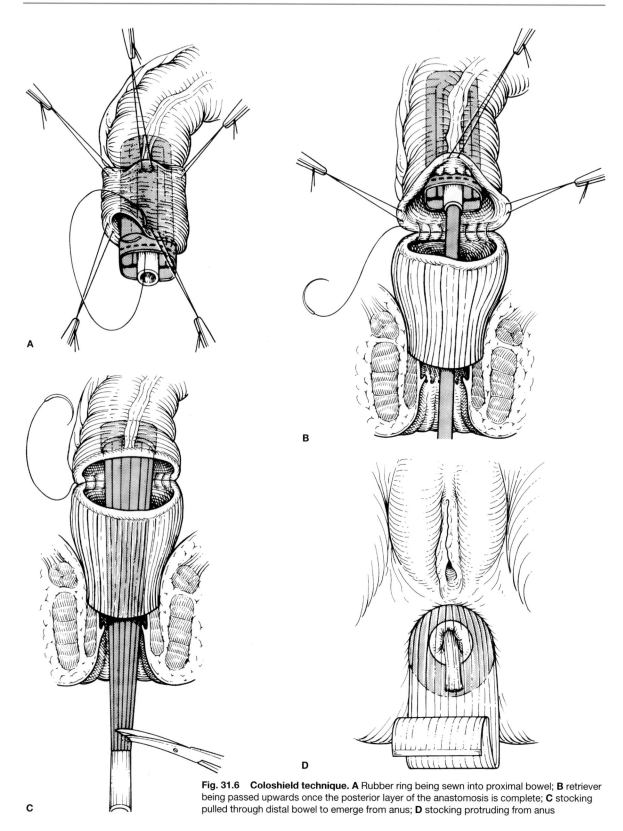

Fig. 31.6 Coloshield technique. A Rubber ring being sewn into proximal bowel; **B** retriever being passed upwards once the posterior layer of the anastomosis is complete; **C** stocking pulled through distal bowel to emerge from anus; **D** stocking protruding from anus

to adhesions, further operation may carry little prospect of success and can be hazardous if the bowel is opened inadvertently. Conservative treatment (nasogastric suction and fluid replacement) sometimes allows obstruction to settle but may have to be abandoned in favour of surgery if obstruction persists or signs develop which suggest strangulation.

Widespread intra-abdominal malignancy. In patients known to have carcinomatosis, intestinal obstruction is treated surgically only if the surgeon, in consultation with the patient and relatives, believes that it is in the patient's best interest. Usually it is not.

Crohn's disease. Crohn's disease of the small intestine is often complicated by bouts of subacute obstruction which frequently resolve on medical management with systemic steroids.

Postoperative obstruction. Distension, vomiting and failure to pass flatus after abdominal surgery are usually due to transient paralytic ileus, but mechanical obstruction can also follow intra-abdominal operations. It is most commonly due to bowel becoming trapped in peritoneal or mesenteric defects. If signs suggesting mechanical obstruction persist for more than 2–3 days, laparotomy is advisable.

Sigmoid volvulus. In many cases it is possible to deflate the sigmoid loop by passing a soft lubricated flatus tube into it through a sigmoidoscope. If this fails or if strangulation is suspected, laparotomy is needed.

PARALYTIC ILEUS

Paralytic ileus may arise as a consequence of peritonitis, pancreatitis or retroperitoneal bleeding, but can also complicate mechanical obstruction. Contributory factors include interference with neural control of the bowel, toxic effects of infection, electrolyte imbalance, hypoxia and shock. In contrast to mechanical obstruction, colic is not a feature of ileus. The abdomen is distended but there may be little tenderness or guarding. Bowel sounds are absent. There is usually copious vomiting or nasogastric aspiration. Plain films show gaseous distension and multiple fluid levels throughout the length of the gut.

Paralytic ileus is treated conservatively (nasogastric aspiration and fluid/electrolyte replacement) unless there is a remediable underlying cause, such as intra-abdominal sepsis. Surgery is normally contraindicated but the patient is reviewed at least twice daily so that a positive decision is made to persist with conservative treatment. Any suggestion of mechanical obstruction, strangulation, or sepsis means that operation should be considered urgently.

PSEUDO-OBSTRUCTION

This is a relatively rare syndrome in which gaseous abdominal distension, obstructive bowel sounds and radiological fluid levels all suggest mechanical intestinal obstruction when no mechanical obstruction is present. It is seen occasionally in patients with major respiratory or renal disease, and may follow major trauma. The fact that gas often extends to the rectum on the plain film suggests the true diagnosis, and an enema using dilute barium will confirm the absence of large bowel obstruction. Treatment is conservative unless the diagnosis remains in doubt or there is anxiety that the distension is so gross as to raise fears of caecal perforation. Colonoscopic decompression of the distended bowel has been successful in some patients.

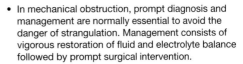

Treatment of intestinal obstruction

- In paralytic ileus, treatment is directed at the underlying cause (e.g. peritonitis, pancreatitis).

- In mechanical obstruction, prompt diagnosis and management are normally essential to avoid the danger of strangulation. Management consists of vigorous restoration of fluid and electrolyte balance followed by prompt surgical intervention.

- Strangulated bowel is blue or black, lacks sheen and peristaltic activity, and has no arterial pulsation in the adjacent mesentery. Strangulated bowel has to be resected with end-to-end anastomosis or exteriorisation of the ends of the divided intestine.

- Situations in which conservative treatment of mechanical intestinal obstruction may sometimes be justifiable include adhesion obstruction, widespread intra-abdominal malignancy, Crohn's disease and postoperative obstruction.

32

Anorectal conditions

CONTENTS

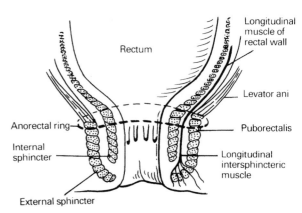

Fig. 32.1   Musculature of the anorectal region.

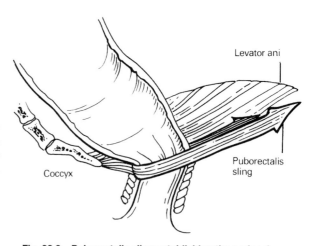

Fig. 32.2   Puborectalis sling establishing the perineal angle.

Surgical anatomy

Musculature

The anal canal is 3–4 cm long and consists of two muscular tubes: the inner tube, which is a continuation of the smooth muscle of the gut, and the outer tube, which consists of a sheath of striated muscle (Fig. 32.1).

Inner tube.   The internal sphincter is the final condensation of the circular layer of gut muscle, and as such is controlled by the autonomic nervous system. The longitudinal muscle of the gut becomes fibrous as it passes between the internal and external sphincters, ending as a series of bands which radiate to the perianal skin (see Fig. 32.1).

Outer tube.   The puborectalis fibres of the levator ani originate from the back of the pubic symphysis and form a U-shaped sling which blends with the outer layer of the bowel as it passes through the pelvic floor. This sling helps to maintain the 80° angle between the axes of the rectum and anal canal (Fig. 32.2) and also compresses the anal canal into an anteroposterior slit.

The lower border of puborectalis is in continuity with the external sphincter (see Fig. 32.1), both muscles being striated and under voluntary control. The *anorectal ring* is the condensed ring of muscle formed by the puborectalis and the upper edges of the internal and external sphincters. The ring can be felt rectally and is vital to continence.

The lining of the anal canal

The anal valves are crescentic mucosal folds which form a serrated or 'pectinate' line around the lumen some 2 cm from the anal verge (Fig. 32.3). The pectinate line corresponds to the line of fusion between endoderm of the embryonic hindgut and ectoderm of the anal pit. The canal above this line has a mucosal lining innervated by the autonomic nervous system, whereas beneath the pectinate line it is lined by modified skin innervated by the peripheral nervous system. Histologically there is a gradual transition from mucus-secreting columnar mucosa to stratified squamous epithelium. Keratinization and epidermal appendages appear only beyond the anal verge.

The mucosa above the pectinate line is thrown into vertical folds, or anal columns, the distal ends of which fuse to form the anal valves. Each valve encloses an anal crypt, and an anal gland opens into the floor of some of the crypts. These glands ramify in the submucosa to reach the internal sphincter, some of them penetrating to the intersphincteric plane (see Fig. 32.3). The glands are important in the spread of anorectal infection.

The submucosa of the anal canal forms three pads of vascular connective tissue, the so-called 'anal cushions'. These lie in the left lateral, right posterior and right anterior positions and impart a Y-shaped configuration to the lumen (Fig. 32.4).

Tissue spaces in relation to the anorectal region

The ischiorectal fossa is the pyramidal space bounded laterally by the side wall of the pelvis, medially by the external anal sphincter and superiorly by the levator

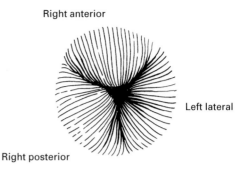

Fig. 32.4 The anal cushions.

ani (Fig. 32.5). The fossa contains fatty connective tissue and is crossed by the inferior rectal vessels. The two fossae communicate behind the anal canal.

The perianal space lies below the inferior margins of the anal sphincters and is loculated by fibrous septae.

The submucous space lies between the internal sphincter and the mucocutaneous lining of the upper two-thirds of the anal canal, and contains the internal haemorrhoidal venous plexus.

The pelvirectal space is a potential space between the upper surface of the levator ani and the pelvic peritoneum, and contains the lateral ligaments of the rectum.

Blood supply

The superior rectal artery is the continuation of the inferior mesenteric artery and forms three branches (two right, one left) which descend from the rectum to the anal canal. The anal canal is also supplied by

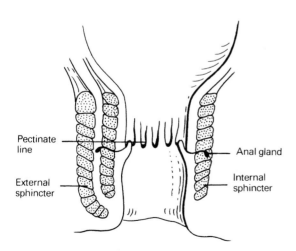

Fig. 32.3 Lining of the anal canal.

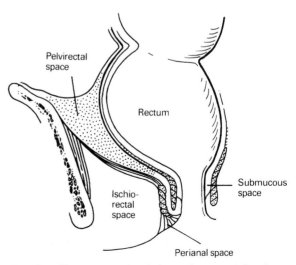

Fig. 32.5 Tissue spaces in relation to the anorectal region.

branches of the internal iliac artery. The middle rectal artery enters the rectum above the levator ani, while the inferior rectal artery traverses the ischiorectal fossa. There are profuse anastomoses between the three rectal arteries.

The superior rectal vein drains upwards into the portal system, while the middle and inferior rectal veins drain laterally into the systemic venous system. Venous anastomoses in the submucosa form the internal haemorrhoidal plexus above the pectinate line, and the external haemorrhoidal plexus below.

Lymphatic drainage

Carcinoma of the rectum spreads upwards along the superior rectal lymphatic vessels, although lesions in the lower extraperitoneal rectum occasionally spread laterally to the internal iliac glands. Metastasis to inguinal glands occurs only when carcinoma involves the skin of the lower anal canal or perianal region (Fig. 32.6).

Surgical physiology

Anal continence

The internal sphincter provides resting anal tone but relaxes following distension of the rectum by flatus or faeces. The external sphincter is contracted voluntarily if defaecation has to be postponed, and, although contraction can only be maintained for a minute or so, the rise in rectal pressure usually abates if the call to stool is resisted.

Continence depends on:

- Intact rectal and pelvic floor innervation to appreciate rectal distension
- Intact anal sensation to determine the nature of the rectal contents
- Intact innervation of anal sphincters and levator ani.

Division of the lower portion of one or both anal sphincters produces only minor defects in continence, but division of the anorectal ring causes disastrous loss of control.

The following mechanical factors may contribute to continence.

- The 80° angle between the rectum and anal canal (see Fig. 32.2) means that increases in intra-abdominal pressure tend to press the anterior rectal wall down onto the anal canal. This prevents inadvertent escape of flatus or faeces when intra-abdominal pressure rises during coughing and exercise.
- The anal canal has been likened to a flutter valve as it passes through the pelvic diaphragm. The canal walls are kept in apposition by the internal sphincter and the puborectalis sling so that continence can be maintained without conscious effort during rises in intra-abdominal pressure. When pressure rises *within the rectum*, the valve opens and contraction of the external sphincter is needed to preserve continence (Fig. 32.7).

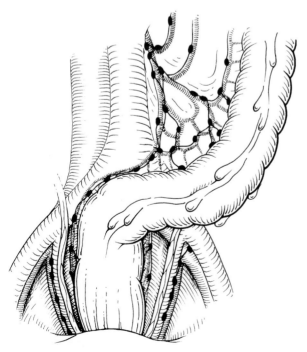

Fig. 32.6 Lymphatic drainage of the rectum.

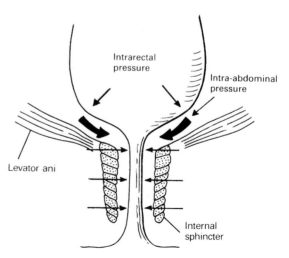

Fig. 32.7 Mechanism of continence.

- The striated muscle of the external sphincter and puborectalis is maintained in a state of tonic contraction. This is important in maintaining the two mechanisms described above.
- The bulk of the anal cushions may contribute to closure. Minor defects in continence occur in about one-quarter of patients following haemorrhoidectomy.

Control of defaecation

An increase in intrarectal pressure is followed, over a few minutes, by relaxation or 'accommodation' of the rectum. During this period there is a feeling of fullness if the rectum is sufficiently distended. At the same time, the internal anal sphincter partly relaxes, allowing rectal contents to reach the upper part of the somatic sensory epithelium. Gas can be detected by a voluntary slight increase in intra-abdominal pressure which allows a small amount of gas to escape. However, if stool is present, the external sphincter is rapidly contracted until the rectum accommodates. During defaecation there is a release of cortical inhibition and a voluntary increase in intra-abdominal pressure. The angle between rectum and anal canal is straightened and the sphincters and pelvic floor relax. Finally, there is reflex contraction of pelvic colon and rectum.

ANAL INCONTINENCE

Anal incontinence may result from any of the following causes.

Anal continence
- Continence depends upon:
  - intact anorectal and pelvic floor sensation
  - intact anal sphincters and levator ani
  - preservation of the anorectal angle
  - the bulk provided by the anal 'cushions'
  - the anal 'flutter valve' effect.

- Incontinence may be due to:
  - congenital abnormalities
  - trauma (obstetric, surgical and accidental trauma)
  - neurological defects (particularly spinal disorders)
  - psychological problems (behavioural difficulty in children, dementia and psychoses)
  - anorectal disease (e.g. prolapse, piles, inflammatory bowel disease)
  - faecal impaction with overflow incontinence
  - diarrhoea with urgency.

Congenital abnormalities. Incontinence is a feature of abnormalities such as anorectal agenesis with rectocloacal fistula.

Trauma. Division of the sphincters and anorectal ring may follow accidental injury, obstetric tears or operative trauma. Denervation may be a long-term consequence of prolonged labour.

Neurological and psychological disease. Various diseases affecting the nervous system (e.g. spina bifida, spinal trauma, spinal tumours, multiple sclerosis, tabes dorsalis) can give rise to incontinence. Incontinence of faeces is a common manifestation of behavioural problems in children, senile dementia and other psychotic illnesses.

Anorectal disease. Rectal prolapse, third-degree piles, chronic inflammatory bowel disease and anorectal cancer may cause incontinence by stretching, infiltrating or destroying the sphincter mechanism.

Faecal impaction. Impaction of faeces leads first to constipation and then to overflow incontinence of faeces with a feeling of incomplete evacuation. Faecal impaction in elderly and bed-bound patients is the commonest cause of incontinence in surgical practice.

Treatment

There is no satisfactory treatment for many causes of incontinence. The management of congenital abnormalities is outwith the scope of this book. Traumatic division of the sphincter mechanism can be repaired surgically under cover of a temporary defunctioning colostomy. If there is gross contamination at the time of injury, it is advisable to limit initial treatment to wound toilet and colostomy, and defer definitive repair until acute inflammation has subsided. Obstetric tears can often be dealt with by primary suture, but may require subsequent repair of the perineum.

Lax anal sphincters may be tightened by suture if the sphincter muscle has been partially or completely divided. A preliminary defunctioning colostomy is advisable. Sphincteroplasty operations are also available to tighten the sphincters and puborectalis muscle. Insertion of an encircling Thiersch wire may be considered in elderly unfit patients, although the results are often disappointing. A permanent colostomy is then required.

Faecal impaction demands manual or instrumental disimpaction followed by enemas and aperients to restore normal bowel action.

HAEMORRHOIDS

Aetiology

Haemorrhoids (piles) remain one of the commonest ailments of Western society, although their aetiology remains uncertain. Piles commonly develop or increase in size during pregnancy and are associated with constipation and straining at stool. There are no valves in the portal venous system, and it may be that increases in intra-abdominal pressure dilate unsupported anal canal veins. Refined low-residue Western diets with a consequent need to strain at stool may be a contributory factor.

However, a number of facts do not support the varicose vein theory of origin. The development of piles in pregnancy could equally be due to increased laxity and vascularity of the pelvic tissues. Piles are not more common in patients with portal hypertension. Rectal cancer is said to predispose to pile formation by obstructing venous drainage, but it is just as likely that these two common conditions coexist.

Alternative explanations for haemorrhoidal formation include hyperplasia of a submucosal vascular network, straining at stool with attenuation of the supporting framework of the anal cushions, and development of constricting fibrous bands within the anal canal.

Classification

Internal piles

These originate as bulges in the upper anal canal and lower rectum. The piles contain the internal haemorrhoidal plexus, but thickened mucosa and connective tissue often contribute to the pile mass. Progressive enlargement involves the skin-lined lower anal canal with its underlying external haemorrhoidal plexus. At this stage the piles become visible externally.

The piles lie in the left lateral, right anterior and right posterior positions relative to the anal canal (see Fig. 32.4). Smaller accessory piles are often present between the three main masses. Piles which bulge into the lumen without prolapsing through the anus are called first-degree, those which prolapse on defaecation but return spontaneously, second-degree, and those which remain prolapsed, third-degree piles. Some long-standing piles cannot be returned to the anal canal and are sometimes called fourth-degree piles.

Thrombosed internal haemorrhoids. This acute painful condition is often described by patients as 'an attack of piles'. It occurs when the anal sphincters contract around prolapsed piles and so prevent their return to the anal canal and obstruct venous return. Congestion and thrombosis follow and the piles become hard and tender, in contrast to uncomplicated third-degree piles. Necrosis may follow. The skin-covered part of the piles and the perianal skin become oedematous and overhanging, hiding the swollen mucosal component. Proctoscopy is usually impossible because of discomfort, and is not needed to establish the diagnosis. The term 'strangulated piles' is commonly used to describe this sequence of events.

External piles

These originate outside the anal canal and are quite distinct from the internal haemorrhoids described above. The term is used to describe anal haematomas and skin tags, but is confusing and best avoided.

Clinical features

Bleeding is traditionally the first symptom, although many patients with prolapsing piles consider prolapse to be their initial complaint. Bleeding is usually first noted as a bright red streak on the toilet paper or stool surface after a bout of constipation, and often increases in frequency and severity until a steady drip or squirting of blood accompanies defaecation. Severe secondary anaemia is however uncommon.

Prolapse produces symptoms in most patients. It is at first transient on defaecation, but occurs with increasing frequency until third-degree piles result.

Mucous discharge occurs when the columnar mucosa of the upper anal canal is exposed. Associated *skin tags* are common and cause excoriation and pruritus.

Pain is rare in uncomplicated piles. Many patients experience discomfort and some consider this to be their main complaint. *Thrombosed piles* can cause severe pain in relation to the pile-bearing areas.

Assessment and diagnosis

A careful history and abdominal examination precedes anorectal examination. Anal bleeding cannot be attributed to piles until other anorectal pathology, particularly a neoplasm, has been excluded.

Inspection of the perianal area is carried out with the patient in the left lateral position. First-degree piles produce no outward abnormality. Separation of the buttocks often reveals the skin-covered component of second-degree piles, and the piles may prolapse when the patient is asked to strain. In prolapsed third-degree piles, the red columnar anal mucosa is usually visible, separated by a furrow from the skin-lined component.

Digital rectal examination may reveal no abnormality, unless the piles are long standing and thickened. Proctoscopy is the key investigation, the piles bulging into the lumen as the instrument is withdrawn. The patient is asked to strain during withdrawal so that vascular engorgement is produced and the degree of prolapse can be determined. Sigmoidoscopy is essential to exclude coexisting rectal pathology which might mimic bleeding from piles. Barium enema is indicated when symptoms cannot be explained by proctoscopic and sigmoidoscopic findings.

With thrombosed piles the skin around the anus is swollen and oedematous in relation to the pile-bearing areas. Gentle separation of these allows a glimpse of the thrombosed pile masses, which may be red, blue or, if necrotic, black.

Treatment of internal piles

Conservative treatment

Small asymptomatic first-degree piles which are discovered as an incidental finding should be left alone. Symptomatic piles merit treatment but there is little place for 'medical' treatment by ointments or suppositories. A high-residue diet or bulk laxative is prescribed to combat constipation, and this may be all that is needed to cure the condition.

Specific treatments

Injection therapy. First-degree piles are easily treated by injection. A trial of injection is also worthwhile in second-degree piles but third-degree piles cannot be cured by this means.

The object of injection therapy is to produce submucosal fibrosis in the upper anal canal and lower rectum, constricting vascular spaces within the pile and decreasing mucosal mobility. A Gabriel syringe is filled with sclerosant (e.g. 5% phenol in almond oil) and, using a proctoscope, 3–5 ml is injected into each pile pedicle at or just above the anorectal ring (Fig. 32.8). Transient deep-seated aching sometimes follows injection of sclerosant but

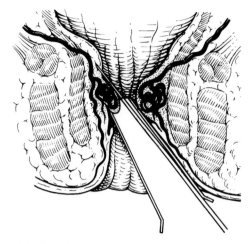

Fig. 32.8 Injection sclerotherapy for haemorrhoids.

the technique is usually painless when performed correctly.

Bleeding should cease within 24–48 hours of successful injection. Injection may be repeated if symptoms recur but operation is then usually advised.

Rubber-band ligation. This technique is a popular alternative to injection. The pile mass is pulled down through a proctoscope and a rubber band is applied around the mucosa-covered part of pedicle using a special applicator (Fig. 32.9). One pile is ligated at each visit, further banding being carried out at 3-week intervals. Approximately one-third of patients require medication for discomfort. Banding is not suitable for the skin-covered component of piles or associated skin tags.

Infrared photocoagulation. A fibreoptic probe connected to a source of infrared radiation is applied to the haemorrhoid and one or two short pulses of irradiation are delivered. This causes coagulation within the haemorrhoid, with consequent reduction in size. The technique can be carried out as an outpatient procedure, is simple and effective and, as the equipment is inexpensive, is steadily gaining in popularity.

Haemorrhoidectomy. Several operations are described to treat internal piles. Most commonly practised is ligation and excision of each pile mass following its dissection from the anal canal (Fig. 32.10).

The plane of dissection passes just within the internal sphincter, which is carefully preserved. Each vascular pedicle is transfixed and ligated, and the piles are excised to leave three raw areas separated by bridges of skin and mucosa. Epithelialization of

Stools should be kept soft (e.g. by methyl cellulose) for 3–4 weeks while epithelialization takes place. Male patients occasionally have difficulty in micturition but catheterization is rarely needed. Reactionary haemorrhage occurs in less than 2% of patients, and secondary haemorrhage 7–10 days after operation in just over 1%. Anal stenosis, fissure, abscess and fistula are rare complications. The late results show that while only 5% of patients have recurrent symptoms, two-thirds still have first-degree piles on proctoscopy. On careful questioning some patients admit to intermittent flatus incontinence or soiling of underwear, but significant faecal incontinence is rare.

Treatment of thrombosed internal haemorrhoids

In the early stages it may be possible to return prolapsed piles to the anal canal and allow the congestion to settle. This is seldom feasible by the time most patients present, although anal dilatation performed under general anaesthesia may promote reduction. Conservative treatment includes bed rest, local application of dressings soaked in hypertonic saline, analgesics and mild aperients.

Resolution takes about 10 days. Although haemorrhoidectomy is usually required at some future date, in some cases the attack of thrombosis will have cured the piles. Immediate haemorrhoidectomy is now seldom undertaken.

Perianal haematoma

This common condition is due to rupture of a vein at the anal verge with haematoma formation. A small painful lump develops rapidly, often after an episode

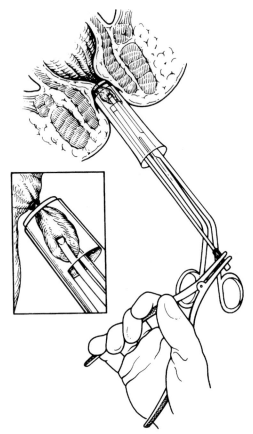

Fig. 32.9   Rubber band ligation of haemorrhoids.

the raw areas takes 3–4 weeks and prevents excessive fibrosis or anal narrowing.

Postoperative pain is common, and considerable discomfort accompanies the first bowel motion.

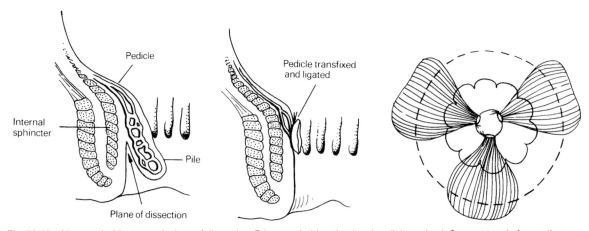

Fig. 32.10   Haemorrhoidectomy: A plane of dissection; **B** haemorrhoid excised and pedicle excised; **C** anus at end of operation showing the three raw areas separated by intact mucosal bridges.

of straining at stool. The lump is tense, blue, well circumscribed and exquisitely tender. The haematoma is readily distinguished from thrombosed internal haemorrhoids by its restricted size, and from perianal abscess by its colour.

Spontaneous resolution takes some days and often leaves a skin tag at the site. Occasionally the haematoma ruptures or becomes secondarily infected.

Evacuation of the haematoma under local anaesthesia is advised to relieve pain and tenderness and speed recovery.

RECTAL PROLAPSE

Three types of rectal prolapse are described.

Type I is an *incomplete, partial* or *mucosal* prolapse in which the mucous membrane lining the anal canal is lax and protrudes through the anus.

Type II is a *complete prolapse* in which intussusception of the rectum results in the whole thickness of the bowel protruding through the anus.

Type III is also a *complete prolapse* involving the whole thickness of the rectal wall, but in this case due to a sliding hernia of the pouch of Douglas. If there is associated vaginal prolapse, the term *procidentia* is applied.

Haemorrhoids
- Internal haemorrhoids originate as bulges within the upper anal canal and consist of thickened mucosa and connective tissue which contains the internal haemorrhoidal plexus.

- Haemorrhoids are usually classified as:
  - first degree (visible in the lumen on proctoscopy but do not prolapse)
  - second degree (prolapse on defaecation but return spontaneously)
  - third degree (remain prolapsed but can be digitally replaced)
  - fourth degree (long-standing prolapse, cannot be replaced in anal canal)

- Manifestations of haemorrhoids include bleeding (usually on defaecation), prolapse, mucus discharge, discomfort and thrombosis.

- Treatment depends on the degree; first-degree piles are usually left alone with advice on avoiding constipation and straining, while symptomatic piles of a higher degree can be treated by injection, banding, photocoagulation or haemorrhoidectomy.

- Thrombosed piles are usually treated conservatively in the first instance but interval haemorrhoidectomy is usually needed to avoid further problems.

Any type of prolapse can occur at any time of life. However, incomplete (type I) prolapse is common in young children, whereas complete (types II and III) prolapse is commoner in adults. Approximately 85% of affected adults are women, and older females are particularly at risk.

Aetiology

Partial prolapse. Prolapse in childhood is favoured if the sacral curve of the rectum is lacking so that the rectum and anus form a vertical tube. Excessive straining at stool is a major factor, and malnourishment contributes by reducing the amount of fat in the supporting ischiorectal and pararectal tissues.

Partial prolapse in adults may complicate haemorrhoid formation or may follow damage to the anal sphincters during labour or anal surgery.

Complete prolapse. Most patients with complete prolapse have deficient muscle tone in the pelvic floor and anal canal, which can now be confirmed by neurophysiological testing. Many female patients have had previous hysterectomy or other gynaecological procedures. Additional factors include lack of fixation of the rectum to its sacral bed, intussusception of the rectum and an abnormally deep rectovaginal or rectovesical pouch.

Clinical features

Prolapse is first noted during defaecation. For a time it reduces spontaneously once straining ceases. Discomfort during defaecation is common, and there may be bleeding and mucus discharge. The prolapse recurs with increasing ease and may be caused by mild exertion such as coughing and walking. The bowel habit becomes irregular, and laxity of the musculature coupled with impaired rectal sensation leads to incontinence of both flatus and faeces. Such incontinence is the main reason for patients seeking help. Associated uterine prolapse compounds the problem by causing incontinence of urine.

The prolapse may not be apparent until the patient is asked to bear down and strain. The anus is usually patulous and can be opened widely simply by drawing the buttocks apart. Digital rectal examination reveals poor sphincter tone, and two or more fingers can be inserted without apparent discomfort. The prolapse appears progressively on straining but seldom protrudes for more than 10 cm. The mucosa is thickened, engorged and corrugated but mucosal folds may be ironed out as the prolapse emerges.

The thickness of the prolapse is judged between finger and thumb to decide whether it is partial or complete. Partial prolapse seldom protrudes for more than 5 cm.

The complications of rectal prolapse include irreducibility with ulceration, bleeding and gangrene, and rarely, rupture of the prolapsed bowel.

The diagnosis of rectal prolapse is usually straightforward. The appearance can be confused with large third-degree piles, and occasionally with prolapse of a rectal neoplasm.

Treatment

Prolapse in children responds to conservative measures in most cases and rarely persists beyond the age of 5 years. Constipation and straining at stool should be avoided, and the buttocks may be strapped together to discourage prolapse during defaecation. If these measures fail, submucosal injection of phenol may be used to fix lax mucosa to underlying tissues.

In adults, the choice of treatment depends on the type of rectal prolapse.

Partial prolapse

Provided sphincter tone is satisfactory, partial prolapse in adults can be treated by excising prolapsing mucosa using a technique similar to that used for the dissection and ligature of haemorrhoids. Patients with poor sphincter tone are unlikely to benefit as their main complaint is incontinence rather than the prolapse. Various methods of improving sphincter tone have been described although none is entirely satisfactory. These methods include voluntary exercise of sphincter muscle, electrical stimulation, and perineorrhaphy to tighten the puborectalis muscle. Education of bowel habit is an important part of treatment, and insertion of a Thiersch wire (see below) may be considered in frail elderly patients but has lost popularity.

Complete prolapse

Various methods are available to treat complete prolapse; none is ideal.

Narrowing of the anus. The simplest form of surgery once consisted of inserting a Thiersch wire of stainless steel or synthetic monofilament material around the anal canal (Fig. 32.11), but this procedure was rarely successful in complete prolapse. The incidence of faecal impaction was high and the procedure is no longer used.

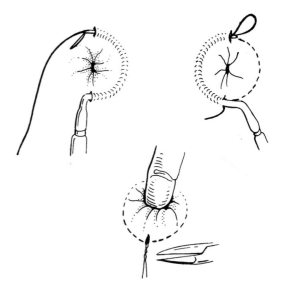

Fig. 32.11 Treatment of rectal prolapse by insertion of a Thiersch wire using an aneurysm needle (the wire is tightened around one finger).

Repair of pelvic structures and fixation of rectum. A variety of repairs can be carried out through the abdomen. These are successful in an anatomical sense in that they prevent further prolapse, but some degree of incontinence persists in about 30% of patients. Most methods include thorough mobilization of the rectum, fixation of the rectum to the sacrum, suture of the levator ani muscles in front of the rectum, and obliteration of the deep pouch of Douglas. Mobilization of the rectum favours extensive adhesion formation and prevents further prolapse by fixing the rectum to the sacrum. Additional fixation can be achieved by attaching a sheet of Ivalon sponge to the front of the sacrum and wrapping this sheet around the mobilized rectum, or by placing non-absorbable sutures between the rectum and periosteum of the sacrum. Anterior restorative resection may be used in some cases. If incontinence persists after a satisfactory anatomical repair, sphincter function may be improved by a *postanal repair*, in which, through an incision posterior to the anus, the posterior part of the sphincters is strengthened by sutures and the margins of the puborectalis are sutured together behind the rectum to increase the angle between the rectum and the anal canal. Abdominoperineal resection of the rectum is a last resort in patients with gross incontinence who fail to respond to less radical measures. In very frail patients a colostomy alone may suffice.

PRURITUS ANI

Aetiology

This common condition occurs most frequently in men between the ages of 30 and 60 years. Causal factors are identified in only 50% of patients. It is assumed that psychogenic problems, chemical irritation by some constituent of faeces, or food allergy are responsible in the remainder. Defined causes of pruritus ani include the following.

Skin disease. Skin lesions may be localized to the perianal area or, as in the case of psoriasis and lichen planus, there may be lesions elsewhere. Contact eczema can be caused by local application of steroid, antibiotic, local anaesthetic or lanolin ointment or creams. Premalignant keratosis is a rare cause of perianal itching.

Infective conditions. Candidiasis must be considered in diabetics and those who have received courses of corticosteroids or broad-spectrum antibiotics. Fungal infections occur occasionally. Threadworms are common in children but not in adults. Anal warts are commonly complicated by pruritus.

Gastrointestinal conditions. Pruritus can be a feature of anorectal disorders which cause a rectal discharge. Such disorders include piles, fissure, fistula, proctitis, polyps and rectal cancer. Frequent bowel movements in the irritable bowel syndrome, ulcerative colitis or malabsorptive disorders also predispose to pruritus.

Miscellaneous conditions. Some drugs such as quinidine and colchicine cause pruritus when taken for prolonged periods. Obesity increases the risk of pruritus.

Clinical features

The itching varies from a minor nuisance to a source of overwhelming misery. The urge to scratch is often irresistible so that the skin is damaged, causing local discomfort or pain. Symptoms are worst after defaecation and at night, regardless of the cause of pruritus.

The perianal skin may show no abnormality on examination, but more often appears raw and excoriated with linear cracks, ulcers and lichenification. Psoriasis and fungal infection often have a well-defined border.

Investigation is aimed at establishing the underlying cause. The entire skin surface is inspected, and proctoscopy and sigmoidoscopy are performed. The urine is examined for glucose. Candidiasis and fungal infection can be confirmed on skin scrapings.

Treatment

Underlying causes such as psoriasis, diabetes and infections are treated in the usual manner. Local abnormalities such as skin tags, fissures and fistulas should be surgically corrected.

If no cause can be defined, a number of useful symptomatic measures can be introduced. First, all local applications are discontinued. Attention to anal hygiene is essential, as there may be primary or secondary sensitivity to faeces or rectal mucus. The region should be washed with lukewarm water in the morning and evening, and immediately after defaecation. Medicated soaps are avoided as their contained antiseptic may cause irritation. Excessive use of any form of soap is discouraged. After washing, the area is patted dry with a soft towel. It must not be rubbed vigorously. Application of talcum powder may be useful in warm weather to combat excessive sweating, and shaving of the perianal skin may be worthwhile. Woollen and nylon underwear favour sweating and should be replaced by cotton mesh garments.

It may be possible to identify certain items of diet which exacerbate pruritus, e.g. beer, red wine, coffee, curries, fruit and milk. Ingestion of mineral oil may favour pruritus by causing anal leakage, and advice on laxatives is essential. Bulk laxatives are preferred as a means of achieving a regular soft motion.

Considerable will power is needed to stop scratching during waking hours. Involuntary scratching during sleep can be reduced by sedation with phenothiazines. Postmenopausal women may benefit from oestrogen therapy, particularly if there is associated genital pruritus.

Continuing support is essential. Regular review ensures that the prescribed measures are being carried out.

Surgical treatment by denervation of the perianal skin through two curved incisions, one on either side of the perianal verge, has been described, but gives no guarantee of success.

ANORECTAL ABSCESS

Aetiology

Anorectal abscesses are a common cause of admission to hospital. They are two or three times more

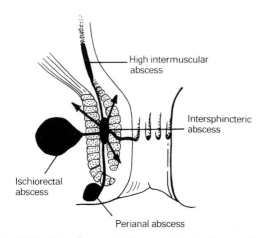

Fig. 32.12 Sites of anorectal abscess with potential origin in an anal gland.

common in males, the highest incidence occurring in the third and fourth decades.

There is no apparent cause for abscess formation in the majority of patients. It has been suggested that infection arises in an anal gland, passes to the intersphincteric space, and may then track:

- Downwards to present as a perianal abscess
- Outwards to form an ischiorectal abscess
- Upwards to produce a high intermuscular abscess (Fig. 32.12).

Intersphincteric abscesses undoubtedly occur, but are less common than this concept suggests.

Underlying diseases such as Crohn's disease, ulcerative colitis, rectal cancer, HIV infection and active tuberculosis should always be considered in patients with recurrent anorectal infection.

Anorectal abscess may lead to the development of a fistula-in-ano or, conversely, may complicate a fistula. In all recurrent abscesses this underlying cause should be kept in mind.

Clinical features

Perianal abscess is common and presents as an acute painful tender swelling at the anal verge. Systemic upset is minimal.

Ischiorectal abscess is also common and produces a brawny diffuse induration lateral to the anus. The swelling is painful and tender but fluctuation occurs late. Systemic upset is pronounced. The swelling may be palpable on digital rectal examination and infection may extend behind the anal canal as a

'horseshoe abscess' involving both ischiorectal fossae.

Intersphincteric abscess is uncommon. Continuous throbbing anal pain is exacerbated by defaecation. There are few external signs unless the abscess is complicated by perianal or ischiorectal suppuration. Discharge into the anal canal leads to the passage of pus and blood. On digital rectal examination there is a boggy tender swelling under the mucosa.

High intermuscular abscess is rare and resembles an intersphincteric abscess in its presentation.

Pelvirectal abscess originates from pelvic sepsis.

Treatment

Perianal and ischiorectal abscesses are incised and drained under general anaesthesia. A specimen of pus is taken for bacteriological examination. The cavity walls are probed gently to detect any communication with the anal lumen. Fistulous connections can be demonstrated in up to one-third of patients but many such 'fistulas' are caused by injudicious probing. Assuming that no communication is detected, the abscess is deroofed by making a cruciate incision and excising the four triangles of skin (Fig. 32.13). The excised skin and a biopsy of the abscess wall are sent routinely for histological examination. A minority of surgeons suture the wound under antibiotic cover.

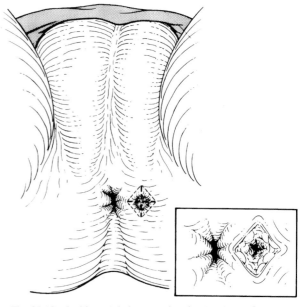

Fig. 32.13 Ischiorectal abscess showing treatment by cruciate incision. Inset: appearance of incision after excision of four skin triangles.

Problems in the treatment of anorectal abscess

Fistula-in-ano. If the internal opening of a fistula-in-ano is demonstrated on exploration and is below the pectinate line, the fistula should be laid open. This should only be performed by an experienced surgeon. If there is doubt about the level of the fistula, treatment should be deferred.

Recurrence. About one-quarter of patients presenting with an anorectal abscess develop recurrent abscess or a fistula, those with ischiorectal abscesses being most at risk. The rate of recurrence is not influenced by the primary treatment, i.e. whether primary suture is carried out or the wound is left to drain and heal by granulation.

Inflammatory bowel disease. Anorectal abscess may be the first manifestation of Crohn's disease, ulcerative colitis or, much less commonly, tuberculosis. These abscesses are characteristically indolent and lined by pale grey granulation tissue. They should be incised and drained. Bacteriological and histological confirmation of the diagnosis is essential. Incision is frequently followed by fistula formation.

FISSURE-IN-ANO

An anal fissure is a tear in the sensitive skin-lined lower anal canal which produces pain on defaecation. The fissure commonly presents as an isolated primary problem but can be associated with other gastrointestinal diseases.

Anorectal infection
- Most cases of anorectal infection are thought to originate in infection of an anal gland.
- Perianal and ischiorectal abscesses are the commonest forms of abscess in the anorectal region.
- Anorectal abscesses (and fissures and fistulae) are commonly associated with underlying Crohn's disease or ulcerative colitis, and may also be associated with rectal carcinoma, tuberculosis and HIV infection.
- Perianal and ischiorectal abscesses are treated by incision and drainage, taking care to exclude underlying bowel pathology or fistula, particularly in patients with recurrent abscesses.

Classification

Primary fissure-in-ano

The aetiology of primary fissure-in-ano is uncertain but many patients first notice symptoms after passage of a hard constipated stool. The superficial fibres of the external sphincter are deficient posteriorly, and this may explain the frequency with which anal fissures occur in the posterior midline.

Secondary fissure-in-ano

Fissures are common in Crohn's disease and ulcerative colitis. Such secondary fissures are frequently multiple, occur at any point on the canal circumference, are broad-based and characteristically indolent. Fissures are a rare complication of anorectal operations such as haemorrhoidectomy.

Pathology of primary fissure

The typical primary fissure (Fig. 32.14) is a longitudinal tear extending from the anal verge to the pectinate line in the posterior midline. In 15% of female patients and in 1% of males the tear is in the midline anteriorly. The tear becomes a canoe-shaped ulcer, the floor of which contains the lower third of the internal sphincter. Inflammation causes swelling of the margins of the fissure, and an oedematous skin tag develops at the anal verge which is known as a *sentinel pile*. The swollen anal valve at the upper extent of the fissure is called a 'hypertrophied anal papilla'. Infection may produce a perianal abscess, incision of which results in a low anal fistula.

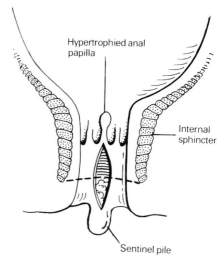

Fig. 32.14 Fissure-in-ano.

Anal fissures may heal spontaneously if untreated, or become chronic with fibrosis of the spastic internal sphincter.

Clinical features

The principal feature of a fissure is severe burning pain on defaecation which may persist for several hours. The pain may be so intense that defaecation is avoided. Bleeding sometimes occurs on defaecation, but is seldom profuse. The sentinel pile and associated serous discharge may cause excoriation and pruritus. Perianal abscesses and anal fistulas can complicate the fissure.

Recurrent or indolent fissures or fissures in an unusual site suggest the possibility of Crohn's disease or ulcerative colitis.

The diagnosis can usually be made on the history alone. Inspection reveals the sentinel pile, and traction on the anal skin brings the lower part of the fissure into view. Digital rectal examination is painful and not often practicable. If the finger can be inserted, sphincter spasm is confirmed and the indurated margins of the fissure are apparent. Maximal tenderness is elicited when the base of the fissure is palpable. Proctoscopy and sigmoidoscopy are essential to exclude other anorectal disease, but must be carried out under anaesthesia.

Treatment

Conservative treatment

Anal fissures can heal spontaneously. Conservative treatment with local anaesthetic ointments and suppositories has usually been tried without success by the time the patient is referred to hospital. Operative treatment allows a full anorectal examination, provides a rapid, more certain cure, and is generally advocated. Chronic fissures are unlikely to heal without operation.

Operative treatment

Under general anaesthesia the patient is placed in the lithotomy position, and the anal canal and rectum are examined thoroughly.

Anal dilatation. The majority of acute fissures respond to dilatation with dramatic relief of pain and spasm and subsequent healing. However impairment of anal control occurs in about a quarter of patients, and this method has now been abandoned.

Lateral subcutaneous internal sphincterotomy. This operation gives a better guarantee of

Fissure-in-ano
- Most anal fissures are primary but fissures are also common as manifestations of Crohn's disease and ulcerative colitis.
- The typical primary anal fissure extends in the midline posteriorly from the pectinate line to the anal verge, and is associated with an oedematous skin tag (sentinel pile) and hypertrophied anal papilla.
- Pain on defaecation is the outstanding symptom of primary anal fissure. Fissures secondary to conditions such as Crohn's disease may be less painful, indolent and multiple.
- Operative division of the lower part of the internal sphincter (lateral subcutaneous internal sphincterotomy) is the treatment of choice.

success for both acute and chronic fissures. A tenotomy knife is introduced through the perianal skin on one side of the anal canal, and the internal sphincter is divided from the pectinate line downwards *without* entering the canal lumen. The procedure gives immediate relief of pain.

FISTULA-IN-ANO

Aetiology

The aetiology of fistula-in-ano is uncertain. It may be that infection commences in an anal gland, spreads to produce an intersphincteric abscess and then tracks into the perianal or ischiorectal region. Surgical incision or spontaneous discharge completes the fistula, which is kept open by continuing infection from the anal lumen.

Anal fistulas have a well-recognized association with Crohn's disease, ulcerative colitis, tuberculosis, colloid carcinoma of the rectum, lymphogranuloma venereum and HIV infection. Carcinoma is a very rare complication of long-standing fistulas.

Classification (Fig. 32.15)

Low anal fistula

This is the commonest anal fistula. The track does not extend higher than the anal crypts and usually enters the bowel at this level. The fistula may traverse both internal and external sphincters as it passes to the exterior, or descend in the intersphincteric plane.

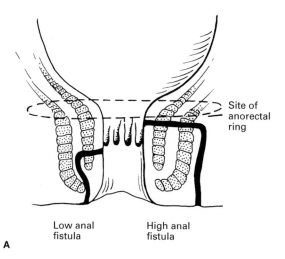

Low anal fistula   High anal fistula

Site of anorectal ring

A

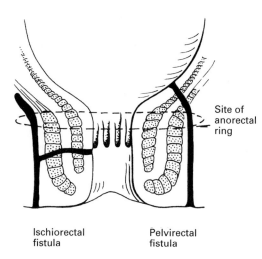

Ischiorectal fistula   Pelvirectal fistula

Site of anorectal ring

B

Fig. 32.15 Types of fistual-in-ano. A: anal fistulas; **B** anorectal fistulas.

High anal fistula

The track extends above the pectinate line but not above the anorectal ring. As with low fistulas, the track may traverse both sphincters or descend between them.

Anorectal fistula

These fistulas are rare. In the *ischiorectal* variety, the track extends above the anorectal ring but does not pass through the levator ani to enter the rectum. The rarer *pelvirectal* fistula does penetrate the levator, entering the rectum above the anorectal ring (see Fig. 32.15).

Goodsall's rule

Fistulas with an external opening in front of a transverse line through the anus generally open into the anal canal at the nearest point on its circumference. Fistulas with external openings behind this line tend to open internally in the posterior midline, and may extend behind the anal canal on both sides, forming a horseshoe fistula (Fig. 32.16).

Clinical features

Fistulas commonly present as abscesses, surgical incision of which completes the fistula. Alternatively, the patient notices a small discharging sinus with excoriation and pruritus. Once the fistula has formed, it is generally painless unless blockage leads to abscess formation.

Examination reveals the external opening or openings. Digital rectal examination may reveal induration along the fistula track, while pressure on the indurated area expresses pus from the external opening. The internal opening may occasionally be seen on proctoscopy, and a malleable probe can be passed carefully along the fistula to define its course. Sigmoidoscopy is performed to exclude associated rectal disease.

Treatment

Fistulas associated with other anorectal disease are usually treated conservatively in the first instance. Those arising de novo rarely close spontaneously and operation is generally advised. The course of the fistula must be determined before embarking on surgery and the anorectal ring must be preserved. Disastrous permanent incontinence follows its inadvertent division.

Low anal fistulas are laid open along their entire length and allowed to heal by granulation and epi-

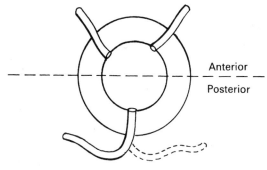

Anterior

Posterior

Fig. 32.16 Goodsall's rule.

thelialization. High anal fistulas and the ischiorectal type of anorectal fistula are treated in the same way provided the surgeon is certain that laying open the fistulas will not divide the anorectal ring. A two-stage procedure is sometimes used, passing a suture along the track and out through the anal canal. The suture is tied at the anal verge and this 'seton' allows fibrosis to occur before dividing the sphincteric muscle.

The rare pelvirectal fistula cannot be laid open without producing incontinence. The alternatives to a difficult formal repair are conservative treatment, long-term defunctioning colostomy, or excision of the rectum with permanent colostomy.

ANAL NEOPLASMS

Anal papillomas (anal warts, condylomata acuminata)

These deserve special mention. They arise from the anus or perianal skin, are often multiple, and often completely surround the anal region. Individual papillomas may be sessile or pedunculated, are often friable and bleed readily, and are usually associated with an offensive irritating discharge. The lesions are due to a viral infection and may present a serious problem in immunosuppressed patients.

Although they are particularly common in male homosexuals, these papillomas must not be confused with the flatter, smoother condylomata lata of secondary syphilis. Dark-ground illumination of the discharge fluid will reveal large numbers of spirochaetes and establish the diagnosis of syphilis.

Treatment

Anal papillomas are treated by local application of podophyllin. Excision or diathermy is needed if this fails. In severe infections, interferon has been used with success.

Squamous cell carcinoma

This lesion accounts for at least 50% of malignant growths arising in the region of the anal canal, but carcinoma of the rectum is about 50 times more common. Squamous carcinoma of the anus is more common in males. The aetiology of anal carcinoma is unknown but chronic irritation or infection may be a predisposing factor.

Clinical features

The patient usually presents with a localized ulcer or raised warty growth with an irregular ulcerated surface. A history of bleeding may give rise to an erroneous diagnosis of haemorrhoids. A profuse discharge results from ulceration and some patients develop incontinence due to involvement of the anal sphincter. Female patients may experience a vaginal discharge due to development of a fistulous communication with the vagina. The lesion is usually indurated, may spread around the anus, and is often fixed to underlying tissues by the time of presentation. Digital rectal examination may prove impossible because of stenosis or discomfort, but it is important to make certain that the lesion does arise from the anus or anal canal and is not a prolapsing or spreading adenocarcinoma of the lower rectum. The inguinal lymph nodes are examined carefully, as they receive lymph from the lower anal canal and perianal region and may be the seat of metastatic spread. Secondary sepsis produces nodes which are soft or firm, in contrast to the stony hard nodes of secondary neoplastic involvement.

The differential diagnosis of anal carcinoma includes anal papillomas, condylomata lata, primary syphilitic chancre, anal fissure, thrombosed piles, and Crohn's disease. The diagnosis must always be confirmed by biopsy.

Treatment

Anal carcinoma may be treated by radium implantation or X-ray therapy, but surgical excision is usually preferred. Abdominoperineal excision of the anus, anal canal and rectum is the treatment of choice, particularly if the lesion extends above the pectinate line. In selected patients there may be a case for wide local excision if the lesion is confined to the anal margin or perianal area.

Treatment of the inguinal lymph nodes is controversial. Some 40% of patients will have nodal metastases at presentation and block dissection of obviously involved nodes is generally recommended once the patient has recovered fully from treatment of the primary anal lesion. If the nodes are not obviously involved, most surgeons would adopt a watching policy rather than 'prophylactic' block dissection with its attendant hazards of sepsis, skin necrosis and lymphoedema. Radiotherapy offers an alternative method of treatment but many surgeons reserve this for patients with fixed inoperable nodes.

Results

The prognosis for patients with anal carcinoma is influenced by the extent of spread, but in general the outlook is less good than that of carcinoma of the rectum. Five-year survival rates of around 50% can be achieved if excision is feasible, but few patients with obvious nodal metastases at presentation survive for more than five years.

Rare malignant tumours

Adenocarcinoma

Primary adenocarcinoma of the anal region is exceptionally rare but the neoplasm may arise in a long-standing fistula-in-ano, in the anal glands, or in the apocrine glands of the skin around the anal margin. Adenocarcinoma of the rectum may extend into the anal region and malignant cells from a colorectal cancer can implant in the raw wound following haemorrhoidectomy.

Primary anal adenocarcinoma is treated in the same way as squamous cell carcinoma, but in general the prognosis is poor.

Basal cell carcinoma

Basal cell carcinoma arising in the anal region is rare. The lesion has the same characteristics as basal cell carcinoma elsewhere and is treated by surgery or radiotherapy.

Malignant melanoma

Malignant melanoma of the anal region is rare.

PILONIDAL SINUS

A pilonidal sinus occurs predominantly in the natal cleft of young adults but can occasionally occur on the hands of barbers and in the periumbilical area.

Typically a post-anal pilonidal sinus starts at an opening some 2 cm posterior to the anus and extends subcutaneously in a headward direction for

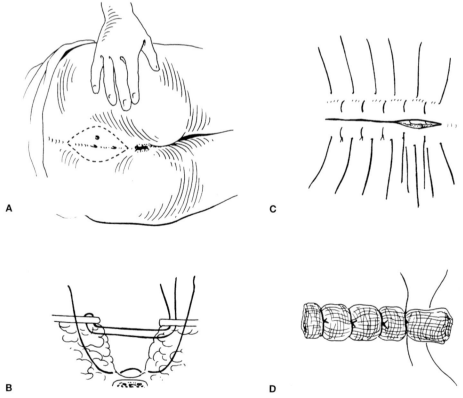

Fig. 32.17 **Treatment of pilonidal sinus: A** elliptical incision to include all sinus openings; **B** insertion of deep tension sutures down to the sacral fascia and placement of sutures in skin edges; **C** skin sutures being tied; **D** deep tension sutures tied over gauze roll to obliterate dead space.

about 2–5 cm, expanding into a cavity. Secondary sinuses may arise from this and open onto the surface above the primary opening.

The opening of the sinus is lined by squamous epithelium but only for a few millimetres. Most of its wall is composed of granulation tissue. A typical feature of the sinus is its content of hairs. These are drawn into the sinus, tips first, and held in its depth by the direction of their scales.

Various theories have been proposed to explain the origin of a pilonidal sinus. It is now generally accepted that the problem is acquired by penetration of hairs and subsequent entry of infection.

Clinical features

A pilonidal sinus does not usually become evident until infected. An acute or chronic abscess then develops, forming either a red tender hot swelling or a chronic discharge from the sinus. If seen in a quiescent phase, the appearance of the external orifice(s) is diagnostic.

Treatment

A pilonidal abscess is drained under general anaesthesia. The abscess cavity is deroofed and thoroughly cleaned out, removing all hair, granulation tissue and debris. It is left open to granulate and will heal over several weeks.

In a quiescent case, the sinus track is either excised or laid open. Excision of the sinus and its ramifications requires wide removal of tissue (Fig. 32.17). Primary suture is preferable but can be difficult if the skin is not to be 'tented' over the underlying cavity. Rotation flaps can be used to facilitate primary healing.

When primary suture is not feasible or has failed, it is necessary to leave the wound open to granulate. Healing may then take many months. For this reason, marsupialization of the sinuses, i.e. laying them open and 'guttering' them by excising the skin edges, is preferred by many surgeons. The wound is left open, the skin edges being held apart by a pack or 'stent' of silicone foam so that they cannot reunite before healing occurs from the depths of the sinus.

Destruction of granulations by injecting phenol into the sinus track has also been reported to control symptoms.

Pilonidal sinuses are prone to recur. It is important that following any operative procedure for a pilonidal sinus the post-anal area is kept clean. In hirsute patients, regular shaving is advised.

33

The liver and biliary tract

CONTENTS

THE LIVER

Anatomy

The liver is the largest abdominal organ, weighing approximately 1500 g. It extends from the fifth intercostal space to the right costal margin. It is triangular in shape, its apex reaching the left midclavicular line in the fifth intercostal space. In the recumbent position the liver is impalpable under cover of the ribs. The liver is attached to the undersurface of the diaphragm by suspensory ligaments which enclose a 'bare area', the only part of its surface without a peritoneal covering. Its inferior or visceral surface lies on the right kidney, duodenum, colon and stomach.

Topographically the liver is divided by the attachment of the falciform ligament into right and left lobes; fissures on its visceral surface demarcate two further lobes, the quadrate and caudate (Fig. 33.1). From a practical standpoint it is the segmental anatomy of the liver, as defined by the distribution of its blood supply, which is important to the surgeon.

Segmental anatomy

The portal vein and hepatic artery divide into right and left branches in the porta hepatis. Occluding either branch at surgery produces an easily visible line of demarcation which runs from the gallbladder bed behind and to the left of the inferior vena cava, thus separating the two hemilivers. Each hemiliver is further divided into four segments corresponding to the main branches of the hepatic artery and portal

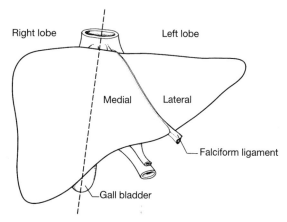

Fig. 33.1   Surgical anatomy of the liver.

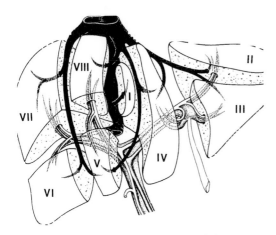

Fig. 33.2 Segmental anatomy and venous drainage.

vein. In the left hemiliver, segment I corresponds to the caudate lobe, segments II and III to the left lobe and segment IV to the quadrate lobe. The remaining segments (V to VIII) comprise the right hemiliver (Fig. 33.2).

Blood supply

The liver normally receives 1500 ml of blood/min and has a dual blood supply: 65% comes from the portal vein and 35% from the hepatic artery. Because of its better oxygenation the hepatic artery supplies 50% of the oxygen requirements.

The principal venous drainage of the liver is by the right, middle and left hepatic veins, which leave the back of the liver to enter the vena cava (Fig. 33.2). In 25% of individuals there is an inferior right hepatic vein and numerous small veins drain direct into the

vena cava from the caudate lobe (segment I). The functional unit of the liver is the hepatic lobule. Sheets of liver cells (hepatocytes) one cell thick are separated by interlacing sinusoids through which blood flows from the 'peripheral' portal tract to the 'central' branch of the hepatic venous system. The lobule forms a many-sided structure at each angle of which is a portal space containing a branch of the portal vein, hepatic artery and bile duct. Bile is secreted by the liver cells into small canaliculi which pass centrifugally through the lobule to drain into bile ductules leading to the right and left hepatic ducts (Fig. 33.3).

JAUNDICE

Jaundice is a yellowish discolouration of the tissues which is most obvious in those containing elastin, such as the skin and sclera. It is due to an increase in the level of circulating bilirubin and becomes obvious clinically when levels exceed 50 μmol/l. Jaundice may result from excessive destruction of red cells (haemolytic jaundice), from failure to remove bilirubin from the bloodstream (hepatocellular jaundice), or from obstruction to the flow of bile from the liver (cholestatic jaundice) (Fig. 33.4). Congenital non-haemolytic hyperbilirubinaemia is a relatively rare cause of jaundice due to defective bilirubin transport; the jaundice is usually mild and transient, the prognosis is excellent and the condition must not be confused with more serious causes of jaundice.

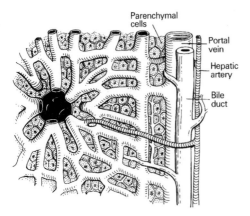

Fig. 33.3 The hepatic lobule: sinusoids drain into the central hepatic vein.

Parenchymal cells

Portal vein

Hepatic artery

Bile duct

Surgical anatomy
- The liver is divisible into right and left hemi-livers (each having four segments) by a line running from the gallbladder fossa to the inferior vena cava.

- Each *lobe* receives a branch of the hepatic artery and portal vein; 65% of liver blood flow and 50% of its oxygen supply are provided by the portal vein.

- The hepatocytes are arranged in lobules, each of which has a central branch of the hepatic vein and peripheral portal tracts (containing a branch of the hepatic artery, portal vein and bile duct).

- Liver anatomy allows the surgeon to perform right hepatectomy, left hepatectomy and extended right hepatectomy (i.e. resecting all of the liver to the right of the falciform ligament). Resection of individual segments is also possible.

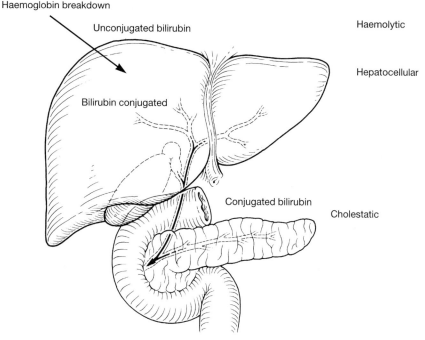

Haemoglobin breakdown

Unconjugated bilirubin

Haemolytic

Hepatocellular

Bilirubin conjugated

Conjugated bilirubin

Cholestatic

Fig. 33.4   Types of jaundice.

To the surgeon the most important type of haemolytic jaundice is that caused by hereditary spherocytosis, in which splenectomy may be necessary (see Ch. 35). Haemolytic jaundice may also occur after blood transfusion and after operative or accidental trauma where haematoma formation produces a pigment load which exceeds hepatic excretory capacity.

Hepatocellular jaundice is usually a medical as opposed to surgical problem although its recognition in patients presenting with abdominal pain is important, since surgical intervention may aggravate the hepatocellular injury.

Cholestatic jaundice due to intrahepatic obstruction of bile canaliculi may be a feature of acute and chronic liver disease and can be caused by drugs (e.g. chlorpromazine). This form of jaundice must be differentiated from that due to extrahepatic obstruction, the cause which has most surgical relevance. Extrahepatic obstruction most commonly results from gallstones or cancer of the head of the pancreas. Other causes include cancer of the peri-ampullary region or major bile ducts, iatrogenic biliary stricture, or extrinsic compression of the bile ducts by metastatic tumour.

Diagnosis

History and clinical examination

An accurate diagnosis of the cause of jaundice must be made as quickly as possible to allow prompt insti-

---

Jaundice

- Jaundice is a yellowish discolouration of the tissues which becomes apparent clinically when serum bilirubin levels exceed 50 μmol/l (normal < 20 μmol/l).

- It may be due to excessive haemolysis, hepatic insufficiency or cholestasis; cholestatic (obstructive) jaundice is the type encountered in surgical practice.

- The two commonest causes of surgical obstructive jaundice are cancer of the head of the pancreas and stones in the common bile duct (choledocholithiasis).

- In cholestatic jaundice the bilirubin has been conjugated by the hepatocytes and is therefore soluble in water and can be excreted in the urine; patients with obstructive jaundice typically have dark urine and pale stools and may have pruritus (thought to be due to accumulation of bile salts).

- Obstructive jaundice is characterized by elevated serum alkaline phosphatase levels in addition to hyperbilirubinameia, and may be accompanied by modest elevations in transaminase (aminotransferase) levels, reflecting liver damage.

tution of appropriate treatment. The age, sex, occupation, social habits, drug and alcohol intake, history of injections or infusions, and general demeanour of the patient must be considered. A history of intermittent pain, fluctuant jaundice and dyspepsia suggest calculous obstruction of the common bile duct, whereas a history of weight loss and relentless progressive jaundice favours a diagnosis of neoplasia. Obstructive jaundice is likely if there is a history of passage of dark urine and pale stools, and if the patient complains of pruritis (due to an inabililty to secrete bile salts into the obstructed biliary system). Hepatocellular jaundice is likely if there are stigmata of chronic liver disease such as liver palms, spider naevi, testicular atrophy, and gynaecomastia. The abdomen must be examined for evidence of hepatomegaly or gallbladder distension, and for signs of portal hypertension such as splenomegaly, ascites, and large collateral veins (caput Medusae) in the abdominal wall.

Biochemical and haematological investigations

Haemolytic jaundice is suggested if there are high circulating levels of unconjugated bilirubin but no bilirubin in the urine. Serum concentrations of liver enzymes are normal in these circumstances and the appropriate haematological investigations should be set in train.

In jaundice due to biliary obstruction, the circulating bilirubin is conjugated by the liver and rendered water-soluble; it can then be excreted in the urine and gives it a dark colour. As bile cannot pass into the gastrointestinal tract, the stool becomes pale and urobilinogen is absent from the urine. Obstruction increases the formation of alkaline phosphatase from the cells lining the biliary canaliculi and produces raised serum levels. In biliary obstruction the rise in serum alkaline phosphatase precedes that of bilirubin and its fall is more gradual once obstruction is relieved. Serum transaminase and lactic dehydrogenase levels also often rise in obstruction. Conversely, swelling of the parenchyma in hepatocellular jaundice frequently produces an element of intrahepatic biliary obstruction and a modest rise in serum alkaline phosphatase concentration.

Serum hepatitis B surface antigen status should be determined in all jaundiced patients. A full blood count and coagulation screen should be undertaken as a matter of routine. The presence of anaemia may signify occult blood loss and a low white cell or platelet count may indicate hypersplenism due to portal hypertension. Prolongation of the prothrombin time may be present in both hepatocellular and cholestatic jaundice but should readily correct with the administration of parenteral vitamin K when jaundice is cholestatic.

Radiological investigations

If the clinical picture and biochemical investigations suggest that jaundice is obstructive, radiological techniques can be used to define the site and nature of the obstruction.

Ultrasonography. This is the key investigation. It is safe, non-invasive and reliable in skilled hands. In the present context, it is used to define whether the patient has duct dilatation or gallbladder distension due to obstruction, and to confirm the need for more invasive investigation. Ultrasonography will also detect gallstones and space-occupying lesions in the liver and pancreas, although overlying bowel gas may prevent a clear view of the pancreas.

Endoscopic retrograde cholangiopancreatography (ERCP). This outlines the biliary and pancreatic systems by injecting dye through a cannula inserted into the papilla of Vater by means of an endoscope passed into the duodenum. It gives more detailed information than ultrasonography and, as will be discussed later, also allows endoscopic treatment of gallstones, biopsy of periampullary tumours and relief of obstructive jaundice by insertion of stents. The investigation may be complicated by acute pancreatitis and prophylactic antibiotics should be administered to reduce the risk of cholangitis. Haemorrhage and perforation are less frequent complications.

Percutaneous transhepatic cholangiography (PTC). Used less often than formerly, it is useful in obstruction of the upper biliary tree. It provides a clear outline of the biliary system by injection of dye through a slim flexible needle passed percutaneously into the liver. While diagnostic cholangiograms can be obtained in virtually all patients with ductal obstruction, the technique may cause bleeding or bile leakage and can be complicated by bacteraemia and septicaemia. Coagulation status must be checked prior to PTC and the procedure should be covered by antibiotic administration (e.g. gentamicin). Facilities for emergency surgery should be available although they are seldom needed.

Computerized tomography (CT). This can be used to identify hepatic, bile duct and pancreatic tumours in jaundiced patients. It often demonstrates the dilated biliary tree to the level of the obstruction and may show dissemination to adjacent lymph nodes.

Other radiological investigations. These are seldom needed. Isotopic liver scanning has been superseded by ultrasonography and CT scanning. Selective angiography is not used to diagnose the cause of jaundice but can be used to assess resectability if there is neoplastic obstruction, and it also identifies vascular anomalies. Barium meal examination and hypotonic duodenography are now obsolete investigations in jaundiced patients given the ready availability of ERCP. Magnetic resonance imaging (MRI) may prove to be useful in future.

Liver biopsy

Liver biopsy is valuable in patients with unexplained jaundice in whom an obstructing lesion has been excluded by ultrasonography. It may be preceded by a CT scan to determine whether metastatic disease is present. If lesions have been identified, a 'targetted' liver biopsy can be conducted under ultrasonic or CT control. Prothrombin time, platelet count and hepatitis B surface antigen (HBsAg) status must always be determined and clotting abnormalities corrected before biopsy is undertaken. In patients with a persistent bleeding disorder, liver biopsy can be undertaken through the hepatic veins employing a transjugular approach.

Laparoscopy

Laparoscopy is used increasingly in the evaluation of liver disease and obstructive jaundice. It is best undertaken under general anaesthesia. In patients with malignant obstruction of the biliary tree, peritoneal dissemination and small hepatic metastases may be apparent.

Laparotomy

Laparotomy is no longer necessary to establish the cause of jaundice and is only undertaken to remove the causal lesion or relieve biliary obstruction. Intraoperative ultrasonography and operative cholangiography may give useful additional information in patients with neoplasia and biliary obstruction. Appropriate pre-operative preparation is particularly important in jaundiced patients (see Ch. 11).

CONGENITAL ABNORMALITIES

Simple biliary cysts are common. They contain serous fluid, are usually solitary and never communicate with the biliary tree. They rarely produce symptoms, are associated with normal liver function and on ultrasound or CT scan have no discernible wall (Fig. 33.5). All cysts tend to recur following aspiration, and sclerosis by alcohol injection is of little value for large symptomatic cysts. Surgical management consists of deroofing and may be undertaken by laparoscopic means. Polycystic disease is a rare cause of liver enlargement and may be associated with polycystic kidneys as an autosomal dominant trait.

Cavernous haemangiomas are one of the commonest benign tumours of the liver and may be congenital. Women are six times as commonly affected as men. Most haemangiomas are small solitary subcapsular growths found incidentally at laparotomy or autopsy, but they are sometimes detected on ultrasound examination as densely hyperechoic lesions which mimic hepatic tumours. These lesions rarely give rise to pain and require resection.

Anatomical abnormalities of the extrahepatic bile ducts are common.

LIVER TRAUMA

After the spleen, the liver is the solid organ most commonly damaged in abdominal trauma, particularly following road traffic accidents. Stab injuries and gunshot wounds of the liver are also increasing in incidence. These are considered in Chapter 14.

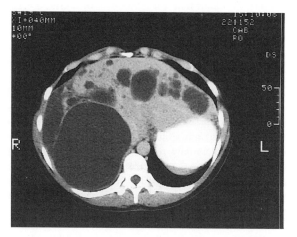

Fig. 33.5 CT scan demonstrating multiple biliary cysts appearing as hypodense areas within both lobes of the liver.

HEPATIC INFECTIONS AND INFESTATIONS

Hepatic abscess

Liver abscesses can be classified as bacterial, parasitic or fungal. Bacterial abscess is the commonest type in Western medicine but parasitic infestation is an important cause worldwide. Fungal abscesses are found in patients receiving long-term broad-spectrum antibiotic treatment or immuno-suppressive therapy, and may complicate actinomy-cosis.

Pyogenic liver abscess

Bacterial infection may gain access through a number of routes. Infection from the *biliary system* is now more common with the increasing use of radio-logical and endoscopic intervention. Infection may spread through the *portal vein* from abdominal sepsis (e.g. appendicitis, diverticulitis), via the *hepatic artery* from a septic focus anywhere in the body, or by direct spread from a *contiguous organ* (e.g. empyema of the gallbladder). Abscess formation may follow blunt or *penetrating injury* and in one-third of patients the source of infection is *indeterminate* (cryptogenic). Anaerobic organisms such as *Streptococcus milleri* are common in cryptogenic infections and those arising from the portal system. Gram-negative bacteria, notably *Escherichia coli*, are present in most cases and are particularly frequent in infections arising from the biliary tree. *Staphylococcus aureus* is invariably the causal organism in abscesses arising from haematogenous spread.

Pyogenic liver abscess is relatively rare. The onset of symptoms is often insidious and the patient may present with a pyrexia of unknown origin. There is sometimes a history of sepsis elsewhere, particularly within the abdomen, and pain in the right hypochon-drium. Other patients present with swinging pyrexia, rigors, marked toxicity and jaundice.

The liver is often enlarged and tender. Plain radiographs may show elevation of the diaphragm, pleural effusion and basal lobe collapse. Leucocytosis is usually present and liver function tests (LFTs) are deranged. Ultrasonography or CT scanning is used to define the abscess (which is often irregular and thick walled) and facilitate percuta-neous aspiration for culture. ERCP may be useful if biliary obstruction is thought to be responsible.

Untreated abscesses often prove fatal because of spread within the liver to multiple sites, septicaemia

and debility. The principles of treatment are percu-taneous drainage of accessible abscesses under ultra-sound guidance and antibiotic therapy selected on the basis of culture of blood or pus. It is unusual to have to resort to formal surgical drainage. Percutaneously or surgically-placed drainage tubes are left in place and the size of the cavity is monitored by serial X-rays following injection of contrast material. Multiple small abscesses may require prolonged treatment with antibiotics for up to 8 weeks.

Amoebic liver abscess

Entamoeba histolytica is a protozoal parasite which infests the large intestine and is endemic in many tropical regions. It is transmitted by cysts that are passed in the stools and which can survive for prolonged periods in moist surroundings. Overcrowding and insanitary living conditions favour ingestion of the cysts, which release tropho-zoites in the intestine. These probably penetrate the mucosa to gain access to the portal venous system and so spread to the liver. The abscess is large and thin-walled, is usually solitary and in the right lobe, and contains brown sterile pus resembling anchovy sauce. The onset of symptoms may be sudden or insidious. Right upper quadrant pain is the most striking symptom and this may be accompanied by anorexia, nausea, weight loss, and night sweats. Tender enlargement of the liver is invariable, although jaundice is uncommon. Other signs include basal pulmonary collapse, pleural effusion and leucocytosis. Ultrasonic and CT liver scans are used to demonstrate the site and size of the abscess which often has undefined margins. The stools should be examined for amoebae or cysts. Direct and indirect serological tests to detect amoebic protein are available.

Early diagnosis and prompt treatment are impor-tant, and treatment may be commenced empirically in areas where the problem is endemic. If untreated, an amoebic abscess may rupture into the peritoneal cavity or into a bronchus. Metastatic brain abscesses have been reported. Treatment consists of adminis-tration of an amoebicide (metronidazole and/or emetine) and usually results in rapid resolution. If there is no clinical response within 72 hours, the abscess should be aspirated by needle puncture although this is rarely necessary. Drainage by open operation is rarely required and even for the few cases of secondary bacterial infection not responding to therapy, percutaneous aspiration should be adequate.

Hydatid disease

This is caused in man by one of two forms of tapeworm, *Echinococcus granulosus* and *E. multilocularis*. The adult tapeworm lives in the intestine of the dog, from which ova are passed in the stool; sheep or man serve as the intermediate host by ingesting ova (Fig. 33.6). The condition is common in sheep-rearing areas, e.g. Greece and Australia, where dogs, sheep and men live in close contact. Ova passed in the dog faeces may contaminate the food or fingers and so be ingested by man. They hatch in the duodenum and the embryos enter the portal venous system and pass to the liver, where they form a hydatid cyst. The cyst wall is surrounded by an adventitial layer of fibrous tissue and consists of a laminated membrane lined by germinal epithelium on which brood capsules containing scolices develop.

The disease may be symptomless, but chronic right upper quadrant pain with enlargement of the liver is the common presentation.The cyst may rupture into the biliary tree or peritoneal cavity, the latter sometimes causing an acute anaphylactic reaction from absorption of foreign hydatid protein. Other complications include secondary infection and biliary obstruction with jaundice.

Eosinophilia is common and serological tests such as the complement-fixation test are available to detect the foreign protein.

Hydatid cysts commonly calcify and may be seen on a plain film of the abdomen. Alternatively, they can be detected by ultrasonic or CT scanning of the liver and are recognizable by their thick wall which may contain multiple daughter cysts. Small calcified cysts may require no treatment in the asymptomatic patient. Large symptomatic cysts are best treated by complete excision of the cyst, together with its contained parasites. At surgery, the liver is isolated by carefully positioned packs soaked in hypertonic saline. The cyst contents are aspirated following puncture with a cannula. Scolicidal agents should never be injected into the cyst since there is invariably a communication with the biliary tree which is then at risk of secondary sclerosing cholangitis. The cyst and its contained daughter cysts are shelled out from the liver, taking care to remove the laminated membrane completely. Great care is taken not to spill the contents in view of the danger of anaphylactic reactions and dissemination of viable scolices. In long-standing cysts, it may be preferable to remove the fibrous ectocyst and minimize the risk of subsequent bile leakage, subphrenic collection and recurrence from contained daughter cysts. Some surgeons advocate packing the residual cavity with the greater omentum.

Mebendazole has been used as an alternative to surgical treatment but its value remains uncertain.

PORTAL HYPERTENSION

Portal hypertension is usually caused by increased resistance to portal venous blood flow, the obstruction being prehepatic, hepatic or posthepatic. Rarely it results primarily from an increase in portal blood flow. The normal pressure in the portal vein varies from 5 to 15 cm water. When the portal venous pressure is consistently raised above 25 cmH$_2$O, there may be serious clinical consequences. The causes of portal hypertension are shown in Table 33.1.

Portal vein thrombosis is a rare cause. It is most commonly due to neonatal umbilical sepsis, though the effects may not be manifest for many years.

By far the commonest cause of portal hypertension is cirrhosis of the liver. This results from chronic liver disease and is characterized by liver cell damage, fibrosis, and nodular regeneration. In micronodular cirrhosis there is an even distribution of nodules a few millimetres in diameter; in macronodular cirrhosis the nodules vary in size and sometimes are very large. Macronodules are

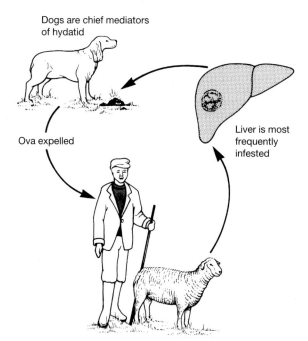

Dogs are chief mediators of hydatid

Ova expelled

Liver is most frequently infested

Fig. 33.6 Life cycle of *Echinococcus granulosus*.

Table 33.1	Causes of portal hypertension
Obstruction to portal flow	
Prehepatic	Congenital atresia of the portal vein
	Portal vein thrombosis
	Neonatal sepsis
	Pyelophlebitis
	Trauma
	Tumour
	Extrinsic compression of the portal vein
	Pancreatic disease
	Lymphadenopathy
	Biliary tract tumours
Intrahepatic	Cirrhosis
	Schistosomiasis
Posthepatic	Budd-Chiari syndrome
	Constrictive pericarditis
Increased blood flow (rare)	
	Arteriovenous fistula
	Increased splenic blood flow in
	hypersplenism

usual in end-stage cirrhosis, irrespective of its aetiology. The fibrosis obstructs portal venous return and portal hypertension develops. Arteriovenous shunts within the liver also contribute to the hypertension.

Alcohol is the commonest aetiological factor in Western countries and is increasing in prevalence. In North Africa, the Middle East and China, schistosomiasis due to *Bilharzia mansonii* is a common cause. In alcoholic cirrhosis the abnormal resistance is predominantly postsinusoidal, as shown by an increase in wedged hepatic venous pressure. The hepatic veins become distorted by regenerative nodules, there is narrowing of the central veins by centrilobular collagen deposition, and swelling of the hepatocytes encroaches on the sinusoidal lumen. In schistosomiasis, granulomas from parasitic involvement are seen in the portal triads, and the hypertension is presinusoidal. Ultimately, as macronodules appear, the obstruction becomes postsinusoidal. Chronic active hepatitis, and primary and secondary biliary cirrhosis are relatively rare causes in this country. In a large number of patients the cause of cirrhosis remains obscure (cryptogenic cirrhosis).

Post-hepatic portal hypertension is rare. It is most frequently due to spontaneous thrombosis of the hepatic veins and this has been associated with neoplasia, oral contraceptive agents, polycythaemia, and the presence of abnormal coagulants in the blood. The resulting Budd-Chiari syndrome is characterized by portal hypertension, liver failure and gross ascites.

Effects of portal hypertension

As a result of gradual chronic occlusion of the portal venous system, collateral pathways develop between portal and systemic venous circulations. Eventually a large proportion of portal venous blood enters the systemic circulation directly and may give rise to portosystemic encephalopathy. Portosystemic shunting occurs:

- In veins at the junction of the oesophagus and fundus of the stomach
- In retroperitoneal and periumbilical collaterals
- In anastomotic veins in the anorectal region (Fig. 33.7).

The most important consequence of shunting is the development of varices in the sub-mucosal plexus of veins in the lower oesophagus and gastric fundus. The oesophageal varices may then rupture to cause acute massive gastrointestinal bleeding. Such bleeding occurs in about 40% of patients with cirrhosis. The initial episode of variceal haemorrhage is fatal in about one-third of patients, and the great majority of those who survive their initial haemorrhage bleed again. Bleeding from retroperitoneal and periumbilical collaterals is troublesome during abdominal surgery and collaterals may develop and cause bleeding at the site of stomas. Anorectal

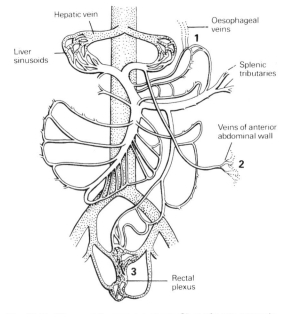

Fig. 33.7 The portal venous system. Sites of portosystemic shunting are marked 1–3. Retroperitoneal communications also exist.

varices are not uncommonly found at proctoscopy but rarely cause bleeding.

Progressive enlargement of the spleen occurs from vascular engorgement and associated hypertrophy. Haematological consequences are anaemia, thrombocytopenia and leucopenia. (The resulting syndrome of *hypersplenism* is discussed in more detail in Ch. 35.) *Ascites* may develop and is due to an increased formation of hepatic and splanchnic lymph, hypoalbuminaemia, and salt and water retention. Increased aldosterone and antidiuretic hormone levels may contribute.

Portosystemic *encephalopathy* is due to an increased level of toxins such as ammonia in the systemic circulation. This is particularly likely to develop where there are large spontaneous or surgically created portosystemic shunts. Gastrointestinal haemorrhage increases the absorption of nitrogenous products and may precipitate encephalopathy.

Clinical presentation

Patients with cirrhosis frequently develop anorexia, generalized malaise and weight loss. Clinical manifestations of liver disease may be present such as hepatosplenomegaly, ascites, jaundice, and spider naevi. The serum bilirubin may be elevated and the serum albumin depressed. Anaemia may be present and the leucocyte count can be raised (or depressed if there is hypersplenism). The prothrombin time and other indices of clotting may be abnormal. Clinical and biochemical parameters are used as the basis of the Child's classification (Table 33.2). Patients allocated to grade A have a good prognosis, whereas those in grade C have a poor prognosis and are not suitable for portosystemic shunting.

Patients with portal hypertension usually present to a surgeon because of:

- Active bleeding from oesophageal varices

Table 33.2   Assessment of patients with portal hypertension by a modification of Child's grading system

Criterion	Points scored		
	1	2	3
Encephalopathy	None	Minimal	Marked
Ascites	None	Slight	Moderate
Bilirubin (µmol/l)	<35	35–50	>50
Albumin (g/l)	>35	28–35	<28
Prothrombin ratio	<1.4	1.4–2.0	>2.0

Grade A = 5–6 points; grade B = 7–9 points; grade C = 10–15 points.

- Consideration for elective surgery after recovery from an episode of acute haemorrhage
- The discovery of varices which have not yet bled.

Patients in this third group are usually kept under supervision although some now recommend prophylactic treatment of varices to avoid future bleeding.

Acute variceal bleeding

Patients presenting with acute upper gastrointestinal bleeding are carefully examined for evidence of chronic liver disease. The liver may be palpably enlarged and firm or nodular, the spleen may be enlarged, and ascites may be present. Jaundice, spider naevi, liver palms, opaque nails, and finger clubbing are also sought. Distended collateral veins may be visible, particularly around the umbilicus, where they give rise to a 'caput Medusae'. Slurring of speech, a flapping tremor or dysarthria may point to encephalopathy, and this may be precipitated or intensified by accumulation of blood in the gastrointestinal tract.

While a barium swallow and meal can detect oesophageal and gastric varices, the key investigation during an episode of active bleeding is endoscopy. This allows detection of varices and defines whether they are or have been the site of bleeding. It is important to remember that peptic ulcer and gastritis are common complaints which occur in 20% of patients with varices. Even though a patient is known to have chronic liver disease and varices, bleeding cannot be assumed to be due to the varices.

Management

The priorities in the management of bleeding oesophageal varices are summarized in Table 33.3.

Active resuscitation. Blood is withdrawn for grouping, cross-matching and a clotting screen; a free-flowing intravenous line is established, a urinary catheter is inserted to measure hourly urine output, pulse rate and blood pressure are monitored, and a central venous line is inserted to monitor central venous pressure. Large volumes of blood may be lost rapidly and the aim is to replace blood loss quickly with a view to urgent endoscopy. Many patients bleeding from varices have coagulation defects from the outset and thrombocytopenia is a common manifestation of hypersplenism. Fresh blood is preferred for transfusion purposes and the advice of the haematologist is sought regarding the use of fresh frozen plasma (FFP) or platelet transfusion.

Endoscopy. This is performed at the earliest

Table 33.3   Priorities in the management of bleeding oesophageal varices

- Active resuscitation
  Group and cross-match blood
  Establish i.v. infusion line(s)
  Monitor: pulse
            blood pressure
            hourly urine output
            central venous pressure
- Assessment of coagulation status
  Prothrombin time
  Platelet count
- Urgent endoscopy
- Control of bleeding
  Tamponade (Minnesota tube) or injection sclerotherapy
  Pharmacological measures (e.g. vasopressin/somatostatin)
- Treatment of hepatocellular decompensation
- Treatment/prevention of portosystemic encephalopathy
- Prevention of further bleeding from varices
  Injection sclerotherapy
  Staple oesophagogastric junction
  Portosystemic shunting/TIPSS
  Liver transplantation

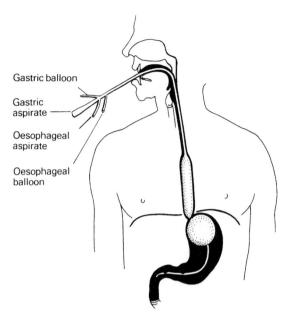

Fig. 33.8   Oesophageal tamponade using a Minnesota tube.

opportunity, and in patients threatened by massive bleeding, active resuscitation is instituted and continued in the endoscopy suite. The tortuous varices are usually in three columns and most prominent in the lower third of the oesophagus. If varices are the source of blood loss, this usually occurs from the lowest few centimetres of the oesophagus. Rarely, bleeding occurs from varices in the gastric fundus.

Control of bleeding. Medical agents used to lower portal venous pressure and arrest bleeding include vasopressin and somatostatin although their value is uncertain. If variceal haemorrhage is apparent at the initial endoscopy, injection sclerotherapy using ethanolamine is now used to arrest the bleeding. If haemorrhage is torrential and prevents direct injection, balloon tamponade is used to stop the bleeding.

The four-lumen Minnesota tube (Fig. 33.8) has largely replaced the three-lumen Sengstaken-Blakemore tube. The four lumina allow:

- Aspiration of gastric contents
- Inflation of a gastric balloon with 150 ml of water to which a radio-opaque dye (Hypaque) has been added so that balloon position can be checked radiologically (this balloon compresses the gastric fundus and oesophagogastric junction, so reducing the flow of blood into the oesophageal varices)
- Inflation of an oesophageal balloon with air to a

pressure of 40 mmHg using a sphygmomanometer (this balloon applies direct pressure to the oesophageal varices)
- Aspiration of the oesophagus and pharynx above the oesophageal balloon, so reducing the risk of aspiration pneumonitis and pneumonia.

Traction is applied to the Minnesota tube by pulling the gastric balloon up against the oesophagogastric junction and taping a spatula to the tube as it emerges from the angle of the mouth. A trained nurse should be in constant attendance, and the pharynx and stomach are aspirated at 15–30 minute intervals. Balloon tamponade arrests bleeding from varices in over 90% of patients, but the tube is not left in place for more than 24–36 hours for fear of causing oesophageal necrosis. Tamponade should be regarded as a holding measure which allows further resuscitation and treatment of hepatic decompensation. Unless more definitive measures are used to prevent further variceal bleeding (see below), two-thirds of individuals rebleed while still in hospital and 90% rebleed within a year.

Further resuscitation and treatment of hepatocellular decompensation. Control of variceal bleeding allows blood loss to be made good and permits full assessment of coagulopathy. An H_2-receptor antagonist (e.g. cimetidine 400 mg i.v. 6-hourly) is prescribed to reduce the risk of bleeding from gastritis or peptic ulceration, and may be combined with instillation of antacids down the gastric lumen of the Minnesota tube. A daily bowel washout is used to evacuate blood from the gut and reduce the risk of portosystemic encephalopathy. This endeavour can be assisted by prescribing aperients such as magnesium sulphate. Alternatively, magnesium trisilicate (30 ml 4-hourly) can be used for both its antacid and aperient properties. Lactulose (15–30 ml 8-hourly) is prescribed to reduce bacterial degradation of blood in the gut lumen and further reduce the risk of encephalopathy. Patients with oesophageal varices due to liver disease frequently have major defects in both the intrinsic and extrinsic clotting systems which may prove refractory to therapy. Vitamin K_1 is prescribed to aid restoration of the extrinsic system, but FFP, factor concentrates, and platelet transfusion may all be required to cover specific procedures such as sclerotherapy or surgery. It should be stressed that these transfusion measures have transient effects on blood coagulation, and that the ultimate coagulation status depends upon restoration of hepatic function.

Prevention of further bleeding

A number of methods are now available to reduce the risk of further variceal bleeding. The method most frequently employed at present is repeated variceal sclerotherapy.

• *Injection sclerotherapy.* Although originally undertaken by means of a rigid oesophagoscope under general anaesthesia, it is now routinely carried out by fibreoptic endoscopy. Injection is repeated at weekly or fortnightly intervals until the varices are completely sclerosed. Following complete ablation, fibreoptic examination is repeated periodically and any recurrent varices are injected. Excessive or too frequent injection may be complicated by ulceration and necrosis, sometimes with a fatal result. Controversy exists as to whether the sclerosant should be injected directly into the varix or into the surrounding mucosa. The increased use of injection sclerotherapy has substantially reduced the number of patients submitted to surgery, and it is most successful in patients with well-preserved liver function. While sclerotherapy reduces the risk of

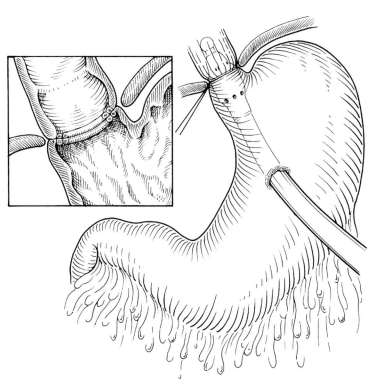

Fig. 33.9 Oesophageal stapling. The gun is inserted through an anterior gastrostomy. A ligature is tied just above the cardia, invaginating a flange of oesophageal wall between the two parts of the gun. Inset: the gun has been fired, simultaneously resecting a full thickness ring of oesophageal wall and anastomosing the cut ends with staples.

further variceal bleeding, it is still uncertain whether it improves long-term survival.

• *Endoscopic banding.* Just as haemorrhoids can be managed by the application of elastic bands, endoscopic applicators are now available which can be used to occlude varices at the oesophagogastric junction. This technique carries less risk of oesophageal ulceration and perforation than sclerotherapy.

• *Surgical disconnection* is usually reserved for patients who continue to bleed despite injection sclerotherapy. The left gastric vein and short gastric veins are ligated and the distal oesophagus is transected and re-anastomosed just above the cardia using a stapling gun (Fig. 33.9). Stapled oesophageal transection is relatively easy to perform and the double row of staples inserted through the full thickness of the oesophageal wall occludes flow into the varices. The procedure is technically more

difficult in patients who have been submitted to repeated injection sclerotherapy and carries considerable morbidity and mortality when employed as a last resort in the emergency situation. It is nowadays more often employed as an adjunct to surgical ligation of gastric varices which have bled and is accompanied by a splenectomy.

• Emergency portosystemic shunting has a high mortality and has been abandoned in most centres. On the other hand, *elective portosystemic shunting* is still used occasionally to decompress the portal system and reduce the risk of further variceal haemorrhage. Portosystemic encephalopathy can be troublesome and it is uncertain whether shunting prolongs life in patients with parenchymal liver disease. In general the operation is only undertaken in patients whose condition is not complicated by jaundice, ascites or encephalopathy and where there is no clear indication for liver transplantation.

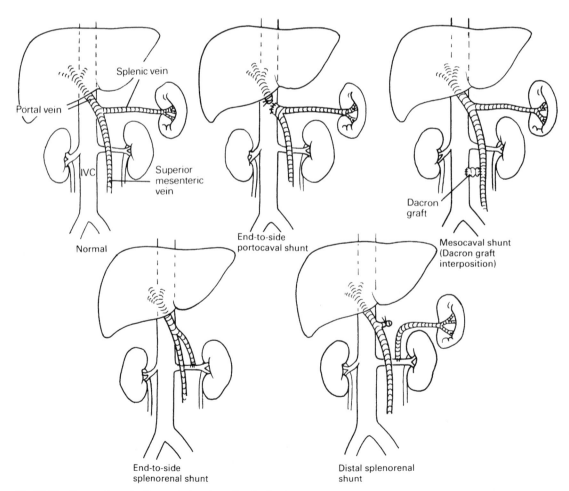

Fig. 33.10   Types of surgically created portosystemic shunts.

Portal venography is essential to define the anatomy of the portal venous system. It can be undertaken by percutaneous transplenic or transhepatic injection of contrast or by examining the venous phase after coeliac angiography. Ultrasonic and CT scans may also be used to examine the portal system.

Types of shunt procedure. There are several anatomical sites at which portosystemic shunts can be performed (Fig. 33.10). In a portocaval shunt the portal vein is anastomosed end-to-side or side-to-side to the inferior vena cava. Mesocaval shunts can be constructed between the superior mesenteric vein and inferior vena cava using autogenous saphenous vein or a synthetic graft; they are easier to perform but have a high incidence of thrombosis.

Splenorenal shunts, between the splenic and renal veins, are most appropriate when there is portal vein obstruction. The distal splenorenal (Warren) shunt selectively decompresses the lower oesophagus and upper stomach and maintains liver blood flow, and is preferred by many surgeons. The incidence of encephalopathy is lower than after other shunt procedures.

The results of shunt surgery are very variable, depending chiefly on the liver function of the patient and the skill and experience of the surgeon. Portosystemic shunts are considered only for patients with well-preserved liver function and who are not candidates for liver transplantation.

There has been considerable recent interest in transhepatic insertion of portosystemic shunts (TIPSS). A metal stent is inserted via the transjugular route using a guidewire passed through the hepatic vein to the intrahepatic branches of the portal vein. Early experience suggests that this is a relatively safe means of decompressing the portal system, since general anaesthesia and laparotomy are avoided. The risk of encephalopathy is similar to that of a surgical portosystemic shunt, and the definitive role of this new form of treatment has yet to be established.

Ascites

Ascites can be controlled by bed rest, salt and water restriction and a diuretic such as the aldosterone-inhibitor spironolactone. If refractory, ascites can be treated by inserting a peritoneojugular (LeVeen) shunt which allows one-way flow between the peritoneum and jugular vein (Fig. 33.11). It is unusual for the shunt to remain patent for more than 12 months but this may suffice for patients with refractory ascites and advanced liver disease who are not candidates for liver transplantation.

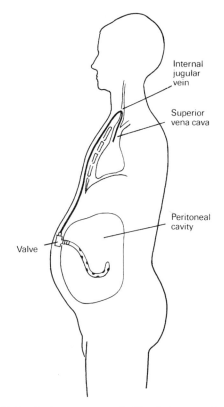

Fig. 33.11 Peritoneo-venous (Le Veen) shunt to relieve ascites.

Encephalopathy

Acute encephalopathy is treated by avoiding protein intake, bowel washouts, and giving oral lactulose to reduce bacterial decomposition of protein in the intestine. In chronic encephalopathy, a low protein (20 g), high calorie (1500 kcal carbohydrate) diet is given daily, with vitamin supplements. Protein intake can be increased by 20 g every 3 days, once encephalopathy is controlled.

TUMOURS OF THE LIVER

Hepatic tumours can be benign or malignant, primary or secondary. Primary tumours may arise from the parenchymal cells, the epithelium of the bile ducts or from the supporting tissues.

Benign hepatic tumours

Cavernous haemangioma is the commonest benign liver tumour. Most are asymptomatic, and are

Portal hypertension

- Portal hypertension is almost always due to obstruction to portal flow (rather than increased inflow) and may be prehepatic, hepatic or posthepatic.

- Cirrhosis of the liver is the commonest cause of portal hypertension in Western medicine and alcoholic cirrhosis is most often responsible.

- Portosystemic shunts develop between gastric and oesophageal veins, in the retroperitoneum and periumbilical area, and occasionally in the anorectum. Varices in the submucosa of the lower oesophagus are a common source of major bleeding, but gastritis (portal gastropathy) can be responsible.

- Child's grading (A, B or C) is based on encephalopathy, ascites, bilirubin and albumin levels, and prothrombin time, and is a valuable prognostic index.

- Variceal bleeding may be controlled by injection sclerotherapy although balloon tamponade (four-lumen Minnesota tube) may sometimes be needed.

- Surgical portosystemic shunts effectively decompress oesophageal varices and reduce rebleeding but can cause encephalopathy and are now seldom used.

- Although injection sclerotherapy (or banding) reduces the risk of rebleeding and may improve survival rates, long-term outcome is determined by the nature and severity of the underlying liver disease.

detected on ultrasonography as a dense hyperechoic lesion or are found incidentally at laparotomy. These lesions rarely reach a sufficient size to produce pain, abdominal swelling or haemorrhage. Heart failure occasionally develops if there is a large arteriovenous communication.

Lesions discovered incidentally at laparotomy should be left alone and needle biopsy can be hazardous. Ligation of the appropriate branch of the hepatic artery may reduce the size of large symptomatic lesions but these should normally be resected by an experienced surgeon.

Biliary hamartomas are small fibrous lesions which are often situated beneath the capsule of the liver. They can be mistaken for a small metastatic tumour unless a biopsy is obtained.

Liver cell adenomas are found almost exclusively in women, and their incidence has increased with the widespread use of high oestrogen-containing contraceptives. The majority present as solitary well-encapsulated lesions but malignant transformation has been reported. They may be asymptomatic but generally present with right hypochondrial pain as a result of haemorrhage within the tumour. Superficial tumours may bleed spontaneously and present with symptoms of haemoperitoneum.

The adenomas may be identified by ultrasonography or CT scanning. LFTs and serum alphafetoprotein levels are usually normal. Percutaneous biopsy should be avoided because of the risk of haemorrhage.

Treatment consists of formal hepatic resection because of the difficulties of differentiating adenoma from a well-differentiated hepatoma.

Focal nodular hyperplasia of the liver is more common in females. The lesion is generally asymptomatic and may regress with time or on withdrawal of the contraceptive pill. Hyperplasia does not undergo malignant transformation and does not require excision unless symptomatic.

Hyperplasia can be differentiated from adenoma by the central fibrous scar which is often visible on ultrasound scanning. Whereas other hepatic lesions produce a filling defect on isotope scan, hyperplastic nodules often produce no filling defect because the isotope is taken up by Kuppfer cells within the lesion.

Primary malignant tumours of the liver

Hepatocellular carcinoma (hepatoma)

Hepatocellular carcinoma (hepatoma) is relatively uncommon in the Western world but is common in Africa and the Far East. Environmental factors are probably important and in American blacks, the incidence is the same as that found in white Americans. In the West, about two-thirds of patients have pre-existing cirrhosis and many others have evidence of hepatitis B infection. In Africa and the East, 'aflatoxin' (derived from the fungus *Aspergillus flavus*, which contaminates maize and nuts) is an important hepatocarcinogen. Viral hepatitis is also an important aetiological factor.

Clinical features. The diagnosis is usually made late in the course of the disease. In non-cirrhotic patients the tumour may have grown to a considerable size before giving rise to abdominal pain or swelling.

In cirrhotic patients, hepatoma may become manifest as sudden deterioration in liver function, often associated with extension of tumour into the portal venous system. Common presenting features include abdominal pain, weight loss, abdominal distension, fever, and spontaneous intraperitoneal haemorrhage. Jaundice is uncommon unless there is advanced cirrhosis. Examination may reveal features of established liver disease and hepatomegaly is invariable.

Liver function is generally deranged. Although early detection of hepatocellular carcinoma in susceptible individuals can be pursued by a policy of serial measurement of alphafetoprotein (an oncofetal antigen) and ultrasonic scanning, this tumour marker is present in only one-third of the white population with hepatocellular carcinoma, compared to 80% of African patients with this disease. Isotope scans are of little value. Chest X-ray may detect pulmonary metastases.

The diagnosis is made on the history and the radiological features of a solid mass lesion in the liver in the absence of primary tumour elsewhere. Percutaneous needle aspiration cytology and needle biopsy for histological confirmation should be reserved for patients who are not being considered for hepatic resection as they carry a small but significant risk of tumour dissemination and haemorrhage.

Abdominal CT scanning is valuable in planning resection and excluding the presence of nodal involvement or peritoneal dissemination of tumour. Hepatocellular carcinoma is seen as an extremely vascular lesion on arteriography and propagation of tumour thrombus along the portal vein or its branches may be demonstrated.

In non-cirrhotic patients, large tumours (particularly those of the fibrolamellar type) may be amenable to extensive liver resection. Cirrhotic patients have less hepatic functional reserve and even those with well-preserved liver function may only tolerate limited segmental or sub-segmental resection of the liver. The only prospect of cure lies in complete surgical resection of the tumour. In cirrhotic patients multicentricity is common and satellite lesions often surround the primary tumour, so that cure is uncommon.

For advanced tumours, hepatic arterial ligation and local infusion of chemotherapeutic agents through a surgically implanted catheter in the hepatic artery may be used. Systemic chemotherapy with doxorubicin (Adriamycin), methotrexate or 5-fluorouracil may have palliative value, although response rates of less than 20% are the norm. More encouraging results have been reported following local embolization of these agents plus lipiodol by selective arteriography (chemoembolization).

The disease is usually advanced at presentation and the 5-year survival rate is less than 10%. Liver transplantation has been used in the treatment of this tumour but recurrence in the transplanted liver and elsewhere is common in immunosuppressed patients. The best results following transplantation are reported in cirrhotic patients undergoing transplantation and in whom an incidental hepatoma has been found on examination of the resected specimen.

Cholangiocarcinoma

This adenocarcinoma may arise anywhere in the biliary tree, including its intrahepatic radicles. It accounts for less than 10% of malignant primary neoplasms of the liver in Western medicine. Risk factors include chronic parasitic infestation of the biliary tree in the Orient, and choledochal cysts (see below).

Jaundice, pain, and an enlarged liver are the common presenting features, although there may be co-existent biliary infection causing the tumour to masquerade as a hepatic abscess. Resection offers the only prospect of cure but is seldom feasible when cholangiocarcinoma arises in the liver substance. Cholangiocarcinoma arising from the extrahepatic bile ducts will be considered later.

Other primary malignant tumours

Angiosarcoma (Fig. 33.12). This is a rare tumour of the liver which may arise after industrial exposure to vinyl chloride or exposure to the previously used radiological contrast medium, Thorotrast.

Haemangioendothelioma. This presents as a diffuse multi-focal tumour and is rarely resectable at presentation.

Biliary cystadenoma. This rare condition of the liver, with a marked female predominance, has a one-in-four risk of malignant transformation.

All of these rare tumours generally present late and resection is seldom feasible. The prognosis is generally poor.

Metastatic tumours

The liver is a common site for metastatic disease. Secondary liver tumours are 20 times more common than primary ones. In 50% of cases the primary tumour is in the gastrointestinal tract; other common sites are the breast, ovaries, bronchus and kidney. Almost 90% of patients with hepatic metastases have tumour deposits in other sites.

Hepatomegaly and tenderness are distinctive

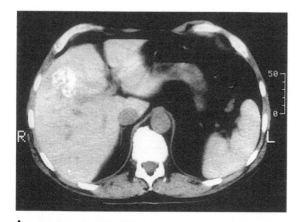

A

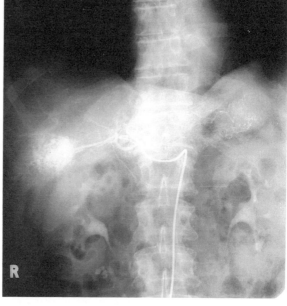

C

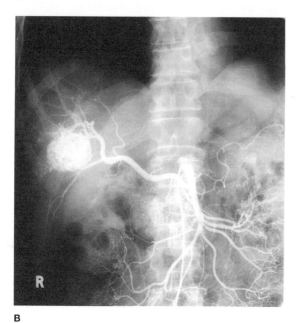

B

Fig. 33.12   A CT scan demonstrating a lesion in segment V. Previous ultrasound guided biopsy had suggested an angiosarcoma; B angiography shows an extremely vascular lesion taking its blood supply mainly from an aberrant right hepatic artery arising from the superior mesenteric artery; C the lesion derives some of its blood supply from the left hepatic artery. The patient underwent a curative resection of the lesion by extended right hepatectomy (segments IV–VIII).

features, and individual deposits may be palpable. The patient is often cachectic, and ascites or jaundice may be present. Pyrexia occurs in up to 10% of patients. LFTs are abnormal, notably the alkaline phosphatase and gamma-glutamyl transpeptidase, which are often raised. Ultrasonic and CT scans may demonstrate multiple filling defects. The diagnosis can be confirmed by aspiration cytology or needle biopsy undertaken under ultrasonic control. Such invasive investigation may be unnecessary when resection is under consideration.

There is no effective treatment for most patients with hepatic metastases. Both lobes of the liver are usually involved, making surgical resection impossible. Hepatic artery ligation, local and systemic chemotherapy, and chemoembolization have given disappointing results.

In some tumours, notably those arising from the colon and rectum, apparently solitary metastases or metastases confined to one lobe may be resected. A careful search for other metastases is required and includes a search for local recurrence of the original primary tumour (e.g. colonoscopy) and dissemination elsewhere (e.g. CT of the thorax and isotope bone scan). In well-selected patients, 5-year survival rates of 30–40% have been reported following resection. Non-curative resection may be considered as a means of palliation in patients with symptomatic hepatic metastases from a carcinoid tumour or sarcoma.

LIVER RESECTION

Resection involves mobilization of the liver from its peritoneal attachments. Following isolation, ligature, and division of the appropriate vessels, the devascularized lobe or segment is separated by careful dissection, which may be facilitated by use of an ultrasonic dissector. Intervening biliary and vascular channels can be defined and divided between ligatures. The hepatic veins or tributaries are controlled by suture ligation following removal of the resected specimen (Fig. 33.12).

Modern techniques of hepatic resection have greatly reduced operative blood loss with subsequent reduction in morbidity and mortality. Adequate drainage of the operating field is essential following resection, since there is a significant risk of bile leakage and intra-abdominal collection.

LIVER TRANSPLANTATION

This is considered in Chapter 15.

THE GALLBLADDER AND BILE DUCTS

Anatomy of the biliary system

The biliary 'tree' consists of fine intrahepatic biliary radicles which drain individual liver segments before forming the right and left hepatic ducts. The left hepatic duct runs a mainly extrahepatic course and joins the right hepatic duct to form the common hepatic duct. This is joined at a variable position by the cystic duct to form the common bile duct which ends at the papilla of Vater, usually in the second part of the duodenum (Fig. 33.13).

The common bile duct is approximately 8 cm long and up to 10 mm in diameter. It lies in the free edge of the lesser omentum before passing behind the first part of the duodenum and through the head of the pancreas. It is usually joined by the pancreatic duct just before entering the duodenum.

The gallbladder lies in a bed on the undersurface of the liver between its right and left halves. It is a muscular structure with a fundus, body and neck. Hartmann's pouch is a dilatation of the gallbladder outlet adjacent to the origin of the cystic duct in which gallstones frequently become impacted. The gallbladder is supplied by the cystic artery, a branch of the right hepatic artery.

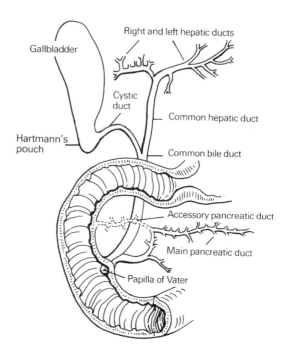

Fig. 33.13   Anatomy of the biliary tree.

Physiology

Bile salts and the enterohepatic circulation

Bile acids are sterols synthesized by the liver from cholesterol. The primary bile acids, chenodeoxycholic and cholic acid, are conjugated with glycine or taurine to increase their solubility in water, and the conjugates (e.g. glycocholic and taurocholic acid) form sodium and potassium bile salts. In the intes-

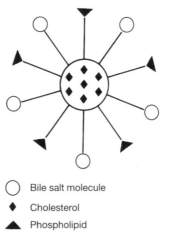

○ Bile salt molecule

♦ Cholesterol

▲ Phospholipid

Fig. 33.14   Cholesterol micelle.

tine, bacterial action produces the secondary bile salts, deoxycholic and lithocholic acid.

Bile salts can combine with lipids to form water-soluble complexes called micelles (Fig. 33.14). Lecithin and cholesterol can be transported from the liver within such micelles. Bile salts are also detergents and reduction in surface tension allows fat to be emulsified in the intestine, thus facilitating its digestion and absorption. On reaching the distal ileum, 95% of the bile salts are reabsorbed, transported back to the liver and passed once again into the biliary system. This enterohepatic circulation (Fig. 33.15) allows a relatively small bile salt pool (2–4 g) to circulate some 6–12 times a day through the intestine. The daily faecal loss equals that of hepatic synthesis (0.2–0.6 g/24 h). When bile is excluded from the intestine, 25% of ingested fat may appear in the faeces and there is a marked malabsorption of fat-soluble vitamins including vitamin K.

The gallbladder has a capacity of 50 ml and can concentrate bile by a factor of ten. It contracts in response to cholecystokinin (CCK), which is released from the duodenal mucosa by the presence of food, notably fatty acids. Gallbladder contraction is accompanied by reciprocal relaxation of the sphincter of Oddi. The secretion of bile is promoted by the hormone secretin. The vagus nerve also stimulates bile secretion and gallbladder contraction.

Bile salts
- The primary bile acids, chenodeoxycholic and cholic acid are conjugated with glycine or taurine and form sodium or potassium bile salts (e.g. sodium taurocholate).

- The bile salts are vital for the excretion of cholesterol in bile; cholesterol is insoluble in water and must be transported in water-soluble complexes (micelles) with bile salts and lecithin.

- Bile salts are detergents and on reaching the intestine they emulsify fat and facilitate the digestion and absorption of fat and fat-soluble vitamins.

- Bile salts must not be confused with bile pigments (e.g. bilirubin) which are waste products and excreted in bile. The small bile salt pool (2–4 g) is conserved by reabsorption of bile salts from the terminal ileum.

- Disease or resection of the terminal ileum prevents the enterohepatic circulation of bile salts and is associated with a high incidence of cholesterol gallstones and diarrhoea (due to cathartic action of bile salts on the colon).

CONGENITAL ABNORMALITIES

Congenital abnormalities of the gallbladder and bile ducts are common. The gallbladder may be absent

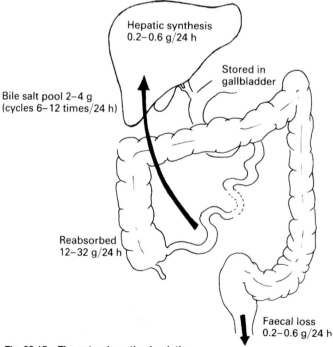

Hepatic synthesis
0.2–0.6 g/24 h

Stored in gallbladder

Bile salt pool 2–4 g
(cycles 6–12 times/24 h)

Reabsorbed
12–32 g/24 h

Faecal loss
0.2–0.6 g/24 h

Fig. 33.15 The enterohepatic circulation.

(agenesis), double, intrahepatic, partitioned with a fold in the fundus (Phrygian cap), or multiseptate. The cystic duct may be absent or join the right hepatic duct rather than the common hepatic duct, and accessory ducts may be present. The cystic artery may be duplicated or may arise from the common hepatic or left hepatic artery. These anomalies are important in that great care must be taken to avoid inappropriate division of major ducts and arteries in the course of cholecystectomy.

Biliary atresia

Failure of development of the duct system occurs once in every 20 000 to 30 000 births and is the commonest cause of prolonged jaundice in infancy. The condition may be acquired after birth, rather than truly congenital, in that it has not been described in autopsies of newborn infants. The site and extent of the atresia are variable and the duct system may be entirely replaced by solid fibrous strands. Fortunately, intrahepatic atresia is rare and the extrahepatic system is usually most affected.

Jaundice usually becomes apparent in the first 2–3 weeks of life and the liver and spleen usually enlarge. LFTs show an obstructive pattern although the serum transaminase levels are often elevated. Liver biopsy reveals cholestatic jaundice but differentiation from neonatal hepatitis is often surprisingly difficult.

In extrahepatic biliary atresia, a Roux loop of jejunum is anastomosed to the intrahepatic duct system in the hilus of the liver (Kasai operation). Delayed treatment may allow cirrhosis to develop, with portal hypertension and ascites. The prognosis for infants with extrahepatic biliary atresia has improved, although recurrent fibrosis and stricture may lead to troublesome cholangitis and abscess formation. Intrahepatic atresia is rarely correctable and liver transplantation may be needed.

Choledochal cysts

Cystic transformation of the biliary tree (choledochal cyst) is rare. It is often associated with an abnormal termination of the common bile duct which enters the pancreatic duct within the head of the pancreas. This may allow reflux into the biliary system resulting in pain, inflammation, calculus formation and malignant transformation. The abnormalities are probably congenital, although diagnosis may be delayed until adult life.

The patient usually presents with intermittent pain and jaundice and may have attacks of pancre-

atitis. Localized abdominal tenderness and a mass may be present in the right hypochondrium. LFTs show a cholestatic pattern, and ultrasonography and cholangiography (ERCP or PTC) establish the diagnosis. Excision of the cyst is indicated in view of the significant risk of malignant transformation. However, the risk of developing intrahepatic cholangiocarcinoma is not completely removed by excision of the extrahepatic biliary tree.

Caroli's disease consists of cystic biliary dilatation which is more marked in the peripheral intrahepatic ducts. Recurring infection may progress to cirrhosis and liver failure. When Caroli's disease is found in association with congenital hepatic fibrosis, portal hypertension is often present. Endoscopic, percutaneous and surgical manipulation of the biliary tree are best avoided and liver transplantation may have a valuable role in management.

GALLSTONES

Pathogenesis

Gallstones are formed from the constituents of bile. The great majority result from failure to keep cholesterol in micellar form in the gallbladder, and pigment stones are less common. Most cholesterol stones become mixed with bile pigments as they increase in size; such 'mixed' stones are much more common than pure cholesterol stones.

Gallstones are common in Europe and North America and less common in Asia and Africa. Their incidence increases with age. In 'developed' countries they occur in at least 20% of women over the age of 40; the incidence in males is about one-third of that in females. The disease has increased markedly in frequency and cholecystectomy is the commonest elective abdominal operation in many Western countries.

Cholesterol stones

Cholesterol stones may occur in both sexes from the late teens onwards but are particularly common in middle-aged, obese, multiparous females. Stone formation is encouraged if bile becomes supersaturated with cholesterol (i.e. lithogenic) either by excessive cholesterol excretion or by reduction in the amount of bile salt and lecithin available for micelle formation. Supersaturation is most likely to occur while the bile is concentrated in the gallbladder, and is favoured by stasis or decreased gallbladder contractility. The formation of cholesterol crystals is the key event, and this 'nucleation' may be due to coalescence of cholesterol molecules or their precipitation around particles of mucus, bacteria, calcium bilirubinate or mucosal cells. Not all individuals with supersaturated bile develop gallstones, so other factors must be implicated. Pure cholesterol stones are yellowish-green with a regular shape but rough surface. They are usually solitary, whereas mixed stones are darker and are usually multiple.

Cholesterol stones are particularly common in some tribes of North American Indians, where more than 75% of women over 40 are affected. Such individuals have a small bile salt pool. Conversely, the high incidence of stones in Chilean women reflects high levels of cholesterol excretion. Obesity and high-calorie or high-cholesterol diets favour cholesterol stone formation by producing highly supersaturated gallbladder bile. Drastic weight reduction and diets designed to lower serum cholesterol levels may also promote stone formation by mobilizing cholesterol and increasing its excretion.

Disease or resection of the terminal ileum and drugs such as cholestyramine favour cholesterol nucleation by reducing the bile salt pool. Hormonal influences are reflected in an increased incidence of stone formation in women taking oral contraceptives or postmenopausal oestrogen replacement. Pregnancy may also have an effect by increasing stasis within the gallbladder. Similarly, after vagotomy the gallbladder becomes flaccid and increases in volume. Hypercholesterolaemia as such is not associated with stone formation.

Pigment stones

Pigment stones consist of calcium bilirubinate and are usually multiple, small and amorphous. Stones found in Occidental patients are usually composed of black pigment, whereas brown pigment stones are common in Orientals. Pigment stones account for 25% of all gallstones in Western patients but for 60% of those in some Oriental countries such as Japan.

Chronic haemolysis favours pigment stone formation by increasing pigment excretion, and stone formation is common in congenital spherocytosis, haemoglobinopathy, and malaria. Cirrhosis and biliary stasis are also important associations. Some patients with brown pigment stones have increased amounts of unconjugated bilirubin in the bile. In Oriental patients this may be due to the action of beta-glucuronidase produced by *E. coli*, an organism which invades duct systems infested with *Clonorchis sinensis* or *Ascaris lumbricoides*.

Pathological effects of gallstones

Acute cholecystitis and its complications

This is usually produced by obstruction of the neck of the gallbladder or cystic duct by a stone. Bacteria are cultured from the bile in approximately one-half of patients with gallstones and unrelieved obstruction in the presence of this infected bile may produce an *empyema*. The thickened gallbladder becomes intensely inflamed, oedematous and occasionally *gangrenous*. The fundus of the distended, inflamed gallbladder may *perforate*, giving rise to localized abscess formation and occasionally to biliary peritonitis. The common organisms implicated in inflammation of the gallbladder are *E. coli, Klebsiella aerogenes* and *Strep. faecalis*. Staphylococci, clostridia and salmonella are occasionally present. These organisms may be cultured from the blood if there is bacteraemia.

Chronic cholecystitis

Repeated bouts of biliary colic or acute cholecystitis culminate in fibrosis, contraction of the gallbladder and chronic inflammatory change with marked thickening of the wall. The gallbladder ceases to function. Chronic inflammatory change may be present in the absence of gallstones as is the case in the gallbladders of typhoid carriers.

Mucocele

A mucocele develops when the outlet of the gallbladder becomes obstructed in the absence of infection. The imprisoned bile is absorbed but clear mucus continues to be secreted into the distended gallbladder.

Choledocholithiasis

When gallstones enter the common bile duct they may pass spontaneously or give rise to obstructive jaundice, cholangitis or acute pancreatitis. Gallstone pancreatitis most commonly occurs when a small stone becomes temporarily arrested at the ampulla of Vater.

Gallstone ileus

This uncommon form of intestinal obstruction occurs when a large gallstone becomes impacted in the intestine. Stones large enough to block the gut are usually too large to pass through the sphincter of

Oddi. They generally gain access by eroding through the wall of the gallbladder into the duodenum.

Carcinoma

The incidence of carcinoma of the gallbladder is increased in patients with long-standing gallstones.

Common clinical syndromes associated with gallstones

The majority of individuals with gallstones are asymptomatic or have only vague symptoms of distension and flatulence. Less than half of such patients develop symptoms or complications from their gallstones within 10 years.

Biliary colic

Biliary colic is due to transient obstruction of the gallbladder from an impacted stone. There is severe gripping pain, often developing after meals or in the evening, which is maximal in the epigastrium and right hypochondrium with radiation to the back.

Gallstones

- Most gallstones form because of failure to keep cholesterol in solution. This can result in pure cholesterol stones, but more commonly the stones also acquire a content of bile pigment as they enlarge, forming 'mixed' stones.

- Pigment stones are the commonest type of stone in some Oriental countries, but are less common in Western society where they are associated with chronic haemolysis, biliary stasis and cirrhosis.

- Only 15% of stones contain enough calcium to be seen on a plain film.

- The majority of individuals with gallstones are asymptomatic and remain so; the presence of gallstones is not in itself an indication for cholecystectomy.

- Gallbladder stones may cause flatulent dyspepsia, biliary colic, acute cholecystitis, and gallbladder cancer (although this is so rare that this consideration does not affect the decision not to treat asymptomatic stones).

- Gallstones which migrate into the bile duct can cause obstructive jaundice, cholangitis and acute pancreatitis, although they often remain asymptomatic.

- Gallstone ileus is a rare form of intestinal obstruction; stones large enough to obstruct the gut are usually too large to pass through the ampulla of Vater and have gained access to the gut by an internal fistula involving the gallbladder.

Though continuous, the pain may wax and wane in intensity over several hours, and vomiting and retching are common. Resolution occurs when the stone falls back into the gallbladder lumen or passes onwards into the common bile duct. The patient then recovers rapidly but repeated bouts of colic are common. In some cases, the obstruction does not resolve and the patient develops acute cholecystitis.

Acute cholecystitis

Acute cholecystitis is a more prolonged and severe illness. It usually begins with an attack of biliary colic, though its onset may be more gradual. There is severe right hypochondrial pain radiating to the right subscapular region, and occasionally to the right shoulder, together with tachycardia, pyrexia, nausea, vomiting, and leucocytosis. Abdominal tenderness and rigidity may be generalized but are most marked over the gallbladder. Murphy's sign (a catching of the breath at the height of inspiration while the gallbladder area is palpated) is usually present. A right hypochondrial mass may be felt. This is due to omentum 'wrapped' around the inflamed gallbladder.

In 85–90% of cases the attack settles within 4–5 days. In the remainder, tenderness may spread and pyrexia and tachycardia persist or worsen. Development of a tender mass associated with rigors and marked pyrexia signals empyema formation. The gallbladder may become gangrenous and perforate, giving rise to biliary peritonitis.

Jaundice can develop during the acute attack. Usually this is associated with stones in the common bile duct but compression of the bile ducts by the gallbladder may be responsible.

Acute cholecystitis must be differentiated from perforated peptic ulcer, high retrocaecal appendicitis, acute pancreatitis, myocardial infarction, and basal pneumonia. Acute cholecystitis can develop in the absence of gallstones (acalculous cholecystitis), although this is rare.

Chronic cholecystitis

Chronic cholecystitis is the most common cause of symptomatic gallbladder disease. The patient gives a history of recurrent flatulence, fatty food intolerance and right upper quadrant pain. The pain is worse after meals and is often associated with a feeling of distension and heartburn.

The differential diagnosis includes duodenal ulcer, hiatus hernia, myocardial ischaemia, chronic pancreatitis, and gastrointestinal neoplasia.

Mucocele

In this condition, the patient often presents with a history of biliary colic and a non-tender piriform swelling in the right hypochondrium. There is little systemic upset and no pyrexia.

Choledocholithiasis

Stones are present in the common bile duct of some 10% of patients with gallstones. There is little muscle in the wall of the bile duct and pain is not a symptom unless the stone impedes flow through the sphincter of Oddi. The vast majority of stones in the common bile duct originate in the gallbladder. 'Primary' duct stones are extremely rare.

Impaction of a stone at the sphincter obstructs the flow of bile, producing *jaundice*, pale stools, and dark urine. Obstruction commonly persists for several days but may clear spontaneously, either as a result of passage of the stone or its disimpaction. Small stones may pass through the common bile duct without causing symptoms.

In long-standing obstruction, the bile ducts become markedly dilated and the diameter of the common bile duct may exceed its upper limit of 10 mm. A totally obstructed duct system becomes filled with clear 'white bile' as back pressure on the hepatocytes prevents clearance of bilirubin and mucus secretion is increased.

Infection of an obstructed biliary tract causes *cholangitis* which is characterized by attacks of pain, pyrexia, and jaundice (the so-called triad of Charcot), frequently in association with rigors. Long-standing intermittent biliary obstruction may lead to secondary biliary cirrhosis.

Acute pancreatitis may be associated with a stone in the common bile duct (see Ch. 34).

Obstructive jaundice due to stones in the common bile duct has to be distinguished from other causes of obstructive jaundice, notably malignant obstruction and cholestatic jaundice. Acute viral or alcoholic hepatitis may occasionally be confused with obstructive jaundice.

Courvoisier's law. Fibrosed gallbladders which contain stones cannot distend when pressure increases in the obstructed biliary tree. Courvoisier's law states that if the gallbladder is palpable in the presence of jaundice, the jaundice is unlikely to be due to stone. This law is not inviolate.

Distended gallbladders are not always easy to feel but can be detected readily by ultrasonic scans.

Other benign conditions of the gallbladder

Cholesterosis

Cholesterosis or 'strawberry gallbladder' is a condition in which the mucous membrane of the gallbladder is infiltrated with lipid and cholesterol. It affects middle-aged and elderly patients of either sex.

Cholesterol stones are found in the gallbladders of half of these patients. Macroscopically the mucosa is brick-red and speckled with bright yellow nodules. Symptoms of acute and chronic cholecystitis may be produced, and cholecystectomy is required in the symptomatic patient.

Adenomyomatosis

This rare condition is characterized by mucosal diverticula (Rokitansky-Aschoff sinuses) which affect particularly the fundus and penetrate the muscular layers to the serosa. Muscular hypertrophy and inflammatory cell infiltrates are present. The gallbladder often contains stones or biliary gravel. The condition is usually apparent on cholecystography and, if symptomatic, may require cholecystectomy.

Acute acalculous cholecystitis

About 5% patients with acute cholecystitis have acalculous inflammation. The condition may be precipitated by major surgery, bacteraemia, trauma, pancreatitis or other serious illness, and may complicate parenteral nutrition. The inflammatory reaction in the gallbladder wall may be intense and severe, leading to gangrene and perforation. In ill patients, percutaneous drainage (cholecystostomy) under ultrasound guidance may be considered but urgent cholecystectomy is often advisable.

Investigation of patients with suspected gallstones

Plain abdominal X-ray

As only 15% of gallstones contain enough calcium to be seen on a plain radiograph, this investigation is seldom used in diagnosis. Gas is occasionally seen outlining the biliary tree if there is a fistula between the biliary tract and the gut. This fistula may have arisen spontaneously, as in gallstone ileus, or have been created surgically, as in choledochoduodenostomy. Previous endoscopic sphincterotomy also allows gas to enter the biliary tree.

Ultrasonography

Ultrasonography using a real-time scanner has become the mainstay of investigation. It permits inspection of the gallbladder, its wall and its contents, and demonstrates dilatation of the intrahepatic and extrahepatic biliary tree. Stones reflect the ultrasonic wave and are thrown into prominence by the acoustic shadow they produce. The technique is extremely accurate in skilled hands. As it does not depend on hepatic excretion of contrast, it can be used both in jaundiced and non-jaundiced patients.

Oral cholecystography

An iodine-containing fat-soluble compound is taken orally, absorbed and excreted in the bile. After some hours the gallbladder becomes opacified and gallstones may be seen as filling defects within it. The technique will not outline the gallbladder when the serum bilirubin concentration is elevated, as sufficient contrast medium is not excreted. In non-jaundiced patients, failure to visualize the gallbladder may reflect obstruction of the cystic duct or the fact that the gallbladder is so grossly diseased that it has ceased to function. Occasionally non-opacification is due to vomiting, diarrhoea, pyloric stenosis or failure to take the tablets. Oral cholecystography is a reliable means of detecting gallstones in non-jaundiced patients but has been largely superseded by ultrasonography.

Intravenous cholangiography

This technique involves intravenous injection of an iodine-containing compound which, within minutes, is excreted into the biliary system. Serial radiographs are taken, but visualization is often poor despite varying the depth of focus (tomography). Absence of gallbladder opacification in the presence of normal liver function indicates that the cystic duct is blocked. The technique is of no value in jaundiced patients and carries a small but definite risk of severe (and even fatal) anaphylactoid reaction. It is now seldom used.

Endoscopic retrograde cholangiopancreatography (ERCP)

Using a side-viewing fibreoptic endoscope, the papilla of Vater may be seen and cannulated. Contrast is then injected to outline the biliary and pancreatic duct systems. If stones are detected in the common bile duct, they can be removed at the same time following endoscopic sphincterotomy.

Percutaneous transhepatic cholangiography (PTC)

In patients with obstructive jaundice the intrahepatic biliary system can be entered percutaneously using a slim flexible needle through which radio-opaque dye is then injected. The site and nature of any obstruction can be defined. Ultrasonography is usually performed first to confirm that there is duct dilatation. PTC is virtually always successful when the ducts are distended and succeeds in two-thirds of patients who do not have a dilated duct system. Leakage of bile or bleeding from the puncture site are now rare complications but antibiotic cover (e.g. with gentamicin) is required and coagulation status must be checked. This investigation is more likely to be employed in the evaluation of malignancy involving the biliary tract.

Isotope scanning

In acute cholecystitis, a gamma-camera was once used to scan the liver and biliary tree following intravenous injection of ^{99m}Tc-labelled HIDA (dimethylacetanilide-iminodiacetic acid). Failure to visualize the gallbladder within 2 hours suggests acute cholecystitis. The technique is no more accurate than ultrasonography and will not outline the biliary tree if the patient has significant jaundice.

Surgical treatment of gallstones

Patients with symptomatic gallstones are usually advised to undergo cholecystectomy to relieve symptoms and avoid complications. Patients with asymptomatic gallstones are treated expectantly, particularly if they are elderly or suffering from medical conditions likely to increase the risk of operating. In younger patients there may be a stronger case for surgery despite the absence of symptoms, particularly if the stones are multiple and likely to cause complications such as acute pancreatitis.

Irrespective of whether open or laparoscopic cholecystectomy is undertaken, the principles of surgical technique remain the same. The gallbladder and its contained stones are removed, while ensuring that no stones remain within the ductal system. 'Open' cholecystectomy may be required if the equipment and expertise for laparoscopic cholecystectomy are not available. A laparoscopic procedure may not be possible in the patient who has previously undergone multiple abdominal operations or who is grossly obese. Pregnancy is considered a contraindication to laparoscopy because of the risk of anaesthetic agents to the developing fetus in the first trimester and because of the risk of spontaneous abortion. There is debate as to whether laparoscopic cholecystectomy should be used in patients with acute complications of biliary disease since the risk of complications is said to be greater than for open cholecystectomy.

Conversion from a laparoscopic procedure to open cholecystectomy should be seen as a limitation of the technique and not as failure of the surgeon. Laparotomy is mandatory when the anatomy in the area of the cystic duct and artery cannot be defined readily, if uncontrolled bleeding occurs, or if the bile duct is injured.

Open cholecystectomy

The gallbladder is now usually approached through a right subcostal rather than a paramedian or midline incision. Following careful inspection and palpation of the abdominal contents to exclude other pathology, the cystic duct and artery are identified. Intra-operative cholangiography is performed by cannulating the cystic duct and taking serial radio-

graphs after injection of contrast. The cholangiogram displays the anatomy of the duct system, identifies ductal stones and confirms that dye passes freely into the duodenum (Fig. 33.16). Once the films have been inspected, the gallbladder is removed after ligation and division of the cystic duct and artery. A retrograde approach in which the gallbladder is mobilized 'fundus first' can be used when inflammation makes visualization of the biliary anatomy difficult.

Some surgeons pursue a policy of selective cholangiography, obtaining a cholangiogram only in patients at high risk of having ductal stones. The presence of such stones may be suspected if there is a history of jaundice or pancreatitis, pre-operative LFTs are abnormal or dilatation of the common bile duct or multiple gallbladder stones have been detected on ultrasound scanning. At surgery, a stone may be palpable in the duct system.

Following removal of the gallbladder, haemostasis

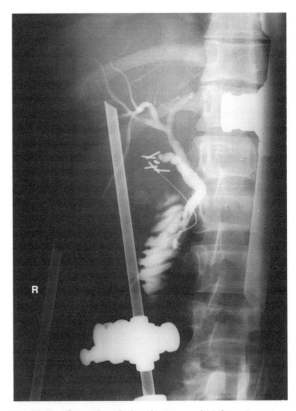

Fig. 33.16 Operative cholangiogram undertaken at laparoscopic cholecystectomy (note the radio-opaque ports). The extrahepatic ducts are not particularly dilated and there is flow of contrast into the duodenum but there is a small solitary radiolucent calculus at the lower end of the common bile duct.

is secured and the wound is closed. Many surgeons leave a drain in the subhepatic space to prevent the development of a collection and to identify leakage of bile.

Laparoscopic cholecystectomy

Access to the peritoneal cavity is obtained through three or four cannulae inserted through the anterior abdominal wall and following insufflation of the peritoneal cavity with CO_2. The gallbladder is retracted by grasping forceps inserted through the most lateral cannula in order to display the structures at the porta hepatis. An excellent view of the operating field is obtained with the laparoscope, and the cystic duct and artery are isolated by dissection with instruments passed through the remaining cannulae. Many surgeons find it difficult to undertake operative cholangiography routinely with this approach and have either abandoned its use or relied upon intravenous cholangiography and/or ERCP in the pre- or postoperative period to exclude the presence of common bile duct stones.

The cystic duct and artery are normally divided between metal clips and the gallbladder is dissected from the liver, employing diathermy or a Neodymium YAG laser. Extraction of the gallbladder through a cannula site may require extension of the incision or tedious removal of individual stones from the gallbladder. Care must be taken to secure haemostasis and many surgeons leave a drain in the subhepatic space.

Exploration of the common bile duct

At open surgery, if stones are present in the duct system, the common bile duct is opened longitudinally between stay sutures (choledochotomy) and the stones are extracted with forceps (Desjardin forceps) or a Fogarty balloon catheter. Following exploration, further check cholangiogram films are obtained or the interior of the duct can be inspected with a rigid or fibreoptic choledochoscope.

The opening in the common bile duct is then closed around a T-tube, the long limb of which is brought out through a stab incision in the abdominal wall (Fig. 33.17). This serves as a safety valve to allow escape of bile if there is temporary obstruction to flow into the duodenum following duct exploration. It also allows installation of iodine-containing dye to obtain a T-tube cholangiogram some 7–10 days following surgery. If this shows free flow of dye into the duodenum and no residual duct stones, the

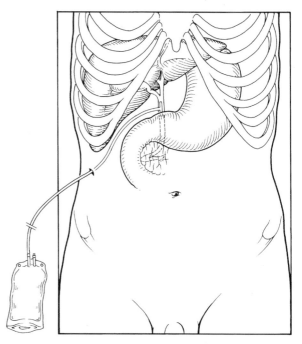

Fig. 33.17   T-tube drainage of the common bile duct.

T-tube can be removed. If at operation there is gross duct dilatation and the bile duct contains multiple stones and debris some surgeons follow duct exploration by anastomosing the common bile duct to the adjacent duodenum (choledochoduodenostomy), but this is rarely necessary.

If at operation a stone is firmly impacted at the lower end of the common bile duct, it may have to be removed through the duodenum. The sphincter of Oddi is incised (transduodenal sphincterotomy) to release the stone, and the operation is completed by suturing the duct mucosa to that of the duodenum (transduodenal sphincteroplasty; Fig. 33.18). Both of these procedures increase the risk of postoperative morbidity and mortality and are only undertaken if the stone cannot be extracted from above.

With the reluctance of some surgeons to perform operative cholangiography during laparoscopic cholecystectomy, increasing reliance has been placed on removing common bile duct stones at ERCP. Other surgeons continue to adhere to the principles employed at open cholecystectomy and explore the common bile duct by means of a choledochotomy or through the dilated cystic duct. Retained stones can be removed with the aid of a small-diameter fibreoptic choledochoscope under direct vision, or by means of a wire basket or an inflatable balloon catheter. The surgeon has the option of leaving a

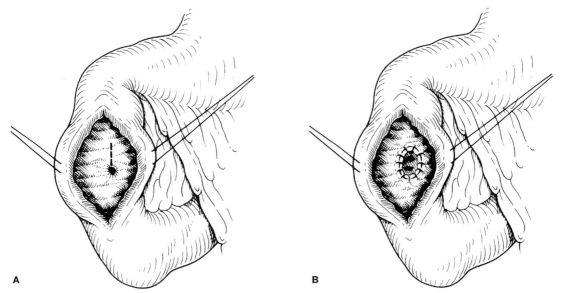

Fig. 33.18 **Transduodenal sphincterotomy and sphincteroplasty. A** Incision of bile duct. **B** Following sphincteroplasty the opening of the pancreatic duct is visible within the open bile duct.

drain in the cystic duct or can oversew the choledochotomy over a T-tube.

Complications of cholecystectomy

The postoperative stay of patients undergoing open cholecystectomy may exceed 7 days. Respiratory complications are not uncommon and there is a significant risk of wound infection (see below). Operative mortality following elective open cholecystectomy is low (0.2%) but is increased tenfold if there is obstructive jaundice or if the common bile duct has to be explored.

Postoperative stay is greatly reduced with laparoscopic cholecystectomy, which in some centres is now undertaken as a day case procedure. Complications resulting from a major abdominal wound are undoubtedly avoided but there is concern regarding the increased incidence of injury to the bile duct. Mortality and morbidity related to the laparoscopic procedure has also been reported. Nonetheless, the advantages to the patient of this minimally invasive technique has led to its widespread adoption by surgeons.

Haemorrhage

This may originate from the cystic artery or gallbladder bed. If the patient becomes shocked and bright red blood issues from the drain, re-exploration is mandatory.

Cholecystectomy
- Cholecystectomy is the standard treatment for symptomatic gallbladder stones; alternatives (stone dissolution, extracorporeal lithotripsy) are now seldom used.

- Open cholecystectomy has been largely superseded by laparoscopic cholecystectomy, but conversion to open operation is still sometimes needed.

- Cholecystectomy now has a low operative mortality (0.2%); inadvertent injury to the bile duct (0.2% incidence) remains the main source of major morbidity.

- Some 10% of patients coming to cholecystectomy have ductal stones, many of which are unsuspected. Opinions vary as to whether intraoperative cholangiography should be undertaken routinely to detect such stones.

- In the era of laparoscopic cholecystectomy there is a growing tendency not to perform routine operative cholangiography, and to extract symptomatic duct stones by non-operative means (i.e. at endoscopic papillotomy).

- If ductal stones cause symptoms they frequently give rise to cholangitis and the triad (Charcot's) of pain, jaundice and fever (often with rigors).

Infective complications

Wound infection with organisms present in the bile (notably *E. coli, Kleb. aerogenes* and *Strep. faecalis*) is common. Its incidence after elective cholecystectomy can be reduced markedly by intravenous administration of a cephalosporin at the time of induction of anaesthesia. A longer course of antibiotics is usually prescribed when operating on patients with obstructive jaundice, cholangitis or complications such as acute cholecystitis or empyema. Collections of bile and/or blood readily become infected after cholecystectomy. Formal drainage may be needed if this progresses to the formation of a subhepatic or subphrenic abscess.

Bile leakage

This may be due to a ligature or clip slipping off the cystic duct, accidental division of an unrecognized accessory duct, damage to the common bile duct, or retention of a duct stone after exploration. If substantial leakage continues, full radiological investigation is indicated and further surgery may be needed.

Retained stones

Even if the bile duct has been explored, the routine postoperative T-tube cholangiogram (see above) may reveal that there is still a stone in the bile duct.

Small stones can sometimes be flushed into the duodenum by irrigating the T-tube with saline and their passage may be facilitated if glucagon is given to relax the sphincter of Oddi. Alternatively, cholesterol stones may be dissolved or made smaller by duct irrigation with volatile agents such as methylterbutyl ether (MTBE). If the duct cannot be cleared by irrigation, stones may be extracted under radiological control. The patient is discharged with the T-tube in place. This is removed 4–6 weeks later and a steerable catheter is passed along its track into the bile duct. A wire basket (Dormia basket) can be passed along the catheter to catch and withdraw the retained calculus (Fig. 33.19).

In some patients, unsuspected stones may be left in the bile duct at cholecystectomy. Such stones may remain asymptomatic but usually give rise to complications such as jaundice, cholangitis and pancreatitis in the months and years following cholecystectomy. ERCP can be used to confirm the presence of such retained stones (Fig. 33.20) and endoscopic papillo-

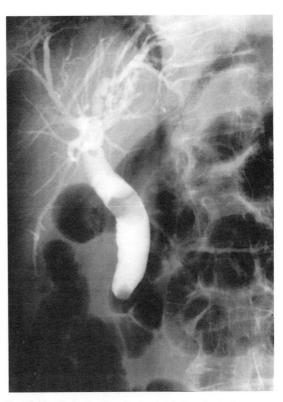

Fig. 33.20 Endoscopic retrograde cholangiography demonstrating multiple stones within the biliary tree. The endoscope has been withdrawn to enable clear visualisation of the lower end of the bile duct which is markedly dilated. These calculi were removed successfully by balloon extraction following sphincterotomy.

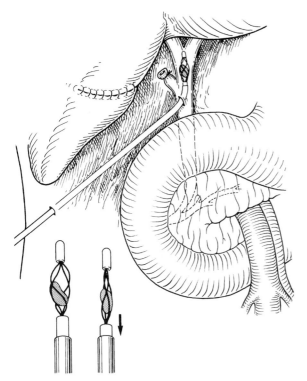

Fig. 33.19 Removal of a retained common bile duct stone.

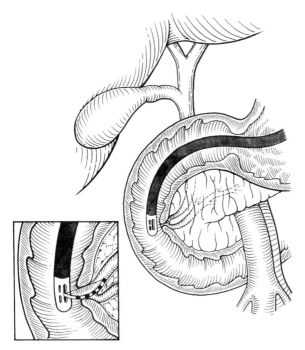

Fig. 33.21 Endoscopic papillotomy to remove retained stones.

tomy is performed to recover them (Fig. 33.21). In this technique a diathermy wire attached to a cannula is passed through the duodenoscope and used to divide the sphincter of Oddi. The stones can then be extracted with a Dormia basket or balloon catheter. The same method can be used to extract stones detected in the immediate postoperative period. If stones are too large to be withdrawn, a catheter can be left in the biliary system (nasobiliary catheter) and the stones can be dissolved (or at least reduced in size) by agents such as MTBE. It is now extremely uncommon to have to operate to retrieve retained bile duct stones.

Bile duct stricture

About 90% of benign duct strictures result from damage during cholecystectomy in which the duct is divided, ligated or devascularized. This last mechanism appears to be a common cause of injury at laparoscopic cholecystectomy. Other causes of injury include division of a ligated common bile duct which has been mistaken for the cystic duct, division of the right hepatic duct below the point of anomalous insertion of the cystic duct, and encirclement of the common bile duct by the ligature or clip used to close off the cystic duct. Strictures only occasionally result from abdominal trauma or erosion of the bile duct by a gallstone.

If the common bile duct is completely occluded, progressive obstructive jaundice develops in the postoperative period. If there is a partial stricture, attacks of pain, fever, and obstructive jaundice signal the development of cholangitis. The serum alkaline phosphatase and transaminase concentrations are usually elevated, and blood cultures may be positive during attacks of fever. If left untreated, persistent cholangitis and obstruction progress to secondary biliary cirrhosis, hepatic abscess formation, portal hypertension, and liver failure.

The site and extent of the stricture must be defined radiologically. After ultrasonography has been performed, PTC and/or ERCP are usually undertaken. Reconstructive surgery is undertaken in a specialist centre and usually necessitates bringing

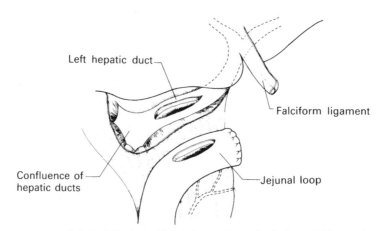

Left hepatic duct

Falciform ligament

Confluence of hepatic ducts

Jejunal loop

Fig. 33.22 Relief of bile duct stricture by anastomosis of a loop of jejunum to the distended biliary tree above the stricture (hepatico-jejunostomy Roux en Y).

up a Roux loop of jejunum and anastomosing this to the distended biliary system above the stricture (Fig. 33.22).

Post-cholecystectomy syndrome

This term is used to embrace a group of complaints such as postprandial flatulence, fat intolerance, epigastric and right hypochondrial discomfort, and heartburn which may follow cholecystectomy. The complaints tend to be more troublesome when cholecystectomy has been performed in the absence of gallstones. Investigations are usually negative but some patients prove to have retained stones or other alimentary disorders such as peptic ulceration, gastritis, and chronic pancreatitis. It is possible that some patients develop pain because of functional abnormalities of the sphincter of Oddi (see below).

Management of acute cholecystitis

Patients with acute cholecystitis are admitted to hospital. The pulse, blood pressure and temperature are monitored, and analgesics, intravenous fluid and a broad-spectrum antibiotic such as a cephalosporin are prescribed. The patient is given nothing by mouth and a nasogastric tube is passed if the patient is vomiting. The majority of patients settle on this regimen within a few days. Failure to settle suggests the presence of an empyema.

Some surgeons delay operation for 2–3 months after the attack in the expectation that the acute inflammatory reaction will have resolved by then, but most now prefer to perform cholecystectomy during the same admission and within 72 hours of the onset of the attack. Provided the operation is carried out by an experienced surgeon and under antibiotic cover, 'early' cholecystectomy is not associated with an increased incidence of complications. The duration of the illness and hospitalization are reduced, and further attacks of acute cholecystitis during the waiting period for elective surgery are averted. It should be noted that this is a planned procedure carried out after appropriate investigation (ultrasonography) and with all facilities, on a routine elective list. 'Emergency' cholecystectomy at the time of admission is not advised except for empyema of the gallbladder or when there is evidence of spreading peritonitis. As mentioned earlier, there is debate about whether laparoscopic cholecystectomy should be used in this context.

If surrounding inflammation makes identification of the relevant anatomical structures difficult, cholecystostomy, i.e. drainage of the gallbladder with

removal of stones, may be performed as an interim measure. Elective cholecystectomy is then usually performed approximately 2 months later.

Acalculous cholecystitis

Patients with an acute attack of acalculous cholecystitis may require urgent cholecystostomy or cholecystectomy. Patients with long-standing symptoms and a radiological diagnosis of cholesterosis or adenomyomatosis are advised to undergo elective cholecystectomy.

Atypical 'biliary' pain

More difficulty arises with patients who have attacks of pain consistent with biliary colic but in whom investigations such as ultrasonography, oral cholecystography and ERCP reveal no abnormality. Some of these patients with 'acalculous biliary pain' may eventually prove to have non-biliary disease such as peptic ulceration, chronic pancreatitis or 'irritable' colon. In the majority, no explanation for the symptoms can be found, although recent evidence suggests that some may be suffering from a functional disorder of the sphincter of Oddi. Endoscopic manometry may be useful in identifying patients who may benefit from endoscopic sphincterotomy.

Laparoscopy or laparotomy are sometimes needed to exclude other pathology, confirm that there are no stones in the biliary tree, and remove the gallbladder as the potential source of symptoms. The results of cholecystectomy in these patients are extremely variable and many continue to have symptoms.

Non-surgical treatment of gallstones

In patients with small non-calcified cholesterol stones in a functioning gallbladder, chenodeoxycholic acid or the more recently introduced ursodeoxycholic acid can be used to expand the bile salt pool and so dissolve the stone(s). Treatment may have to continue for at least a year, during which time the patient remains at risk of the complications of gallstones. Diarrhoea and disordered LFTs are dose-related side-effects and gallstones may reform on stopping treatment. For these reasons, dissolution therapy has not become popular.

Percutaneous extraction or dissolution of gallstones with MTBE is possible but the efficacy and complications of this approach have yet to be evaluated. Destruction of stones by extracorporeal shock wave lithotripsy has also been used and is effective in selected patients in combination with oral dissolution therapy.

The popularity of non-surgical treatments has greatly declined with the advent of laparoscopic cholecystectomy.

OTHER BENIGN BILIARY DISORDERS

Asiatic cholangiohepatitis

There has been a decline in the incidence of this condition which occurs in the Far East and is particularly common in coastal Chinese communities. Suppurative cholangitis develops and pigment stones form in the intrahepatic and extrahepatic biliary tree. Deconjugation of bilirubin glucuronide by bacteria may be implicated in stone formation, and E. coli and Strep. faecalis can often be isolated from the bile and portal blood.

The clinical features are those of obstructive jaundice, pain and fever, and liver abscesses may form. Cholangitis is treated with antibiotics and stones within the duct can be removed by percutaneous, endoscopic, and operative means. Ductal obstruction may be treated by choledochoduodenostomy or hepaticojejunostomy. A limb of the Roux loop of jejunum may be left in a subcutaneous position to facilitate subsequent percutaneous manoeuvres to treat residual or recurrent calculi. Hepatic resection may be indicated if suppuration and obstruction have led to regional destruction of liver tissue.

Primary sclerosing cholangitis

Both intrahepatic and extrahepatic bile ducts may become indurated and irregularly thickened in this condition. There is a marked chronic inflammatory cell infiltrate and fibrous narrowing of the biliary tree. The aetiology of the condition is unknown but it may have an immunological basis. Over three-quarters of patients also suffer from ulcerative colitis, and other associated conditions include retroperitoneal fibrosis, immunodeficiency syndromes and pancreatitis. Bile duct carcinoma can develop and obstruction can give rise to bacterial cholangitis and secondary biliary cirrhosis.

The condition frequently affects young adults and gives rise to intermittent attacks of obstructive jaundice, pruritis and pain. ERCP and liver biopsy are the mainstays of diagnosis. Treatment is generally unsatisfactory, and colectomy does not improve the cholangitis in patients with ulcerative colitis.

Corticosteroids and D-penicillamine have been used but have no proven value. The outlook is extremely variable and in some the disease appears to remit. Duct strictures can sometimes be treated by surgical bypass or insertion of stents but such manoeuvres may compromise the ability to undertake successful liver transplantation which offers the only prospect of cure.

TUMOURS OF THE BILIARY TRACT

Carcinoma of the gallbladder

Carcinoma of the gallbladder is rare and is almost invariably associated with the presence of gallstones. The condition is four times as common in females as in males. About 90% of lesions are adenocarcinomas, the remainder are squamous carcinomas.

Direct invasion commonly obstructs the bile duct or porta hepatis and early lymphatic and haematogenous dissemination is common. Initial symptoms are indistinguishable from those of gallstones but jaundice is unremitting. A mass is frequently palpable. Many tumours are detected incidentally at the cholecystectomy for treatment of gallstones. Some surgeons recommend an aggressive approach of segmental resection involving segments IV, V and VI of the liver with dissection of the regional lymph nodes. Tumours presenting with jaundice cannot be cured by resection and palliation by endoscopic or percutaneous insertion of a stent or surgical bypass is required.

The 5-year survival rate is less than 5%.

Carcinoma of the bile ducts

Cholangiocarcinoma is a relatively uncommon cancer which affects the elderly and may be increasing in frequency. The tumour may arise at any site within the biliary tree and can be multifocal. Sclerotic lesions involving the confluence of the hepatic ducts (Klatskin tumour) pose considerable problems in management. The lesions are said to be slow-growing but this has been overemphasized. Cholangiocarcinoma may develop in patients with underlying primary sclerosing cholangitis or choledochal cyst.

Clinical features

Progressive obstructive jaundice, often preceded by vague dyspeptic pain, is the usual presenting feature. The gallbladder may become obstructed because of

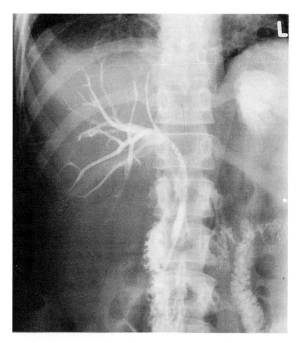

Fig. 33.23 Percutaneous transhepatic cholangiogram demonstrating a stricture at the confluence of the hepatic ducts. This lesion has the typical appearance of a cholangiocarcinoma and has been managed by percutaneous insertion of a stent.

cystic duct involvement and mucocele or empyema can develop. Anorexia and weight loss are common. Pruritus is often particularly distressing.

Management

The diagnosis of malignant obstruction may be made on the history and clinical findings. The presence of intrahepatic duct dilatation and a collapsed gallbladder on ultrasound scan are highly suggestive of a tumour involving the common hepatic duct. Resectability is best assessed by CT scanning (to exclude the presence of hepatic metastases and nodal involvement) and angiography (to assess vascular invasion). PTC may assist the surgeon in planning resection.

Carcinoma of the common bile duct is treated by the Whipple operation (see p. 511) if the tumour is localized and the patient is fit for radical resection. Long-term survival following this procedure is considerably better in patients with cholangiocarcinoma than in those with carcinoma of the head of the pancreas.

Carcinoma of the upper biliary tract is resectable in only 10% of patients, some of whom may require hepatic resection to achieve satisfactory clearance of tumour. Following resection, the remaining biliary tree is anastomosed to a Roux loop of jejunum. In the majority of patients not submitted to resection, palliation can be achieved by insertion of a stent by endoscopic or percutaneous transhepatic techniques (Fig. 33.23). Most stents are liable to occlusion, exposing the patient to repeated attacks of cholangitis and/or jaundice. Some surgeons prefer to palliate patients surgically and implantation of a stenting tube at operation has largely been replaced by intrahepatic anastomosis of a Roux loop of jejunum to the segment III duct in the left lobe of the liver. Although decompression of only one-half of the biliary tree is achieved, this operation provides effective palliation in the short-term. Few patients with cholangiocarcinoma survive for more than 18 months.

34
The pancreas

CONTENTS

Surgical anatomy

The pancreas develops from separate ventral and dorsal buds of endoderm which appear during the fourth week of fetal life. The ventral pancreas develops in association with the biliary tree, and its duct joins the common bile duct before emptying into the duodenum through the papilla of Vater (Fig. 34.1). During gestation the duodenum rotates clockwise on its long axis, and the bile duct and ventral pancreas pass round behind it to fuse with the dorsal pancreas. Most of the duct which drains the dorsal pancreas joins the duct draining the ventral pancreas to form the main pancreatic duct (of Wirsung); the rest of the dorsal duct becomes the accessory pancreatic duct (of Santorini) and enters the duodenum 2.5 cm proximal to the main duct. In fetal life the common bile duct and main pancreatic duct are dilated at their junction to form the ampulla of Vater. In extrauterine life, only 10% of individuals retain this ampulla, although the great majority still have a short common channel between the two duct systems.

The pancreas is deep-seated and inaccessible. It lies retroperitoneally, behind the lesser sac and stomach. The head of the gland lies within the C-

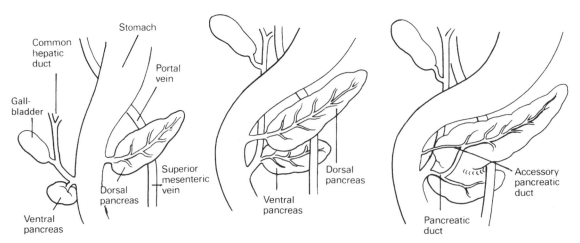

Fig. 34.1   The development of the pancreas.

loop of the duodenum with which it shares a blood supply from the coeliac and superior mesenteric arteries (Fig. 34.2). The superior mesenteric vein runs upwards to the left of the uncinate process, and joins the splenic vein behind the neck of the pancreas to form the portal vein. The body and tail of the pancreas lie in front of the splenic vein as far as the splenic hilum, and receive arterial blood from the splenic artery as it runs along the upper border of the gland. The intimate relationship of the friable pancreas to these major blood vessels explains why bleeding is so problematic after pancreatic trauma. The close association between the common bile duct and the head of pancreas explains why obstructive jaundice is so common in cancer of the head of the pancreas, and why gallstones frequently give rise to acute pancreatitis.

Surgical physiology

Exocrine function

The pancreas secretes 1–2 litres of alkaline (pH 7.5–8.8) enzyme-rich juice each day. The enzymes are synthesized by the acinar cells and stored there as zymogen granules. Trypsin is the key proteolytic enzyme; it is released in an inactive form (trypsinogen) and is normally only activated within the duodenum by the brush border enzyme enterokinase. Once trypsin has been activated, a cascade is established whereby the other proteolytic enzymes become activated in turn. Lipase and amylase are secreted as active enzymes. The alkaline medium required for the activity of pancreatic enzymes is provided by the bicarbonate secreted by the ductal epithelium.

Pancreatic secretion is stimulated by eating. Hormonal and neural (vagal) mechanisms are involved. Food entering the duodenum (notably fat and protein digestion products) releases cholecystokinin (CCK) which stimulates pancreatic enzyme secretion while at the same time causing the gallbladder to contract and increase bile flow into the intestine. Acid in the duodenum releases the hormone secretin which stimulates the pancreas to secrete watery alkaline juice.

Endocrine function

The islets of Langerhans are distributed throughout the pancreas. Although they account for only 2% of the weight of the gland, they receive 10% of its blood

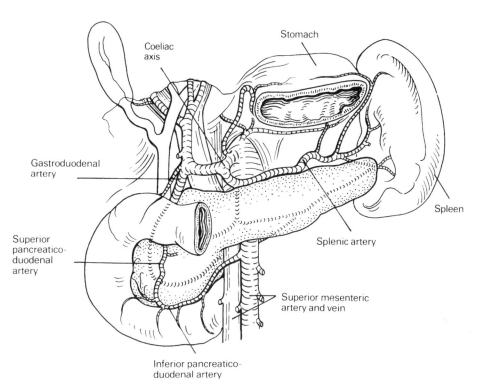

Fig. 34.2 Anatomical relationships of the pancreas.

supply. Interaction between the endocrine and exocrine pancreas is facilitated by the close proximity of islets and acini, and by a local 'portal' system in which blood draining from the islets enters a capillary network around neighbouring acinar cells before entering the tributaries of the portal vein. Four types of islet cells are recognized: A cells produce glucagon, B cells insulin, D cells somatostatin and PP cells pancreatic polypeptide. Glucagon and insulin have well-established physiological roles; the function of the other islet products is uncertain but somatostatin and pancreatic polypeptide may serve as local (paracrine) regulators, rather than as circulating (endocrine) messengers. Gastrin-producing (G) cells are not normally found in the pancreas except in the rare Zollinger-Ellison syndrome (Ch. 28).

Pancreatic pain

The parasympathetic nervous system has no role in the perception of pancreatic pain. Painful stimuli from the pancreas are transmitted by sympathetic fibres which travel along the arteries of supply to the coeliac ganglion, and from there to segments 5 to 10 of the thoracic spinal cord via the greater (and lesser) splanchnic nerves.

CONGENITAL DISORDERS OF THE PANCREAS

Annular pancreas

This rare cause of duodenal obstruction results from failure of rotation of the ventral pancreas.

Pancreas divisum

In approximately 5% of individuals, the ducts draining the dorsal and ventral pancreas fail to fuse, giving rise to pancreas divisum. This means that the secretions of the larger dorsal pancreas have to drain to the duodenum through the smaller accessory duct. The suggestion that pancreas divisum can predispose to acute and chronic pancreatitis is now generally discounted.

Heterotopic pancreatic tissue

Rests of pancreatic tissue may be found at a variety of sites within the gut wall, but are commonest in the duodenum, stomach and proximal small bowel.

Most remain asymptomatic but they can cause ulceration, bleeding and obstruction.

Cystic fibrosis (mucoviscidosis)

Cystic fibrosis affects sweat glands, pancreas and bronchial mucous glands. Meconium ileus can produce surgical problems by giving rise to intestinal obstruction in neonates.

PANCREATITIS

Pancreatitis may be acute or chronic. After an attack of acute pancreatitis the gland usually returns to anatomical and functional normality, whereas chronic pancreatitis is associated with permanent derangement of structure and function. Some patients suffer from recurrent acute pancreatitis, enjoying relatively normal health between attacks.

Acute pancreatitis

Acute pancreatitis is a common cause of emergency admission to hospital. Britain has 50–100 new cases per million of the population each year, and the incidence is rising, possibly as a result of increasing alcohol consumption. The disease is relatively rare in children but all adult age groups may be affected. Roughly one in four patients prove to have severe disease, and of these, one in four will die.

Aetiology

Conditions associated with the development of acute pancreatitis are listed in Table 34.1; gallstones and alcohol are of overriding importance.

Gallstone pancreatitis. Gallstones are present in some 50% of patients who develop acute pancreatitis in Britain. Most of these patients have many small stones in the gallbladder, a wide cystic duct, and a common channel between the common bile duct and main pancreatic duct (Fig. 34.3). It is now believed that stones impact transiently in the common channel and so promote reflux of bile into the pancreatic duct and/or impair the normal flow of pancreatic juice. Stones ranging in diameter from 1–12 mm have been recovered from the faeces in the days following an attack of acute pancreatitis, supporting the concept of transient impaction. It has also become apparent that many patients with 'idiopathic acute pancreatitis' are actually suffering from pancreatitis caused not by stones *per se* but by

Table 34.1 Causes of acute pancreatitis	
Non-traumatic causes (75%)	
Major factors	Biliary tract disease (50%)
	Alcohol (20–30%)
Minor factors	Viral infection (mumps, Coxsackie)
	Drugs (e.g. steroids)
	Hyperparathyroidism
	Hyperlipidaemia
	Scorpion bites (Trinidad)
	Hypothermia
	Pancreatic cancer
	Periarteritis nodosa
	Previous Polya gastrectomy
Traumatic causes (5%)	
	Operative trauma
	Blunt or penetrating injury
	Investigation (ERCP or angiography)
Idiopathic (20%)	

debris containing microcrystals of cholesterol and calcium bilirubinate granules (so-called biliary sludge). The causal significance of gallstones and biliary sludge in acute pancreatitis is underlined by the fact that further attacks are exceptional once biliary tract disease has been eradicated.

Alcohol-associated pancreatitis. The proportion of cases of acute pancreatitis linked to alcohol varies in different parts of the world. In Scotland the figure is around 30%, whereas in some parts of France and North America it may be as high as 50–90%. The mechanism responsible is uncertain. Alcohol may cause secretion of unduly viscid juice with formation of protein plugs and impairment of flow, and may also generate toxic free-radicals which directly damage the gland. Alcohol-associated pancreatitis frequently causes permanent damage to the gland with progression to chronic pancreatitis.

Pathophysiology

Pancreatic inflammation ranges in severity from mild oedema to severe necrosis and haemorrhage. In general, *oedematous* pancreatitis is usually mild and settles on conservative treatment, whereas *necrotizing* pancreatitis is frequently severe, often leading to complications, need for operation and death.

The exact mechanism responsible for acute pancreatitis remains uncertain. Reflux of duodenal juice and/or bile into the pancreatic duct, and obstruction to the flow of pancreatic juice may trigger premature activation of pancreatic enzymes within the duct system. Intraduct activation of trypsin, chymotrypsin, phospholipase, catalase and elastase may then unleash a chain reaction of cell necrosis, further enzyme release, and changes in the microcirculation. Rupture of the duct system permits autodigestion of the gland. Continued release of activated proteolytic enzymes is responsible for increased capillary permeability, protein exudation, retroperitoneal oedema, and peritoneal exudation. Vasoactive kinins such as kallikrein are also released and activated macrophages may release cytokines such as tumour necrosis factor (TNF), and interleukins 1 and 6 (IL1, IL6).

Profound hypovolaemic shock may follow the fluid, protein and electrolyte loss which results from altered capillary permeability, while metabolic upsets result from cytokine release. Endotoxin can be detected in the systemic circulation in many

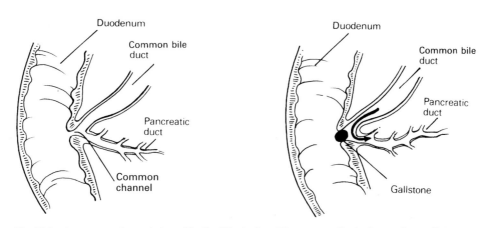

Fig. 34.3 A common channel shared by the bile duct and the pancreatic duct may allow gallstone pancreatitis.

patients, indicating that bacteria and their products may also be implicated in the circulatory upset. Other factors which contribute to the systemic upset include acute renal failure (possibly due to a combination of hypovolaemia, endotoxaemia and local intravascular coagulation), adult respiratory distress syndrome (ARDS) (due to altered permeability in pulmonary capillaries), consumptive coagulopathy, and altered liver function (due to hepatocyte depression and/or obstruction of the common bile duct by a gallstone or pancreatic oedema).

Clinical features

Severe or agonizing constant pain in the epigastrium with radiation through to the back is usually prominent. Pain can also be experienced in either hypochondrium. Nausea, vomiting and retching are often marked.

Clinical examination often reveals much less tenderness, guarding and rigidity than might have been expected from the patient's history. Shock is often present in severe pancreatitis. Bruising around the umbilicus (Cullen's sign) or brawny discolouration of the flanks (Grey-Turner's sign) are uncommon, relatively late signs of severe pancreatitis. Obstructive jaundice may be apparent in patients with pancreatitis due to an impacted gallstone, but is usually transient. A pleural effusion may be detected in about 20% of cases, and is almost always left-sided; it probably represents the effect of inflammation tracking retroperitoneally to involve the pleura.

Diagnosis

The key to the diagnosis of acute pancreatitis is a high index of suspicion and measurement of the serum amylase concentration. Previous attacks of flatulent dyspepsia, biliary colic or jaundice may suggest biliary pancreatitis. Alcohol intake should be documented carefully.

The normal range for serum amylase is 100–300 iu/l and values above 1000 iu/l strongly support the diagnosis of acute pancreatitis. Hyperamylasaemia reflects rupture of acinar cells and parts of the ductal system with release of amylase into the circulation. The serum amylase levels usually rise rapidly (within 6 hours) but are often raised only transiently, returning to normal within 48 hours. Serum lipase levels also rise in acute pancreatitis, the rise being slower but more sustained.

As shown in Table 34.2 a number of other conditions can produce hyperamylasaemia, although the

Table 34.2 Non-pancreatic disorders capable of causing hyperamylasaemia

- Acute cholecystitis
- Perforated duodenal ulcer
- High intestinal obstruction
- Mesenteric vascular occlusion
- Bowel strangulation
- Dissecting aortic aneurysm
- Ruptured aortic aneurysm
- Ruptured ectopic pregnancy

rise is seldom as high as 1000 iu/l. Most conditions causing such 'false positive' rises in serum amylase demand prompt surgical intervention, whereas surgery is usually avoided whenever possible in the early stages of acute pancreatitis. If there is significant diagnostic doubt, urgent ultrasonography or computerized tomography (CT) scanning may reveal the true diagnosis; some surgeons occasionally use diagnostic peritoneal lavage in this situation, the diagnosis of pancreatitis being confirmed by the return of amylase-rich fluid and the absence of bile, blood or intestinal content. False negative results occur in 5–10% of cases of acute pancreatitis, in that the patient is seen before (exceptional) or after the hyperamylasaemia has occurred. There is no correlation between the height of the serum amylase level and the severity of the attack; some of the most severe attacks are accompanied by relatively modest hyperamylasaemia. Macroamylasaemia is a rare cause of confusion in which persistent hyperamylasaemia results from amylase being bound to globulin and forming a complex too large to be excreted by the kidney. It is found in 1–2% of the normal population and in a similar proportion of patients with acute pancreatitis.

There are no pathognomic radiological signs of acute pancreatitis on plain films of the chest or abdomen. A left-sided pleural effusion is seen in 20% of cases and pulmonary oedema may be present in patients with ARDS. A bowel empty of gas except for a 'sentinel loop' of jejunum may reflect local ileus, and in some cases gas is seen in the hepatic and splenic flexures but not the transverse colon, the 'colon cut-off' sign. Radio-opaque gallstones may be seen in some patients with gallstone pancreatitis.

Ultrasonography may reveal swelling of the pancreas with peripancreatic fluid collections and oedema, and may detect gallstones. CT scanning is not usually performed as part of the initial diagnostic assessment but may also reveal pancreatic and peripancreatic swelling, development of necrosis (see below) and the presence of gallstones. Gastrografin studies are not normally indicated unless ulcer perforation cannot be excluded; the examination often shows widening of the duodenal C-loop by an inflamed head of pancreas, oedematous and coarse duodenal folds, and the 'reversed 3 sign' in which duodenal oedema produces the appearance of retraction of the papilla of Vater.

Assessment of severity

The severity of an attack of pancreatitis can be assessed at the time of admission in a number of ways. It may be obvious clinically from the shocked state of the patient that the attack is severe, or formal 'prognostic factor scores', such as the Glasgow system, can be employed (Table 34.3). Urea and electrolyte measurements reflect the state of hydration and are helpful in managing fluid and electrolyte balance. Liver function tests (LFTs) may show hyperbilirubinaemia and elevation of liver enzymes, particularly in patients with gallstone pancreatitis. Hyperglycaemia and glycosuria can occur transiently in severe disease. Arterial blood gas analysis may reveal severe hypoxia. Moderate polymorphonuclear leucocytosis is common. Serum calcium levels may fall in severe disease. At one time it was believed that this reflected formation of calcium soaps following fat necrosis within the abdomen, but it is now recognized that much of the fall reflects the drop in serum albumin levels caused by protein exudation. Marked reduction in the level of ionized calcium is unusual and frank tetany is exceptional.

Progress can be monitored by regular clinical evaluation, and a rising APACHE II score or a rising level of C-reactive protein (see below) may help to identify patients in need of urgent investigation and surgical intervention. If deterioration occurs, endoscopic retrograde cholangiopancreatography (ERCP) and endoscopic papillotomy may be considered in

patients thought to have gallstone pancreatitis, or CT scanning may be indicated to detect pancreatic necrosis.

Treatment

There is no specific treatment for acute pancreatitis and most attacks settle on conservative management.

Conservative treatment
- *Pain relief.* Severe pain requires the administration of opiates; pethidine is frequently prescribed.
- *Treatment of shock.* Large volumes of crystalloid solution, plasma or dextran may be needed to maintain circulating blood volume. Oxygen is essential in shocked patients in whom pulse, blood pressure, urine output and central venous pressure should be monitored (see Ch. 3).
- *Suppression of pancreatic function.* The patient is forbidden to eat or drink. A nasogastric tube may relieve vomiting but there is no evidence that routine nasogastric intubation is beneficial.
- *Other measures.* Broad-spectrum antibiotics should be prescribed only if there is a specific indication such as cholangitis. Diabetes mellitus is rarely precipitated by acute pancreatitis and it is extremely uncommon to have to initiate insulin therapy. Attempts to 'rest' the pancreas by pharmacological means have proved disappointing and it remains to be seen whether somatostatin analogues will be of value as inhibitors of secretion. Peritoneal lavage with isotonic crystalloid solutions was once advocated as a means of removing enzymes and vasoactive substances from the peritoneal cavity and so preventing their absorption. However, recent trials have not shown any reduction in mortality or morbidity in patients with severe acute pancreatitis.

Endoscopic treatment. When gallstones are suspected to be the cause of acute pancreatitis, consideration may be given to the endoscopic retrieval of such stones from the biliary tree by a basket or balloon following endoscopic sphincterotomy. When patients are admitted with a mild attack of pancreatitis, there is no need to institute such active therapy; in most cases the offending gallstone will pass on into the duodenum spontaneously. In patients with severe disease which does not settle promptly on conservative management, endoscopic stone retrieval may abort the attack and reduce morbidity and mortality.

Surgical treatment. Acute pancreatitis is managed conservatively whenever possible but

Table 34.3 Glasgow system used to predict severity of acute pancreatitis. Factors are assessed within 48 hours of admission and three or more positive criteria indicate the presence of severe disease	
Age	>55 years
White cell count	>15 x 10^9/l
Blood glucose (no diabetic history)	>10 mmol/l
Serum urea (no response to i.v. fluids)	>16 mmol/l
Pa$_{O_2}$	< 60 mmHg (8 kPa)
Serum calcium	< 2.0 mmol/l
Serum albumin	< 32 g/l
Serum lactate dehydrogenase	> 600 iu/l
Serum aspartate aminotransferase	> 100 u/l

surgery is indicated under the following circumstances.

1. *When the diagnosis is uncertain.* If alternative causes of hyperamylasaemia are suspected, laparotomy is occasionally needed to confirm the diagnosis. If acute pancreatitis is present, no further action is usually needed, although when gallstones are found, consideration should be given to cholecystectomy.

2. *When the patient fails to improve on conservative management or deteriorates.* If the general condition and other indices (e.g. APACHE II score or C-reactive protein level) are deteriorating, the presence of pancreatic and peripancreatic necrosis must be suspected. A dynamic CT scan is obtained urgently, the term dynamic reflecting the fact that contrast is injected into the circulation so that it can be seen whether all of the pancreas enhances (and therefore has a blood supply and is not necrotic). If there is extensive necrosis and particularly when there is evidence of infected necrosis (gas visible radiologically or a positive culture on needle aspiration), urgent laparotomy is usually needed. Necrotic pancreatic and peripancreatic tissue is removed from the lesser sac by blunt dissection with a finger, and after thorough debridement, drains are inserted so that lavage can continue in the postoperative period to wash out any further necrotic material. Alternatively the wound can be left open so that repeated debridement can be carried out more easily. A gastrostomy is usually inserted at the time of necrosectomy so that the patient does not have to suffer the discomfort of prolonged nasogastric intubation in the days or weeks that may elapse before duodenal ileus resolves. A feeding jejunostomy may also be inserted so that feeding can continue without reliance on total parenteral nutrition. As might be expected, the mortality of necrotizing pancreatitis is higher (10% or more) than that of oedematous pancreatitis (2% or less).

3. *When gallstones are present.* In the past, patients thought to have gallstone pancreatitis were allowed to settle on conservative management before being investigated radiologically, and were then admitted for elective biliary surgery some 6–8 weeks later. Modern practice favours 'early' eradication of gallstones in the course of the first admission with pancreatitis. Ultrasonography is used to confirm the presence of stones and surgery is undertaken once the attack of acute pancreatitis has settled. In patients with severe disease who fail to settle promptly, ERCP may both confirm the presence of stones and allow their removal following endoscopic

sphincterotomy, thus permitting resolution of the attack. It cannot be overemphasized that patients who have had an attack of gallstone pancreatitis should not be allowed to have another because of failure to eradicate gallstones. When biliary surgery is undertaken it consists of cholecystectomy with operative cholangiography to ensure that there are no stones in the duct system which also require removal.

4. *When complications develop* (see below).

Complications of acute pancreatitis

Pancreatic pseudocyst. A pancreatic pseudocyst is a collection of pancreatic secretions and inflammatory exudate. In contrast to a true cyst, the collection has no epithelial lining and is surrounded by inflammatory tissue. Pseudocysts form most commonly in the lesser sac or in the adjacent retroperitoneum. Small pseudocysts are usually asymptomatic and resolve spontaneously. In about 10% of patients, larger collections persist and can pose problems.

- *Clinical features.* Pseudocysts typically do not declare themselves for some 2–3 weeks after the episode of pancreatitis. Persistent or intermittent abdominal discomfort and grumbling hyperamylasaemia usually signal their presence, and larger collections may compress neighbouring structures to cause vomiting and obstructive jaundice. Ultrasonography is of great value in monitoring the progress of inflammation and in detecting pseudocyst formation. Some cysts become so large that they are palpable and, in some cases, visible.

- *Treatment.* The presence of a pseudocyst is not in itself an indication for surgical treatment. Treatment is indicated only if the pseudocyst is enlarging, and aims to avoid infection of the contents, haemorrhage or rupture. It normally consists of drainage of the pseudocyst into a Roux loop of jejunum (pseudocyst-jejunostomy), the stomach (pseudocyst-gastrostomy) or duodenum (pseudocyst-duodenostomy), whichever appears most appropriate (Fig. 34.4). As the tissues holding the sutures must be firm, it is desirable to allow the pseudocyst some 4–6 weeks to 'mature' if possible. Ultrasound-guided puncture of the pseudocyst and insertion of a catheter for external drainage offers an alternative to surgical drainage, particularly in ill patients. However, this approach may allow infection to supervene and is sometimes followed by development of an external pancreatic fistula.

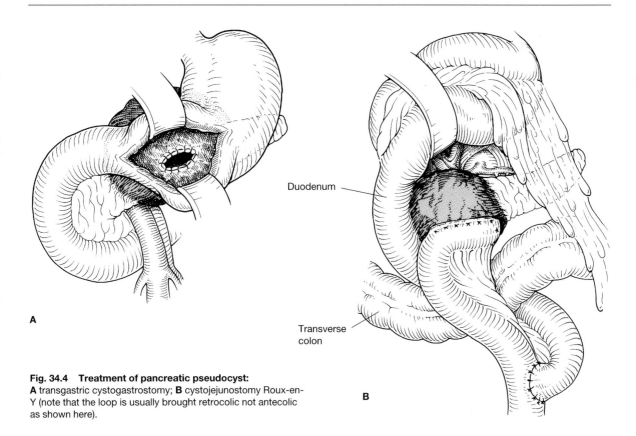

A

Duodenum

Transverse
colon

B

Fig. 34.4 Treatment of pancreatic pseudocyst:
A transgastric cystogastrostomy; **B** cystojejunostomy Roux-en-
Y (note that the loop is usually brought retrocolic not antecolic
as shown here).

Pancreatic abscess. The presentation often resembles that of pancreatic pseudocyst but the patient is usually more ill, and has pyrexia and leucocytosis. The presence of an abscess is confirmed by ultrasonography. Treatment consists of adequate external drainage under antibiotic cover, and this can be achieved by laparotomy or by percutaneous drainage under ultrasound control.

Progressive jaundice. Persistent or progressively deepening jaundice suggests that a gallstone is impacted at the lower end of the biliary tree or that the bile duct is compressed by pancreatic inflammation or pseudocyst formation. ERCP can be used to define the problem and remove any impacted stones following endoscopic sphincterotomy. Alternatively, calculous obstruction can be dealt with by cholecystectomy, operative cholangiography and extraction of any duct stones.

Persistent duodenal ileus. Protracted ileus usually reflects continuing pancreatic inflammation. In the absence of an indication for operation (e.g. pancreatic necrosis, pseudocyst formation), conservative management is instituted and nutritional status maintained by tube feeding (nasoenteric fine-bore

tube) or parenteral nutrition while the pancreatitis is resolving.

Gastrointestinal bleeding. Severe acute pancreatitis may be complicated by bleeding from gastritis, erosions or duodenal ulceration and prophylactic H_2-receptor antagonists are advisable in all such cases. If bleeding develops, the guidelines for investigation and management are as outlined in Chapter 28. On rare occasions, laparotomy (preceded if possible by angiography) is required urgently for massive intraperitoneal bleeding due to erosion of blood vessels by the inflammatory process.

Prognosis

Following resolution of the acute attack, prognosis depends on the aetiological factor involved. The biliary tree must be fully investigated in all cases as gallstone pancreatitis has an excellent long-term outlook once cholecystectomy has been carried out and gallstones have been cleared from the biliary tree.

The prognosis in alcohol-associated pancreatitis is

Acute pancreatitis

- Acute pancreatitis is defined as an attack of pancreatic inflammation after which the gland returns to anatomical and functional normality.

- Gallstones (50% of cases) and alcohol (30% of cases) are the outstanding causes of acute pancreatitis.

- In one in four cases the attack is severe as assessed by prognostic factor scoring; in one in four patients with severe pancreatitis the attack proves fatal.

- In most cases the pancreatic inflammation is mild and *oedematous* and settles on conservative management. *Necrotizing* pancreatitis is frequently severe, and often leads on to complications, need for surgery and death.

- Severe attacks of gallstone pancreatitis can often be aborted if a stone occluding the lower end of the biliary tree can be removed by endoscopic papillotomy. Once gallstones have been eradicated, recurrent attacks of gallstone pancreatitis are exceptional.

less favourable. Many patients are unwilling or unable to abstain from drinking and suffer further attacks of acute pancreatitis with progression to chronic pancreatitis.

Chronic pancreatitis

Aetiology

Chronic pancreatitis is a relatively rare disease but its incidence may be increasing with the growing problem of alcoholism. Although alcohol is much the commonest aetiological factor, being implicated in some 70–80% of cases, the factors which predispose some patients to develop chronic pancreatitis are poorly understood. Smoking appears to be an important co-factor. In parts of equatorial Africa, the Middle East and India, adolescents and young adults may suffer from so-called tropical pancreatitis. This was once thought to be a consequence of malnutrition but it is now thought that toxins in dietary staples such as cassava are responsible and that malnutrition is a result rather than a cause of the condition. Rare causes of chronic pancreatitis include hyperparathyroidism, traumatic duct strictures, gallstones and pancreas divisum, although the significance of the last factor is still uncertain.

Pathophysiology

Secretion of an unduly viscid pancreatic juice may allow protein plugs to form in the duct system and these plugs subsequently calcify to form duct stones. Impaired flow of pancreatic juice then leads to inflammation, stricture formation in the duct system and progressive replacement of the gland by fibrous tissue. Loss of acinar tissue is reflected eventually by steatorrhoea and, in time, loss of islet tissue may lead to diabetes mellitus.

Clinical features

Pain is the outstanding feature in most cases. It is characteristically epigastric with marked radiation through to the back, and is often eased by leaning forwards or getting down on all fours. Some patients experience marked pain in one or both loins and gain relief by lying on one side. In some cases the pain is precipitated by eating or the patient learns to avoid certain foods, notably fatty foods. Application of heat sometimes brings relief and permanent discolouration of the skin may reflect continued use of heat pads or hot water bottles. Progressive use of powerful opioid analgesics can result in drug addiction.

Weight loss is usual and reflects a combination of inadequate intake and malabsorption. Steatorrhoea is common, the bowel motion being pale, bulky, offensive, floating on water, and difficult to flush. Diabetes mellitus develops in about one-third of patients but islet function is often preserved for some years following the onset of exocrine insufficiency.

Other less common manifestations of chronic pancreatitis include transient or intermittent obstructive jaundice, duodenal obstruction and splenic vein thrombosis (leading to splenomegaly, hypersplenism and gastric and oesophageal varices).

Investigation and diagnosis

Abdominal plain films and CT scans may reveal the speckled calcification typical of chronic pancreatitis. Ultrasonography and CT scanning can be used to detect pancreatic enlargement and may also reveal pseudocysts, dilatation of the pancreatic duct, and splenomegaly. ERCP is of great value and must always be performed if operation is contemplated. The architecture of the pancreatic duct is revealed and any compression of the biliary tree can be evaluated. When investigating these patients it must be borne in mind that cancer of the pancreas may block the duct system and cause pancreatitis and that the two conditions can co-exist.

Pancreatic endocrine function is assessed by measurement of random blood glucose levels, supplemented if necessary by a glucose tolerance test.

Exocrine function can be measured in a multitude of ways but insufficiency may not be detectable until 90% of the pancreatic parenchyma is destroyed. Furthermore, function tests do not differentiate between chronic pancreatitis and pancreatic cancer. If necessary, faecal fat excretion can be measured over 3–5 days while the patient's fat intake is controlled at 100 g/day (normal individuals excrete less than 5 g/day), or fat absorption can be measured by isotopic labelling of dietary fat. In practice, the key question is: does the patient have clinically obvious steatorrhoea? Duodenal intubation studies aimed at measuring pancreatic secretion after food or hormonal stimulation are now seldom employed.

Management

The diagnosis of chronic pancreatitis is not in itself an indication for surgery. Considerable clinical judgement is needed to determine the need for, and timing of, operation. In most cases, intractable pain is the cardinal indication for surgery; operation does not restore pancreatic endocrine and exocrine function and at best merely slows their decline.

Conservative management. This consists of encouraging abstinence from alcohol, relief of pain, treatment of exocrine and endocrine insufficiency, and attempts to improve nutritional status. Relief of pain is notoriously difficult; opiates are avoided if possible but their use may prove essential. Coeliac plexus block is rarely of value and at best provides relief for a few weeks or months. Diabetes mellitus is treated by appropriate means (diet, oral hypoglycaemic agents or insulin). Steatorrhoea is treated by pancreatic exocrine supplements and modern position-release preparations (e.g. Creon) minimize enzymic degradation of the supplements by acid and pepsin during their passage through the stomach.

Surgical treatment. This is indicated if pain is intractable, when neighbouring structures such as the common bile duct, duodenum, portal or splenic vein are compressed, when pseudocysts or abscesses develop, or when cancer cannot be excluded.

In general, the objective of surgery is to relieve pain or compression while at the same time conserving as much pancreatic tissue and function as possible. In about one-third of cases the pancreatic duct system is sufficiently dilated to allow these objectives to be achieved by a drainage operation. Demonstration of ductal anatomy is essential in determining the most appropriate option and operative pancreatography is mandatory if ERCP has not been successful. The method of drainage used depends on the extent of the obstruction. There is

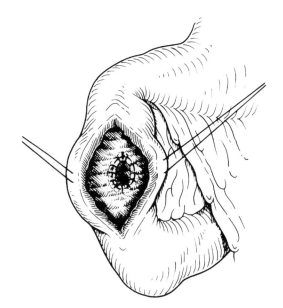

Fig. 34.5 Sphincteroplasty.

rarely a single area of narrowing close to the sphincter of Oddi so that sphincteroplasty (Fig. 34.5) rarely suffices. More frequently there are multiple strictures throughout the length of the duct, which must be slit open so that a Roux loop of jejunum can be brought up and anastomosed to the entire length of the pancreatic duct as a longitudinal pancreaticojejunostomy (Fig. 34.6). Approximately 70% of patients remain pain-free or substantially improved when assessed 5 years after this operation, and avoidance of resection often means that pancreatic function does not worsen appreciably. As with all aspects of chronic pancreatitis, the results of pancreaticojejunostomy are better in patients who continue to abstain from alcohol.

If drainage is not feasible, part or all of the pancreas will have to be resected. This is a more difficult undertaking and may precipitate endocrine and exocrine insufficiency or compound existing insufficiency. In a few patients, chronic pancreatitis is confined to the distal part of the gland so that distal pancreatectomy is appropriate. In many patients, the disease is more severe in the head of the gland and the Whipple operation (pancreaticoduodenectomy, see p. 511) is indicated. In some patients, the entire pancreas appears to be so diseased that total pancreatectomy is undertaken. This must be regarded as a last resort procedure given the permanent brittle diabetes and exocrine insufficiency which follow, and careful patient selection is vital. As with drainage operations, approxi-

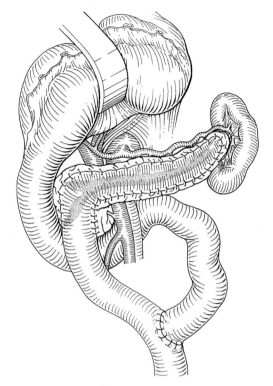

Fig. 34.6 Pancreatic duct decompression by longitudinal pancreatico-jejunostomy.

mately 70% of patients are pain-free or substantially improved when assessed 5 years following resection.

NEOPLASMS OF THE PANCREAS

Neoplasms of the exocrine pancreas are common and are almost always malignant whereas neoplasms of the endocrine pancreas are rare and may be benign.

NEOPLASMS OF THE EXOCRINE PANCREAS

Benign pancreatic neoplasms such as cystadenomas frequently remain asymptomatic until their size causes pressure on surrounding structures. Resection of the affected part of the pancreas is usually needed but the prognosis thereafter is excellent.

Malignant neoplasms of the pancreas are almost invariably ductal adenocarcinomas. Acinar cell carcinomas, cystadenocarcinomas and sarcomas are all rare.

Chronic pancreatitis
- Chronic pancreatitis is defined as pancreatic inflammation in which the pancreas does not return to anatomical and/or functional normality.

- The disease is frequently, but by no means invariably, associated with alcohol abuse, and is characterized by blockage of the pancreatic duct system by protein plugs in which calcification occurs.

- Other causes of chronic pancreatitis include hyperparathyroidism, cholelithiasis, duct obstruction due to trauma, mucoviscidosis, haemochromatosis, pancreas divisum and nutritional disorders.

- Pain is the cardinal symptom in chronic pancreatitis; other symptoms include weight loss, steatorrhoea, obstructive jaundice and diabetes mellitus.

- Surgery is indicated if pain cannot be controlled by conservative means or if complications ensue. If the pancreatic duct system is distended, pancreaticojejunostomy is the operation of choice; if the duct system is not distended, partial or even total pancreatectomy may be necessary.

Adenocarcinoma of the pancreas

Aetiology

The cause of pancreatic cancer is unknown. It is increasing in frequency and is now the fourth commonest cause of cancer death in males and sixth commonest in females in many Western countries. It accounts for about 10% of all cancers of the alimentary system.

Men are more commonly affected than women and the peak incidence lies between 55 and 70 years of age. Factors thought to increase the risk of pancreatic cancer include tobacco smoking and a high-fat, high-protein diet.

Pathology

The great majority of adenocarcinomas arise from ductal rather than acinar tissue. The head of the gland is more often affected than the body or tail. The cancer spreads locally and disseminates to lymph nodes around the gland. Regardless of the site of origin, spread outwith the reach of surgical cure is usual by the time the disease is diagnosed. It is hardly surprising that 90% of patients are dead within a year of the diagnosis being made and that survival beyond 5 years is truly exceptional.

Cancer arising from the periampullary region, distal common bile duct and duodenum has a much better outlook than cancer of the pancreas. It may be that biliary obstruction occurs so early that the tumour is discovered at a stage where resection is still curative.

Clinical features

Obstructive jaundice, with passage of dark urine and pale stool, is the common presenting feature of cancer of the head of the pancreas. It is usually progressive, in contrast to the intermittent jaundice of calculous obstruction. Pruritus is frequently troublesome. In keeping with Courvoisier's law (p. 490), the gallbladder is frequently palpable in patients with obstructive jaundice due to pancreatic cancer, but is often felt more laterally than might be expected from its usual surface markings. When cancer arises in the body and tail of the pancreas, jaundice is more likely to be due to liver metastases or the involvement of nodes in the porta hepatis.

Weight loss is invariable and may be the first symptom. It reflects a combination of inadequate intake, malabsorption and depressed liver function. Cancer of the pancreas was once said to cause painless obstructive jaundice but this is not true. Most patients have ill-defined upper abdominal pain or discomfort and neoplastic infiltration can cause severe back pain.

Pancreatic insufficiency is common in that diabetes mellitus or impaired glucose tolerance is present in one-third of patients. Steatorrhoea due to impaired digestion and absorption of fat is common and the associated failure to absorb the fat-soluble vitamin K may cause coagulopathy.

Thrombophlebitis migrans is a late manifestation in some patients but is not specific for this form of cancer.

Investigation and diagnosis

In patients with jaundice, its obstructive nature is confirmed by examination of the urine, stool and blood (see Ch. 3). Ultrasonography will detect dilatation of the biliary tree, exclude gallstones, and may show the mass lesion in the pancreas or reveal liver metastases. CT scanning may be used for the same purposes, but is no more accurate than ultrasonography in assessing the pancreatic tumour. If biliary obstruction is present, cholangiography is used to define the site and nature of the obstruction; in general ERCP is preferred to percutaneous transhepatic cholangiography as it causes less discomfort, displays both pancreatic and biliary duct systems and readily allows therapeutic intervention

such as stent insertion (see below). A common finding in pancreatic cancer is the 'double duct sign' in which both the pancreatic duct and common bile duct are narrowed as they pass through the neoplasm. Endoscopy also allows lesions in the gastroduodenal lumen to be biopsied and pancreatic juice and bile can be sampled for cytological examination.

Pancreatic function tests are of no value in diagnosis. A number of circulating tumour markers (e.g. CA 19–9) have been described in pancreatic cancer, but their lack of sensitivity and specificity has prevented their use in screening and diagnosis.

Every effort should be made to obtain cytological or histological confirmation of the malignant nature of any mass lesions revealed radiologically. This is particularly important if surgery is not contemplated as a number of benign lesions (e.g. chronic pancreatitis) can masquerade as malignancy, while a number of malignancies (e.g. lymphoma) that can mimic pancreatic cancer have a far better prognosis if recognized and given appropriate treatment. Pancreatic tissue can be obtained safely by percutaneous fine-needle aspiration or Tru-cut needle biopsy under ultrasound or CT scan guidance.

If radical surgery is contemplated, selective angiography is used in some centres to display the vascular anatomy and detect invasion of major vessels, such as the portal vein, that would preclude resection. Alternatively, laparoscopy can be used to exclude dissemination of disease (peritoneal seedlings or liver metastases) that would prevent radical surgery.

Management

Surgical resection offers the only prospect of cure but only about 10% of patients are candidates for radical surgery. In most cases, the presence of advanced disease, advanced age or intercurrent disease means that palliation is the objective of management.

Curative treatment. The standard operation of radical pancreaticoduodenectomy (Whipple's procedure) entails block resection of the head of pancreas, distal half of stomach, duodenum, gallbladder and common bile duct. Reconstruction is achieved by anastomoses between the jejunum and the pancreatic remnant, common hepatic duct and gastric remnant respectively (Fig. 34.7). The operation aims to eradicate the cancer and yet retain enough pancreas to sustain endocrine and exocrine function. The procedure used to carry a prohibitively high operative mortality but in specialist hands

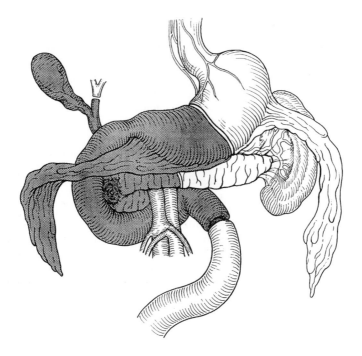

A

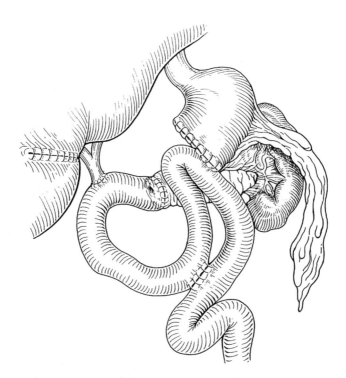

B

Fig. 34.7 Whipple procedure showing: A the area resected and B the anastomoses performed. (The gallbladder is usually removed.)

this should now be less than 1–2%. Although 5-year survival rates of 20% have been reported in a series of selected patients, overall survival rates are little better than those obtained by palliative surgery and cure remains exceptional. Attempts to improve the radicality of resection by removing all of the pancreas have proved disappointing; total pancreatectomy offers no advantage in terms of operative mortality or long-term survival and also confers permanent diabetes and exocrine insufficiency.

The prospects for patients with cancer of the periampullary region, distal common bile duct or duodenum are less gloomy, with 5-year survival rates ranging from 20–40%.

Palliative treatment. Relief of jaundice, pruritus, pain and duodenal obstruction are the objectives of palliative treatment. In the past, operation was usually undertaken to bypass the obstructed biliary system (cholecystojejunostomy or choledochojejunostomy) and gastrojejunostomy was carried out to treat or prevent blockage of the duodenum by continued tumour growth. In many cases, operation can now be avoided by insertion of a prosthetic stent following endoscopic papillotomy. If this fails it may still be possible to avoid surgery by inserting the stent by the percutaneous transhepatic route. Stenting suffers from the disadvantages that it cannot deal with or prevent duodenal obstruction, and that the stents frequently encrust and block after about 3 months so that their replacement becomes necessary.

Mean survival following palliative intervention is only about 4 months and few patients live for more than a year. Prolonged survival raises doubt about the diagnosis of cancer, underlining the need to have cytological or histological confirmation of the diagnosis in all patients.

Although there is evidence that survival rates can be improved by radiotherapy and/or chemotherapy, the benefits obtainable with currently available regimens does not justify their use outwith the context of controlled clinical trials. Pain relief is a vital part of the management of advanced pancreatic cancer, and coeliac plexus block should be considered if pain cannot be controlled by appropriate analgesic therapy.

NEOPLASMS OF THE ENDOCRINE PANCREAS

These rare neoplasms may give rise to defined syndromes due to oversecretion of peptide products,

---

Pancreatic cancer

- Ductal adenocarcinoma of the pancreas is predominantly a disease of the aging population and has shown a threefold increase in incidence during this century.

- Aetiological factors include a high-fat, high-protein diet and smoking, and one-third of patients have abnormal glucose tolerance.

- As the head of the pancreas is the commonest site for tumour formation, obstructive jaundice is commonly the presenting complaint. Other features include weight loss, steatorrhoea and diabetes mellitus.

- Late presentation is the rule and 90% of patients are dead within a year of diagnosis.

- Only 10% of patients are potential candidates for curative resection (Whipple's operation) and overall 5-year survival rates are close to zero.

- Endoscopic stenting now offers an alternative to palliative surgical bypass of the obstructed biliary system but duodenal obstruction by tumour is also a problem in 10–20% of patients.

---

but some tumours which appear histologically to be of neuroendocrine origin neither contain identifiable products on immunohistochemistry nor give rise to circulating products. The commonest islet cell tumour is the insulinoma which has an annual incidence of 1 per million of the population. It arises from B cells and results in oversecretion of insulin with episodes of hypoglycaemia. Gastrinomas arise from G cells and give rise to the Zollinger-Ellison syndrome (see Ch. 28). Tumours of the A cells producing glucagon are known as glucagonomas, while excessive secretion of vasoactive intestinal peptide (VIP) from vipomas produces pancreatic cholera (see below). Some tumours may produce more than one peptide or the pattern of secretion may vary with time. A proportion of patients have tumours and/or hyperplasia of the parathyroid glands or anterior pituitary gland and are regarded as suffering from multiple endocrine neoplasia type I (MEN I; see p. 257).

Insulinoma

Insulinomas are usually single, small (less than 2 cm in diameter), benign tumours which may affect any part of the pancreas. Multiple insulinomas are usually associated with MEN I. Less than 10% of insulinomas are malignant but such tumours are often larger than 2 cm in diameter.

Clinical features

Unlike normal islet cells which secrete appropriate amounts of insulin in response to changing glucose concentrations, insulinomas secrete insulin autonomously and inappropriately. The resulting hypoglycaemia may give rise to mild symptoms, but over the years there is gradual intellectual and motor impairment with insidious personality changes. More severe attacks of hypoglycaemia can produce sweating, palpitations, tremulousness and a wide variety of transient psychoneurological symptoms with episodes of bizarre behaviour. Because of memory lapses, the patient may not recall these events and the diagnosis only comes to light when the patient is found in hypoglycaemic coma. Attacks are typically precipitated by fasting and relieved by taking glucose. Many patients become obese because of the associated hunger. Some patients are misdiagnosed as suffering from psychiatric illness, epilepsy, alcoholism or brain tumours, and it is not unusual for 2–3 years to elapse between the first symptom and establishment of the correct diagnosis.

Diagnosis

The diagnosis of insulinoma demands a high index of suspicion and rests on:

1. The demonstration of hypoglycaemia after fasting (blood glucose concentration of less than 2.2 mmol/l after an overnight 12–14 hour fast).
2. The confirmation that hypoglycaemia is due to inappropriate insulin secretion.

Insulin is not normally detectable when glucose levels are subnormal, but in patients with insulinoma, serial plasma insulin levels remain inappropriately high in the face of falling glucose levels.

Factitious hypoglycaemia caused by insulin injection is a rare problem which is occasionally encountered in members of medical and nursing staff. It can be excluded by measuring C-peptide levels at the same time as insulin levels are determined. One molecule of C-peptide is normally produced for every molecule of endogenous insulin. If exogenous insulin is being administered, there is no corresponding C-peptide production.

Once the presence of an insulinoma has been confirmed, a variety of methods can be used to localize the tumour(s). Ultrasonography, CT scanning and selective angiography are successful in less than 50% of cases due to the small size of the tumour. Selective venous sampling from a catheter inserted into the portal and splenic veins through the liver allows plotting of the concentration of insulin at various sites and may define the point at which excess secretion is entering the venous system. Although successful in some 90% of cases, the method is invasive and in some centres is not used routinely. Endoscopic ultrasonography has been introduced recently and appears to offer a safe, accurate method of localization.

Treatment

Surgical removal of the tumour is the treatment of choice although patients can be controlled temporarily by diazoxide (a diabetogenic antihypertensive drug; 5 mg/kg daily in three divided doses given orally). At laparotomy, the pancreas is exposed fully and carefully palpated. Most insulinomas can be enucleated but resection of the affected part of the pancreas is occasionally necessary. If the tumour cannot be found, distal pancreatectomy used to be recommended in the mistaken belief that insulinomas were more common in the body and tail of the gland. If no tumour is found it is better to close the abdomen, control hypoglycaemia with diazoxide, and carry out interval selective venous sampling or endoscopic ultrasonography in order to localize the lesion for reoperation.

If a malignant insulinoma is found confined to the pancreas, resection is indicated. Chemotherapy using streptozotocin may prove useful if there is unresectable or metastatic disease. Symptoms of hyperinsulinism can be controlled by diazoxide if necessary.

Glucagonoma

Excessive glucagon production may give rise to a syndrome of necrotizing dermatitis, painful glossitis, stomatitis, bowel upset, weight loss, diabetes mellitus and anaemia. Plasma levels of glucagon are raised and the tumour may be defined by CT scanning or angiography.

Resection of the tumour (which is sometimes benign) often reverses these effects. Streptozotocin may be beneficial in patients with non-resectable tumours and the somatostatin analogue, octreotide (initially 50 μg twice daily by subcutaneous injection) may help to control symptoms.

Vipoma

Vipomas may be solitary and benign but half are malignant. Oversecretion of VIP causes a syndrome of profuse watery diarrhoea, hypokalaemia and achlorhydria also known as 'pancreatic cholera'. The systemic upset may be profound with daily loss of 5

Insulinoma

- Insulinoma is the commonest endocrine tumour of the pancreas (but is still rare, having an annual incidence of 1 per million of the population).

- The diagnosis of insulinoma is often delayed as the episodes of hypoglycaemia (usually precipitated by fasting and relieved by food) are often misinterpreted (e.g. as due to brain tumour, psychiatric upset, epilepsy).

- The diagnosis is confirmed by demonstrating that fasting produces hypoglycaemia in association with inappropriately *high* insulin levels.

- Measurement of C-peptide levels (one molecule of C-peptide is released for every molecule of insulin) excludes factitious hypoglycaemia.

- Most insulinomas are small benign tumours which may be difficult to locate; they are usually treated by enucleation.

litres or more of potassium-rich stool, and production of marked metabolic alkalosis. The patient may be confused and ileus and abdominal distension may lead to intestinal obstruction being suspected. Alternatively, symptoms may be intermittent and the diagnosis so delayed that malignant tumours have metastasized by the time they are discovered.

Diagnosis rests on a high index of suspicion, recognition of the typical syndrome and the detection of increased levels of VIP in the circulating blood. The tumours are often large and demonstrable on CT scanning and angiography.

Adequate fluid and electrolyte replacement is essential before surgery. The aim of surgery is to remove the tumour although this may necessitate total or subtotal pancreatectomy. In the case of solitary tumours, surgery may be curative. In unresectable cases and those with metastases, streptozotocin or the somatostatin analogue, octreotide, may be useful in controlling symptoms.

35
The spleen

Anatomy

The spleen is a friable blood-filled organ lying in the left upper quadrant of the abdomen, protected by the ninth, tenth and eleventh ribs. It weighs about 150 g, has an ellipsoid or 'coffee bean' shape and lies with its long axis along the line of the tenth rib. The convex outer surface of the spleen lies against the diaphragm and its lower pole rests on the splenic flexure of the colon below. Its concave inner surface is related to the fundus of the stomach, the tail of the pancreas and the upper pole of the right kidney. It has a fibrous capsule and, except at its hilus, is covered by peritoneum which is reflected as ligaments running to adjacent organs. These are the lienorenal, lienogastric and lienocolic ligaments. The phrenicocolic ligament, which runs between the splenic flexure of the colon and the undersurface of the diaphragm, provides additional support.

The splenic artery is a branch of the coeliac axis (Fig. 35.1), which carries 40% of the splanchnic blood flow into the spleen. Venous blood drains into the portal venous system via the splenic vein. The splenic vessels are closely related to the pancreas; the artery runs within the lienorenal ligament and

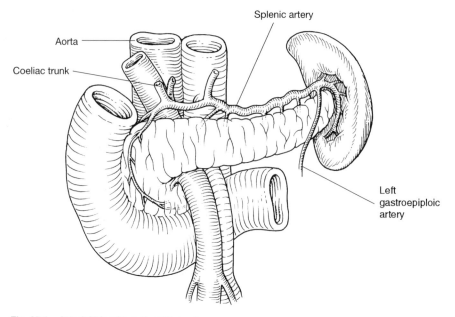

Fig. 35.1   Arterial blood supply of the spleen.

Aorta

Coeliac trunk

Splenic artery

Left gastroepiploic artery

branches reach the splenic hilus, the only part of the spleen without a peritoneal covering. Further branches continue as the short gastric vessels which run within the lienogastric ligament to the upper part of the greater curvature of the stomach. Both the lienogastric and lienorenal ligament and their contained vessels must be divided during splenectomy.

Some 25% of the lymphoid tissue of the body is contained within the spleen and forms its *white pulp*, which consists of lymphoid follicles (Malpighian bodies) and lymphatic tissue, containing lymphocytes, macrophages and plasma cells. These cells migrate to the spleen from the bone marrow, and 30–50% of them are thymus-dependent. The *red pulp* is a loose honeycomb of reticular tissue which contains the splenic sinusoids. The blood vessels are carried into the pulp along fibrous trabeculae which are continuous with the capsule. The arterioles first traverse white pulp, where they are surrounded by lymphoid tissue, and then flow into the red pulp and sinusoids (Fig. 35.2). It is uncertain whether blood flows through the pulp spaces on its way to the sinusoids or enters the sinusoids directly and then meanders slowly backwards and forwards through the pulp. Erythrocytes move in and out of the pulp tissue so that 1% of the body's red cells and 20–30% of the platelets are sequestrated at any given moment.

The pulp of the spleen is not provided with lymphatic vessels and those present are confined to the capsule and trabeculae. Lymph nodes close to the hilus thus receive more lymph from the stomach than the spleen and drain to nodes along the splenic artery.

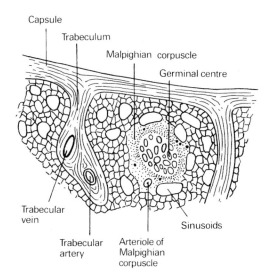

Fig. 35.2   Architecture of the splenic pulp.

Labels: Capsule; Trabeculum; Malpighian corpuscle; Germinal centre; Trabecular vein; Trabecular artery; Arteriole of Malpighian corpuscle; Sinusoids

Normally the spleen is impalpable and cannot be percussed. When enlarged, it extends downwards and medially below the costal margin. It is then best palpated bimanually, with the patient lying on his right side with the left side turned slightly forwards. The distinctive notch on its antero-inferior border may then be felt. On percussion an enlarged spleen causes dullness over the ninth rib in the midaxillary line. Splenic enlargement can also be detected by soft tissue X-ray or a splenic scintiscan (using ^{99m}Tc-labelled sulphur colloid which is taken up rapidly by the reticuloendothelial cells), but splenomegaly is normally confirmed by ultrasonic or computerized tomography (CT) scan.

Function

Haemopoiesis.   The spleen is a source of red blood cells and granulocytes in fetal life. Thereafter extramedullary haemopoiesis occurs only in the myeloproliferative syndromes.

Filtration of blood cells.   Normal blood cells pass through the spleen unchanged. Abnormal and ageing cells are trapped. Following splenectomy there is an increased number of misshapen red cells in the peripheral blood, some containing nuclear remnants (Howell-Jolly bodies) and others containing clumps of iron (siderocytes). It has been estimated that 20 ml of red cells are phagocytosed daily. White cells and platelets, particularly when coated with antibodies, also are removed.

Immunological function.   The spleen is an important site for effecting both cell-mediated and humoral immunity. Particulate antigens are filtered off and immunoglobulins (particulary IgM) and phagocytosis-promoting peptides (tuftsin) are produced. Following splenectomy, immunological responses are impaired.

Storage function.   In dogs the spleen acts as a reservoir for blood and in states of shock empties by contraction of its muscular capsule to provide an 'autotransfusion'. This is not a function of the spleen in man.

Endocrine effects.   There is some evidence that the spleen exerts a humoral effect on the bone marrow, stimulating erythropoiesis and depressing white cell and platelet counts.

INDICATIONS FOR SPLENECTOMY

While the recommendation to remove the spleen often comes from the haematologist, the surgeon must be aware of the indications for splenectomy and the criteria which should be fulfilled before accepting a patient for operation. The common indications are outlined below.

Trauma

In recent years there has been an increasing tendency to avoid unnecessary laparotomy in trauma patients thought to have minor splenic injury. In those patients submitted to laparotomy, splenectomy is indicated only if the organ cannot be conserved by the use of haemostatic agents, local suturing or partial splenectomy. Spleens involved by pathological conditions such as portal hypertension, polycythaemia and infective mononucleosis are prone to rupture on slight trauma. It must also be appreciated that, following rupture, temporary improvement in the clinical state may precede sudden deterioration. Awareness and careful observation are critical, particularly in patients with suspected or known splenic trauma such as subcapsular haematoma, which can lead to 'delayed rupture'. Splenic injuries are considered in more detail in Chapter 14.

Haemolytic anaemias

Hereditary spherocytosis

This congenital disease is transmitted as an autosomal dominant trait and the red blood cells are spherical rather than biconcave, unduly fragile, and less able to withstand the effects of passing through the splenic pulp. Excess haemolysis results in anaemia, jaundice and splenic enlargement. It is a disease of remissions and relapses with 'haemolytic crises' requiring transfusion. Pigment gallstones occur in 30–60% of cases.

Splenectomy is indicated in all cases when health is impaired. However, it should not be performed before the age of 3–4 years. If gallstones are present, cholecystectomy is carried out simultaneously.

Acquired haemolytic anaemias

Excess haemolysis may occur following exposure to agencies such as chemicals, drugs, infection, or extensive burns, or it may be an autoimmune phenomenon. In the last case the red cells are coated with an autoantibody which can be detected by agglutination when antihuman globulin is added to a suspension of the patient's red cells (positive Coomb's test).

Autoimmune haemolytic anaemia affects predominantly middle-aged women and causes severe haemolytic crises superimposed on a background of mild anaemia. Treatment consists of steroids, but if this fails to control the disease and excess sequestration of red cells has been demonstrated, splenectomy may be required.

The purpuras

Idiopathic thrombocytopenic purpura (ITP)

This disease of unknown aetiology is characterized by a low platelet count and short platelet life-span despite plentiful megakaryocytes in the bone marrow. Cyclical bleeding from the gastrointestinal tract and other sites is associated with petechiae and ecchymoses. Platelet counts are below $50 \times 10^9/l$, bleeding time is prolonged, clotting time is normal, and capillary fragility is increased. The spleen is palpably enlarged in only 2–3% of patients and dense adhesions may form around it.

Clinical course. The disease may be chronic or acute. In the *acute* form there is usually a short history of a preceding illness. Spontaneous remission is common and the response to steroids or splenectomy is excellent. The *chronic* form is characterized by a course of remissions and relapses which may last several years. Its response to steroids is poor and the outcome after splenectomy less satisfactory.

Choice of treatment. The acute form of the disease is treated initially with steroids. A rapid increase in the platelet count is associated with a good prospect of complete and lasting remission when therapy is stopped. If steroid therapy does not result in rapid remission, splenectomy is advised. Splenectomy is the treatment of choice for patients with the chronic form of the disease. Steroids have been advocated to provide temporary improvement before surgery but the increased risks of infection and the free availability of blood products has rendered this unnecessary.

Because of the high incidence of spontaneous remission, splenectomy is not advised for acute ITP in children.

Secondary thrombocytopenia

Splenectomy is contraindicated in secondary haemorrhagic purpuras, although it may be advised if hypersplenism is associated with secondary thrombocytopenia.

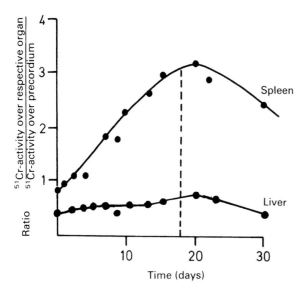

cating a large mass of lymphoid tissue puts the patient at long-term risk from serious bacterial infection. For this reason, antibiotics are generally administered pre-operatively and are often continued into the postoperative period. Splenectomy must not be undertaken lightly and the haematologist will take into account the degree of cytopenia, the extent of splenic enlargement, the amount of discomfort caused, and the incidence of recurrent infections from leucopenia. Isotopic studies to measure the rate of sequestration of red cells in the liver and spleen are usually performed and operation is advised only if the spleen-to-liver ratio exceeds 2:1 (Fig. 35.3). This is calculated from the 'half-life' of ^{51}Cr-labelled autologous red cells as measured by radioactivity over the spleen and liver relative to the precordium.

Fig. 35.3 Measurement of the rate of red cell destruction in the liver and spleen using 51Cr-labelled autologous erythrocytes. Radioactivity is measured over the spleen and liver, and in each compared with that over the precordium. The relative role of the spleen in red cell destruction is determined by the spleen-to-liver ratio, which in this case is 3.2:0.8 = 4.0:1.0.

Hypersplenism

This syndrome consists of splenomegaly and pancytopenia in the presence of an apparently normal bone marrow and the absence of an autoimmune disorder. There is sequestration and destruction of blood cells in the spleen, affecting predominantly white cells and platelets.

Hypersplenism may complicate a number of inflammatory conditions (e.g. rheumatoid arthritis), infections (e.g. malaria), and myeloproliferative and lymphoproliferative disorders. In portal hypertension, splenic congestion frequently leads to splenomegaly and hypersplenism.

The effects of hypersplenism include expansion of the total blood volume to fill the increased vascular spaces of the enlarged spleen and splanchnic bed. There is increased pooling of cells within the enlarged spleen and excess destruction, possibly induced by metabolic damage due to the cells being packed together in the enlarged spleen. In the peripheral blood there is anaemia, leucopenia and thrombocytopenia, but marrow turnover is increased, with reticulocytosis and leucoerythroblastosis. Increased amounts of urobilinogen are present in the urine.

Removal of a grossly enlarged spleen carries appreciable morbidity and mortality, and by eradi-

Segmental portal hypertension

A localized form of portal hypertension associated with hypersplenism and oesophago-gastric varices may follow occlusion of the splenic vein. Thrombosis may result from acute or chronic pancreatitis, or the vessel may become compromised by direct invasion from a carcinoma of the pancreas. Gastric varices are particularly prominent in this condition and often communicate directly with short gastric veins. Acute variceal haemorrhage in this situation is best managed by splenectomy with ligation of the vessels on the greater curvature of the stomach. Recurrent haemorrhage is unusual following surgery and the prognosis is favourable, given that there is often no associated liver disease.

Proliferative disorders

Myelofibrosis

This condition was once believed to be due to obliteration of the blood-forming elements in the bone marrow by fibrosis. The resulting gross enlargement of the spleen was thought to be a secondary phenomenon to provide a site for extra-medullary haemopoiesis. Splenectomy was thought to be contraindicated.

It is now recognized that the condition is due to an abnormal proliferation of mesenchymal elements in the bone marrow, spleen, liver, and lymph nodes, and that extramedullary haemopoiesis occurs at many sites. Contrary to previous belief, splenectomy does not lead to a lethal aplastic anaemia but decreases transfusion requirements. By relieving the discomfort of a grossly enlarged spleen, it also improves symptoms. However, careful haematological studies are indicated before it is advised.

Lymphomas

In non-Hodgkin's lymphoma, splenectomy is now only indicated in the rare event that a primary neoplasm is confined to the spleen. However, in both myelo- and lymphoproliferative conditions splenectomy may be indicated to reduce transfusion requirements when hypersplenism is a problem.

Other tumours

Apart from lymphomas and leukaemias, tumours of the spleen are rare. Haemangiomas (capillary or cavernous) may reach sufficient size to cause splenic enlargement with a consumptive coagulopathy and haemorrhagic tendency. Most haemangiomas are recognized at operation, when the spleen should be removed.

Miscellaneous conditions

Cysts of the spleen

Cysts of the spleen are rare. They are usually single but occasionally multiple. Single cysts may be congenital, degenerative or parasitic.

Congenital cysts are due to an embryonic defect and result in a dermoid-like lesion. They are lined by flattened epithelium and contain thin blood-stained fluid or thick creamy material, sometimes with hair and teeth.

Degenerative cysts result from liquefaction of an infarct or haematoma. The wall is fibrous and often calcified and the cyst is filled with brownish fluid or paste-like material.

Parasitic cysts are usually acquired through contact with dogs and are due to infection with *Echinococcus granulosus* (hydatid disease).

Splenic cysts normally cause no symptoms and are often discovered fortuitously when splenic enlargement is found on clinical examination or abnormal calcification is shown on abdominal X-ray. The lesion may be recognized by CT or ultrasound scan, investigations which are usually sufficient to characterize the nature of the cyst. Intervention is not indicated for small congenital or degenerative cysts and needle aspiration is not advised, since the cyst may be parasitic. Large symptomatic cysts are treated by splenectomy.

Abscess of the spleen

A splenic abscess is rare. It should be suspected when progressive splenic enlargement is associated with bacteraemia and abscess formation at other sites. Splenectomy, although desirable, may not prove feasible. Drainage of the abscess may be the only possible method of treatment.

Splenic artery aneurysm

This is a relatively common complication of atherosclerosis in elderly patients. The calcified wall of the aneurysm is visible on X-ray and there is obvious calcification of the tortuous splenic artery. The presence of a small uncomplicated atherosclerotic aneurysm is not necessarily an indication for surgical treatment, particularly since this lesion often affects elderly, frail patients. Bleeding can, however, occur and operation is then mandatory.

Rarely, a congenital aneurysm affects the splenic artery. Such aneurysms are more common in women and may rupture during pregnancy. An asymptomatic congenital aneurysm may be discovered on abdominal X-ray as a thin calcified ring shadow. Because of the risk of rupture, it should be treated electively. As most congenital aneurysms lie close to the splenic hilus, splenectomy is usually required.

Other indications for splenectomy

Removal of the spleen may be required as part of other surgical procedures, such as radical gastrectomy for carcinoma and less frequently for certain types of splenorenal shunt.

SPLENECTOMY

Pre-operative preparation

Routine pre-operative preparation is as for any abdominal operation, but particular attention must be paid to the full blood count and coagulation status. In the presence of any bleeding tendency, transfusion of blood, fresh frozen plasma, cryoprecipitate or platelets may be required to bring the coagulation profiles to as near normal as possible before surgery. For thrombocytopenia, platelets should be available to cover the operation and the postoperative phase.

Accessory spleens in the splenic hilus, splenic pedicle or omentum, may account for relapse of the condition for which the splenectomy was performed.

Scintiscanning after administration of ^{51}Cr-labelled red cells may be used to detect functioning accessory splenic tissue so that it can be removed at the time of primary surgery.

The degree of splenic enlargement should be known before operation. If in doubt, the surgeon should request a CT scan. A massively enlarged spleen, particularly if due to tropical disease, may give a spurious impression of mobility despite gross adhesion formation. This results from movement of the attenuated diaphragm. Where there is reason to suspect that blood loss during surgery may be considerable, pre-operative selective embolization of the splenic artery may minimize intra-operative haemorrhage.

Prophylactic antibiotics should be administered with the pre-medication because of the increased risk of infection. As the stomach is handled during splenectomy, a nasogastric tube should be inserted.

In cases of suspected splenic trauma, laparotomy is normally undertaken through a long, vertical incision. For an elective splenectomy, access is usually gained by a left subcostal incision but occasionally a thoraco-abdominal incision is necessary to remove a large spleen. Laparoscopic splenectomy is now favourable.

Technique

A normal-sized non-adherent spleen is removed after first mobilizing it medially by division of its lateral peritoneal attachments. The splenic artery and vein are then doubly ligated and divided. Finally, the lienogastric ligament with its contained vessels is divided between ligatures.

When the spleen is enlarged or adherent, preliminary mobilization may not be possible, and the vascular pedicle is dissected first. The lienogastric ligament is first divided between ligatures. The splenic artery is then identified at the upper border of the pancreas and doubly ligated and divided. Alternatively, it may first be ligated in continuity so that the spleen shrinks in size, allowing it to be mobilized and vessels to be ligated close to the splenic hilus.

If there are any adhesions between the spleen and the diaphragm, it is advisable to ligate and divide its vascular supply before interfering with them.

Postoperative course and complications

Drainage of the abdomen is not normally required after removal of a normal-sized spleen. After removal of an enlarged organ, bleeding from the pedicle should not occur if the splenic vessels have been doubly ligated, but oozing from multiple adhesions and the cut edge of the peritoneum is common. This should be controlled by electro-cautery or, if large collateral vessels are present, by oversewing of the peritoneal edge. Any bleeding tendency increases the likelihood of this complication. Hypotension and circulatory collapse within 48 hours of surgery indicate the need to re-explore the abdomen. Drains are not used (since they may actually increase the incidence of subphrenic sepsis) unless there is a possibility that the tail of the pancreas has been injured or there is persistent oozing due to a coagulation defect.

Pancreatitis occasionally follows splenectomy. This is due to handling and bruising of the tail of the pancreas during mobilization of the spleen. Serum amylase levels should be monitored in the immediate postoperative period. Pancreatic fistula formation is uncommon, although gastric fistula (involving the greater curvature of the stomach) can follow injury to the greater curvature of the stomach when the short gastric vessels are ligated in the lienogastric ligament.

Left lower lobe collapse or atelectasis is the most frequent complication of splenectomy but usually responds to conservative measures. Atelectasis and pleural effusion may also be manifestations of a subphrenic abscess and this possibility must be con-

---

Splenectomy

- The spleen is the intra-abdominal organ most frequently ruptured during blunt trauma. Rupture is particularly liable to occur if the spleen is pathologically enlarged.

- Other indications for splenectomy include hereditary spherocytosis, acquired haemolytic anaemia, idiopathic thrombocytopenic purpura, hypersplenism, and myeloproliferative disorders such as myelofibrosis.

- Following traumatic rupture or laceration of the spleen there is now increased emphasis on splenic conservation (rather than splenectomy) whenever this is safe and feasible.

- Splenectomy in childhood (and to a lesser extent in adult life) carries an appreciable risk of overwhelming post-splenectomy sepsis, and pneumococcal infection is frequently responsible.

- If splenectomy is unavoidable, the patient should receive polyvalent anti-pneumococcal vaccine (before splenectomy if possible) and may benefit from prophylactic penicillin. The duration of penicillin therapy is uncertain but the risk of sepsis is greatest in the first few years after splenectomy.

sidered. Subphrenic abscess may arise from pancreatic or gastric injury, inadequate haemostasis or inappropriate use of drains.

Following splenectomy there is a transient increase in the platelet and white cell count. This predisposes to venous thrombosis. In patients with portal hypertension, splenectomy may be complicated by splenic vein thrombosis with propagation of clot into the portal vein. Low-dose heparin is advised in all patients undergoing splenectomy.

Loss of lymphoid tissue reduces immune activity and impairs the response to bacteraemia. There is a deficiency in the production of phagocytosis-promoting peptides and immunoglobulin. The risk of overwhelming post-splenectomy sepsis is greatest when splenectomy is performed in childhood, but a slightly increased incidence of death from pneumonia, complicated by disseminated intravas-cular coagulation and adrenal failure, has also been reported in adults. As most infections occur within 3 years of splenectomy, some surgeons advise prophylactic penicillin for this period. Although this is mandatory in young children, no clear benefit has been shown in adults. Polyvalent anti-pneumococcal vaccine may also be given before elective splenectomy to minimize the risk of serious infection, but it is not wholly effective and should not be given to patients younger than 2 years of age. Prophylactic antibiotics given postoperatively become especially important in this age group, and it may be advisable to continue treatment indefinitely.

Splenectomy should be avoided if at all possible in all young children. Lacerations should be sutured and, even when the spleen is ruptured, a partial splenectomy is preferable to total splenectomy if this is feasible.

Section 8
UROLOGICAL SURGERY

36
Urological surgery

CONTENTS

INVESTIGATION

History

Most patients who present to a urological clinic have signs or symptoms which suggest an abnormality in the urinary tract. Thus, any patient with blood in the urine (haematuria), *irrespective of other symptoms*, requires a full urological investigation. There are also patients who present in other clinics complaining of symptoms which may be due to urological problems, e.g. backache from metastatic prostatic carcinoma, fever of unknown origin from renal carcinoma, lethargy and anaemia due to obstructive renal failure or headaches from hypertension of renal origin. Since common things occur commonly, an elderly male complaining of difficulty in passing urine *probably* has outflow tract obstruction due to benign enlargement of the prostate. But the patient may also recently have been prescribed a diuretic, so causing the change in his urinary habits.

Environmental factors must not be ignored. In some parts of the world, bilharziasis is a common cause of haematuria. In the industrialized world, the patient may have been exposed to certain carcinogenic agents which, years later, cause bladder cancer.

Urinary tract symptoms

The site of *pain* must be accurately defined. Pain in the 'side' could originate from the chest, loin or spinal column. Renal pain occurs in the renal angle, i.e. the angle between the 12th rib and the sacrospinalis muscles. Ureteric pain (or colic) may start in the renal angle but typically radiates forwards and downwards into the groin and to the testes or labia. When the bladder is obstructed acutely, there is characteristic severe central lower abdominal pain. Chronic bladder obstruction may produce only a vague lower abdominal ache even though the bladder is grossly distended. Bladder abnormalities and prostatic diseases may also cause ill-defined perineal or penile pains. A prostate which is grossly enlarged can encroach onto the rectum and cause rectal symptoms, including *tenesmus*. The recognition of penile and testicular pain is usually easy.

Frequency of micturition is recorded numerically. Thus D/N = 6/3 indicates that the frequency by day is six times and that by night three times. A *poor stream* and *dribbling* are characteristic of mechanical obstruction in the outflow tract. *Urgency* describes the sudden uncontrollable urge to empty the bladder. This may be associated with incontinence (*urge incontinence*). *Stress incontinence* indicates involuntary loss of urine due to stress such as straining to lift, running or even laughter. *Dysuria* is painful micturition which is often described as burning or scalding.

Patients may use a wide range of phrases to describe alterations in urinary habits. The interrogation must aim to reveal whether the patient is describing obstruction (e.g. poor stream), detrusor contraction (e.g. urgency), infection (e.g. frequency, dysuria) or a more sinister sign of malignancy (e.g. dark, discoloured or brown urine).

Examination

Examination should be full and not confined to the urinary system. Thus, cardiological, neurological and gynaecological problems may be associated with urinary signs and symptoms. Since many urological patients are elderly, they must be assessed as to their fitness for further investigations and operative treatment. For example, the cardiovascular state may be relevant to subsequent investigations (e.g. those requiring an anaesthetic) or treatment (e.g. administration of oestrogens for carcinoma of the prostate).

Physical examination of the *kidneys* is difficult. The patient must be able to relax the abdominal muscles so that the kidney can be lifted with one hand behind the loin and palpated by the other hand pressing downwards (Fig. 36.1). The *ureter* cannot be palpated even though it does pass close to the posterior fornix of the vagina. The *bladder*, if enlarged, is central and rises out of the pelvis; it is dull to percussion, and in a patient with chronic retention who is lying flat and relaxed it is visible. Abnormalities of adjacent abdominal organs must be sought. For example, a mass in the iliac fossa could be ovarian.

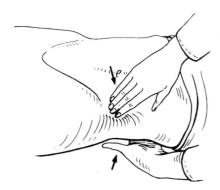

Fig. 36.1 Bimanual palpation of the right kidney.

In the male, the groins, hernia sites, cords, testes and epididymes, are examined both with the patient standing up and lying down. The penis should always be examined. If it is uncircumcised, it must be confirmed that the foreskin retracts and that the glans and meatus are normal.

In the female, the vulva, urethra and vagina must be examined; a speculum examination should be carried out if there is any suspicion of vaginal or cervical abnormality. A full pelvic bimanual examination, whether in males or females, is best carried out under general anaesthesia with a muscle relaxant.

A rectal examination is mandatory not only to examine the prostate but also to detect abnormalities of the anal margin (e.g. haemorrhoids, fissures) and lower rectum (e.g. carcinoma).

Routine investigations

Urine

Routine examination of the urine consists of testing for protein and sugar with proprietary test-papers. Testing for protein is used as a simple guide to glomerular function. Provided that there is no urinary tract infection, normal urine is almost protein-free. A protein leak of more than 150 mg/24 h requires further investigation of the kidneys. Detection of sugar in the urine may point to diabetes, and urinary symptoms may be related to this. Screening for urinary tract infection may also be done by dipstix.

The routine *microscopic examination* of a fresh specimen of urine is no longer carried out but is limited to special circumstances, e.g. to detect casts or tubular epithelial cells associated with renal parenchymal disease, to detect crystals that are often present in patients with renal calculi or to detect ova in a patient suspected of having bilharziasis.

Urine cytology for malignant cells is a useful examination both in the diagnosis and in the follow-up of bladder (urothelial) cancers.

For *microbiological examination* of the urine, a fresh sample must be collected in a sterile container. In order to avoid contamination by normal urethral flora, the patient is asked to pass some urine into the toilet, then, without interrupting the flow, the next part into a special container, and the remainder into the toilet — hence the term *midstream specimen* of urine (MSU). If it is necessary to store the specimen, it should be kept at 4°C. To rule out possible contamination during the collection of midstream specimens, fine-needle suprapubic aspiration of a full bladder may be required in difficult cases. To detect organisms the microbiologist cultures the urine in a suitable medium, and then determines the sensitivity of any organism to antimicrobial agents.

Blood

A guide to overall renal function is provided by measuring blood urea or creatinine. Urea is the major end-product of protein metabolism but its blood level may be influenced by diet and urine flow rate. As the blood urea concentration does not start to rise unless the glomerular filtration rate is halved, considerable renal damage can exist in the presence of a normal blood urea. Measurement of serum creatinine is preferred since it is stable, independent of urine flow and little influenced by diet. Measurement of creatinine clearance using the formula UV/P, where U is the creatinine concentration in the urine, V the volume of urine (in ml) over a timed period, and P the creatinine concentration in blood, is required only in patients whose kidneys are failing so that the clinician can estimate when more active treatment is needed.

The blood chemistry may also be examined to exclude a metabolic disorder (see below). The haemoglobin should be checked and will be low in a patient with chronic renal disease. The erythrocyte sedimentation rate (ESR) can be markedly raised in idiopathic retroperitoneal fibrosis, a cause of ureteric obstruction.

A search for tumour secretory products (*tumour markers*) in the blood may help to diagnose and monitor malignant disease. In tumours of the testis, human chorionic gonadotropin and alphafetoprotein are valuable tumour markers. Prostate specific antigen (PSA) is a marker for prostate cell activity and is not specific for prostate cancer; nevertheless it is a valuable marker for both the diagnosis and follow-up of this cancer.

Intravenous urography

The basic radiological investigation of the urinary tract is *intravenous urography* (IVU). A plain X-ray of the abdomen and pelvis is obtained first to show the areas of the kidneys, ureters and bladder. In addition to the lumbar spine and pelvis, opacities such as stones in the region of the urinary tract will be shown. An iodine-containing contrast material is then injected intravenously and serial X-rays are taken as the contrast is excreted.

The concentration of contrast is influenced by the urine flow, which in turn depends on the hydration of the patient. Routine preparation for an IVU should include fluid restriction for 12 hours. As faeces within the large bowel will obscure the radiographic outline of the urinary tract, an aperient may be given on the day before the X-ray.

An IVU demonstrates the renal pelvis and calyces and the rate of emptying from the kidneys. The calibre of the ureters is seen as contrast passes down to the bladder. Once the bladder has filled with contrast, the patient empties the bladder and a 'post-micturition' film is taken to show the efficiency of bladder emptying and to indicate the amount of residual urine.

Delayed excretion of the contrast is a sign of obstruction somewhere in the urinary tract. Delayed films, taken up to 24 hours after contrast injection, may then give added detail of the affected kidney and ureter.

Special investigations

To define the ureter, pelvis and calyces more clearly, a *retrograde ureteropyelogram* may be necessary. This involves retrograde injection of contrast material through a ureteric catheter placed in the lower ureter (Fig. 36.2). With improved technology, direct vision by a ureteroscope is now preferred for examining the ureter.

Abnormalities of the renal vessels, such as stenosis of the renal artery, or an aneurysm can be demonstrated by *renal angiography*. A catheter is passed into the aorta via a femoral artery up to the level of the renal arteries, where contrast media is injected and serial films are taken. Renal angiography is now rarely used in the assessment of renal tumours, CT being the preferred method of imaging.

To define the bladder, detect ureterovesical reflux or examine the bladder neck and urethra, a *micturating cystourethrogram* (MCU) is required. The bladder is filled with contrast material (via a catheter) and emptying is then studied by X-ray screening. An *ascending urethrogram*, in which contrast medium is injected into the urethra, can be used to define strictures, but is less useful than an MCU.

Ultrasonography

The main use of ultrasound in the urinary tract is to distinguish between solid tumours and cysts of the kidney. Other uses include the detection of perirenal collections of fluid which may occur around a transplanted kidney, and the characterization of masses in

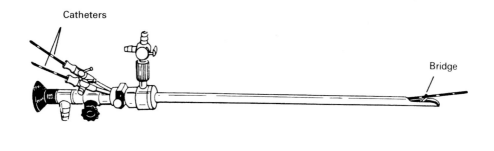

Catheters

Bridge

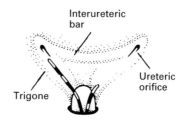

Interureteric bar

Ureteric orifice

Trigone

Fig. 36.2 Cystoscope and ureteric catheterization.

the pelvis. Ultrasound is of limited value in determining the size or spread of tumours.

Nuclear imaging

Radiolabelled substances are used for two main purposes.

1. *Detection of metastases in bones.* (^{99m}Tc)-labelled methylene diphosphonate (MDP) is the most reliable marker for detecting metastases from carcinoma of the prostate.

2. *Measurement of renal function.* MAG3 is now used extensively: it is excreted by the proximal tubules rather than by glomerular filtration. Diethylenetetramine pentaacetic acid (DTPA) is reserved for patients in whom there is renal failure. Dimercaptosuccinic acid (DMSA) is concentrated in the renal tubule. As only 5% is excreted, static imaging can be carried out some 2–3 hours after injection. Parenchymal defects such as scars, haematoma, lacerations or ischaemia may be demonstrated. Differential renal function can be quantified from measuring the DMSA concentration in each kidney.

Urodynamic studies

Maximum urinary flow rate during micturition can be measured by a flow meter. The normal flow rate in males is 15–30 ml/s and in females 20–40 ml/s. It is important to measure flow rate when the voided volume is at least 150 ml, otherwise the values may be misleading and reflect bladder dysfunction rather than outflow obstruction. A flow rate of less than 6 ml/s for a voided volume of 150 ml or more is abnormal. The urinary stream may be so poor that quantification is unnecessary, but in a proportion of patients with equivocal urinary symptoms, the flow rate can help to determine the degree of obstruction.

For additional information, measurements of flow rate are combined with *cystometry*. This provides a measure of the residual urine, the capacity of the bladder, the capacity at which a desire to void occurs and the detrusor pressures when the bladder is full and at maximum flow rate. Detrusor muscle pressure is recorded continuously, and any spontaneous contractions during bladder filling may indicate an unstable bladder (a cause of urgency and urge incontinence). The pressures along the urethra may also be measured (urethral pressure profile).

These measurements are of particular value in distinguishing between bladder and urethral abnormalities in an incontinent patient. They also help to distinguish between neurological, pharmacological and mechanical causes of outflow tract symptoms.

Semen analysis

Microscopic examination of the semen is a basic investigation in infertile males. The specimen is collected 3 days after the last ejaculation and is examined within 2 hours. Normal semen has a volume of 2–6 ml and a sperm concentration of $20–120 \times 10^6$/ml. More than 60% of the sperms are motile at 2 hours.

The morphology, biochemistry and viability of the sperm may also be studied. In selected cases, immunological tests may help to determine the cause of infertility.

Biochemical screening for stones

The main metabolic causes of urinary tract stones are hyperparathyroidism, idiopathic hypercalciuria, hyperoxaluria and cystinuria. All patients with urinary tract calculi should be screened for such an underlying metabolic abnormality. Serum calcium, phosphate, oxalate and uric acid are measured. More detailed investigation requires 24-hour collection of urine for determination of calcium, phosphate, oxalate and uric acid excretion. The composition of passed or removed stones should be analysed to determine their metabolic type.

URINARY TRACT OBSTRUCTION: OUTFLOW TRACT

The outflow tract extends from the bladder neck through the urethra to the external urinary meatus. In older males it is most commonly obstructed by benign hyperplasia of the prostate; in younger males the obstruction may be due to a stricture. Carcinoma of the prostate is a less frequent cause.

Benign prostatic hyperplasia

From about the age of 40 years the prostate undergoes progressive change in size and consistency. Enlargement results from hyperplasia of periurethral glandular tissue forming adenomas in the central zone of the prostate. These characteristically form lateral 'lobes', and often a 'middle lobe'. The normal prostatic tissue is gradually compressed to form a shell or capsule around these adenomas. There is considerable variation in the growth rates of the adenomas and in the proportion of stromal and epithelial tissue. A prostate that has been previously infected or has a preponderance of stromal tissue is firm and fibrous on rectal examination. Adenomas with epithelial preponderance can grow to large discrete masses weighing more than 100 g and on examination have a characteristic rubbery consistency. These changes are generally referred to as benign prostatic hyperplasia (BPH) (Fig. 36.3).

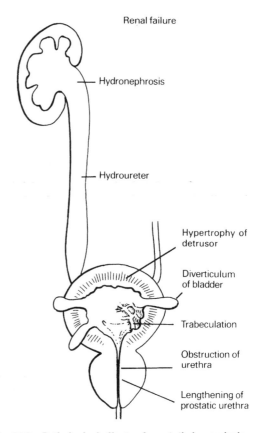

Fig. 36.3 Pathological effects of prostatic hyperplasia.

The enlarging adenomas lengthen and obstruct the prostatic urethra, interfere with the sphincter mechanisms of the internal meatus, and lead to the signs and symptoms of prostatic obstruction. To overcome increasing outflow resistance, the detrusor muscle hypertrophies. The muscle bands form trabeculae between which saccules form diverticula. Occasionally a diverticulum may become quite large, even larger than the bladder. Bladder diverticula empty poorly and are liable to the three main complications of urinary stasis: infection, stones and tumour.

With progressive inability to empty the bladder completely (chronic retention), the risk of urinary infection and stone formation increases. Bladder stones have become rare in Western countries but are often seen in areas of poor nutrition and especially in children. Eventually the residual urine volume may exceed 1 litre, leading to progressive obstruction and dilatation of the ureters (hydroureter) and pelvicaliceal system (hydronephrosis) ultimately leading to obstructive renal failure.

Clinical features

The pathological changes at the bladder neck produce signs and symptoms which correlate poorly with the size of the prostate. Frequency, urgency and dysuria are common. Nocturia may become increasingly troublesome. The force of the stream is noticeably weaker and, with straining in an attempt to empty the bladder, vessels at the bladder neck may bleed. These clinical features may be separated into two main groups: those that are due to obstruction (slow stream and hesitancy) and those that are due to an unstable detrusor muscle (urgency and urge incontinence). These latter irritative symptoms alone are not an indication for prostatectomy.

Increasing frequency may deceive the patient into thinking that he is passing an adequate amount of urine whereas the bladder may be full though painless. The frequency may progress to dribbling incontinence. Such patients are liable to develop the signs and symptoms of obstructive uraemia, including drowsiness, anorexia and personality changes.

Some patients suddenly stop passing urine (acute retention). Urinary infection, cold weather, anticholinergic drugs or excessive alcohol intake can cause sufficient congestion of the bladder neck to tip the balance from difficult micturition to acute painful retention. If obstruction has already led to chronic retention of urine, acute-on-chronic obstruction may occur. If the patient has a bladder stone, he may have obstructive symptoms during micturition and there may also be bladder pain at the end of micturition.

Examination of a patient with symptoms of prostatism reveals little except enlargement of the gland on rectal examination. The enlargement is symmetrical and smooth, with a median groove between the two lateral 'lobes'. The consistency of an adenoma is described as rubbery. Asymmetry or hard consistency raises the suspicion of malignancy.

In a patient with acute painful retention of urine, the size of the prostate is more difficult to determine. This is partly due to the pelvic discomfort but also to the fullness of the bladder, which changes the normal relationship of the prostate to the lower rectum so that the gland appears to be larger than it is. In patients with chronic retention, the painless, enlarged bladder rises out of the pelvis, almost to the umbilicus. Even if it is not visible, the overlying area will be dull on percussion. In addition, the patient with chronic retention may be ill from obstructive uraemia.

Investigation

All patients must have basic assessment of renal function, and haemoglobin and serum electrolyte estimations. As symptoms of dysuria and frequency may be related principally to urinary infection (which will have to be treated), the urine must be cultured in all cases. PSA is measured as a routine; although the range of normal is given as $0 – 4$ ng/ml, prostate cancer can occur with values within this range, also BPH can cause elevated values. The interpretation of the significance of a raised PSA will depend on the age of the patient and on the size of the prostate. If the digital rectal examination is suspicious of malignancy then a needle biopsy of the prostate is always indicated. An IVU or an ultrasound is necessary to detect the secondary effects of obstruction on the bladder (e.g. diverticula, stones) and upper urinary tract, and especially to assess the volume of residual urine after micturition. A urine flow rate measurement is useful to quantify a reduction in the urinary stream. The patient may also complete a symptom score sheet to quantify the degree of inconvenience or bother.

In some patients, especially the elderly, neurological or pharmacological causes of the changes in micturition must be considered. A pressure flow urodynamic assessment may be necessary.

Treatment

The main clinical issue is to decide whether or not the patient requires treatment. Patients can be divided into three clinical groups, each requiring a different approach to management.

- *Symptomatic only.* The patient's assessment of the severity of symptoms is influenced by his age, the social inconvenience caused and by their frequency and progression. Thus, a young man may be greatly inconvenienced by symptoms that are quite acceptable to one who is elderly. If the exact role of the prostate in causing symptoms is difficult to determine, urodynamic studies may be helpful, especially if the symptoms appear to be irritative rather than obstructive.

Once it is established that the prostate is the principal problem, prostatectomy (TURP or open) has been the standard recommendation. Few patients are unfit for this operation and only if there is a history of myocardial infarction within the last 3 months should operation be deferred. In recent years a number of alternative treatments have been recommended. These include thermotherapy, laser ablation, focused ultrasound, stents and drugs. Drugs include alpha-adrenergic blockers to relax the smooth muscle of the bladder neck and prostate capsule, and 5 alpha-reductase inhibitors which block the intra-prostatic development of dihydro-testosterone from testosterone and leads to a reduction in prostate size. All of these new procedures or treatments are still under evaluation and are not yet standard management.

• *Acute retention.* This is an emergency usually requiring admission to hospital. If there is a history of prostatism, conservative measures to encourage micturition (e.g. sedation, a warm bath) only delay inevitable catheterization.

A self-retaining Foley catheter (size 16 Fr) is passed using strict asepsis and connected to a closed drainage system. If it is not possible to pass a urethral catheter, the bladder is entered directly by puncture with a trocar/cannula (suprapubic cystostomy). A specimen of urine is cultured and antibiotics are given if there is microbiological evidence of an infection.

If the history of urinary symptoms is short, then the catheter can be removed after 12 hours following which normal voiding may occur though this is unpredictable. If retention recurs then routine preoperative investigations are performed and definitive treatment carried out.

• *Chronic retention.* It is essential to determine whether the patient has any of the complications of obstruction, especially renal damage. Though the upper urinary tracts may be dilated, renal function is not necessarily impaired.

If the patient is well, with no haematological or biochemical disturbance, there is no indication for preliminary bladder drainage and prostatectomy may be planned in the usual way.

If the patient is uraemic, his general fitness for operation must be assessed. Uraemia alone is not a contraindication but hyperkalaemia, dehydration or other evidence of fluid and electrolyte disturbance must be corrected by intravenous fluids. The bladder is catheterized and prostatectomy is carried out as soon as the patient is judged to be fit. It is not necessary to wait unduly long for the blood urea to return to normal, as the risk of infection from prolonged catheterization may be a more serious hazard.

Relief of chronic obstruction is almost always followed by a diuresis due partly to an osmotic (urea) diuresis and partly to renal tubular changes resulting from back pressure. These losses can be detected by accurate intake/output fluid charts. The blood pressure should be monitored and intravenous fluid replacement may be necessary.

Prostatectomy may be performed by open or closed (endoscopic) techniques.

Open prostatectomy. Earlier open procedures used a transvesical approach in which the bladder was opened and the adenomatous obstruction enucleated from the capsule. Later, a retropubic approach was used in which the adenoma was enucleated through a transverse incision in the prostatic capsule (Fig. 36.4).

These open procedures are now reserved for very large adenomas or when another procedure, such as removal of a bladder diverticulum, is required. Apart from the length of hospitalization (7–10 days) and the presence of an abdominal wound, enucleation of some of the smaller adenomas may damage the external sphincter mechanism and cause inconti-

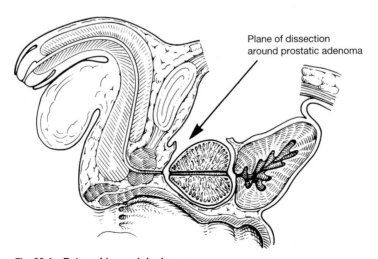

Plane of dissection around prostatic adenoma

Fig. 36.4 Retropubic prostatectomy.

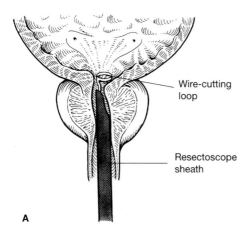

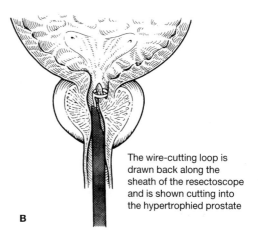

Wire-cutting
loop

Resectoscope
sheath

The wire-cutting loop is
drawn back along the
sheath of the resectoscope
and is shown cutting into
the hypertrophied prostate

A

B

Fig. 36.5 Transurethral resection of the prostate.

nence. This is a particular problem with more fibrous glands and those that contain a focus of cancer.

Closed (endoscopic) prostatectomy (transurethral resection, TUR). The prostate is removed piecemeal by electroresection using an instrument called a resectoscope (Fig. 36.5).

The advantages of this approach are patient acceptance, short hospitalization (3–5 days), and the precision of removal of the obstructing tissue. However, serious damage can be inflicted on the prostatic sphincter mechanism by inexpert use of the resectoscope. Also, a prolonged resection can result in excessive absorption of irrigating fluid and electrolyte imbalance (TUR syndrome). Retrograde ejaculation is a common sequel to any operative procedure on the prostate (and bladder neck) and all patients should be advised pre-operatively of this effect.

If the patient has a bladder stone, this may be crushed with a lithotrite or removed by suprapubic lithotomy. If there is a diverticulum with a narrow neck, this should be removed through a suprapubic transvesical approach. If the diverticulum is shallow with a wide neck, then prostatectomy only is required.

Postoperative care

After either form of prostatectomy, the bladder must be drained freely by a urethral catheter while the prostatic bed heals and bleeding stops. After TUR the catheter is normally removed on the 3rd postoperative day; after an open procedure, because of the bladder or prostate incision, it is usually left until the 5th postoperative day.

The main postoperative hazard is bleeding. In an open procedure, blood vessels at the bladder neck are sutured, but bleeding within the capsule is less easy to control. In a TUR, coagulation of the blood vessels is more precise but not always complete. If postoperative bleeding is excessive, clot may lead to obstruction (clot retention). The hazard can be minimized by ensuring a good flow of urine by giving diuretics or by continuous irrigation through a three-way urethral catheter.

The results of all forms of prostatectomy continue to improve but TUR has the lowest morbidity and mortality (1%) and requires a shorter hospital stay (50% less) than other procedures.

Obstruction due to prostatic carcinoma

Carcinoma of the prostate is discussed in detail later in this chapter.

Bladder neck obstruction

Occasionally the obstruction to the outflow tract appears to be at the bladder neck. The prostate is often quite small, giving rise to the expression 'prostatism without a prostate'. The cause may be an infective condition such as prostatitis or schistosomiasis, or a neurological disorder, such as diabetes or a prolapsed intervertebral disc. More commonly, the obstruction is due to failure of the bladder neck to open when the detrusor contracts (dyssynergia).

Characteristically, bladder neck dyssynergia is found in younger middle-aged men, i.e. at an age when benign prostatic hyperplasia is not expected. The urinary stream is poor, though the patient may have thought it normal, and there may be frequency and urgency.

The muscular dysfunction that causes dyssynergia may be improved by alpha-adrenergic blocking drugs. Endoscopic incision or excision of the bladder neck is preferable to long-term drug treatment, but surgery is contraindicated if the risk of retrograde ejaculation and therefore infertility is of concern to the patient.

Urethral obstruction

Lesions of the urethra may be congenital, traumatic, infective or malignant. Each may result in outflow tract obstruction (Fig. 36.6). Foreign bodies, including urinary stones, may also cause obstruction. Any of these causes may be complicated by infection, with periurethral abscess, fistulas and stones as late complications.

Congenital lesions. Congenital valves in the posterior urethra occur only in boys. They lie at the level of the verumontanum and may cause gross obstructive changes in the bladder and upper urinary tracts at birth. Increasingly, this diagnosis is being established during pregnancy by ultrasound examination. If the diagnosis is established after birth, it is confirmed by micturating cystourethrography and treatment consists of endoscopic incision of the valves.

Diverticula of the urethra are rare causes of obstruction. More commonly, diverticula of the urethra are secondary to obstruction in women.

Urethral trauma. An important late sequel of urethral trauma is a stricture whose severity is related to both the site and the extent of injury. Thus, a posterior urethral stricture that follows

major trauma to the pelvis may be surrounded by dense fibrous tissue, whereas a stricture of the bulb of the urethra may be surrounded by healthy tissues. The former requires major reconstructive surgery, but the latter can be readily managed by urethral dilatation or incision.

It must be remembered that rough inexpert use of any instrument (including a catheter) in the urethra can be followed by stricture formation.

Infective lesions. In the male, the principal organism responsible for inflammatory change, scarring and stricture of the urethra is *Neisseria gonorrhoeae*. The periurethral glands of the bulb of the urethra are the main site of infection and when treatment is inadequate, stricture formation in this area is likely.

Long-term use of a self-retaining catheter, although not necessarily associated with infection, can also cause an inflammatory reaction in the urethra. This may result in a stricture, most commonly at the external meatus.

The foreskin may cause problems due to infection (balanitis), narrowing of the orifice (phimosis), or by becoming retracted and stuck (paraphimosis).

In the female the paraurethral glands, sometimes called the 'female prostate', may be the site of chronic inflammation. The urethra becomes narrow, and these women experience recurring infective symptoms or obstructive symptoms without infection, the so-called *urethral syndrome*. Urethral stenosis and incomplete bladder emptying are but part of this difficult clinical problem. In some women symptomatic relief may follow urethral dilatation or urethrotomy.

Tumours of the urethra. Transitional cell tumours, which may be associated with bladder

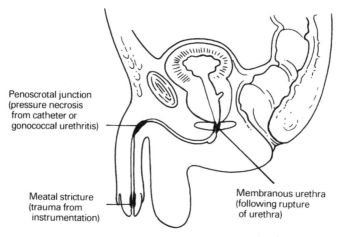

Penoscrotal junction
(pressure necrosis
from catheter or
gonococcal urethritis)

Meatal stricture
(trauma from
instrumentation)

Membranous urethra
(following rupture
of urethra)

Fig. 36.6 Common sites and causes of urethral stricture.

tumours, and squamous carcinoma of the distal urethra are uncommon tumours which may cause obstructive symptoms.

Clinical features

The change in micturition due to urethral narrowing may be indistinguishable from that which occurs with BPH. However, stricture should be considered if there is a history of urethral infection, instrumentation or trauma.

The external meatus must always be examined and, if present, the foreskin retracted for full inspection. The urethra is palpated. It is possible for a stone to be lodged in the urethra yet the patient still passes urine, though with difficulty. In women, the urethra is best examined during cystourethroscopy under general anaesthesia; the urethra can then be palpated against the shaft of the cystoscope.

Investigation

An IVU may show only incomplete bladder emptying while an ascending urethrogram may not show the posterior urethra adequately because of spasm. A micturating cystourethrogram is preferred. Urodynamic assessment of the *urethra and bladder* may be indicated, especially when neurological and mechanical problems coexist.

The final investigation to assess a urethral lesion is urethroscopy. This procedure should be considered as a cystourethroscopy since both urethra and bladder are always examined. The site and character of the lesion is determined and the degree of narrowing is measured.

Treatment

Many simple strictures are treated easily by repeated dilatation with plastic or metal bougies, or may be incised under direct vision using a urethrotome. Most simple short strictures in the region of the bulb respond well but recurrence may require operative reconstruction (urethroplasty). In this procedure a strip of full-thickness skin is used to restore the normal calibre of the urethra.

A long persistent stricture of the anterior urethra may require two-stage plastic reconstruction. A tight fibrous post-traumatic stricture of the membranous urethra may require excision of the scar tissue and urethral reconstruction. Stenosis of the meatus is treated by meatoplasty.

If the foreskin cannot be retracted normally (phimosis), and especially if infections are trouble-some, circumcision is recommended. If paraphimosis is present without gross oedema, it may be possible to reduce it manually, compressing the glans to allow the constricting band to be drawn forwards. Otherwise it is necessary to incise the constricting band. Circumcision may be carried out at a later date (see p. 549).

URINARY TRACT OBSTRUCTION: UPPER TRACT

The upper urinary tract includes the pelvicalyceal system and ureters. As with any tubular structure, obstruction may be due to extrinsic, intrinsic or intraluminal causes (Table 36.1).

In the kidney, stones within the pelvicalyceal system and congenital abnormality of the pelvi-ureteric junction (PUJ) are the main causes of obstruction; both cause hydronephrosis.

More rarely, a sloughed renal papilla or blood clot (from a tumour) may obstruct either kidney or ureter.

During pregnancy there is a physiological dilatation of the ureters due to progesterone, which reduces smooth muscle tone.

Renal and ureteric calculi

Stones which form in the kidney are of two main types: infective and metabolic.

An *infective* stone is whitish and chalky and crumbles or breaks easily. It is composed mainly of calcium, ammonia and magnesium phosphates. Such stones develop wherever drainage is impaired and are usually associated with an anatomical abnormality such as a diverticulum or with long-term recumbency or paraplegia. Their formation indicates

Table 36.1 Causes of obstruction of urinary tract
Extrinsic
Retroperitoneal fibrosis
External pressure (e.g. carcinoma of the cervix, prostate)
Intrinsic
Transitional cell tumours
Tuberculosis/bilharziasis
Ureterocele
Ectopic ureter
Intraluminal
Calculi

an established infection which cannot be eradicated by antibiotics alone. As the stone enlarges, drainage is further impaired and there is progressive damage to the kidney.

A *metabolic* stone, commonly of calcium oxalate, is usually hard and dark with an irregular sharp surface. It develops as a result of an abnormality of the composition of the urine. There may be abnormal concentration of normal constituents (e.g. due to dehydration), excess excretion of normal constituents (e.g. calcium in hyperparathyroidism, or uric acid in gout) or the urine may contain abnormal constituents (as in cystinuria). It is likely that several aetiological factors must occur together or in sequence for a stone to form. As indicated above, all patients with urinary calculi should be screened for metabolic abnormalities.

Up to 80% of the stones seen in the UK are mixed calcium oxalate/phosphate stones. Some 10% are magnesium ammonium phosphate stones with a variable proportion of calcium. Most of the remainder are uric acid stones. Cystine and xanthine stones are rare.

Clinical features

Renal pain, renal colic or ureteric colic are characteristically unilateral. Renal pain is dull and aching while ureteric colic is acute and severe and occurs in waves which pass down the line of the ureter. A stone may cause bleeding or there may be symptoms of urinary tract infection. However, a stone in the kidney may remain silent, even one large enough to fill the pelvis and calyces (a 'staghorn' calculus).

Investigation

An IVU usually provides all the necessary information on the position of the stone(s). Routine haematological and biochemical tests are needed to assess renal function and to exclude metabolic causes of stones. A urine sample is cultured to determine if there is infection. If an obstruction is acute, relief of the obstruction is the prime clinical need; if it is chronic and has caused renal damage, the surgical approach depends on the function of the affected kidney. This is best determined by radioisotope methods.

Treatment

Symptomatic treatment should be instituted as soon as the diagnosis is confirmed. IM diclofenac is the most effective analgesic but pethidine is an alterna-

tive. Antispasmodics may assist the passage of the stone. The likelihood of spontaneous passage depends on the size of the stone and on its smoothness. A stone of less than 0.5 cm in diameter should pass down the ureter. If it becomes fixed (causing increasing hydroureter and hydronephrosis), if the urine is infected, or the patient has increasing pain and fever, the stone must be removed.

A stone in the lower ureter may be disintegrated under vision using a ureteroscope with either laser, electrohydraulic or pneumatic lithotripsy. A stone basket may be used but only under fluoroscopic control. Stones in the upper ureter can be pushed into the renal pelvis and broken up by extracorporeal shock wave lithotripsy (ESWL). Some lower ureteric stones can also be treated by ESWL. It is now rare to remove a ureteric stone by a direct surgical approach (ureterolithotomy).

Stones within a kidney can be the cause of renal destruction especially if the urine is infected. If the damage is severe so that the kidney contributes <10% of total renal function, then a nephrectomy is recommended. A stone in the kidney that is too large to pass down the ureter (more than 0.5 cm) can be treated by percutaneous nephrolithotomy (PCNL) or ESWL. Larger stones can be treated by ESWL alone but are generally managed by a combination of these techniques. It is now rare to require open surgery (pyelolithotomy or nephrolithotomy) for kidney stones.

Pelviureteric junction obstruction (Idiopathic hydronephrosis)

Narrowing at the junction between the renal pelvis and the ureter is a common cause of hydronephrosis. As the aetiology is obscure, the term 'idiopathic' hydronephrosis is appropriate. Electron microscopy of the narrow area shows normal muscle cells with normal innervation, but the muscle bundles are separated by an excess of collagen fibres which may prevent relaxation of the segment. The abnormality is likely to be congenital, is often bilateral, and is seen in very young children. Gross hydronephrosis may, however, present at any age.

Clinical features

Idiopathic hydronephrosis may produce a large painless mass in the loin; in its grossest form the volume of urine in the hydronephrotic sac may simulate free fluid in the peritoneal cavity. The more usual moderate hydronephrosis causes ill-defined renal pain or ache which may be exacerbated by drinking large volumes of liquid and the patient may regard these symptoms as 'indigestion'. Rarely, there may be no symptoms.

Investigation

An IVU, with or without delayed films, provides sufficient information in many cases. The calibre of the ureter is normal. There are a few patients in whom there is doubt as to whether the dilatation of the pelvis and calyces is truly obstructive in nature. Methods to resolve this include urography and renography during induced diuresis, and antegrade pressure/flow measurements.

Treatment

Operation (pyeloplasty) is designed to remove the obstructing tissue and refashion the pelviureteric junction (PUJ) so that the lower part of the renal pelvis drains freely into the ureter (Fig. 36.7). Occasionally, an aberrant vessel to the lower pole of the kidney crosses the PUJ and gives the appearance of having caused the obstruction (though this is unlikely); in this situation, the PUJ is reconstructed in front of the vessels. Endoscopic alternatives to pyeloplasty are being developed and may give good results.

It is not possible to predict the degree of recovery of renal function after relief of obstruction but it is generally felt that a kidney contributing less than 10% of total renal function should be removed.

Retroperitoneal fibrosis

Fibrosis of the retroperitoneal connective tissues may encircle and compress the ureter(s), causing hydroureter and hydronephrosis. Fibrosis occurs in three groups of conditions.

Idiopathic. In this, the largest group, the fibrosis extends across the pelvic brim to involve the ureters and vena cava. The aetiology is unknown though it may be associated with methysergide or analgesic abuse. Mediastinal fibrosis and Dupuytren's contracture may coexist.

Malignant infiltration. The fibrosis contains malignant cells which have metastasized from primary sites such as breast, stomach, pancreas and colon.

Reactive fibrosis. Radiotherapy to pelvic organs, resolving blood clot after major vascular or other surgical procedures, or extravasation of sclerosants (e.g. phenol for a nerve block) can lead to fibrotic change in the retroperitoneum.

Since the gross appearance of all three groups of fibrosis may be similar, biopsy of the tissue is essential for diagnosis.

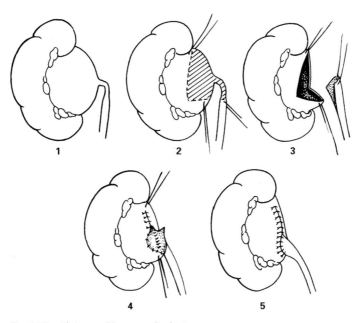

Fig. 36.7 Anderson-Hynes pyeloplasty.

Clinical features

Ureteric obstruction may cause symptoms similar to idiopathic hydronephrosis, namely, ill-defined renal pain or ache. Some patients complain of low backache.

Investigation

An IVU shows hydronephrosis and usually hydro-ureter down to the level of the obstruction. The anatomy of the ureter is often hard to define and a retrograde ureteropyelogram may be required. It is rarely necessary to pass a ureteric catheter up to the kidney although it is characteristic of retroperitoneal fibrosis that a ureteric catheter will pass easily through what appears to be a severe obstruction.

A markedly raised ESR is found in more than 50% of cases with idiopathic fibrosis.

Treatment

The relief of obstruction may be difficult. The ureter is dissected out of the fibrous sheet of tissue (ureterolysis) and wrapped in omentum to prevent further involvement. Although obstruction may regress with steroids, these agents are reserved for recurrent obstruction.

Transitional cell tumours

Though most commonly arising in the bladder, transitional cell tumours may occur in any part of the urothelium. During endoscopy, a tumour of the lower ureter may be seen protruding through the ureteric orifice. Tumours higher in the ureter are often detected late, and change in the IVU may not be obvious until there is significant obstruction. The tumour may bleed and clot may cause colic and obstruction.

Although a transitional cell tumour in the upper urinary tract may appear suitable for local excision, radical excision (nephroureterectomy) is recommended because of the difficulties of follow-up examination of this area. Conservative surgery may be considered in the elderly and is necessary in those with bilateral upper tract tumours.

Miscellaneous causes

Congenital abnormalities

A *ureterocele* develops behind a pin-hole ureteric orifice; the intramural part of the ureter dilates,

bulges into the bladder and can become very large. Incision of the pin-hole opening relieves the obstruction.

An *ectopic ureter* occurs with congenital duplication of one or both kidneys (duplex kidneys). Developmentally, the ureter has two main branches and, if this arrangement persists, the two ureters of the duplex kidneys may drain separately into the bladder (Fig. 36.8). One ureter enters normally on the trigone, while the ectopic ureter (from the upper renal moiety) enters the bladder or, more rarely, the vagina or seminal vesicle.

A ureter that is ectopic and drains into the bladder is liable to have an ineffective valve mechanism so that urine passes *up* the ureter on voiding (vesicoureteric reflux). Reflux can occur in normally sited ureters if the normal intramural ureter fails to act as a valve. The pressure of refluxing urine behaves as an intermittent obstruction which in children may lead to serious renal damage. Vesicoureteric reflux is treated by reimplantation of the ureter with the formation of an effective valve.

In primary obstructive *megaureter* there is dilatation of the ureter in all but its terminal segment

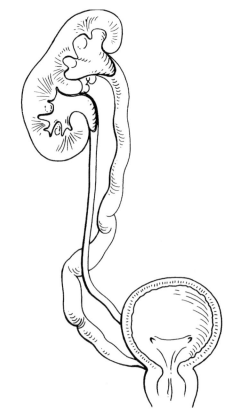

Fig. 36.8 Duplex kidney.

without obvious cause and without vesicoureteric reflux. There are normally no ganglionic cells in the ureter so that megaureter cannot be due to neuromuscular inco-ordination. Radiographic and pressure/flow studies may be needed to determine whether there is obstruction to urine flow. Narrowing of the ureter and reimplantation may be necessary.

Infections

Tuberculosis of the urinary tract is a rare cause of stricture of the ureter and even complete obstruction. This process may be silent and 'autonephrectomy' may be detected at a later date.

Bilharziasis affecting the urinary tract is common in parts of Africa and the Middle East. Ureteric fibrosis and obstruction are part of the process that can affect the whole of the urinary tract. Many patients present in such an advanced state of the disease that surgical treatment is not feasible.

Both infections require specific drug treatment. When the ureters are involved and obstructed, a variety of reconstructive surgical procedures may be

---

Urinary tract obstruction
- Common causes of obstruction of the outflow tract are:
  - benign prostatic hyperplasia
  - prostatic cancer
  - bladder cancer involving the bladder neck
  - bladder-neck obstruction (dyssynergia, infection, neurological disorders)
  - urethral obstruction (congenital posterior urethral valves, blocked urinary catheter, trauma, infection).

- Common causes of obstruction of the upper urinary tract are:
  - renal and ureteric calculi (80% are calcium oxalate/phosphate stones)
  - pelviureteric junction obstruction (idiopathic hydronephrosis)
  - retroperitoneal fibrosis (idiopathic/malignant infiltration/radiotherapy)
  - transitional cell carcinoma (with or without bleeding and clot)
  - congenital abnormalities (e.g. ectopic ureter, ureterocele)
  - infections (notably bilharziasis and tuberculosis).

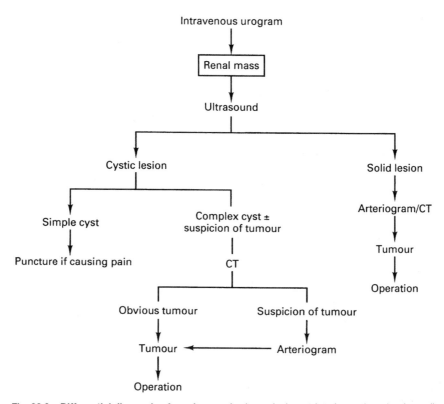

Fig. 36.9 Differential diagnosis of renal mass. Angiography is restricted to patients in whom all imaging methods (including MRI) have proved equivocal or if partial nephrectomy is considered.

used to conserve renal function and correct obstruction and/or reflux.

RENAL CYSTS

Simple cysts of the kidney are usually single. They are almost always asymptomatic and are often found incidentally on IVU or ultrasound. The differential diagnosis between a cyst and a renal carcinoma must then be made. Ideally, a cyst should be diagnosed and treated at the same session in the radiology department (Fig. 36.9). Fluid from the cyst is examined cytologically and if there is any suspicion of tumour cells, the cyst must be explored. Malignant change in a cyst can occur but is very rare.

Polycystic kidney disease is a congenital anomaly (dominant) that affects both kidneys and often leads to chronic renal failure in middle life. Despite their very large size the cystic kidneys cause few symptoms. Infection or bleeding into a cyst can occur and may require exploration to relieve symptoms. The condition may cause haematuria.

TUMOURS OF THE URINARY SYSTEM

Benign renal adenomas are small and usually incidental findings. Haemangiomas are a rare cause of dramatic haematuria.

Primary renal malignant tumours are nephroblastoma (or Wilms' tumour) in children and renal carcinoma in adults. Metastases from other tumour sites may occasionally be found in the kidney.

Nephroblastomas

These tumours usually occur in children under 4 years of age, and account for 10% of all childhood malignancies. The tumour is probably derived from embryonic mesodermal tissue and microscopically has a mixed appearance of spindle cells, epithelial cells and muscle fibres. Growth is rapid and there is early local spread, including invasion of the renal vein. Invasion of the renal pelvis occurs late, so that haematuria is not common. Distant metastases most commonly appear in the lungs, liver and bones. Tumours presenting in the first year of life have a better prognosis.

Clinical features

The cardinal sign is a large abdominal mass which is often first noted when the baby is bathed. Some of the unusual clinical features associated with a renal carcinoma in adults, such as fever or hypertension, may be present.

Investigation

An IVU and chest X-ray are essential. The main differential diagnosis is from neuroblastoma affecting the adrenal, but other causes of a large kidney, such as hydronephrosis and cystic disease, must be considered. The tumour is bilateral in 5–10% of cases.

Treatment

Transabdominal nephrectomy with wide excision of the mass is carried out after preliminary ligation of the renal pedicle. This is followed by radiotherapy and chemotherapy using actinomycin D and vincristine. As a result of this treatment, the 5-year survival rate has improved from 10% to 80%.

Renal carcinoma

This is the commonest malignant tumour of the kidney. The incidence in males is three times greater than in females, and most patients are over 40 years of age. The tumour arises from renal tubules. Haemorrhage and necrosis gives a characteristic mixed golden yellow and red appearance to the cut surface. Microscopically there are clear and granular cell types; the former are more common. There is early spread of the tumour into the renal pelvis, causing haematuria. Invasion of the renal vein, often extending into the inferior vena cava, also occurs early. Direct spread into perinephric tissues is common, so that the whole fascial envelope and kidney should be removed 'en bloc'. Lymphatic spread occurs to para-aortic nodes, while blood-borne metastases (which may be solitary) may develop almost anywhere in the body.

Clinical features

The triad of pain, haematuria and a mass is an important but late feature. A remarkable range of systemic effects may occur early, including fever, a raised ESR, polycythaemia, disorders of coagulation, and abnormalities of plasma proteins and liver function tests. The patient may present with pyrexia of unknown origin (PUO) or, rarely, with neuromyopathy.

Systemic effects may be due to tumour secretion of products such as renin, erythropoietin, parathormone and gonadotropins. The effects disappear when the tumour is removed but may reappear when metastases develop, and so can be used as markers of tumour activity.

Investigation

The investigation of renal carcinoma is as for any space-occupying renal lesion or mass. The main differential diagnosis is from a simple renal cyst. The sequence of investigations used is that which gives the maximum information with the least number of tests and which facilitates the diagnosis and treatment of simple renal cysts (Fig. 36.9). The tests most commonly used are ultrasonography, needle aspiration and CT scanning (Fig. 36.10).

Additional staging information about the extent of spread into the renal vein, lymph node enlargement and lung metastasis is best obtained by CT.

Treatment

Radical nephrectomy, that includes the perirenal fascial envelope and ipsilateral para-aortic lymph nodes, is performed whenever possible. Pre-operative radiotherapy is of no benefit but postoperative radiotherapy may be given if surgical excision is incomplete. Infarction of the kidney by renal artery embolization at the time of arteriography can be used to reduce the vascularity of the tumour mass and to facilitate removal of larger tumours. There is no effective chemotherapy for these tumours, although some are believed to be hormonally sensitive.

Because of the unusual features associated with renal carcinomas, nephrectomy should always be considered. Not only may systemic effects disappear, but there may even be regression of a solitary metastasis. Solitary metastases tend to remain single for long periods and excision or radiotherapy is often worthwhile.

Urothelial tumours

The urothelium, or transitional cell lining of the urinary tract, extends from the renal papilla to the external urinary meatus. Approximately 8000 patients present annually with tumours arising from this source in the UK. The incidence of these tumours is increasing, possibly due to environmental carcinogens.

The high incidence of urothelial cancer in workers in certain chemical, dyestuff and rubber-moulding industries led to the identification of carcinogens (naphthylamines and benzidine) which are now banned. Carcinogens associated with hairdressing and leather work have also been suspected. Smoking and analgesic abuse are associated with an increased incidence of urothelial cancer.

The vast majority of urothelial tumours occur in the bladder.

Pathology

Almost all tumours are transitional cell carcinomas. Squamous carcinoma may occur in urothelium

Renal carcinoma
- Renal carcinoma is much the commonest malignant renal tumour and is three times commoner in males.

- The carcinoma arises in the renal tubules and spreads early to the renal pelvis and produces haematuria. Later spread involves the renal vein (with bloodstream dissemination), perinephric invasion and lymphatic spread.

- The clinical presentation is very varied. The triad of pain, haematuria and a mass may be late features, and early systemic effects include fever, polycythaemia, disordered coagulation and PUO.

- The key investigations are ultrasonography with needle aspiration, chest X-ray, CT scan and isotope bone scanning.

- Treatment consists of radical nephrectomy; postoperative radiotherapy may be used if surgical excision is incomplete. The natural history of renal carcinoma is very variable and excision or irradiation of solitary metastases may be worthwhile.

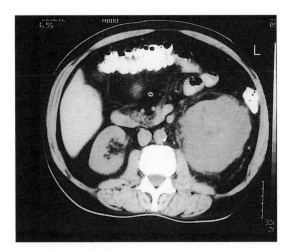

Fig. 36.10   CT showing tumour of left kidney.

that has undergone metaplasia, usually due to chronic inflammation or irritation due to a stone or bilharziasis. An adenocarcinoma is a rarity but may occur in a urachal remnant in the dome of the bladder or from local infiltration, e.g. bowel cancer.

The appearance of a transitional cell tumour ranges from a delicate papillary structure to a solid ulcerating mass. The appearance correlates well with subsequent behaviour, in that papillary tumours are relatively benign while those which ulcerate are mostly malignant.

A *biopsy* is essential to confirm the diagnosis, determine the degree of cell differentiation (i.e. the *grade*) and determine the depth to which the tumour has penetrated the bladder wall (i.e. the *stage*).

The TNM system of tumour classification is also applicable to bladder tumours. Assessment of the *primary tumour* (T) is of prime clinical importance and requires bimanual examination under anaesthesia to judge the degree of penetration through the bladder wall. This is especially important for T2 and T3 tumours (see Fig. 36.11). Involvement of *regional and juxtaregional lymph nodes* (N) is assessed by both clinical examination and radiography, including urography and CT scan. Assessment of *distant metastases* (M) requires clinical examination and radiography.

Histopathological examination allows much more accurate assessment of the tumour and is of great help when deciding the best form of treatment. Biopsy gives accurate information on superficial tumours but invasive tumours cannot be assessed precisely without examining the full thickness of the bladder wall.

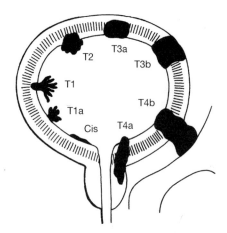

Fig. 36.11 T-categories of bladder tumour. Cis = carcinoma-in-situ.

Clinical features

More than 80% of patients have haematuria, which is usually painless. It should be assumed that such bleeding is from a tumour until proved otherwise. In women, symptoms of cystitis are so common that occasional bleeding may be thought to be part of an infective problem. In men, symptoms of prostatism are common and may include bleeding.

Bleeding at the end of micturition, and especially passage of pink/red urine, suggests that the site of bleeding is in the bladder; uniformly dark-coloured urine suggests that the source is in the upper tract.

A tumour at the lower end of a ureter or a bladder tumour involving the ureteric orifice may cause obstructive symptoms, but usually there are few complaints apart from discoloration of the urine. Examination is usually unhelpful. Rectal examination detects only advanced tumours.

Investigation

The urine may contain obvious blood. Cytological examination may lead to diagnosis but histology and bimanual examination are essential for estimating the stage and grade of the tumour: cytology of the urine can be useful in the follow-up of patients with bladder cancer.

Because upper tract tumours are much less common, they may be overlooked in the presence of an obvious bladder tumour. Both may occur together and the whole of the urothelium must be examined on the intravenous urogram. If there is any suspicious defect in the ureter, a retrograde ureteropyelogram is necessary.

Cystourethroscopy and examination under anaesthesia are the basic investigations for all suspected bladder tumours. With the patient under relaxation anaesthesia, the bladder and tumour are examined bimanually to determine the depth of spread. The physical features of the tumour(s) are noted, the normal bladder mucosa is inspected and biopsies are taken from the tumour and any suspicious area.

Treatment

Upper tract tumours. The management of these tumours is discussed on page 539.

Superficial bladder tumours (Ta, T1). Small superficial tumours can be treated by endoscopic diathermy alone but whenever possible a biopsy followed by transurethral resection of the tumour (TURT) is recommended. Larger and even multiple superficial tumours can also be treated effectively by

TURT. Occasionally a tumour in the upper half of the bladder is best treated by open operation, provided that at least 2 cm of healthy bladder wall can be included (partial cystectomy); in that site transurethral resection is awkward and even unsafe.

Histological examination may show that an apparently superficial tumour has invaded superficial bladder muscle (T2). Provided the resection has been complete and the tumour is well or moderately well differentiated, no further treatment is indicated. If the tumour is poorly differentiated and the exact depth of invasion cannot be determined, it should be treated as an invasive tumour (see below).

Intravesical chemotherapy (e.g. epirubicin, mitomycin C) is useful to treat multiple low-grade bladder tumours and to reduce the recurrence rate of low-grade superficial tumours. Regular check cystoscopies are required and recurrences treated either by extensive diathermy or by cystectomy.

Carcinoma-in-situ (Cis) may occur in association with a proliferative tumour (often in an apparently normal mucosa), or as a separate entity, when there may be only a generalized redness (*malignant cystitis*). Untreated patients with Cis have a high risk of progression to invasive cancer. The tumour responds well to intravesical Bacille Calmette-Guérin (BCG) treatment but if there is any doubt about the response, and especially if there is any pathological evidence of progression, more aggressive treatment is needed (see below).

Invasive bladder tumours. The management of invasive (T3) tumours is debated. The combination of a short course of radiotherapy followed by total cystectomy is recommended for patients under 65 years of age. The morbidity and mortality associated with such a radical procedure increases with age and a radical course of radiotherapy may be a better option in older patients. Unfortunately this may not always cure the tumour and 'salvage' cystectomy may be needed for recurrence or for symptoms such as intractable bleeding.

Cystectomy always necessitates diversion of the urine. In an ileal conduit (or uretero-ileostomy) the ureters are implanted into a short segment of ileum which then opens onto the abdominal wall as an ileostomy (Fig. 36.12). In some countries where an 'ostomy' is not acceptable, the ureters can be implanted into the sigmoid colon (ureterosigmoidostomy), but renal infection and metabolic disturbances can be serious complications. Other methods for bladder replacement have been developed and may be suitable for younger patients.

An invasive T4 tumour, fixed to the pelvis or surrounding organs, is inoperable and only palliative treatment can be given.

The place of adjuvant chemotherapy is not yet established. Both cisplatin and methotrexate have an effect on transitional cell cancer but response rates in the treatment of metastatic disease are modest (about 20%).

The prognosis of bladder tumours depends on

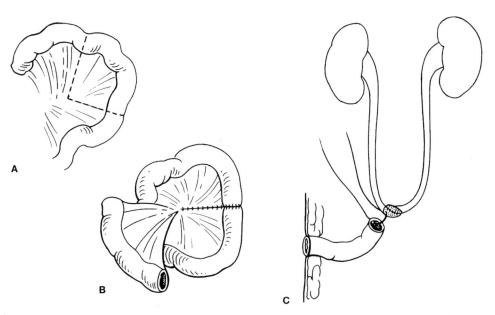

Fig. 36.12 Ileal conduit urinary diversion: **A & B** isolation of segment of ileum; **C** uretero-ileal anastomosis.

tumour stage and grade. The 5-year survival rate varies from 20–30% in those with deep muscle invasion to 50–60% in those with mucosal tumours. Overall about one-third of patients survive for 5 years.

Invasive tumours sometimes develop in the posterior (prostatic) urethra and require aggressive combination treatment.

Carcinoma of the prostate

In the UK this is the third most common malignancy in males, arising in over 10 000 new patients each year and increasing in frequency. It is the second commonest cause of cancer death in men in the UK. The tumour is common in northern Europe and the US (particularly in the black-skinned) but rare in China and Japan. It rarely occurs before the age of 50 and is uncommon before the age of 60. The mean age at presentation is approximately 70 years. The aetiology is unknown but hormonal and possibly viral factors are implicated.

Almost all malignant tumours of the prostate are carcinomas. If a prostate is examined by serial section, a small malignant focus is detected in almost all men over the age of 80 years. Thus, there is a very high incidence of histological prostate cancer and many men will die with a cancer of the prostate but not *from* that cancer. It is estimated that the incidence of focal histological cancer in men aged 50–75 is approximately 40%, whereas the incidence of clinical prostate cancer is approximately 8% – one-quarter of whom will die from that cancer.

The TNM system is used in classification:

T0 No evidence of primary tumour.
T1 Incidentally diagnosed tumour, not palpable and not visible by imaging (small-volume tumour T1a, large-volume tumour T1b, detected because of a raised PSA only T1c)
T2 Tumour confined within the prostate.
T3 Tumour extends through the prostate capsule.
T4 Tumour fixed or invades adjacent structures.

Metastatic spread to pelvic lymph nodes occurs early. One-third of clinically localized tumours at the time of presentation will have spread to regional nodes. Metastases to bone, mainly the lumbar spine and pelvis, are common; more than half of all new cases have such metastases.

Clinical features

Most patients present with 'prostatic' symptoms of frequency, urgency and dysuria. One-quarter present with acute retention. Occasionally the tumour extends posteriorly around the rectum and causes alteration in bowel habit.

Symptoms and signs due to metastases are much less common and include back pain, weight loss, anaemia and obstruction of the ureters.

On rectal examination the prostate feels nodular and stony hard. The diagnosis must never be made on clinical grounds alone; many irregular prostates, even with nodules, are not malignant. Conversely, 10–15% of malignant prostates are not palpably abnormal on rectal examination.

Investigation

Since most patients present with outflow tract obstruction, an IVU and serum creatinine determination are used to assess the urinary tract. An X-ray of the pelvis or lumbar spine (to investigate backache) may show osteosclerotic metastases as the first evidence of prostatic malignancy.

Whenever possible, the diagnosis is confirmed by needle biopsy (either transperineal or transrectal) of a suspicious part of the prostate or by histological

---

Urothelial tumours
- The urothelium or transitional cell epithelial lining of the urinary tract extends from the renal papilla to the external urinary meatus.
- The incidence of urothelial cancer is increasing, possibly because of increasing exposure to occupational carcinogens, smoking and analgesic abuse.
- Almost all urothelial cancers are transitional cell tumours and the vast majority occur in the bladder. Squamous cancers are rarer and are associated with chronic irritation or inflammation (e.g. calculi and bilharziasis). Adenocarcinomas are extremely rare.
- Frank haematuria is present in 80% of cases.
- Transitional cell cancers of the bladder are treated as follows:
  - carcinoma in situ (Tis) may respond to intravesical BCG but is unpredictable and may require more aggressive treatment
  - superficial tumours (T1,T2) are usually treated by transurethral resection ± intravesical chemotherapy
  - invasive T3 tumours may be best dealt with by radiotherapy followed by total cystectomy (or by radical radiotherapy)
  - invasive T4 tumours with fixation to the pelvis or surrounding organs are dealt with by palliative radiotherapy.

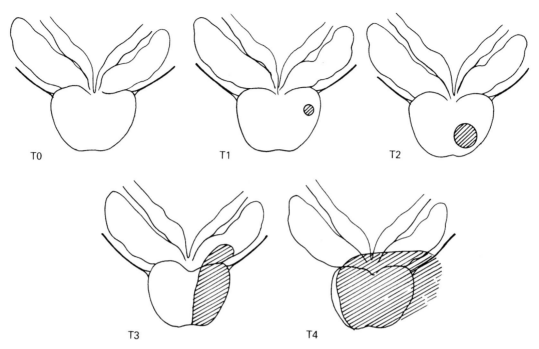

Fig. 36.13 T-categories of prostatic carcinoma. T0 = no evidence of primary tumour; T1 = incidentally diagnosed, not palpable; T2 = palpable tumour confined within prostate; T3 = extending beyond prostate capsule; T4 = fixed — or invades adjacent structures.

examination of tissue removed by endoscopic resection if this is needed to relieve outflow obstruction.

The patient is assessed for distant metastases by a radioisotope scan. PSA is now the main serum marker for the detection of prostate cancer. High levels (e.g. >100 ng/ml) almost always indicate distant bone metastases. PSA is also the main test for monitoring response to treatment and for disease progression. A bone scan may be carried out at follow-up to localize and define the extent of metastases.

There is no non-invasive method of staging pelvic lymph nodes. Patients considered suitable for either radiotherapy or radical surgery as primary treatment should have the pelvic lymph nodes staged either by open or by laparoscopic surgery.

Treatment

Prostatic cancer, like breast cancer, is sensitive to endocrine influences. Management is best considered in four clinical groups:

Incidental or focal cancer. Such patients will usually have had a prostatectomy and the diagnosis of cancer is made incidentally on histological examination. With increasing use of PSA, a raised value may be the only abnormality that leads to the diagnosis of cancer confirmed by a needle biopsy. A patient with a small focus of well-differentiated carcinoma may be managed by a watch-and-wait policy because treatment is rarely required for these tumours and the patient has a normal life expectancy. A large tumour with a less well-differentiated cell pattern may progress; either radical surgery or radiotherapy is recommended for a man with a life expectancy of more than 10 years.

Organ confined cancer; no evidence of bone metastases. If the general health of the patient is good then either radical surgery or radiotherapy should be considered. Endocrine treatment is kept in reserve until there is evidence of tumour progression.

Metastatic prostate cancer. Approximately half of the men with prostate cancer will have metastatic disease at the time of diagnosis. The basis of treatment is either androgen depletion by surgery (orchiectomy) or androgen suppression by drugs (gonadotrophin-releasing hormone analogues with or without an antiandrogen).

Secondary treatment. A small proportion of patients fail to respond to endocrine treatment. A larger number respond for a year or two, but then the disease progresses. Other oestrogens or progesterones are of limited value but chemotherapy with 5-fluorouracil, cyclophosphamide or nitrogen mustard may be effective. Radiotherapy is effective treatment for localized bone pain. For severe generalized bone pain, hemi-body radiotherapy, hypophysectomy or strontium-89 may give effective palliation but the basis of treatment remains pain control by analgesia.

Prognosis

The life-expectancy of a patient with an incidental finding of focal carcinoma of the prostate is that of the normal population. With tumours localized to the prostate, a 10-year survival rate of 50% can be expected but if metastases are present this falls to 10%.

Testicular tumours

Tumours of the testes, although uncommon, occur mainly in men between the age of 20–40 years. In the UK there are over 1000 new cases per year and the incidence is increasing. These tumours secrete 'tumour markers' which provide good indices for both diagnosis and prognosis. Seminoma and teratoma account for 85% of all tumours of the testis. Malignant lymphoma, yolk-sac tumours, interstitial cell tumours and Sertoli cell/mesenchyme tumours make up the remainder.

Seminoma. This tumour arises from seminiferous tubules and is of relatively low-grade malignancy. The cut surface has a uniformly grey appearance. Microscopically, the cell type varies from well-differentiated spermatocytes to undifferentiated round cells. Metastases occur mainly via the lymphatics and may involve the lungs.

Teratoma (non-seminomatous tumour). This tumour arises from primitive germinal cells. It may contain cartilage, bone, muscle, fat and a variety of other tissues and is classified according to the degree of differentiation. Well-differentiated tumours are the least aggressive; at the other extreme, trophoblastic teratoma is highly malignant. Occasionally, teratoma and seminoma occur in the same testis.

Clinical features

The history is often vague and symptoms may be attributed to an injury or there may be pain and swelling suggesting inflammation. The patient may wrongly have received treatment for 'acute epididymitis'. Very rarely, patients with teratoma may complain of gynaecomastia.

Irrespective of the history, any new painless testicular lump in a young man must be regarded with suspicion. A hydrocele in a young man also demands investigation and testicular tumours may be accompanied by blood-stained effusion in the tunica vaginalis.

The peak age for a teratoma is 20–30 years and for a seminoma 30–40 years, but either may occur at any age.

Investigation

As soon as a tumour is suspected, and before orchiectomy, serum levels of alphafetoprotein (AFP) and the beta-subunit of human chorionic gonadotropin (HCG) should be determined. The levels of these 'tumour markers' are increased in extensive disease.

Testicular ultrasound is very useful in assessing abnormalities within the scrotum. Accurate staging is based on CT scans of the lungs, liver and

---

Prostatic cancer

- In the UK this is the third commonest cancer in men, presents at a mean age of 70, and is increasing in incidence.

- The carcinoma may be incidental (i.e. found incidentally on histological examination), clinical (prostatism and a hard craggy prostate) or occult (metastatic disease).

- Metastatic spread may occur early; one-third of clinically confined cancers have spread to lymph nodes while more than half of all new cases have bony spread (to lumbar spine and pelvis).

- Treatment of prostatic cancer varies:
  - *Incidental or focal cancer.* If well differentiated, then normal life expectancy can occur with a watch-and-wait policy. If the cancer contains undifferentiated cells then either radical surgery or radiotherapy is considered.
  - *Localized cancer with no evidence of bony metastases* is treated by either radical surgery or radiotherapy, keeping endocrine therapy in reserve.
  - *Metastatic cancer* is treated by androgen depletion (orchiectomy) or androgen suppression (gonadotropin-releasing hormone analogues).

- The overall 5-year survival rate is 25% but tumours localized to the prostate carry a 10-year survival rate of 50%.

retroperitoneal area, and an assessment of renal and pulmonary function.

Tumours are staged according to the following classification:

I No evidence of metastases
II Metastases confined to abdominal nodes
III Involvement of supra- and infradiaphragmatic lymph nodes, no extralymphatic metastases
IV Extralymphatic metastases.

Treatment

Through an inguinal incision the cord is ligated and divided at the internal ring and the testis is removed. Subsequent treatment depends on the histological report. Radiotherapy is the treatment of choice for early stage seminoma since this tumour is very radiosensitive.

The management of a teratoma depends on the stage of the disease. Early disease confined to the testes may be managed without further treatment provided that there is close surveillance for at least 2 years; tumour progression is treated by chemotherapy. More advanced cancers are managed initially by chemotherapy, usually the combination of bleomycin, etoposide and cisplatin. The place of retroperitoneal lymph node dissection is now less certain because of the effectiveness of chemotherapy.

AFP and beta-HCG each offer a valuable means of monitoring response to treatment and detecting recurrent disease. Both markers should be monitored in all patients with testicular tumours for at least 2 years after they are considered to be tumour-free.

CT, in addition to being useful in staging, can be used to follow the response of enlarged lymph nodes to treatment.

Prognosis

The 5-year survival rate for patients with seminoma is 90–95%. The more variable prognosis of teratomas depends on tumour type, stage and volume. With more favourable tumours the 5-year survival rate may be as high as 95% but in more advanced cases 60–70% is more usual.

Carcinoma of the penis

This uncommon tumour is generally attributed to poor hygiene associated with a non-retractile

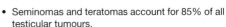

Testicular tumours

- In the UK there are about 1000 new cases of testicular tumour per year and the age group 20–40 is predominantly affected.

- Seminomas and teratomas account for 85% of all testicular tumours.

- Seminomas arise from the seminiferous tubules, are of relatively low-grade malignancy, spread predominantly via the lymphatic system and are very sensitive to radiotherapy.

- Teratomas arise from germinal cells, their differentiation reflects their aggressiveness (well-differentiated tumours are the least aggressive), and they are not radiosensitive.

- Treatment consists of orchiectomy with division of the spermatic cord at the level of the deep inguinal ring. Radiotherapy is used if the tumour proves to be a seminoma, whereas chemotherapy (bleomycin, etoposide and cisplatin) is used for teratomas that are advanced or recurrent.

- Seminomas have a 5-year survival rate of 90–95% while teratomas have a more varied prognosis (60–95% 5-year survival rate).

foreskin. It is very rare in circumcised men and occurs only in the elderly.

The cancer may be either a papillary or an ulcerating squamous cell carcinoma. Local spread occurs early and the tumour may ulcerate and fungate. Lymphatic spread to inguinal lymph nodes is common but infection of the tumour may also lead to inguinal node enlargement.

Clinical features

The patient may present with a purulent or blood-stained discharge. Unfortunately, many patients do not seek help until the lesion is advanced and ulcerating, and some present only when much of the penis is already destroyed and inguinal lymph nodes are involved.

Treatment

The diagnosis must be confirmed by biopsy. Early tumours respond dramatically to bleomycin. An initial circumcision is required to keep the tumour area clean and treat any infection. Advanced tumours require partial amputation and bilateral block dissection of the inguinal lymph nodes. Inoperable tumours are treated by palliative radiotherapy.

TRAUMA

Kidney and renal pedicle

Open injuries.   The kidney and renal pedicle may be injured by a gunshot or stab wound. Inadvertent damage during percutaneous needle biopsy can cause severe bleeding and rarely an arteriovenous fistula. Open lacerations of the parenchyma, collecting system or pedicle are usually associated with other injuries within the abdomen.

Closed injuries.   These are of two main types.

Direct blunt injury may be caused by a fall against the edge of the bath (or similar hard object) or by a blow or kick in the loin. These injuries are commonly associated with fractured ribs and, if on the right side, with injury to the liver.

Major renal trauma may occur as a result of rapid deceleration, as in aircraft or road accidents. The pedicle is injured rather than the kidney. Deceleration injuries to the pedicle may cause intimal tears, spasm or thrombosis of the vessels.

The late effects of renal trauma include perirenal collection of urine (urinoma), scarring of the kidney, or renal artery stenosis (hypertension). Hydronephrosis may be an early or late complication.

Clinical features

While a gunshot wound is obvious, a penetrating knife wound may appear trivial even if it involves several important deep structures.

Commonly, the patient presents with a history of injury (sometimes trivial) to the loin followed by haematuria. Usually, the worse the haematuria, the worse the renal damage. Thus, a bruise or contusion of the kidney causes mild haematuria, a laceration moderate haematuria, while a fragmented kidney causes gross haematuria. Severe injuries are characterized by a mass in the loin which is increasing in size, and signs of shock. These patients may have injuries to other organs. Damage to the renal pedicle may cause few signs or the patient may be severely shocked.

Investigation

Urgent intravenous urography is indicated to determine the extent of renal damage. A shocked patient must be resuscitated but urographic information about the other kidney must always precede emergency surgery.

With mild contusion the urogram may be normal.

With increasing damage there is distortion of the renal outline and calyces, and extravasation of contrast. Non-visualization of the kidney implies serious damage to the pedicle and is an indication for angiography. Angiography is also helpful in assessing parenchymal/vascular damage in patients who are likely to need surgical exploration.

A renal scan using technetium-labelled dimercaptosuccinic acid and ultrasonography are of more help in the follow-up of an injured kidney than in immediate care.

Treatment

Renal contusion is managed conservatively by bed rest and observation.

Lacerations which are part of an open injury are explored to determine the extent of the damage. Those due to closed injury may be treated conservatively at first, but should be explored if haematuria persists or loin swelling increases. Severe lacerations with fragmentation of the kidney must be explored.

The extent of operation depends on the severity of the laceration. Whenever possible, partial rather than total nephrectomy is carried out.

Ureter

Open injuries.   A ureter is occasionally damaged by a knife or a bullet, but always in association with other injuries.

The principal cause of injury to a ureter is inadvertent damage during an operation involving the colon, rectum, bladder, major abdominal blood vessels and, most commonly of all, the uterus. The proximity of the ureter to these organs means that it is frequently affected by direct spread of a variety of pathological conditions. Surgical damage may lead to complete or partial obstruction with subsequent hydronephrosis, or to a urinary fistula. A fistula may occur immediately (if damage is not recognized at operation) or later (if the injury to the ureter causes late necrosis). Urine may leak to the skin (cutaneous fistula), form a 'urinoma' or, after a gynaecological operation, leak through the vagina (ureterovaginal fistula).

Closed injuries.   The ureter is occasionally damaged in major road traffic accidents.

Clinical features

The patient may complain of renal pain after an operation but even a completely obstructed kidney may cause few symptoms. If there is infection in the obstructed kidney, the patient may be extremely ill with pain, fever and rigors. Any excessive 'watery' discharge from a wound is suspicious.

Investigation

A rapid way to determine whether a watery discharge is urine or serum is to measure its concentration of urea. Alternatively, intravenous methylene blue quickly appears in a urinary leak. An IVU will show the side of the damage and after ureteric injury there is always some hold-up in the contrast on the affected side. This differs from the urogram in a patient with a *vesicovaginal* fistula, where the upper tract is usually normal.

If there is still uncertainty as to whether a vaginal leak is from the ureter or bladder, discoloration of a vaginal swab after intravesical instillation of methylene blue will confirm that the leak is from the bladder.

Occasionally, cystoscopy and ureteric catheterization are indicated.

Treatment

Early exploration of the wound is advised to avoid infection. Provided it has sufficient length, a damaged lower ureter can be reimplanted directly into the bladder. If the ureter is short, the gap may be bridged by a tube of bladder (Boari flap) (Fig. 36.14) or by drawing up the bladder and fixing it to the psoas muscle (psoas hitch).

If the ureter is too short for these procedures, it may be joined to the other ureter (ureteroureterostomy). However, if there is infection, or the patient has a poor prognosis because of the underlying disease, it may be best to remove the kidney or embolize the renal artery.

Bladder

Open injuries. The bladder may rupture as a result of a penetrating injury to the lower abdomen. In this case the bladder, urethra and rectum are all likely to be damaged. The bladder may also be injured in the course of extensive cancer operations in the pelvis. Occasionally, a large inguinal or femoral hernia may include bladder in the medial wall of the sac, and may be damaged during repair of the hernia. Unrecognized damage during surgical procedures may lead to a wound fistula, a vesicovaginal fistula or a vesicocolic fistula.

Closed injuries. Intraperitoneal rupture typically occurs in a patient who has been drinking alcohol, has a full bladder and is assaulted and kicked in the abdomen. The dome of the bladder ruptures and urine extravasates into the peritoneum (Fig. 36.15a), causing intestinal ileus and abdominal distension.

Extraperitoneal rupture is usually due to a major road traffic accident in which the pelvis has also been fractured (Fig. 36.15b), but may follow endoscopic resection of the prostate or a bladder tumour.

Clinical features

The ileus and distension that occur with intraperitoneal rupture of the bladder are often detected late because of the circumstances surrounding the injury. However, the patient will soon note that he is not passing urine and seeks advice.

Extraperitoneal extravasation of urine, if part of a

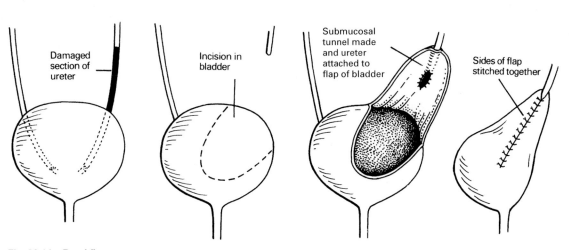

Fig. 36.14 Boari flap.

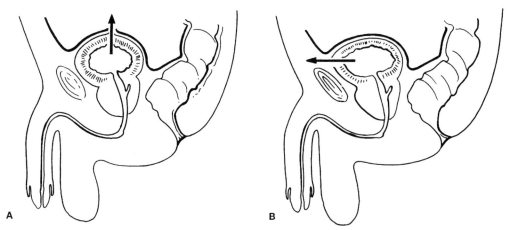

Fig. 36.15 Rupture of the bladder: A intraperitoneal; **B** extraperitoneal.

major accident, adds to what already are severe pelvic symptoms. When the leak occurs during an endoscopic procedure, the patient later complains of suprapubic pain with varying degrees of lower abdominal tenderness.

Investigation

Generally, the circumstances of the bladder injury establish the diagnosis. If confirmation of bladder injury is required, water-soluble contrast is injected via a urethral catheter and the bladder examined on the X-ray screen.

Treatment

Intraperitoneal rupture demands laparotomy. The bladder rupture is oversewn, the viscera are examined for other injuries and drainage by a urethral catheter is established. Extraperitoneal rupture of the bladder may require surgical exploration to remove blood and serum, correct bony injuries, close the tear and establish bladder drainage.

If urine has extravasated during any pelvic operation, a urethral catheter to keep the bladder empty is usually all that is needed. Very rarely a suprapubic drain is required.

Urethra

Open injuries. Penetrating injuries resulting in damage to the anterior or posterior urethra are rare.

Closed injuries. Damage to the *anterior urethra* is typically due to falling astride a hard object, although a kick can cause a similar injury. There may be contusion or laceration, and a laceration may be partial or complete.

The mechanism of injury to the *posterior urethra* is similar to that of extraperitoneal rupture of the bladder, e.g. a road traffic accident. For such an injury to damage the urethra, a fracture of the pubis or fracture-dislocation of the pelvis must occur. Both posterior urethra and bladder are damaged in 10% of cases. The urethral rupture may be partial or complete.

Injury to the posterior urethra may also be iatrogenic. Inexpert instrumentation can tear the mucosa and cause a false passage and subsequent stricture formation.

Clinical features

Anterior urethral injuries are usually located at the bulb so that the patient presents with a perineal haematoma. If this haematoma becomes infected, there may be sloughing of the skin, urethra and even scrotal tissues.

Because of the mechanism of injury, patients with posterior urethral tears are usually shocked and require resuscitation before a detailed assessment can be made. If the patient has passed clear urine, the bladder and urethra are probably intact. If there is blood at the external meatus, urethral injury must be suspected. A distended bladder can occur because of spasm of the urethral sphincter or because of a torn posterior urethra.

Investigation

If the physical signs suggest an *anterior* urethral injury and the patient has passed clear urine, no further steps need be taken. If there is blood at the external meatus or the urine is blood-stained, a urethrogram using water-soluble contrast material may demonstrate the extravasation.

There is a strongly held view that any investigative procedure of the *posterior* urethra is dangerous and may worsen the urethral injury. A catheter should never be passed in the emergency room 'just to see'. If the patient passes clear urine, nothing further should be done. If the urine is blood-stained, retrograde urethrography may be carried out. The radiological distinction between an extraperitoneal bladder rupture and rupture of the membranous urethra may be difficult. Catheterization for these injuries is best carried out at the time of other surgical procedures with full aseptic precautions.

Treatment

All patients with an injury to the bulb of the urethra have a perineal haematoma. This will resolve if the injury is only a contusion but prophylactic antibiotics are indicated. A large haematoma may need to be drained if the urethra has been lacerated. The extent of injury should be defined and the urethra repaired if possible. The bladder is drained by a urethral or suprapubic catheter.

Treatment of a posterior urethral injury depends on the expertise available. It is quite acceptable to perform a suprapubic cystostomy and deal with the injury to the urethra at a later date. If laparotomy is necessary for other reasons, this may give an opportunity to pass a catheter. If the rupture is incomplete, the catheter will act as a splint. If the rupture is complete, the ends of the urethra can be approximated and splinted by the catheter.

The late complication of these injuries is stricture and impotence.

EXTERNAL GENITALIA

Penis

Circumcision

The foreskin is normally non-retractile in the first few months of life. By the end of the first year, half will retract but it may be 3–4 years before all do so. Provided the parents are reassured, there is no reason, *apart from religious grounds*, to remove the foreskin within the first few years of life.

In some children the foreskin remains non-retractile and has to be treated by division of preputial adhesions or circumcision. Otherwise, secretions collect under the foreskin, leading to infection (balanitis) and narrowing of the orifice (phimosis). In those whose foreskin can retract, but not easily, pain during intercourse may be a problem in later years. If there are difficulties in keeping the glans and coronal sulcus clean, accumulated secretions may predispose to carcinoma of the penis.

If a poorly retracting foreskin remains retracted, it can act as a tight band and cause engorgement and oedema of the glans (paraphimosis). This demands urgent treatment. It may be possible to compress the glans and draw the foreskin forwards, but if this fails, the tight band must be incised under general anaesthesia. Later elective circumcision is advocated.

Congenital abnormalities

Hypospadias. Failure of fusion of embryonic folds results in abnormal placing of the external urinary meatus on the ventral surface of the penis. The opening may be coronal, penile, scrotal or even perineal. With opening in these latter sites, the corpus spongiosum is scarred and fibrosed, leading to a ventral curvature or *chordee* of the penis.

The aim of treatment is to correct the chordee by excising the fibrosis and then to perform a plastic surgical operation to make a new urethral opening in the normal position on the glans. This procedure should be completed before the boy goes to school.

Epispadias. In this condition, the external urinary meatus opens on the dorsal surface of the penis. The extent of the malformation varies from a penile abnormality to a gross failure in development of the bladder and urethra. Severe deformity results from extension of the cloacal membrane onto the lower abdominal wall, preventing the two halves of the wall from closing over the developing bladder. As a result, the mucosa of the bladder and the ureteric orifices are exposed and form the infra-umbilical part of the abdominal wall (exstrophy). The urethra lies opened out and the testes are undescended; additional abnormalities include separation of the symphysis pubis and rectal prolapse.

Reconstruction of these deformities is not always successful and urinary incontinence may remain a major problem and require urinary diversion.

Disorders of erection

Priapism. In this condition there is a maintained erection, unassociated with sexual desire. It occurs in association with leukaemia, disorders of coagulation, renal dialysis and sickle-cell trait, and is believed to be due to sludging of venous blood in the sinuses of the corpora cavernosa. Thus the painful erection affects the corpora cavernosa but not the corpus spongiosum or glans.

Non-operative methods to relieve the congestion such as spinal anaesthesia, heparinization and aspiration of the thickened blood are ineffective. Insertion of a venous shunt (e.g. saphenous vein to corpus cavernosum or corpora cavernosa to corpus spongiosum) carried out within 6–12 hours, gives satisfactory results and the patient can achieve normal erections subsequently. If treatment is delayed or incomplete, the erectile tissue is damaged and the patient will be impotent.

Priapism may also occur as a complication of intracavernosal self injection for impotence. Treatment by aspiration and intracavernosal phenylephrine will usually correct this type of priapism.

Peyronie's disease. This is the occurrence of a hard fibrous plaque (or plaques) in the wall of a corpus cavernosum causing lateral curvature of the penis. The cause is obscure but is possibly related to trauma leading to the formation of hard scar tissue in a corpus cavernosum. In addition to the deformity, the patient complains of pain during intercourse.

Various treatments including cortisone injections, vitamins and radiotherapy have met with little success. Excision of the plaque with replacement by a dermal patch graft, or excision of a wedge of tissue on the convex (opposite) border of the penis may prove effective.

Impotence

Impotence may be psychogenic, organic or drug-induced. Although loss of libido may be due to a generalized illness or endocrine disease, the majority of patients who complain of impotence have a psychosexual disturbance.

Psychogenic causes can be established from a careful history that includes details of sexual habits. However, it is important to exclude organic causes so that the correct advice may be given.

Organic impotence may occur with diabetes mellitus or neurogenic disorders, after major pelvic injury or operations, or with vascular disease of the pelvic vessels (e.g. Leriche syndrome), priapism and Peyronie's disease. Most of these conditions cause irreversible impotence, but angiography may help to define a treatable abnormality.

Drug-induced impotence occurs in patients receiving oestrogens for prostatic cancer. In addition, some antihypertensive drugs may cause loss of erection or inability to ejaculate. Drugs such as barbiturates, benzodiazepines, corticosteroids, phenothiazines and spironolactone may all affect libido.

Medical treatment is by intracavernosal injection of papaverine or prostaglandin E. Vacuum devices or implantation of prostheses into the corpora cavernosa are effective alternatives to self injection.

Scrotum

Examination of the scrotal contents should follow a simple routine. With the patient supine, the configuration of the scrotum and the scrotal wall is first observed. The contents of the scrotum are then palpated between the thumb and index and middle fingers. In sequence the testes, head, body and tail of the epididymis, the cord and the external inguinal ring are checked. With the patient standing and the doctor seated, examination of the contents is repeated, specifically excluding an inguinal hernia and a varicocele.

Undescended testes (cryptorchidism)

Normally both testes should be in the scrotum within 6 months of birth. However, the testes may be excessively mobile and readily retract towards the external inguinal ring or into the inguinal canal, especially when the patient is examined in a cold room. Such *retractile* testes may easily be misdiagnosed as being incompletely descended. Care must be taken to examine the baby in a warm room or after a bath.

Undescended testes are of two types: incompletely descended and ectopic.

Incomplete descent of the testis. Such a testis is arrested in its normal pathway to the scrotum. Usually this is within the inguinal canal, more rarely within the abdomen. The testis is smaller than normal and cannot be palpated. Its ability to produce sperm is doubtful.

As the spermatic cord is short, such testes are difficult to bring down into the scrotum by operation (orchiopexy). If this can be carried out before the age of 2–4 years, the testis may be of some use; otherwise it should be removed.

Occasionally, an incompletely descended testis is situated just inside the external inguinal ring through which it can be coaxed (*emergent testis*). Testes that remain incompletely descended have a 1 in 77 chance of becoming malignant: the risk is greater if the testis is retained in the abdomen. Laparoscopy is used increasingly to locate and remove an intra-abdominal testis.

Ectopic testis. It is important to distinguish an ectopic from an incompletely descended testis. An ectopic testis has developed normally but after passing through the external inguinal ring its further descent is impeded. It either remains in the superficial inguinal pouch (common) or is transposed to perineal, femoral or prepubic sites (rare).

Because an ectopic testis is normal in size, it is palpable and its cord is normal. Orchiopexy is achieved without difficulty. Provided this is done early, preferably before the age of 6 years, spermatogenesis is believed to occur normally. However, even if the diagnosis is not made until later (frequently just before puberty), orchiopexy should still be performed.

Orchiopexy consists of mobilizing the testis and its cord and placing the testis in the scrotum. Various methods are used to stop the testis from retracting towards the inguinal canal. The simplest is to place the testis in a pouch between the dartos muscle and scrotal skin (Fig. 36.16).

As indicated above, mobilization of an ectopic testis and placement in a dartos pouch is easy. Because of the shorter cord, an incompletely descended testis can be brought into the scrotum only with difficulty.

Torsion of the testis

Torsion is due to an abnormality of the visceral layer of the tunica vaginalis which completely covers the testis so that it is suspended within the parietal layer and can twist the cord. Torsion is a surgical emergency. Delay in diagnosis or treatment may lead to loss of the testis.

Characteristically the patient, usually a teenager, presents with an acutely tender, swollen testis of sudden onset. There may be a history of minor trauma or previous episodes of pain in the testis due to partial torsion. On examination there is a red, swollen hemiscrotum which is usually too tender to palpate. Misdiagnosis of the swelling as epididymo-

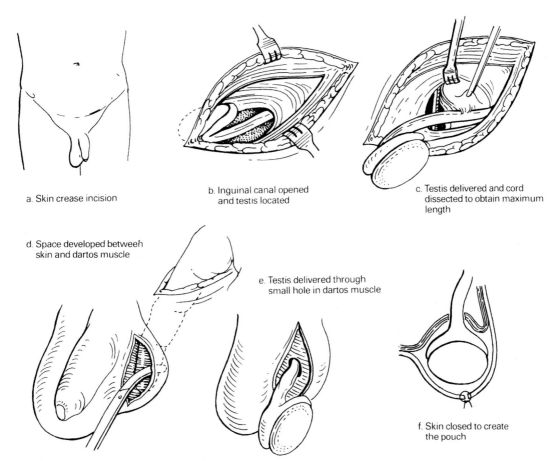

a. Skin crease incision

b. Inguinal canal opened and testis located

c. Testis delivered and cord dissected to obtain maximum length

d. Space developed between skin and dartos muscle

e. Testis delivered through small hole in dartos muscle

f. Skin closed to create the pouch

Fig. 36.16   Dartos pouch fixation of testis.

orchitis, which is rare in teenagers, is a serious error.

The scrotum must be explored as soon as possible so that the twist can be reversed and the blood supply restored. If this is not done within 12–18 hours, the testis infarcts and must be excised. If the testis is viable, it is fixed by suture or by creating a dartos pouch. Since the underlying abnormality of the tunica is bilateral, the other testis must be fixed to its parietal tunica vaginalis *at the same time*. Otherwise, torsion may occur later on that side with disastrous effects on fertility.

Hydrocele

This is a common condition, especially in older men, in which fluid collects in the tunica vaginalis, resulting in an enlarged but painless scrotum. The inconvenience of its size usually leads the patient to seek advice.

The cause of most hydroceles is unknown (idiopathic). The fluid is straw-coloured and protein-rich. In some patients it develops as a reaction to epididymo-orchitis. Rarely, it may develop with a malignant testis (secondary hydrocele) and the fluid may then be blood-stained.

On examination of the scrotum there is a smooth oval swelling above which a normal spermatic cord can be palpated. The fluid around the testis transilluminates when a torch is held against the scrotum, but in long-standing hydroceles this may be difficult to elicit owing to fibrosis and thickening of its wall. It is important always to seek this physical sign and also to examine the neck of the scrotum carefully to exclude an inguinal hernia as the cause of the swelling.

It may be possible to palpate the testis and confirm that it is normal, but this is unusual as it lies behind and is enveloped by the hydrocele. If there is any doubt about the diagnosis then an ultrasound study should be done. If ultrasound is not available, then the fluid is aspirated and the testes re-examined to exclude a tumour. If there is still doubt, exploration is indicated to exclude a testicular tumour.

Injury to the scrotum may result in a swelling that resembles a hydrocele but does not transilluminate because the tunica has filled with blood (*haematocele*).

Aspiration alone does not cure an idiopathic hydrocele and the tunica soon refills. It is possible to obliterate the sac by injecting a sclerosant after aspiration, but preferably it should be excised or everted so that recurrence is prevented.

If the hydrocele fluid becomes infected, incision and drainage of the pus are necessary. Similarly, a haematocele may require treatment by incision and drainage.

Varicocele

The veins of the pampiniform plexus are dilated and tortuous, producing a swelling in the line of the spermatic cord which resembles a 'bag of worms'. It is more common on the left side because of the right-angled drainage of the testicular vein into the renal vein, which renders it more liable to stasis. In some men, varicocele is associated with infertility. A dragging sensation in the scrotum may cause concern.

Treatment is by ligation of the spermatic vein: this may be done surgically at the internal inguinal ring or laparoscopically or radiologically by embolization.

Cyst of the epididymis

Cysts in the epididymis arise from diverticula of the vasa efferentia. The distinction between a cyst of the epididymis and a hydrocele is easy. Epididymal cysts are almost always multiple and therefore nodular on palpation; they are located above and behind the testis, which is palpably separate from the cysts, and always transilluminate brightly.

A solitary epididymal cyst may even resemble a testis, so giving rise to fables of three testes.

Sometimes the fluid within an epididymal cyst is opalescent and contains sperms (it is then called a *spermatocele*). Usually the fluid is clear.

It is best to leave these cysts alone unless increasing size warrants excision. Careful dissection is needed to remove the cyst completely. Often several other little cysts are present which, if not removed, will eventually increase in size and produce a so-called recurrence. If all the cysts are removed, the pathway for sperm will almost certainly be damaged. Bilateral operation can result in sterility.

Epididymo-orchitis

Acute epididymo-orchitis is usually the appropriate term as both testis and epididymis are involved in the acute inflammatory reaction. Further, the spermatic cord is often thickened (funiculitis). After infection has subsided, the epididymis alone may remain thickened and irregular, so that chronic epididymitis may be diagnosed. Thus a late effect of tuberculosis is an irregularly hard (craggy) epididymis.

Apparent involvement of the testis alone may be a feature of viral infections such as mumps orchitis.

The usual cause of epididymo-orchitis is bacterial spread, either from infected urine or from gonococcal urethritis. The affected side of the scrotum is swollen, inflamed and very tender. In all cases the urine or urethral discharge must be cultured. Sometimes there is no evidence of a bacterial cause and a viral aetiology is then likely.

Treatment consists of antibiotics, bed rest and a scrotal support. The choice of antibiotic depends on the results of culture and sensitivity determination of the organism responsible. If there is any doubt about the diagnosis, the testis should be explored.

Abscess formation is now rare, but if signs of localization or fluctuation develop, the pus should be drained. An important late complication of epididymo-orchitis is infertility.

Infertility

The investigation and management of infertility requires assessment of both partners, but only aspects of male infertility will be discussed here. While more patients are being referred for investigation, management of infertility is still very limited in its success. Often it consists only of clarifying the diagnosis and appropriate counselling.

A detailed history is essential, particularly with regard to factors that may contribute to an abnormal sperm count. These include operations (e.g. for hernia), infections such as mumps, tuberculosis, and gonorrhoea, and drugs (nitrofurazone, cyclophosphamides and possibly some tranquillisers). Excessive smoking, alcohol intake, obesity and working in a hot environment may all suppress spermatogenesis. The patient should be asked about any psychosexual problems, including impotence or premature ejaculation.

Physical examination may be entirely normal. Body build and hair distribution are noted. Testicular size is a crude but useful guide to spermatogenic potential. For example, a tall male with female hair distribution and pea-sized testes almost certainly has Klinefelter's syndrome. Examination of the scrotum may reveal dilated spermatic veins (varicocele).

The principal investigation is analysis of seminal fluid. The values given as 'normal' are only a guide, for pregnancy can occur with low sperm concentrations (oligozoospermia). However, the lower the concentration of sperms, the less the chance of pregnancy.

If a patient has no sperm (azoospermia), it is necessary to distinguish between obstruction and primary failure of spermatogenesis. This may be possible by measuring plasma gonadotropins (FSH). A normal value indicates obstruction which is usually in the epididymis. In these patients the testes are also normal in size. More detailed tests such as immunological compatibility and chromosome analysis may be necessary.

Management

There is no treatment for a patient with azoospermia due to primary spermatogenic failure. Testicular biopsy to confirm the diagnosis is all that is possible.

Azoospermia due to obstruction may be treated by bypass (epididymovasostomy). This may be successful if the obstruction is in the tail of the epididymis, but if it is elsewhere in the epididymis or vasa efferentia, the results are generally poor but new microscopically assisted in vitro fertilization techniques now offer a chance of success.

Patients with oligozoospermia are initially advised to reduce weight, improve dietary and smoking habits, and (if possible) adjust their occupation or working environment. It is important to ensure that the patient understands the basis of reproductive biology and especially the timing of intercourse in relation to the menstrual cycle. These measures alone often lead to a successful pregnancy.

The role of a varicocele as a cause of infertility is debatable. There is evidence that some varicoceles affect testicular temperature, and therefore spermatogenesis, and ligation of these veins is practised to avoid this effect. Most series have shown improvement in semen analysis following the ligation, but none of these studies is controlled.

Drug treatment for oligozoospermia is disappointing; clinical trials are in progress but no one treatment can at present be recommended. If infertility is due to antisperm antibodies, courses of high dose steroids may be of use.

Vasectomy and vasectomy reversal

Bilateral ligation of the vasa deferentia, in the neck of the scrotum, is now widely practised as a form of permanent contraception. This is usually done as an outpatient procedure under local anaesthesia. Each vas is divided and ligated, and the ends are separated in order to avoid recanalization.

It is essential to repeat the semen analysis 6–8 weeks postoperatively to confirm azoospermia. Two negative tests are required for assurance that fertilization cannot occur but the patient is still warned of the very rare chance of recanalization.

Reversal of a vasectomy may be requested, usually because of remarriage. Reported pregnancy rates vary from 50% to 80% following microsurgical repair.

DISORDERS OF CONTROL OF MICTURITION

Anatomy of the outflow tract

The *fundus* of the bladder consists of interlacing bundles of smooth muscle, the detrusor, which do not lie in defined layers. During the storage phase the detrusor stretches to accommodate the increased volume of urine but without an increase in intravesical pressure (compliance).

The *trigone* forms the base of the bladder and includes both ureteric orifices and the internal urethral orifice. It has two muscle layers:

1. The superficial trigonal muscle which merges with the ureteric muscle and extends down into the proximal urethra.
2. The deep trigonal muscle to which is attached the detrusor muscle.

The proximal urethral sphincter mechanism (bladder neck sphincter) in the male consists of specially adapted fibres of detrusor muscle arranged in a circular fashion at the bladder neck. These detrusor fibres are richly supplied with sympathetic nerves and close tightly with ejaculation to prevent retrograde passage of sperm.

The *distal urethral sphincter mechanism* (external sphincter) consists of intrinsic urethral (striated) muscle which surrounds the urethra distal to the verumontanum and forms the external urethral sphincter.

In the female the external urethral sphincter extends over the length of the urethra but is most prominent around the middle third.

Neurological control of micturition

The *parasympathetic* fibres arise from S2–4 as preganglionic axons, relay through the pelvic ganglia and, as postganglionic nerves, supply the detrusor muscle. These (cholinergic) nerves stimulate detrusor contraction.

Sympathetic fibres arise from T11–L1 and relay in the pelvic ganglia. Their exact role in the control of micturition unclear. It is known that alpha-adrenergic receptors and their nerve terminals are found mainly in the smooth muscle of the bladder neck and proximal urethra, whereas beta-receptors are found in the fundus of the bladder. The alpha-receptors respond to noradrenaline by stimulating contraction, while the beta-receptors relax the smooth muscle. It is possible that the sympathetic neurones play a role in both urethral closure and detrusor relaxation during the filling phase of the micturition cycle.

The distal sphincter mechanism is innervated from the sacral segments S2–4 by somatic motor fibres which reach the sphincter either by the pelvic plexus or via the pudendal nerves. Afferent nerves are carried in both the parasympathetic and pudendal pathways and transmit sensory impulses from the bladder, urethra and pelvic floor. These sensory impulses not only pass to the cerebral cortex and the micturition centre but also to the cord as part of the spinal cord reflexes. Thus bladder filling stimulates afferent impulses which stimulate pelvic floor contraction, so adding to urethral compression.

Cortical control is a basic part of the micturition cycle described below. The higher centres suppress detrusor contractions and their main function is to inhibit micturition until it is appropriate to micturate. Afferent impulses pass to the brain via the posterior columns and lateral spinothalamic tracts. Thus bladder sensation is transmitted bilaterally and is lost only when both tracts are divided. The higher centres are situated in the pons, anteromedial aspect of the frontal lobe, the cingulate gyrus and the paracentral lobule.

The micturition cycle

The micturition cycle, has three phases.

Storage (or filling) phase. Because of the high compliance (elasticity) of the detrusor muscle the bladder fills steadily without a rise in intravesical pressure. As the bladder volume increases, stretch receptors in the bladder wall are stimulated and once a threshold is reached there is the desire to void, which marks the end of this phase.

Postponement (or inhibitory) phase. Voluntary control is now exerted over the desire to void, which disappears temporarily. Compliance of the detrusor allows further increase in capacity until the next desire to void. Just how often this desire needs be inhibited depends on many factors, not the least of which is finding a suitable place in which to void.

Emptying (or micturition) phase. The act of micturition is initiated first by voluntary and then by reflex relaxation of the pelvic floor, followed by reflex detrusor contraction. These actions are coordinated by the micturition centre in the pons along spino-bulbo-spinal pathways. Intravesical pressure remains greater than urethral pressure until the bladder is empty.

The normal control of micturition requires co-ordinated reflex activity of autonomic and somatic nerves, as described above. These responses depend on normal anatomical structures and normal inner-vation. There are thus two main types of disorders of micturition: structural and neurogenic. Examples are extensive carcinoma of the prostate that has damaged the sphincter mechanism (structural) and spinal cord injury that has damaged the innervation (neurogenic).

DISORDERS OF MICTURITION

Disorders of micturition occur when there is either underactivity or overactivity of the bladder or urethral sphincter. The causes may be either struc-tural or neurogenic.

Structural disorders

Investigation

Abnormalities of function of the lower urinary tract are notoriously difficult to assess because there is frequently dual underlying pathology. For example, incontinence in an elderly man may be due to cortical deficiency resulting from cerebral degenera-tion but could also be due to chronic outflow tract obstruction resulting from prostatic hyperplasia.

The history is important but may be deceptive, mainly because different abnormalities can produce similar symptoms. The exact character of the urinary abnormality must be determined so that structural causes can be separated from neurological causes. Details of drug treatment are noted. Diuretics and drugs with anticholinergic side-effects may tip the balance when there is already dysfunction. Urine is tested for glycosuria and infection.

In addition to intravenous urography there is now a range of more specific methods for assessing micturition but not all are required for a diagnosis. Their value lies in resolving specific clinical ques-tions relating to management. These methods in-clude radiology (cystourethrography), urodynamic studies (uroflowmetry, cystometrography and urethral pressure measurement) and direct inspection (cysto-urethroscopy and pelvic examination under anaes-thesia).

A full history and physical examination, with cysto-urethroscopy and bimanual examination remain the basic initial investigation of structural disorders.

Structural causes of incontinence in males

Operation. Disordered control of micturition occurs in 3–5% patients after prostatectomy. In this operation the bladder neck sphincter is deliberately excised posteriorly but the external sphincter is carefully preserved. Any damage to the external sphincter can lead to difficulties with continence.

Other procedures on the urethra, such as repeated dilatations for urethral stricture or urethroplasty, may be followed by incontinence.

Stress incontinence occurs with any sudden increase in abdominal pressure, as with coughing. Since the damage to the sphincter is mild, it usually responds to physiotherapy.

Urge incontinence is not due to sphincter weakness but to involuntary contractions in an uninhibited or unstable bladder. Removal of the prostatic obstruc-tion alone is usually sufficient to correct urgency and urge incontinence, but antispasmodics may be necessary.

It must be emphasized that continence requires normal cortical control and this may be impaired in an elderly patient. Possible abnormalities of both structure and innervation need to be considered in these patients.

Disease. *Carcinoma of the prostate* may involve adjacent urethral structures. Repeated transurethral resections for recurring obstruction may be neces-sary. The net effect is to convert the posterior urethra into a rigid tube so that dribbling incontinence occurs, i.e. leakage of urine during the storage phase. An indwelling catheter or condom incontinence appliance may be necessary.

Benign prostatic enlargement may induce urgency with or without other obstructive symptoms. An early sign of benign enlargement, 'post-micturition dribble', is probably due to a small amount of urine being trapped between the proximal and distal mechanisms. A similar complaint may occur with prostatitis and early outflow changes of bilharziasis. Chronic retention with overflow or dribbling incon-tinence is dealt with on page 529.

Chronic illness and debility, especially in the elderly, may lead to incontinence because of poor tone in the periurethral striated muscle of the pelvic floor. This may be worsened by loss of cortical inhibition of micturition.

Structural causes of incontinence in females

Incontinence is more prevalent than generally suspected. As many as 50% of nulliparous young women may have some degree of stress incontinence and in approximately 20% this may occur daily. Overall, approximately 10% of women aged 15–64 years are incontinent twice or more per month. This figure rises rapidly in older patients and in geriatric units. Only a proportion of younger women seek advice, either because of embarrassment or because of stoical acceptance of some incontinence as a normal event.

Childbirth and operations. Multiparous women commonly lose some of the tone in the pelvic floor muscles with each pregnancy. Symptoms may range from occasional stress incontinence to dribbling incontinence. Examination shows weakening of the pelvic floor muscles and anterior vaginal wall (*cystocele*). It is important to distinguish stress incontinence from urge incontinence. The former responds to surgical procedures designed to support the bladder neck and strengthen the anterior vaginal wall, while the latter should be treated by drug therapy. Stress incontinence is characterized by an involuntary loss of urine during coughing, laughing, sneezing or any other activity that raises the intra-abdominal pressure suddenly. A cough, however, may stimulate involuntary detrusor contractions, which cause motor urge incontinence. This differential diagnosis can be made only by urodynamic assessment. Urge incontinence may thus be motor, due to unstable detrusor contractions, or sensory, in which infection or stones produce excessive sensory stimulation.

In parts of the world where obstetric services are poor, prolonged labour may lead to a *vesicovaginal fistula*, which presents as continuous dribbling incontinence. The association with delivery is usually clear, but a small fistula may be missed. Investigation of dribbling incontinence must distinguish between urethral damage and a fistula. Treatment consists of closing the fistula through a vaginal or suprapubic approach.

Hysterectomy may also be followed by urinary incontinence, suggesting damage to the ureter(s) at operation. Again, the association of an operation with incontinence should suggest the diagnosis of *ureterovaginal fistula*. Investigations are directed at establishing which ureter has been damaged. Treatment consists of reimplanting the ureter into the bladder.

Disease. *Cystitis* is common in women and in addition to causing frequency, urgency and dysuria, sometimes causes sensory urge incontinence. Treatment of both the infection and bladder spasm is required.

Chronic interstitial cystitis (Hunner's ulcer) is a chronic inflammatory condition which, in addition to causing frequency and dysuria, may also cause urgency and urge incontinence. Treatment is often unsatisfactory. Hydrostatic dilatation may be effective or the condition may respond to steroids.

The *urethral syndrome* is characterized by symptoms of cystitis in the absence of infection. There may be some incontinence. These patients often have a degree of urethral stenosis and urethral dilatation or incision may be successful. However, the urethral syndrome usually responds to regulation of micturition habits and careful perineal hygiene.

Dribbling incontinence in a child should raise the suspicion of an *ectopic ureter* in which the lower of the two ureters opens outside the control of the urethral mechanism. The abnormal ureter must be relocated in the bladder.

Carcinoma of the cervix or its treatment by radiotherapy may cause vesicovaginal fistula and incontinence.

Neurogenic disorders

A full history, including an interview with relatives, is required. Examination must include assessment of the plantar reflexes and sensation and tone of the anal canal. Glycosuria and urinary infection should be excluded.

Urodynamic, radiological and electromyographic studies may all be required.

Aetiology of abnormal micturition

Impaired cortical control. Diseases affecting the frontal lobe can alter the pattern of micturition by increasing or decreasing the frequency or affecting the social awareness of incontinence. Lesions such as cerebral thrombosis or cerebral degeneration may produce incontinence by failing to inhibit the postponement phase of micturition. The paracentral lobule controls the activity of skeletal muscle, so that lesions in this area may cause sustained pelvic and perineal muscular contraction. It must be remembered that a disorder of micturition may be accentuated by or even be due to the physical inability to prepare for micturition.

Emotional states may affect the postponement of micturition, giving rise to 'giggle' incontinence and possibly to enuresis in some patients. Incontinence with epilepsy is also due to a loss of inhibitory control. Excessive *sensory stimuli*, as with the pain of cystourethritis in women, may cause 'sensory urge incontinence'.

Drugs including alcohol may alter cortical control

of micturition. Sedatives can affect the postponement phase and precipitate incontinence, especially at night. The intoxicated patient may lack the mental alertness to maintain continence or may continually suppress the desire to void, leading to prostatic congestion and retention.

Damage to the spinal cord. Two aspects of disease or injury to the spinal cord influence disordered micturition, namely the level of the disease and the completeness of the damage.

Injury at or below the spinal reflex centre (S2, 3, 4) may be due to a fracture of the spine at the level of T12 and L1 which damages the conus medullaris, a central prolapsed intervertebral disc leading to cauda equina injury, or spinal stenosis. The bladder distends without sensation and the external sphincter is flaccid, and the cystometrogram is flat. The patient develops retention with overflow, but emptying is possible with abdominal straining or hand pressure.

Injury above the sacral segments (upper motor neurone lesions) includes fractures of the cervical spine or gunshot wounds. Tumours such as angiomas may compress the cord or it may be injured during surgical removal of the tumour. Diseases affecting the spinal cord include multiple sclerosis, transverse myelitis, and cervical cord stenosis.

If the central connections are disrupted, the patient develops a reflex bladder with impaired or absent cortical control. The bladder fails to empty completely, because of the unco-ordinated action of the detrusor and sphincter, and develops a thick, trabeculated wall. Usually the central connections are not completely disrupted and there may be some sensation and some cortical inhibition.

Damage to pelvic nerves. Operation may interrupt the autonomic pathways, especially when dissection involves the side walls of the pelvis, as in radical dissection of the rectum or the uterus. Similarly, aneurysm surgery may disrupt neural pathways in the pelvis.

Diseases affecting the autonomic system, principally diabetes mellitus, also affect the control of micturition.

With the loss of sensation and contraction, the bladder becomes an atonic sac, prone to the complication of stasis infection. The external sphincter remains closed by uninhibited tonic contractions, but the internal sphincter is partly open since it partly depends on detrusor activity.

Causes within the bladder. Primary failure of the detrusor has been described but is usually a sequel of chronic overdistension.

Atonic myogenic bladder is caused by prolonged outlet obstruction and is found in the late stages of bladder decompensation. The commonest cause is silent prostatic obstruction, where progressive loss of the desire to void results in overflow incontinence. In women, conscious postponement can lead to a large, atonic bladder.

Principles of management of disorders of micturition

- The diagnosis must be as complete as possible. More than one mechanism may account for disordered micturition. A urodynamic assessment is mandatory in all patients with a suspected or proven neuropathic bladder.
- Infection is the single most sinister complication and every effort must be made to prevent it.
- Renal damage (from vesicoureteric reflux) and chronic infection are the most serious complications of bladder and urethral dysfunction, and their prevention takes priority.
- Early management of spinal injury consists of continuous bladder drainage with a fine urethral catheter. Infection must be avoided.
- If there is evidence that the spinal reflex is intact, reflex activity may return to the bladder. Reflex activity leads to unco-ordinated micturition.

Micturition

- Micturition requires parasympathetic (S2–4) innervation of the detrusor, sympathetic innervation (T11–L1) of the bladder neck and proximal urethra, and somatic innervation (S2–4) of the bladder, pelvic floor and urethra.

- Structural causes of disordered micturition in the male include prostatic enlargement, prostatectomy (dribble, stress and urge incontinence) and chronic illness/debility.

- Structural causes of disordered micturition in the female include childbirth, surgery, radiotherapy and cystitis (infection, chronic interstitial cystitis and urethral syndrome).

- Neurogenic causes of disordered micturition are:
  - impaired cortical control,
  - alcohol abuse and drugs
  - spinal cord damage (at/below T12–L1 – flaccid bladder with overflow; above T12–L1 – reflex bladder with reduced cortical control which fails to empty)
  - pelvic nerve damage (surgery, diabetic autonomic neuropathy)
  - atonic myogenic bladder (prolonged outlet obstruction).

The bladder becomes thick-walled and sacculated and there is vesicoureteric reflux.

- In the absence of reflex activity, a large atonic bladder must be expressed manually. If this is unsatisfactory then clean intermittent self catheterization (CISC) is a very successful option. If CISC fails, the distal urethral mechanism can be incised to allow complete bladder emptying.

- For severe reflux and recurrent urinary infections, urinary diversion is indicated.

- Carefully selected cases may be treated by an artificial sphincter whose opening and closing is controlled by the patient. If the patient is not suitable for such a device, and especially in women in whom incontinence is difficult to control, early urinary diversion may be needed.

Section 9
NEUROLOGICAL SURGERY

37
Neurosurgery

CONTENTS

Although there is evidence that primitive man trepanned skulls and that in medieval times crude attempts were made at trepannation, tumour removal and nerve section, surgical neurology is a relatively new specialty. Conditions which may require neurosurgical intervention may affect the central nervous tissue itself, the coverings of the nervous tissue such as the meninges, or the bony compartments containing the nervous system. The signs and symptoms produced may be *generalized* (e.g. headache, vomiting, alterations in conscious level) due to increase in intracranial pressure, or *localized* (e.g. paralysis, sensory defect) because of damage to a specific area from trauma, local pressure, ischaemia or haemorrhage.

Increased intracranial pressure

The central nervous system (CNS) is enclosed in a rigid bony framework, and increases in mass content produced by tumour, haemorrhage, oedema or failure to reabsorb cerebrospinal fluid (CSF) result in an increase in pressure within the framework, particularly within the cranium. In children, the ununited cranium permits expansion of intracranial contents with smaller increases in intracranial pressure than in adults, although in certain situations hydrocephalus results (see p. 567).

Intracranial pressure normally fluctuates throughout the day and increases during coughing, defaecation or any circumstances which increase intrathoracic pressure. Such transient rises do no harm; only sustained increases produce disorders.

Increases in intracranial pressure lower perfusion pressure (i.e. intracerebral arterial pressure minus intracranial pressure), but autoregulatory processes initially maintain an effective perfusion pressure of above 40 mmHg. Intracranial vessels dilate as extracranial pressure increases, resulting in increased cerebral flow. If raised intracranial pressure (ICP) is unrelieved, bradycardia, hypertension and respiratory abnormalities (e.g. apnoea) develop with eventual progression to irreversible oedema, vasoparalysis and death.

Pressure may not increase uniformly throughout the intracranial and spinal cavities, producing distortion of vessels and local ischaemia. Marked displacement of intracranial structures may lead to three major types of herniation.

Transfalcine herniation. The cingulate gyrus herniates beneath the free edge of the falx. The anterior cerebral artery may be compressed sufficiently to produce medial hemisphere infarction, but otherwise there are no obvious clinical signs except deterioration in conscious level.

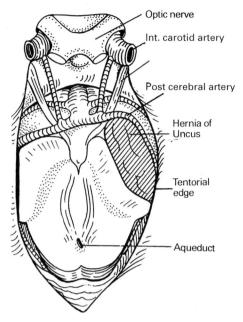

- Optic nerve
- Int. carotid artery
- Post cerebral artery
- Hernia of Uncus
- Tentorial edge
- Aqueduct

Fig. 37.1 Transtentorial herniation.

Transtentorial herniation. The medial part of the temporal lobe is pushed down through the tentorial notch to become wedged between the tentorial edge and the midbrain (Fig. 37.1). The opposite cerebral peduncle is pushed against the sharp tentorial edge, and the midbrain and uncus become wedged at the tentorium. The aqueduct is compressed, obstructing flow of CSF, and venous obstruction produces midbrain haemorrhage. The condition of the patient rapidly deteriorates. Epidural haematomas, or tumours or contusions of the temporal lobe are the usual causes.

Upward herniation is less common, but sometimes occurs with posterior fossa tumours. The pons and superior cerebellum become impacted at the tentorium.

Foraminal herniation. The cerebellar tonsils and medulla are displaced downwards through the foramen magnum, and cerebellar impaction occurs, causing medullary compression (Fig. 37.2). This may follow lumbar puncture and removal of CSF (also known as coning) in patients with raised intracranial pressure. Deterioration with loss of consciousness and decerebration is rapid. Thus, lumbar puncture should *not* be performed in patients suspected of having increased intracranial pressure.

Signs and symptoms of increased intracranial pressure

The principal symptoms are headache, vomiting and visual disturbance (Hippocratic triad), and papilloedema may be detected. Clinical suspicion should be aroused by any one of these signs or symptoms.

Headache is common but not invariable in patients with tumour. It is usually generalized, dull and aching, and may be exacerbated by straining, coughing or defaecation. It is classically worse in the morning, when it may be accompanied by vomiting.

Nausea or vomiting is more common in posterior fossa tumours than supratentorial lesions and may

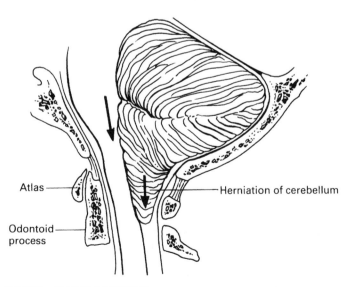

- Atlas
- Odontoid process
- Herniation of cerebellum

Fig. 37.2 Foraminal herniation.

be due more to medullary displacement than to generalized increase in pressure.

Visual disturbance in the form of transient *amblyopia* or blurred vision may occur in one or both eyes, particularly during straining or stooping. In the early stages of *papilloedema*, the retinal veins appear full and there is blurring of the nasal margin of the optic disc. Later, the disc becomes reddened and congested, with haemorrhagic streaks radiating from its edges, and filmy exudates form. Papilloedema is often present or more marked in one eye, but this is usually of no localizing significance.

Weight loss and anorexia may be present and usually indicate the presence of a tumour.

Bradycardia and *mild hypertension* are common in the later stages. *Intellectual deterioration* and *disorders of consciousness* occur as intracranial pressure rises progressively.

Assessment of consciousness level

Swelling, ischaemia or displacement of brainstem structures result in dysfunction of the reticular activating system in the brainstem which is concerned with consciousness. Continuing brainstem compression leads to deterioration of consciousness, coma and death.

Assessment of consciousness level is invaluable in the observation of patients with neurological disorders, where even minor changes in consciousness level may signal the need for urgent treatment.

The most useful coma classification is the Glasgow coma scale (GCS) (Table 37.1). This records the patient's responses to stimulation in terms of verbal response, motor response and pupillary reaction.

Focal signs of intracranial lesions

Compression or destruction of parts of the brain often produces subtle signs and symptoms long before there is evidence of increased intracranial pressure. The following signs are general pointers to the site of the pathology but are not specific. Displacement and the resulting ischaemia frequently produce symptoms from parts of the brain distant to the causative lesion.

Frontal lobe. Lesions of the frontal lobe are associated with intellectual and emotional changes, and may cause expressive dysphasia (dominant lobe lesion) and focal epilepsy. Contralateral faciobrachial weakness occurs in convexity lesions, and contralateral lower limb weakness in medial lesions. Lateral gaze paralysis with the eyes deviated to the

Table 37.1	Glasgow coma scale	
Eyes open	spontaneously	4
	to verbal command	3
	to pain	2
	no response	1
Best motor response		
to verbal command	obeys verbal command	6
	localizes pain	5
	flexion withdrawal	4
to painful stimulus	abnormal flexion (decorticate rigidity)	3
	extension (decerebrate rigidity)	2
	no response	1
Best verbal response	orientated and converses	5
	disorientated and converses	4
	inappropriate words	3
	incomprehensible sounds	2
	no response	1
Total number of points (minimum 3, maximum 15)		—

side suggests a destructive lesion on that side, while lateral gaze fixation with the eyes deviated to the side is more likely to be due to an irritating lesion on the opposite side. Urinary and faecal incontinence and anosmia may develop as the disease progresses.

Parietal lobe. Convexity lesions cause contralateral faciobrachial sensory loss, while medial lesions are associated with sensory loss in the lower limb. Astereognosis and sensory epilepsy also point to parietal lobe damage. Dominant lobe lesions produce receptive and global aphasia.

Occipital lobe. Patients with occipital lobe lesions may develop dyslexia (dominant lobe) and homonymous hemianopia.

Temporal lobe. Lesions in the temporal lobe may produce emotional changes, temporal lobe epilepsy, memory loss, receptive auditory disorder and homonymous quadrantanopia.

Cerebellum. Ipsilateral weakness, hypotonia, ataxia, dysmetria, and nystagmus all suggest a cerebellar lesion.

Brainstem. Lesions of the brainstem are commonly associated with cranial nerve palsies, and long-tract motor and sensory signs.

Cerebellopontine angle. Functional disturbance may develop in all or some of the 5th–12th cranial nerves. Weakness of the contralateral arm and/or leg and ipsilateral ataxia may also occur.

Basal tumours. Anosmia (unilateral or bilateral), optic nerve atrophy and paresis of eye movement suggest a basal tumour.

Pituitary or ***parapituitary tumours.*** Patients with such tumours may show early signs of visual disturbance and endocrine abnormalities.

Reaction of CNS to injury or infection

The reaction of the CNS to injury is similar to that of other tissues. Oedema is, however, more prominent because damage to the blood–brain barrier allows albumin, sodium and water to pass into the extracellular fluid (ECF). Oedema may be exacerbated by a number of factors, including a rise in Pa_{CO_2}. The injured area becomes surrounded by glial cells which phagocytose dead neurones and other material, and localize infection. Fibrosis (gliosis) or scarring is the final outcome.

Oedema may result in loss of function of involved neural cells, with recovery as it resolves. Irritation of cells may also result from oedema, or from their involvement in the scar process, leading to epilepsy, or pain if pain fibres are involved. Replacement of destroyed neurones by regeneration is not possible in the central nervous system.

Investigation of neurological disorders

A detailed history and careful examination are essential if the investigations available are to be used rationally.

A *full blood count* is needed in all patients. Severe anaemia and/or abnormal liver function should arouse the suspicion of metastatic disease, while polycythaemia in a patient with posterior fossa symptoms suggests cerebellar haemangioblastoma. A raised white count suggests infection. In patients with suspected pituitary tumours hormonal estimations should be made.

Lumbar puncture and *CSF examination* may help to confirm the diagnosis of meningitis, subarachnoid haemorrhage, or neoplasm. The investigation should not be carried out if raised ICP is suspected because of the risk of foraminal herniation and cerebellar coning.

Plain radiography

X-rays of the *skull* or *spine* are obtained routinely. Metastatic disease of the spine or skull is often clearly seen. A narrowed intervertebral disc space

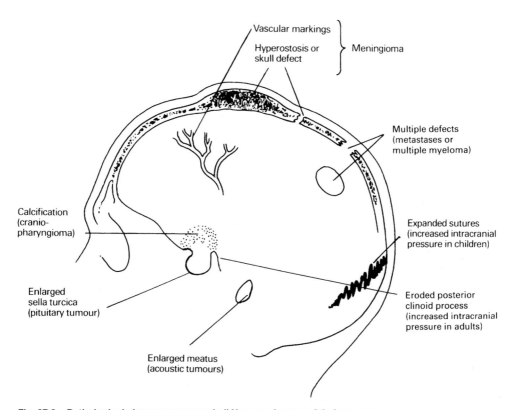

Fig. 37.3 Pathological changes seen on skull X-ray and some of their causes.

confirms prolapse of an intervertebral disc. Congenital disorders may be revealed by the abnormal shape of the skull. Raised ICP in children produces expansion of the sutures, while in adults the posterior clinoid processes are thinned. Enlargement of the sella turcica or internal auditory meatus may be due to pituitary or acoustic tumours respectively, while the vascular markings of the skull may be enlarged in the region of vascular tumours such as meningioma. Bony erosion or overgrowth (hyperostosis) are other features of meningioma. Calcification of the pineal gland or choroid plexus may reveal displacement of these structures, while abnormal calcification may develop within certain cysts or tumours (Fig. 37.3).

A *chest X-ray* should always be obtained. About 25% of cerebral tumours are secondary deposits from lung cancer. The chest X-ray may also reveal metastases from other primary sites.

Contrast radiology

Dye may be injected to outline the spinal cord and nerve roots (*myelography* or *radiculography*; Fig. 37.4) or the cerebral ventricles (*ventriculography*; Fig. 37.5). The ventricles and basal systems may also be filled with air injected via

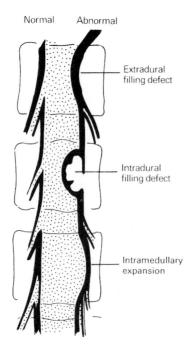

Fig. 37.4 Myelographic appearances of normal and abnormal spinal canal.

Normal   Abnormal

Extradural filling defect

Intradural filling defect

Intramedullary expansion

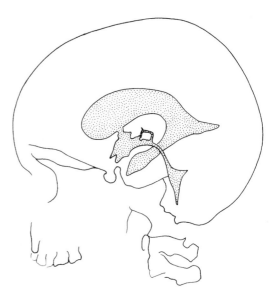

Fig. 37.5 Contrast radiology: normal ventriculogram.

lumbar puncture (*pneumo-encephalography*). This technique is contraindicated if raised intracranial pressure is suspected. Ventriculography or pneumo-encephalography are unnecessary if modern imaging techniques such as computerized tomography (CT) or magnetic resonance imaging (MRI) scans are available. *Angiography* may reveal lesions such as aneurysms and arteriovenous malformations, and display the relationship of important arteries to tumours.

Other imaging techniques

Computerized tomography (CT) is a non-invasive and accurate diagnostic technique (Fig. 37.6A). Ventricular enlargement and displacement, and the extent of tumours and abscesses with their associated oedema can be clearly shown. Haemorrhages and clots show up as dense areas, and the presence of even small haemorrhages and associated oedema may indicate subarachnoid haemorrhage. Intravenous contrast injection may 'enhance' the density of some lesions such as tumours.

Cerebral isotope scanning. This investigation has generally been supplanted by CT or MRI scanning. Technetium-99 was usually used as a marker. Vascular tumours such as meningiomas, metastases and some gliomas are readily revealed, but the vascularity of the neck muscles tends to obscure posterior fossa tumours. Isotope scanning does not provide as good anatomical detail as CT, but is a valuable method of assessing tumour vascularity

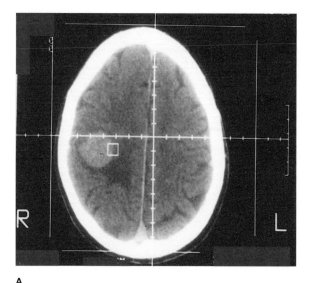

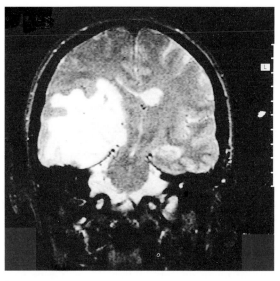

A

B

Fig. 37.6   A CT scan of brain tumour, probably, a metastasis. A ruled grid has been superimposed to provide accurate coordinates for stereotactic incision. **B** MRI scan of an extensive temporal lobe glioma demonstrated by a coronal reformation.

following radiotherapy or chemotherapy, and may be used to study cerebral blood flow and CSF flow.

Magnetic resonance imaging (MRI) and *positron emission tomography* (PET) scanning are new developments which provide additional information on certain brain lesions. (Fig. 37.6B)

Electrophysiological measurements

Electroencephalography (EEG) is less used than formerly, except in epilepsy. *ICP monitoring* is of some value in assessing the response to treatment of raised ICP.

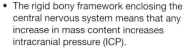

CONGENITAL LESIONS

Congenital malformations of the central nervous system are relatively common. Although genetic counselling and advances in intrauterine diagnosis are reducing the number of babies born with severe defects, minor defects continue to occur. The role of viral infection and ingestion of certain drugs and toxic substances during pregnancy is well established, and therapeutic abortion may be considered in some cases. Children with mild defects who are likely to live independent lives should be offered immediate surgical treatment. Those with major defects are often denied surgery because it is thought unlikely that they will be able to live independent

Intracranial pressure
- The rigid bony framework enclosing the central nervous system means that any increase in mass content increases intracranial pressure (ICP).

- Increased ICP lowers perfusion pressure and if unrelieved, leads progressively to bradycardia, hypertension, respiratory abnormalities (e.g. apnoea), irreversible oedema, vasoparalysis and death.

- The principal symptoms of raised ICP are headache, vomiting and visual disturbance (blurring of vision). Papilloedema may be apparent.

- If ICP is not increased uniformly, intracranial structures may be displaced. There are three major forms of herniation: transfalcine, transtentorial and foraminal.

lives. Unfortunately some children survive with much greater defects than if surgery had been undertaken. Currently, simple corrective surgery at least is offered to all, except those with severe defects associated with bladder abnormalities.

Spinal defects

These are common. *Dysrhaphism*, due to defective closure of the neural tube, includes spina bifida occulta, simple meningocele and meningomyelocele. Closure of the neural tube begins in the mid-dorsal region and extends cranially and caudally. Thus, thoracic defects are rare, cervical defects uncommon, and lumbar/lumbosacral defects are common.

Spina bifida occulta

This common condition is not usually associated with neurological defect. The overlying skin may be hairy or dimpled, or have an associated fat pad. Occasionally a fibrous band tethers the cord, producing increasing symptoms as the vertebral column grows and the spinal cord 'ascends' the vertebral canal. The onset of paraesthesia or sphincter disorders is usually due to an associated lesion such as a cord lipoma, or to *diastemyelia* where the cord is split by a projection from the posterior surface of a vertebral body. A sinus may connect the skin and spinal canal in a few cases and is a rare cause of meningitis in children. Plain X-rays may reveal an abnormality of the lamina or failure of fusion of the laminar arches.

Patients with neurological disorders require surgical treatment. Paraesthesia, backache and sphincter disorder due to tethering by a fibrous band may be dramatically relieved by dividing it. Splitting of the cord by a bony spur can be dealt with by careful removal of the spur. Intraspinal lipomas are often diffuse. Although removal has been facilitated by microscopic techniques, severe neurological disturbances may result.

Simple meningocele

The defect is usually lumbar and results from failure of fusion of laminae (Fig. 37.7A). The subarachnoid space is distended and protrudes through the defect. The arachnoid fuses with the skin, forming a membrane to which nerve roots may adhere. The cord, however, is normal and usually there are no neurological abnormalities.

Meningomyelocele

The condition occurs most commonly in the lumbar region. Spinal nerve roots and the cord adhere to the membrane because of distension of the central canal and may be exposed on the surface (Fig. 37.7B). Craniocerebral malformations such as hydrocephalus are commonly associated.

There is usually serious motor and sensory loss affecting the lower limbs and sphincters due to involvement of the cauda equina. Bladder paralysis is of the lower motor neurone type with paralysis of the detrusor muscle and pelvic floor musculature.

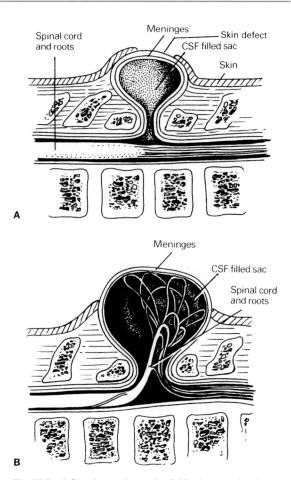

Fig. 37.7 A Simple meningocele. B Meningomyelocele.

These patients often require complex corrective procedures, and urinary continence is difficult to achieve.

Syringomyelia and syringobulbia

Distension of the central canal of the cord or paraventricular extension of the fourth ventricle results in syringomyelia or syringobulbia respectively. Most believe that the conditions result from failure of closure of the connection between the fourth ventricle and the central canal, coupled with failure of development of exit foramina in the membrane around the cerebellar tonsils.

Symptoms, which are steadily progressive, appear in the third decade and affect men more commonly. In the cord, distension of the central canal gradually compresses and destroys the decussating pain and temperature pathways, producing 'dissociated sensory loss' (loss of pain and temperature sensation but not of touch) over the upper part of the body, most often in the fingers. Pain, however, is a common presenting symptom. Trophic lesions develop on the hands and arms due to loss of pain sensation. The small muscles of the hand are often involved early, with deformity and wasting. Ultimately the long tracts become involved, producing paresis and sensory changes below the level of the lesion. Denervation arthritis (Charcot's joints) may occur.

The condition is treated by creating an opening in the membrane around the cerebellar tonsils to allow drainage of CSF. Occasionally a persisting communication with the central canal may be plugged. A posterior fossa approach is used. Isolated cysts of the cord can be drained by direct puncture either by laminectomy or percutaneously. Orthopaedic deformities may require correction, e.g. arthrodesis of unstable joints.

Malformations of the skull

These are less common than spinal defects.

Meningocele and encephalocele

Protrusion of the meninges (meningocele) or of the meninges and brain (encephalocele) through a skull defect occurs most commonly in the occipital region, and is usually associated with other abnormalities such as hydrocephalus and mental retardation.

Craniostenosis

Premature fusion (before 4 years of age) of one or more skull sutures restricts the growing brain and increases intracranial pressure. Associated ophthalmic disorders such as exophthalmus are common. Severe cases are treated by excising the fused sutures and lining their edges with dura or plastic material to retard re-union and allow the brain to expand.

Orbital hypertelorism

This malformation is produced by overgrowth of anterior fossa structures resulting in widening of the intercanthal distance and persistence of clefts and fusion lines. In its most advanced form this produces gross malformation requiring excision of the central sutures and transposition of the lateral masses.

Epidermoid cysts

These contain cheesy debris and arise from skin which has been engulfed by bone. They expand the bone and erode the skull, producing a characteristic scalloped lytic area.

Miscellaneous malformations

Malformations associated with autosomal abnormalities (e.g. Down's syndrome, microencephaly, macroencephaly, porencephaly) are not correctable. Tuberous sclerosis is a form of neuroectodermal dysplasia associated with mental retardation and epilepsy in which astrocytes form pale firm 'tubers' in the cortex and subependyma which occasionally become malignant. Angiomatous malformations of the skin (usually in the distribution of the ophthalmic branch of the trigeminal nerve), or of the retina and meninges (Sturge-Weber syndrome) may be associated with epilepsy and mental retardation.

Hydrocephalus

CSF is produced by the intraventricular choroid plexus. It passes from the lateral ventricles via the narrow foramen of Munro into the slit-like third ventricle and then through the aqueduct of the upper brainstem into the widening fourth ventricle. From here the fluid passes via 'exit foramina' in the lower part of the fourth ventricle into the cisterna magna, thereafter flowing over the surface of the brain and spinal cord to be absorbed by cerebral veins and arachnoid granulations. Hydrocephalus results when the rate of production of CSF exceeds that of absorption, and is usually associated with increased intracranial pressure. Though a choroid plexus papilloma may oversecrete CSF, much the commonest cause of hydrocephalus is obstruction to flow with failure of CSF to reach sites of absorption (Fig. 37.8).

Obstruction may be congenital, due to failure of communications between ventricles (as in aqueduct stenosis), or acquired as a result of tumour or fibrosis after infection or haemorrhage. For simplicity, acquired hydrocephalus is also considered in this section. Obstruction within the ventricular system leads to *non-communicating* or *internal hydrocephalus*. In *communicating* or *external hydrocephalus* the ventricular system is patent, but absorption by the arachnoid granulations is prevented by blood or fibrosis, or occasionally by their failure to develop.

Hydrocephalus usually presents at birth or in early infancy with characteristic enlargement of the head. Presentation in later childhood or in adult life is associated with the signs and symptoms of raised intracranial pressure.

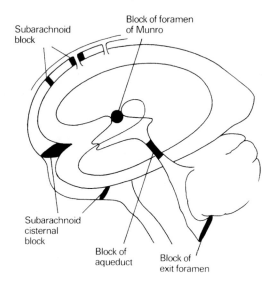

Fig. 37.8 Hydrocephalus: sites of CSF blockage.

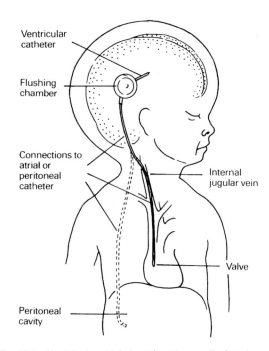

Fig. 37.9 Ventriculo-atrial shunt (continuous line) and ventriculo-peritoneal shunt (interrupted line) to relieve hydrocephalus.

If the cause of hydrocephalus can be removed (e.g. cysts, thin membranes, certain tumours), this should be done after preliminary drainage of the ventricles via a right frontal burr hole. Lumbar puncture should be avoided because of the risk of medullary 'coning'. If the cause cannot be removed, a ventricular shunt may be inserted (Fig. 37.9). A catheter is introduced into a lateral ventricle and tunnelled subcutaneously into the neck, where it is inserted into the internal jugular vein and passed into the superior vena cava or right atrium (ventriculo-atrial shunt). Alternatively, the catheter can be tunnelled to the peritoneal cavity (ventriculo-peritoneal shunt). The catheter has a one-way valve to prevent reflux of blood, and a chamber which may be compressed to prevent clotting and encourage flow. Despite this, blockage is frequent, especially in children, necessitating revision or replacement of the catheter.

Cerebral palsy

Cerebral palsy may result from agenesis, birth injury or infection. There is often a history of neonatal distress, cyanosis and feeding difficulties. Although many patients have normal intelligence, mental subnormality is common and signs of retarded development become apparent as the child grows. Spasticity and athetoid movements become marked, and the abnormal movements may be so violent that the patient cannot sit up. Joint contractures may develop. In milder cases, the patient has a character-istic 'scissor' gait with adduction of the legs and equinovarus posture.

Treatment consists of physiotherapy and special education in mild cases, but major disability often progresses so that the patient becomes helpless and unable to dress or feed himself. Joint deformities may be relieved by tendon transposition or neurec-tomy. Stereotactic destruction of thalamic or cerebellar nuclei is successful in relieving lower limb spasticity, and to a lesser degree spasticity of the upper limbs.

DEGENERATIVE DISEASES OF THE VERTEBRAL COLUMN

Degenerative changes in the intervertebral discs are common at all levels. Intervertebral discs have three parts: the *cartilage end plates* which adhere to the cancellous bone of adjacent vertebral bodies; the central semifluid *nucleus pulposus* which is relatively incompressible and inelastic, and the slightly elastic *annulus fibrosus* which surrounds and retains it and which regulates and restricts movement of the spine. The disc is subject to severe and repeated compres-sion, and the nucleus pulposus may protrude

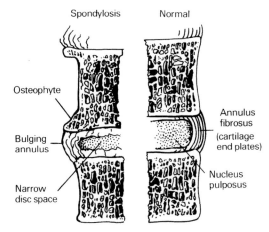

Fig. 37.10 Intervertebral disc of normal spine and in spondylosis.

through the cartilage end plate or horizontally through the annulus fibrosus. Horizontal protrusion usually occurs in a posterolateral direction and may compress the cord or nerve roots.

Herniation of the nucleus pulposus is usually gradual and intermittent so that symptoms remit between exacerbations. Acute herniation may result from severe trauma with flexion injury. The annulus fibrosus ruptures, allowing posterior (central) protrusion of the nucleus with sudden severe neurological deficit.

If the nucleus pulposus has lost substance by protrusion or desiccation (as occurs in advancing age), the fibres of the annulus fibrosus bulge outwards and the 'disc space' narrows. Strain on the apophyseal joints then results in osteophyte formation around the joints and disc margin, and narrowing of the intervertebral foramina. This condition is known as *spondylosis* (Fig. 37.10). With continuing degeneration, osteophytes may protrude on the cord or nerve roots.

Spinal *osteoarthritis* is a disorder affecting the posterior apophyseal joints and producing back pain without distant radiation. It should be distinguished from spondylosis (which depends on disc degeneration) although the two frequently coexist in older patients.

Cervical spine

Cervical spondylosis

Degenerative changes in the cervical spine are common and may start as early as adolescence. Compression of a nerve root in an intervertebral foramen produces pain, usually in the neck but often radiating to the shoulder or arm, and exacerbated by rotation of the neck. The most commonly affected level is C5–6.

Plain X-ray of the spine shows narrowing of one or more disc spaces and foramina with osteophyte formation. Myelography may demonstrate nerve compression, and in severe cases compression of the cord (Fig. 37.11). MRI scanning is increasingly used to demonstrate the soft and hard tissues without the hazard of contrast injection.

Treatment is initially conservative and comprises physiotherapy, neck traction and a supporting cervical collar. For more severe compression with weakness and paraesthesia, decompression is required. Through an anterior approach a central core of disc and related vertebra is removed and the lateral portion of the disc is curetted away. A dowel of bone taken from the iliac crest is then hammered in to stabilize the two vertebrae (Fig. 37.12).

Acute cervical disc prolapse

Acute prolapse is uncommon and fortunately most protrusions are small. The patient experiences sudden acute neck pain radiating down the arm in the area supplied by the involved root or roots. Symptoms usually resolve following conservative management with analgesics, neck traction and use of a cervical collar. Persistence of symptoms is an indication for surgery, and patients with major prolapse and long-tract signs (which may include quadriparesis) require urgent operation.

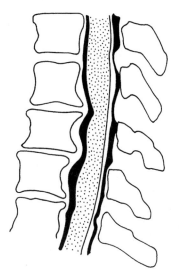

Fig. 37.11 Cord compression by cervical spondylosis.

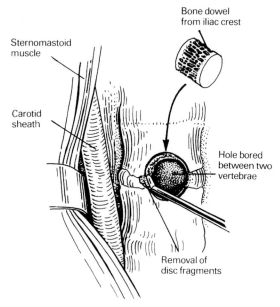

Sternomastoid muscle

Carotid sheath

Bone dowel from iliac crest

Hole bored between two vertebrae

Removal of disc fragments

Fig. 37.12 Anterior cervical decompression and fusion.

The disc fragments may be removed through a posterior approach or, less commonly, by anterior decompression; this is usually accompanied by vertebral fusion.

Thoracic spine

Thoracic disc degeneration with formation of osteophytes and foraminal narrowing is relatively common, although surgical treatment is seldom required.

Acute disc prolapse is uncommon. It requires urgent surgery because the narrow calibre of the vertebral canal in the thoracic region favours cord compression. Acute pain in the distribution of the segmental nerves may be accompanied by paraparesis or paraplegia. An anterolateral or posterolateral approach is used to avoid injuring the compressed cord.

Lumbar spine

Disorders of the lumbar spine are extremely common. Low backache (*lumbago*), with pain radiating down one or both legs (*sciatica*) may be caused by a variety of conditions. Metastases from lung, breast or prostatic cancer should always be considered, but degenerative disease of the vertebrae and discs accounts for the majority of cases.

Lumbar spondylosis

As a result of bulging of the annulus fibrosus, osteophytes form at the disc margins. Posterior osteophyte formation reduces the diameter of the vertebral canal, while additional stress on the posterior joints results in hypertrophy of the bone and ligaments, reducing the canal laterally. There is thickening of the laminar arch, and the ligamentum flavum degenerates, losing its elasticity and tending to buckle on extension. All lumbar vertebrae may be affected, but severe changes usually occur only at the lower lumbar level. Radiculography confirms the diagnosis.

Most patients can be managed conservatively with exercise and support, but those with severe symptoms require decompression by laminectomy.

Acute lumbar disc prolapse

Acute disc prolapse is most common in the fourth and fifth decades and occurs more frequently in men. It is often associated with degenerative spinal disease elsewhere. Trauma which subjects the disc to torsional stress (e.g. twisting while carrying heavy weights) may precipitate rupture of the annulus fibrosus, allowing protrusion of the nucleus pulposus.

Rupture through the central portion of the annulus may compress the roots of the entire cauda equina, causing severe back pain (without a predominant root involvement), urinary retention and weakness below the knees. This *cauda equina syndrome* requires urgent surgical relief.

More commonly the prolapse occurs posterolaterally and compresses and angulates the nerve emerging at that level. The commonest levels for prolapse are L4–5 and L5–S1. Prolapse above L4–5 becomes less common as one ascends. Most patients recover on conservative management, but those with symptoms persisting for more than 6 weeks should be offered surgery.

Signs and symptoms. Pain is the predominant symptom, and is exacerbated by coughing and sneezing. Tendon jerks and muscle power are diminished according to the site of the lesion. Straight leg raising stretches the sciatic nerve and pulls on nerve roots, resulting in pain if the roots are stretched over a disc protrusion. Straight leg raising is measured in degrees and reflects the amount of root compression. The limit of straight leg raising is normally 80–90°, but it may be reduced to less than 30°. Dorsiflexion of the foot at the limit of straight leg raising often exacerbates the pain. Examination of the back usually reveals flattening of the lumbar spinal curve and mild lumbar scoliosis, concave to the side of the lesion. This scoliosis is exaggerated when the patient is asked to bend forward.

L5–S1 prolapse compresses the root S1 and produces pain which radiates down the back of the thigh and lateral aspect of the leg onto the lateral border of the foot. Sensory changes may be detected in this distribution. The ankle jerk is diminished or absent, and plantar flexion of the foot is weak, so that the patient has difficulty in standing on his toes.

L4–L5 prolapse compresses the root of L5, causing pain which radiates down the back of the thigh and then passes from the lateral aspect of the leg to the dorsum of the foot and into the great toe. Sensory changes may also be detected in this distribution. The ankle jerk is normal, but dorsiflexion of the foot is weak.

L3–L4 prolapse compresses the root of L4 and produces pain and sensory disturbance down the front of the thigh and medial aspect of the leg on to the medial malleolus. The knee jerk is diminished or absent, and there is quadriceps weakness.

Investigation. Full examination of the abdomen (including rectal examination) is imperative as retroperitoneal or pelvic pathology may also produce severe back pain with radiation if nerves become involved.

The diagnosis is often apparent from the history and physical examination, although some difficulty may arise when an adjacent root is involved in addition to the root at the level of the prolapse. Posteroanterior and lateral X-rays of the lumbar spine are essential and often show narrowing of the involved disc space. Radiculography is indicated if the diagnosis remains in doubt.

Treatment. Immediate strict bed rest is mandatory. The patient should lie flat and should not sit up for meals, although he may be allowed up for toilet purposes. Most patients improve within 2–3 weeks and are allowed up after 4 weeks.

Patients with major protrusions are unlikely to respond and should be offered early surgery. Any patient who has not progressed satisfactorily after 6 weeks' bed rest also requires operation. The prolapsed material is removed through a posterior approach. Microdiscectomy is performed through a small incision using a microscope. Little if any part of the lamina is removed and the limited nature of the operation ensures a quick recovery. The results are good for those with acute prolapse, though pain may recur if there is generalized spinal disease.

Spondylolisthesis

Spondylolisthesis is caused by a bilateral defect in the pars interarticularis of the neural arch of the fifth lumbar vertebra (spondylolysis) which allows the anterior part of the vertebra (comprising body, pedicles, transverse processes and superior articular facets) to slide forward on the sacrum.

Spondylolysis is probably not a congenital defect although there is an inherited tendency in some patients, and signs and symptoms may appear in childhood, most often between 10 and 15 years of age. Vertical stresses on a weakened neural arch may be responsible for the slipping, while in adults it may follow stress fracture in mature bone or facet deficiency due to degenerative joint disease.

In children, the condition is usually painless, though a prominent lumbar lordosis may be detected. The normal presenting symptom in adolescents or adults is backache exacerbated by exercise. Sciatica may develop as a result of S1 root pressure. The diagnosis is confirmed radiologically.

Symptomatic younger patients are treated by lumbosacral fusion, but, as this is a major undertaking, older and less fit patients are usually managed with a spinal brace.

Spinal stenosis

This is a congenital generalized narrowing of the vertebral canal. Symptoms do not occur until middle life, and are associated with other degenerative changes, such as spondylosis, which are more likely to produce symptoms. Several nerve roots are often affected.

Treatment is similar to that of spondylosis, although decompression by laminectomy (with or without fusion) is more frequently necessary.

VASCULAR DISORDERS

The metabolic demand of the brain is greater than that of any other organ and requires a considerable blood supply. The cerebral blood flow of 800 ml/min (16% of cardiac output) is provided by two systems: the carotid arteries, which supply the forebrain, and the vertebral arteries, which supply the hindbrain. The two systems communicate freely in the circle of Willis (Fig. 37.13), and occlusion of a major artery may be compensated for by anastomotic flow.

The common carotid artery divides into the external carotid artery, which supplies the soft tissues of the head and the dura, and the internal carotid

Acute lumbar disc prolapse

- The condition is most common in the fourth and fifth decades, and men are most often affected.

- The annulus fibrosus ruptures allowing protrusion of the central nucleus pulposus. The prolapse most commonly occurs posterolaterally and compresses and angulates the spinal nerve(s) it as leaves the spinal canal. Less commonly the disc ruptures posteriorly with compression of the cauda equina.

- The commonest levels for prolapse are L4–5 and S1–2.

- Pain is the predominant symptom and is exacerbated by coughing and sneezing. Tendon jerks and muscle power are diminished, straight leg raising is restricted (e.g. from 80–90° to 30°), and lumbar lordosis is flattened with scoliosis concave to the side of the lesion.

- Most cases settle on conservative therapy but those with major protrusions or persistence of symptoms beyond 6 weeks should be considered for removal of the prolapsed material using a posterior approach.

- The cauda equina syndrome (severe back pain, urinary retention and weakness bilaterally below the knees) requires urgent surgical relief.

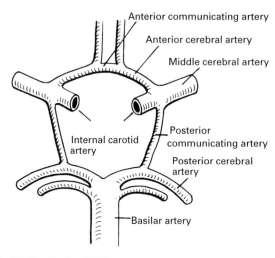

Fig. 37.13 Circle of Willis.

artery, which enters the skull to supply the brain. After passing through the carotid sinus, the internal carotid artery divides into the anterior cerebral artery and the middle cerebral artery. The two vertebral arteries join within the skull to form the basilar artery, which supplies the cerebellum and brainstem and then divides into the posterior cerebral arteries, which pass through the tentorium to supply the occipital lobe and the posterior two-thirds of the medial aspect of the hemisphere.

Disorders of the CNS resulting from vascular disease are due mainly to occlusion or haemorrhage.

Occlusive vascular disease (see also Ch. 21)

Symptoms most often result from occlusive disease of *extracranial* vessels. The lumen of the carotid or vertebral vessels may be narrowed or occluded by arteriosclerotic changes, particularly at the carotid bifurcation or at the level of entry into the skull. While arteriosclerotic disease may be widespread in the cerebral vessels, *intracranial occlusion* is usually embolic.

Transient ischaemic attacks (TIA)

Small thrombi and platelet aggregates attached to atheromatous plaques, and occasionally small portions of the plaques themselves, may embolize and lodge in small intracranial vessels, producing sudden and alarming symptoms which are often transient. Sudden occlusion of the carotid artery commonly causes ipsilateral blindness and contralateral weakness, with associated speech disorder if the dominant hemisphere is affected. Auscultation over the carotid bifurcation reveals a bruit in 70% of patients, and ophthalmodynometry may show lower pressure on the affected side. The extent of the lesion can be revealed by angiography, although this is not without risk.

About 50% of patients with TIA will have a major stroke within 5 years if the primary lesion is not treated. Stenotic lesions in the neck arteries are relatively easy to remove; those arising in the aortic arch are more difficult. Gentle handling of the carotid artery is essential to avoid dislodging thrombi. If the pressure in the distal carotid artery is less than 50 mmHg, a bypass is used to lessen the risk of postoperative stroke. The value of carotid endarterectomy is debated, many contending that aspirin therapy is equally effective. Where there is major occlusion, however, the hazard of endarterectomy is outweighed by the poor prognosis if nothing is done.

Unfortunately many of these patients suffer from generalized arteriosclerotic disease and a high proportion die from myocardial infarction within a few years of surgery.

Cerebral thrombosis

Stenotic lesions may progress to complete occlusion, with thrombus extending up the carotid tree. If the collateral circulation is defective, cerebral infarction occurs. In the past, extracranial–intracranial anastomosis was commonly advocated to improve the precarious circulation. However, it is now believed that this is of no value in this context.

Haemorrhage

Intracranial haemorrhage may be intracerebral, subarachnoid, subdural or extradural. Extradural and subdural haemorrhage usually result from trauma and are considered in Chapter 14.

Intracerebral haemorrhage

Intracerebral haemorrhage is relatively common in the middle-aged and elderly. The risk is particularly high in patients with hypertension and diabetes. In hypertension the perforating arteries of the middle cerebral arteries develop micro-aneurysms which rupture and tear open the internal capsule. Intracerebral haemorrhage may also be due to rupture of 'berry' aneurysms deep within the brain, arteriovenous malformations, or trauma producing brain lacerations.

The onset is abrupt and the majority of patients become comatose with stertorous respiration and flaccid hemiparesis. One-third of patients die within 3 days, but some survive with partial recovery of function.

Emergency removal of acute intracerebral haematomas is rarely successful since bleeding continues. If patients survive the initial haemorrhage, evacuation of clot through a burr hole may result in marked improvement.

Subarachnoid haemorrhage

In more than 50% of patients, haemorrhage is due to rupture of an aneurysm, while in 15% arteriosclerotic disease is the cause. Arteriovenous malformations, trauma, tumour or infection account for the remainder.

Intimal proliferation with degeneration of the internal elastic lamina produces weakness of arterial walls, particularly at sites of congenital weakness in the circle of Willis. Failure of the media to develop allows the intima to bulge and form an aneurysm. The majority of aneurysms occur in the anterior portion of the circle of Willis; only 15% are sited in the posterior portion. About 15% of patients have more than one aneurysm.

Although 10% of patients present with symptoms due to local pressure effects (e.g. 3rd cranial nerve palsy in posterior communicating artery aneurysm) or with signs suggesting tumour, the majority have no symptoms until the aneurysm ruptures. Sometimes the patient has pre-ictal symptoms of vague headache or neck pain, while the first haemorrhage (ictus) may be relatively minor and pass unrecognized.

Rupture of the aneurysm into the subarachnoid space produces sudden severe headache, neck stiffness and photophobia. Kernig's sign indicates meningism. The patient's conscious level is affected in varying degrees, ranging from mild disorientation to deep coma, and sudden death may occur. These symptoms, apart from meningism, are mostly due to vasospasm. The focal signs depend on the vessels affected. For example, rupture of a middle cerebral artery aneurysm commonly produces faciobrachial paresis. Associated rupture into brain substance is more serious than subarachnoid haemorrhage, and is the usual cause of sudden death.

Diagnosis and assessment. The diagnosis is confirmed by lumbar puncture. The fluid is evenly blood-stained, in contrast to a 'traumatic tap', which progressively clears. Oxyhaemoglobin appears within a few hours of haemorrhage, giving an orange colour to the supernatant fluid. By 3 days bilirubin (due to red cell breakdown) is present and gives the supernatant fluid a characteristic yellow colour.

A special grading system (Botterell) is used to assess the patient (see Table 37.2).

Patients in group A have a much better prognosis and are fit for definitive surgery directed at the aneurysm. Patients in group B may sometimes be improved by removing intracerebral clot.

Table 37.2	Botterell's grading system	
Group A		
Grade 1	Conscious, with or without signs of subarachnoid blood.	
Grade 2	Drowsy, without significant neurological deficit.	
Group B		
Grade 3	Drowsy and confused or with mild neurological deficit.	
Grade 4	Major neurological deficit and generally deteriorating, possibly the result of intracerebral clot.	
Grade 5	Moribund or nearly so, with vegetative disturbance and extensor rigidity.	

Skull X-rays usually show no abnormality, although a giant aneurysm may erode a clinoid process or have a calcified wall. A CT scan may reveal a large aneurysm but is more useful in detecting oedema or intracerebral haemorrhage. Angiography is sometimes deferred until the patient is in group A and has no evidence of vasospasm. Although the clinical picture may point to the site of the aneurysm, it is important to have a complete picture of the cerebral circulation, as aneurysms are commonly multiple (Fig. 37.14).

Management and prognosis. Mortality is high in the first week but falls steadily thereafter. Without operation, 60% of patients die within 2 months, and of those who survive the first haemorrhage, 50% die within 5 years if not treated. Thus, surgical treatment should always be considered and it has been suggested that the best time to operate is during the second week following the first haemorrhage, provided the patient is in group A. Others believe that operation should be performed immediately after diagnosis.

While awaiting surgery the patient is confined to bed and given oxygen. Sedation may be required. If neurological signs are present, dexamethasone (10 mg initially and 4 mg 6-hourly thereafter) is given. Hypertension is treated by hypotensive drugs, the aim being to reduce blood pressure by 10%.

Most aneurysms are now treated by a direct approach. Using the operating microscope, the neck of the aneurysm is exposed and a special clip applied (Fig. 37.15). The wall of the aneurysm can be strengthened by coating it with plastic material or by wrapping it in gauze to cause a fibrous reaction. The mortality rate of operation (less than 5%) is substantially less than that of non-operative treatment, but vasospasm can result in brain oedema, requiring

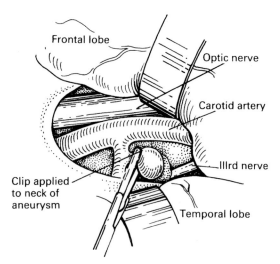

Fig. 37.15   Treatment of internal carotid aneurysm by clipping the neck of the aneurysm.

energetic treatment with steroids and other anti-oedema agents.

Common carotid artery ligation may be the procedure of choice for aneurysms within the cavernous sinus or for giant aneurysms of the carotid system, provided angiography has revealed a satisfactory cross-circulation. The procedure is normally performed under local anaesthesia so that speech, behaviour, sensation and motor function can be monitored after clamping the common carotid artery. If these remain satisfactory for 5 minutes, the vessel is ligated and the clamp removed.

Advances in anaesthesia and microsurgical techniques have permitted many giant aneurysms previously considered inoperable to be excised. The aneurysmal sac may also be obliterated by intra-arterial embolization of balloons or metallic spirals.

Arteriovenous malformations

These congenital malformations may occur close to ventricular walls, in the substance of the brain, or on the cerebral cortex. They vary in size from small lesions undetectable by conventional angiography to large masses occupying major portions of brain. The lesions frequently bleed and are the commonest source of subarachnoid haemorrhage in younger patients. They may also cause epilepsy. Once bleeding has occurred, the risk of re-bleeding is high. Within 10 years 20% of patients die and a further 30% suffer severe disability from recurrent haemorrhage. The prognosis improves with increasing age at the first bleed.

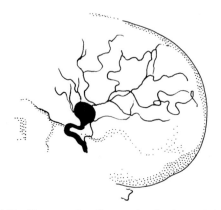

Fig. 37.14   Diagram of angiogram showing internal carotid aneurysm.

Arteriovenous malformations are best demonstrated by angiography, although CT scans enhanced by contrast media will reveal moderate-sized to large lesions. Calcification may be apparent on plain X-rays. Occasionally a bruit may be heard.

The lesion may be locally excised or removed by block resection (lobectomy). Pre-operative embolization of feeding vessels with small plastic spheres may facilitate resection, and small anomalies may be sealed completely. Stereotactic radiotherapy is an increasingly popular alternative to resection.

Spinal arteriovenous malformations

These lie over the posterior surface of the cord and form loops of vessels which may involve cord substance. Thrombosis frequently occurs, producing cord ischaemia. Symptoms are often progressive, and include pain, weakness and ultimately paraplegia. Excision using the operating microscope is the only available treatment, but its long-term value is uncertain.

INFECTION

Infection of the CNS and its coverings acquires surgical importance if it produces a mass (abscess or

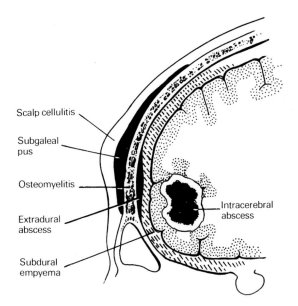

Fig. 37.16 Types of cranial infection.

oedema), hydrocephalus or osteomyelitis, or if it occurs as a result of a breach in or absence of the coverings of the brain (Fig. 37.16).

Intracranial infection

Osteomyelitis of the skull

Bone may become infected by penetrating wounds, during surgery, by local extension (from sinuses, the middle ear or mastoid), or by blood-borne infection. Pus may track into the subgaleal space or involve the overlying scalp to produce 'Pott's puffy tumour', and there is often an associated small extradural abscess. The infection is difficult to eradicate and may require removal of large areas of calvarium and their subsequent replacement by an acrylic plate.

Extradural abscess

Extradural abscess is usually secondary to osteomyelitis and most often occurs close to the middle ear, mastoid air cells or paranasal sinuses. Trauma is another cause. Pus may infiltrate the pericranium to produce Pott's puffy tumour and frequently breaks through the dura to produce meningitis, subdural empyema or cerebral abscess.

Systemic upset is usually severe. There is local tenderness, and focal neurological signs may result

---

Vascular disorders and the central nervous system

- Symptoms due to occlusive vascular disease most often originate from blockage of extracranial vessels by atherosclerosis. Intracranial occlusion is usually embolic.

- Transient ischaemic attacks are associated with a 50% risk of major stroke within 5 years unless treatment is instituted (e.g. by carotid endarterectomy or aspirin therapy).

- Intracranial haemorrhage may be extradural, subdural, subarachnoid or intracerebral. Extradural and subdural haemorrhage are usually the result of trauma; subarachnoid bleeding is due to rupture of an aneurysm in at least 50% of cases, and intracerebral bleeding is frequently associated with hypertension and diabetes mellitus (and the rupture of a deep microaneurysm).

- Surgical treatment of intracerebral bleeding is rarely successful.

- Patients with subarachnoid haemorrhage from an aneurysm should be considered for clipping of the aneurysm to avoid recurrent bleeding.

from thrombophlebitis of superficial cortical veins. Facial nerve paralysis is frequent when mastoiditis is the source.

Treatment involves giving large doses of antibiotics, drainage, excision of infected bone, and drainage of infected sinuses or mastoid air cells.

Subdural empyema

Subdural empyema (pus within the subdural space) is commoner than cerebral abscess in the Western world. It may follow penetrating wounds or surgery, but is most commonly associated with paranasal or ear infection which has spread along emissary veins or via dural sinuses.

Pus may spread over the whole hemisphere, beneath the falx to involve the opposite hemisphere, or beneath the tentorium. It may accumulate in multiple sites, making treatment difficult. Although accumulation of pus exerts pressure on the brain, symptoms are largely due to venous thrombosis. Patients may present with disordered consciousness, paresis and epilepsy, or with signs of meningitis. Spread of infection is reflected in altering localizing signs. Deterioration of consciousness in patients with a history of frontal sinusitis or ear infection should arouse suspicion of subdural empyema.

Plain X-ray of the skull may reveal opaque air sinuses, but the diagnosis is confirmed by angiography or CT scan. Immediate treatment is indicated. Multiple burr holes are made to drain the pus, and catheters are inserted through which antibiotics are instilled 4-hourly in addition to systemic administration. The common infecting organisms are staphylococci and streptococci, which determines the choice of antibiotic until bacteriological reports are available. Occasionally, a large area of skull may have to be removed to achieve adequate decompression. Anticonvulsant treatment is continued indefinitely. Despite these measures, the mortality is 20–35%, and residual paresis and epilepsy are common.

Cerebral abscess

Although the brain is relatively resistant to infection, abscess formation may occur, particularly if there has been previous haemorrhage, trauma or anoxia. Initially there is a cerebritis (encephalitis) following which the brain necroses to form pus surrounded by a tough glial capsule which is resistant to passage of antibiotics.

Abscesses occur, in descending order of frequency, as a result of:

- Direct extension from the paranasal sinuses, mastoid or middle ear
- Haematogenous spread, most commonly in patients with bronchiectasis or lung abscess, or in patients with cyanotic heart disease with a right-to-left shunt
- Direct penetrating trauma.

The presentation is often acute, with high fever, progressive disturbance of consciousness, and evidence of increasing intracranial pressure. If the abscess is chronic and walled off, systemic signs of infection may be minimal and the patient presents with signs of a slowly expanding localized mass.

Diagnosis requires a high degree of suspicion and is confirmed by CT scanning.

Treatment. Urgent treatment is essential. In the acute stage of encephalitis, systemic antibiotics in high doses and anti-oedema agents are administered in an effort to localize the infection. Once localization has occurred, the abscess is drained through burr holes and a catheter is inserted so that antibiotics can be instilled regularly. Alternatively, the abscess is tapped every few days with a brain cannula. Systemic antibiotics are continued for 10 days while the size of the cavity is monitored by CT scanning. If the patient does not become rapidly more alert following drainage of an abscess, excision is indicated. Encapsulated abscesses and cerebellar abscesses are excised.

Nearly 50% of patients with cerebral abscess develop epilepsy, and anticonvulsants are continued indefinitely. With early diagnosis, the mortality is low. The overall mortality rate of 30–50% reflects failure to make an early diagnosis.

Infections of the spine

Tuberculosis

Tuberculosis of the spine is still relatively common in Third World countries. The bovine bacillus, from infected milk, is the usual agent and most commonly affects the thoracic spine.

Infection initially affects the anterior border of one or more vertebral bodies where it causes caseous necrosis. It then spreads through the disc space to affect the adjacent vertebrae. The disc space narrows because of loss of fluid. A paraspinal abscess develops which may compress the cord and nerve roots, and the disc may sequestrate into the abscess. The anterior part of the vertebral body may collapse if there is sufficient damage, producing angulation (kyphosis) of the spine and, in severe forms, a gibbus. In 10% of patients angulation is severe enough to produce cord compression and paraplegia.

The patient presents with back pain, limitation of spinal movement and systemic signs of infection. Cord compression produces neurological deficits. Spinal X-rays show narrowing and irregularity of the disc space with erosion of the vertebral body, and a paravertebral abscess may be seen as a soft tissue mass. Angulation is seen with more advanced disease.

Early treatment carries a good prognosis, and even if cord compression has occurred from an epidural abscess, the chances of recovery are usually good. The late form of Pott's paraplegia is due to ischaemic changes in the cord and carries a poor prognosis for recovery. If tuberculosis is suspected, chemotherapy is instituted and the patient is nursed in bed in a plaster cast. Once adequate chemotherapy has been given, the diagnosis is confirmed by biopsy, infected material is removed and, if necessary, the spine is stabilized by bone grafting.

The presence of pus or signs of compression are indications for urgent drainage. All necrotic material is removed and bone grafts (from rib or iliac crest) are inserted to stabilize the spine.

Osteomyelitis of the spine

The usual infecting organism is *Staphylococcus aureus*. The infection most often arises as a result of haematogenous spread from boils, dental root infections, tonsillitis or otitis media, but may follow local trauma or operation.

The infection is most common in adolescence and early adulthood, and is much more common in males. In contrast to spinal tuberculosis, the lumbar region is most frequently infected, the illness is usually more acute and severe, and large paravertebral abscess and vertebral collapse are rare. Radiological signs are absent in the first 10–14 days, but signs of bone erosion and regeneration and loss of disc space begin to appear thereafter.

Treatment consists of immobilization in a plaster cast and administration of large doses of the appropriate antibiotic, as determined by culture of material from the primary site or by blood culture. Any associated abscess should be drained via an anterolateral approach and the area debrided. If the resultant defect is large, bone grafting may be required.

Epidural abscess

Epidural abscess may arise from haematogenous spread or local spread of a vertebral infection.

The patient develops severe pain and signs of cord compression, with retention of urine. Plain X-rays are usually normal in the absence of an established bone infection, but myelography confirms the compression.

Antibiotics and urgent evacuation of the pus are indicated. In the absence of local bone infection, a laminectomy approach is used, but an anterolateral approach can be used if the abscess is secondary to vertebral infection.

NEOPLASMS

Tumours arising from the skull

Osteoma

This relatively common benign tumour is usually solitary. It commonly arises in a paranasal sinus or in the orbit. Osteomas usually grow outwards to produce a palpable hard mass but may grow inwards to compress the underlying brain and meninges. Osteomas within a sinus may produce obstruction and sinusitis, while those in the orbit may cause proptosis and diplopia.

Symptomatic osteomas should be excised.

Chordoma

These rare malignant neoplasms are thought to arise from remnants of the notochord. They occur in the spheno-occipital region of the skull or the sacrococcygeal region of the spine. They are highly vascular, firm grey tumours which slowly erode bone and may invade the optic chiasma, sella and cavernous sinus or displace the pons. Complete surgical removal is rarely possible, but radiotherapy may slow growth and prolong life.

Glomus jugulare tumours

These tumours arise in the middle ear and invade the posterior fossa. They often present with bleeding from the ear and are visible as a soft fleshy red mass protruding through the drum. Invasion of the internal jugular vein is common. Invasion of the middle ear produces tinnitus, deafness and facial paresis, while intracranial growth produces signs and symptoms of a cerebellar pontine angle tumour.

Radical excision of the petrous and occipital bones followed by irradiation is indicated.

Histiocytosis

Histiocyte-containing tumours (eosinophilic granuloma, Hand-Schuller-Christian disease and Letterer-Siwe disease) may develop in infancy or childhood and erode the skull or spine. Radiotherapy may be helpful in some cases.

Multiple myeloma

Myeloma usually occurs after the age of 50 years and is twice as common in males. The tumour is multicentric and may involve other bones as well as the skull. The condition may be confused with metastases from a primary solid tumour. Systemic cytotoxic chemotherapy is indicated.

Paget's disease (osteitis deformans)

This condition of unknown aetiology produces thickening, softening and deformity of bone which later densely scleroses. Both sexes are equally affected and the condition usually begins between the fourth and sixth decades. The skull is most frequently affected and is enlarged and thickened. Encroachment on the optic or auditory foramina may produce visual or auditory disturbance. Sarcomatous change occurs in 10% of patients.

Management is usually confined to pain relief. Entrapped nerves may require surgical decompression, while radiotherapy is effective for localized pain. Calcitonin is used increasingly in systemic management.

Metastatic tumour

The skull is a common site for metastases from cancers of the lung, breast, prostate, thyroid and kidney. The lesions are usually osteolytic, although metastases from breast and prostate may be osteoblastic. Local radiotherapy may be indicated for a rapidly enlarging metastatic tumour.

Intracranial tumours

Primary intracranial tumours show a bimodal age incidence, with a small peak at 6–7 years of age, a decline until puberty, and thereafter a progressive rise to a maximum in the fifth decade. Both sexes are equally affected. Apart from certain tumours such as cholesteatomas and craniopharyngiomas, which arise from cell remnants, their cause is unknown.

They rarely metastasize, and death usually results from continued growth within the confined space of the skull.

About 50% of intracranial tumours are metastatic, the most frequent primary sources being lung and breast.

Intracranial tumours may present with general or localized effects. Diagnosis is easy when tumours are large, but early diagnosis while the tumour is still small facilitates treatment and improves prognosis. CT scanning and angiography (Fig. 37.17) are essential investigations. A biopsy should be obtained if at all possible by stereotactic techniques so that appropriate treatment can be instituted. Cell culture is important for immunological investigation and determination of sensitivity to treatment.

Tumours arising from the meninges

Meningiomas. These account for 20% of all brain tumours. They arise from arachnoidal cells and are most commonly close to intracranial sinuses. About 90% occur in the supratentorial region. They are slow-growing and often highly vascular, deriving their blood supply from meningeal vessels. They are usually rounded or bossellated and embedded in the brain, but tumour cells may invade bone or spread widely over the dura (meningioma en plaque). The overlying skull may be rarefied or thickened with production of a palpable mass.

The parasagittal region is the commonest site for supratentorial meningiomas, and their proximity to the motor cortex results in focal seizures, particularly in the leg. They frequently invade the sagittal sinus.

Meningiomas are treated by surgical excision. If the sagittal sinus is involved, it is resected and replaced with a vein graft to reduce the risk of recurrence.

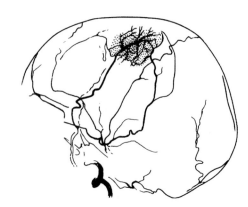

Fig. 37.17 Angiographic appearance of meningioma.

Pituitary and parapituitary tumours

Pituitary tumours account for 15% of all intracranial tumours. They produce effects due partly to endocrine change and partly to local pressure (Fig. 37.18). The management of functioning pituitary tumours is dealt with in Chapter 19.

Craniopharyngioma. These tumours develop in remnants of Rathke's pouch and present in childhood or in later life. Most are multicystic and they may reach a large size. The majority lie anterior to the pituitary stalk, although some may occur within the sella.

Visual field defects occur early from compression. Progressive growth results in hypopituitarism due to hypothalamic involvement, and eventually causes signs and symptoms of raised intracranial pressure.

Complete surgical removal is the treatment of choice for small solid tumours. If the tumour is large, and particularly if it is cystic, stereotactic puncture and aspiration of the cyst contents followed by radiotherapy is safer and more effective.

Cholesteatoma. These tumours, not to be confused with cholesteatoma of the middle ear, are pearly-white and glistening, and composed of layers of large finely granular cells. They may arise in the suprasellar region but are most commonly found in the posterior fossa at the cerebellopontine angle or within the fourth ventricle or cerebellum.

Complete removal is seldom possible, but partial removal often prolongs survival.

Neurinomas

Neurinomas of the cranial nerves account for about 5% of primary intracranial tumours and affect almost exclusively the acoustic nerve. Bilateral tumours may occur in generalized neurofibromatosis but are rare.

The tumour develops within the internal auditory meatus, which it erodes and expands. The 8th and 7th cranial nerves become stretched over the tumour as it grows into the cerebello-pontine angle (Fig. 37.19). Early symptoms are due to 8th nerve involvement and include progressive nerve deafness, tinnitus and vertigo. Further growth results in 7th nerve compression and facial weakness, while upward extension may damage the trigeminal nerve and lead to diminished facial sensation. Large tumours eventually compress the pons and cerebellum and cause ataxia and nystagmus, while gradual displacement of the brainstem angulates the aqueduct and fourth ventricle to produce internal hydrocephalus. The neurinoma may reach a large size before the patient is first seen by the surgeon. Patients with early symptoms are frequently misdiagnosed as having Ménière's disease.

Plain X-rays show enlargement of the internal auditory meatus, while the tumour itself is usually clearly demonstrated by CT scanning.

Treatment consists of surgical removal via a posterior fossa approach. It is usually possible to preserve the facial nerve if the operating microscope is used and the effects of nerve stimulation are carefully observed.

Intracerebral tumours

Metastatic tumours

Metastatic tumours are found in about 20% of autopsies in patients with cancer and in 50% are

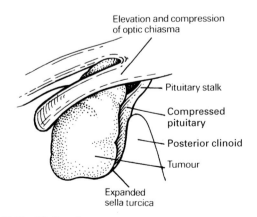

Fig. 37.18   Pituitary tumour.

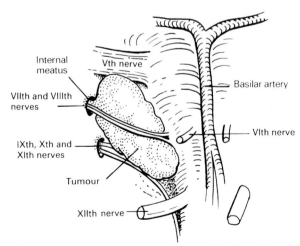

Fig. 37.19   Right acoustic tumour in the cerebellopontine angle seen from the front.

multiple. Because of breakdown in the blood–brain barrier they are usually associated with considerable oedema. About 80% of patients have papilloedema.

Multiple metastases are best treated by cytotoxic therapy or hormonal manipulation, if appropriate (e.g. breast cancer). Whole-brain radiotherapy may produce some improvement, while gross oedema can be reduced by steroids such as dexamethasone. If a metastasis is single and accessible, the patient is otherwise well, and there is no evidence of wide extension of the primary tumour, surgical removal may be considered. The surgical mortality is less than 10% and survival ranges from 3 to 12 months, although in patients without a demonstrable primary tumour the median survival is about 2 years.

Gliomas

Gliomas arising from the supporting cells of the brain (the glia) are the commonest primary brain tumour and account for 25% of all intracranial tumours. Astrocytomas are often initially slow-growing, but may be rapidly invasive (glioblastoma multiforme). The less common oligodendrogliomas are slow-growing, sometimes become calcified, and have less tendency to infiltrate the brain.

Complete removal of gliomas is difficult and is often prevented by infiltration of the tumour. The cerebellar astrocytoma of childhood is an exception in that removal is usually feasible and curative. Gliomas confined to a single lobe may be removed by lobectomy. Recurrence is common despite postoperative radiotherapy, but may take several years to become manifest. Unfortunately, many gliomas occupy vital cerebral areas, for example the speech area, so that radical removal would produce unacceptable brain damage, in this case aphasia and hemiplegia. Judicious use of radiotherapy, steroids, chemotherapy and immunotherapy is preferable and prolongs useful independent life for many months. Hydrocephalus may be treated by appropriate shunts, while aspiration of unresectable cystic tumours usually results in considerable improvement.

Some gliomas present with rapid onset of coma and decerebration. Prompt administration of anti-oedema agents, and ventricular drainage to relieve hydrocephalus may improve the patient's condition and allow appropriate investigation and treatment.

Ependymomas

Ependymomas arise from ependyma in the walls of the ventricles, and from ependymal remnants in the central canal. They are most common in the fourth ventricle and produce hydrocephalus. They may emerge from the fourth ventricle into the cisterna and spread over the brainstem, producing multiple cranial nerve palsies. With the operating microscope many of these tumours can now be safely and completely removed.

Medulloblastomas

These malignant tumours of childhood arise from the roof of the fourth ventricle and, like ependymomas, tend to seed through the CSF pathways, so that the presenting symptoms may be due to lumbar or sacral root lesions. Treatment consists of partial removal followed by radiotherapy to the entire CNS.

Spinal tumours

Primary spinal tumours are about one-sixth as common as intracranial tumours. Two-thirds are

---

Tumours affecting the skull and its contents

- Common tumours involving the skull are osteomas and metastatic deposits. Less common tumours include deposits of multiple myeloma, histiocytosis, glomus jugulare tumours and chordomas.

- Intracranial tumours have a bimodal age distribution (peaks at 6–7 years and fifth decade). Almost 50% of intracranial tumours are metastatic (most common primary sources are lung and breast).

- Meningiomas account for 20% of intracranial tumours (90% of meningiomas are supratentorial), grow slowly, can cause focal seizures, and are treated by excision.

- Pituitary and parapituitary (craniopharyngioma and cholesteatoma) account for 15% of all intracranial tumours. Pituitary tumours may be functional, both types can cause pressure effects and both types are best removed surgically.

- Neurinomas of the cranial nerves account for 5% of all intracranial tumours, Acoustic neurinomas develops in the internal auditory meatus and involve the 7th and 8th cranial nerves to cause deafness, tinnitus, vertigo and facial weakness. Involvement of the 5th nerve may cause loss of facial sensation.

- Primary intracerebral tumours may arise from the supporting cells of the brain (gliomas), from the walls of ventricles (ependymomas) and from the roof of the fourth ventricle (medulloblastomas).

benign, and many of the remainder are radio-sensitive to varying degrees and have a better prognosis than intracranial lesions. Metastatic tumours are as common as primary tumours.

The majority of spinal tumours arise in relation to the coverings. The commonest early symptoms are pain due to root displacement and associated mild spastic paraparesis, more marked in one leg, which may drag during walking. Bladder function is usually impaired. Intrinsic tumours of the cord (intra-medullary tumours) account for only 5% of spinal tumours and, in contrast to extramedullary tumours, usually present with sensory symptoms due to involvement of the decussating spinothalamic pain and temperature fibres.

Clinical differentiation between intra- and extra-medullary tumours is not always easy. Plain radiology and myelography are needed to make the distinction.

Epidural tumours

Epidural tumours account for more than half (55%) of all spinal tumours. About 90% are malignant and 75% are the result of metastatic spread from a primary site elsewhere.

Lymphoma is the commonest non-metastatic tumour, but leukaemic infiltration and myeloma may also involve the epidural space and produce cord compression. Metastatic deposits in the vertebrae may be the first manifestation of the disease, and tumour cells may enter the epidural space. These lesions most commonly affect the thoracic spine, and symptoms progress rapidly.

Treatment consists of decompression, laminectomy and removal of the epidural tumour, followed by local radiotherapy and systemic treatment appropriate to the primary disease. In extensive vertebral involvement, it may be necessary to excise the affected bone and replace it with bone grafts secured or stabilized by metal rods, plates and screws.

Intradural tumours

Intradural tumours account for 45% of all spinal tumours. The great majority are extramedullary rather than intramedullary. Nearly all intradural tumours are primary tumours and more than half are benign. Progression tends to be slow, in contrast to epidural lesions.

Extramedullary tumours. Meningiomas and schwannomas are the common lesions. Meningi-omas are ten times as common in females. They are firm hemispherical tumours occurring most commonly in the thoracic region. They usually present after the age of 40 years and compress the cord and nerve roots. Surgical removal confers an excellent prognosis.

Schwannomas affect the sensory roots more commonly than the motor roots. They tend to grow out through the intervertebral foramen and expand, producing a 'dumb-bell' tumour. They are as common as meningiomas. The much less common neurofibroma occurs as part of generalized neuro-fibromatosis. The prognosis is excellent following removal of the tumour, although the attached nerve root may have to be resected.

Intramedullary tumours. Ependymomas are the commonest intramedullary lesion and usually affect the conus and filum terminale. They arise at the centre of the cord and expand slowly rather than invade. Complete removal is often possible and is followed by a good prognosis.

Gliomas, usually astrogliomas, are most often found in the thoracic region. They infiltrate the cord to produce a fusiform swelling. They can seldom be removed completely but with microscopic techniques, incomplete removal followed by radiotherapy may allow survival for 5 years or longer.

Tumours affecting the spinal cord
- Primary tumours affecting the spinal cord are one-sixth as common as intracranial tumours; two-thirds are benign and the remainder have a better prognosis than intracranial tumours because they are often radiosensitive.
- Metastatic tumours involving the spinal cord are as common as primary tumours.
- Spinal cord tumours can be classified as epidural (55%) or intradural (45%); intradural tumours are usually extramedullary (meningiomas and schwannomas) and are rarely intramedullary (ependymomas, gliomas).
- Epidural tumours are malignant in 90% of cases and may arise primarily (e.g. lymphoma) or from metastatic disease (eg. vertebral metastases). Treatment consists of decompression by laminectomy and removal of the tumour if possible; radiotherapy and/or systemic chemotherapy may be helpful. Extensive vertebral disease may require bone grafts and fixation.
- Intradural tumours are frequently benign, cause compression of the cord and nerve roots and have an excellent prognosis if removed.

MISCELLANEOUS CONDITIONS

Disorders of movement

Parkinson's disease

Parkinson's disease affects 0.1% of the population overall, with an incidence of 1% in those over 50 years of age. The characteristic histological features are depigmentation of the substantia nigra and the presence of inclusion bodies in many neurones of the brainstem nuclei and spinal cord grey matter.

The cause is unknown in 80% of cases (idiopathic parkinsonism). Postencephalic parkinsonism usually becomes manifest 10–20 years after an attack of encephalitis. Blepharospasm and oculogyric crises are particularly common in this form of the disease. Arteriosclerotic parkinsonism occurs in older patients and is often of sudden onset. Psychotropic drug-induced parkinsonism may follow administration of drugs such as the phenothiazines. The condition regresses in two-thirds of patients following withdrawal of the drug.

The onset of tremor, akinesia or bradykinesia, and rigidity may be sudden or insidious. Common early complaints include a painful limb, clumsiness or weakness. The tremor is often unilateral and affects distal muscles. The fully developed clinical picture is unmistakable with the mask-like face, flexed posture, festinating gait and tremor. Swallowing becomes difficult, leading to drooling and aspiration, and weight loss is common. Idiopathic parkinsonism is progressive, leading to death or severe disability in 15–20 years.

The majority of patients are treated medically, surgery being reserved for patients with severe tremor. Stereotactic radiofrequency lesions are made in the *nucleus ventralis lateralis* of the thalamus, which is an important relay centre of the motor system. Results are good.

Chorea

Chorea causes rapid and purposeless involuntary contractions of facial or limb muscles at rest which also interfere with voluntary movement. Chorea may follow thrombosis of brainstem vessels. *Huntington's chorea* is an autosomal dominant disorder associated with progressive dementia in adult life. There is widespread neuronal loss in the cortex, caudate and putamen. Although stereotactic thalamotomy will relieve chorea, it is rarely undertaken.

Choreoathetosis

Choreoathetosis with spasticity is common in young patients with cerebral palsy. Stereotactic dentato-tomy converts the spastic paresis into a flaccid one, improves speech and feeding, and allows the limbs greater facility.

Torsion dystonia

This disease is characterized by sustained muscle contractions, which may be spasmodic or continuous. It usually results from birth injury or cerebral anoxia, but is occasionally inherited. Partial forms are relatively common in adults (e.g. orofacial dyskinesia and dystonia or torticollis). A good response is often obtained by stereotactic thalamotomy or dentatotomy.

Epilepsy

Onset of epilepsy at any age requires investigation to determine its cause. This is particularly important in *late-onset epilepsy*, which is often due to a tumour or vascular lesions which may be relieved by surgery. Epilepsy may continue after removal of the cause, but is then usually easier to control by anticonvulsants.

Idiopathic epilepsy can usually be managed satisfactorily by drugs, but if control cannot be achieved, surgery is considered after accurate localization of the focus of discharge. A cortical lesion may be carefully excised, using electrocorticography to ensure that the whole of the epileptic focus is removed.

Temporal lobe epilepsy is not infrequently associated with definite, though small, cortical or subcortical haematomas. If the focus is well-localized, temporal lobectomy gives excellent results.

Intractable grand mal seizures sometimes respond to stereotactic thalamotomy.

Psychiatric disorders amenable to surgery

Surgical treatment of mental disorder was discredited by the indiscriminate use of gross frontal leucotomy and is only now regaining reputable status. Full co-operation with the referring psychiatrist is essential, and surgery is only recommended after frank discussion with the patient and his or her relatives. In the UK the provisions of the Mental Health Act (1983) must be considered.

Intractable anxiety states which do not respond to

medical treatment may be improved by a discrete stereotactic leucotomy which interrupts white matter pathways from various parts of the limbic lobe, such as the orbital frontal gyri.

Aggressive disorders, particularly those associated with temporal lobe epilepsy, may respond to stereotactic amygdalotomy.

Hyperactivity of severe grade is difficult to manage, but stereotactic hypothalotomy is sometimes useful.

INTRACTABLE PAIN

Intractable pain (i.e. pain not responding to conservative measures) requires careful assessment before recommending procedures which themselves may be extensive or hazardous. A detailed history and clinical examination are essential, and factors which exacerbate the pain should be noted. It is important to determine whether the pain is in any way related to anxiety or drug dependence and whether it is a means of seeking attention. Many hospitals operate special 'pain clinics' where patients are examined and their problems are discussed by a team of physicians, surgeons, anaesthetists and psychiatrists before management is initiated.

Intractable pain may be iatrogenic. Careful attention to surgical technique and adequate reassurance and information both before and after the operation reduces this risk. Adequate pain relief should always be provided during the painful early postoperative period, but powerful analgesics (which carry a high risk of addiction) are rarely required for more than 48 hours.

Some patients seeking pain relief merely require reassurance while others need a change in their drug regimen. A third group merit specific treatment of an underlying cause. Surgical procedures to relieve pain should not incapacitate the patient and should aim to secure complete and long-lasting relief. Patients with incurable malignant disease in whom survival is likely to be short are not usually considered for surgical procedures, provided their pain can be controlled by drugs without severe side-effects. Patients with a longer life expectancy and those in whom life expectancy is shortened by analgesic drugs should be offered surgery. The success rate is high in patients with malignant disease, possibly because they die from the disease before the pain recurs. In patients with pain from benign disease the success rate is lower (except in those with clear-cut conditions such as trigeminal neuralgia).

Table 37.3 Surgical treatment of intractable pain	
Peripheral procedures	Central procedures
Neurectomy	*Spinal cord*
Surgical posterior rhizotomy	Spinothalamic tractotomy (cordotomy)
Intrathecal chemical rhizotomy	Myelotomy
Epidural techniques	*Brainstem*
	Spinothalamic tractotomy
	Thalamus
	Thalamotomy

The procedures available for surgical pain relief are summarized in Table 37.3.

Peripheral procedures

Peripheral neurectomy

Most nerves are mixed nerves so that peripheral neurectomy produces not only anaesthesia but also paresis and loss of all sensation. Facial pain is an exception, as neurectomy can be limited to purely sensory fibres. Splanchnicectomy, now usually performed chemically by local injection of alcohol, is sometimes helpful in the management of intractable upper abdominal pain such as that due to pancreatic cancer.

Posterior rhizotomy

Posterior rhizotomy (division of nerve roots) is a satisfactory procedure for pain syndromes due to direct nerve involvement, but because of the extensive overlap of dermatomes (especially on the trunk) several nerve roots have to be divided to obtain a relatively small area of anaesthesia. Surgical rhizotomy requires extensive laminectomy and is now often replaced by *percutaneous rhizotomy*. Electrodes are introduced percutaneously into the appropriate intervertebral foramina, and the roots are destroyed by electro- or radio-frequency coagulation. The procedure may be repeated, and is suitable for patients in poor general condition. Percutaneous rhizotomy carries a greater risk of motor root injury than surgical rhizotomy.

Intrathecal chemical rhizotomy

This is suitable for patients with pain involving a large area or multiple sites. Injection of alcohol carries a high risk of paresis so that its use is restricted to those already paralysed. Phenol produces fewer unwanted side-effects and may control pain for many months. Hypertonic saline is the safest of all, but pain relief rarely lasts for more than 3 months. It is therefore most suitable for patients with a short life expectancy.

Intrathecal steroids

Local intrathecal injection of steroids is sometimes effective in chronic back pain (particularly chronic lumbar pain from arthritis) and severe continuous pain following laminectomy. The effect is unpredictable, but some patients obtain relief of pain for a few weeks. The effect is presumed to be due to a local anti-inflammatory action but there may be a placebo effect.

Epidural anaesthesia

Epidural anaesthesia has become increasingly popular in recent years and an epidural catheter can be left in situ postoperatively so that analgesia may be topped up, avoiding the need for systemic opiates. When used for intractable pain, epidural anaesthesia provides only temporary relief.

Recent demonstration of the presence of morphine receptors within the cord has stimulated the use of epidural morphine in the management of postoperative and chronic pain.

Central procedures

Spinothalamic tractotomy (cordotomy)

Spinothalamic tractotomy (Fig. 37.20) gives excellent pain relief in patients with malignant disease when life expectancy exceeds 6 months. It is less satisfactory for pain due to benign causes. Cordotomy removes pain and temperature sensation but preserves touch. It is usually performed at the cervical level, but section at C1 is required to obtain analgesia of arm and shoulder.

The procedure is usually performed percutaneously, using rough aiming or a stereotactic technique. Local anaesthesia is used so that the patient can be assessed during the operation and thus reduce the risk of damage to motor tracts and to bladder and respiratory fibres.

Myelotomy

Bilateral cordotomy carries a high risk of respiratory or bladder dysfunction and is very rarely indicated.

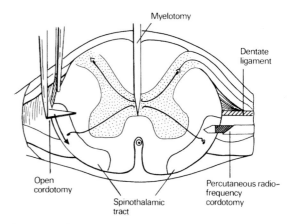

Fig. 37.20 Spinal cord tractotomy and myelotomy for intractable pain.

However, bilateral analgesia can be produced by cutting the cord longitudinally in the midline and thus dividing the decussating fibres (see Fig. 37.21). This is done as an open procedure in the lumbar region and is useful for intractable pain following abdominoperineal excision of the rectum. Cervical myelotomy for pain arising at higher levels

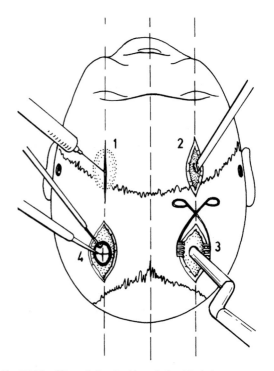

Fig. 37.21 Sites of standard burr holes. Technique: (1) infiltration and incision; (2) scraping away the pericranium; (3) drilling of cranium; (4) incision of dura.

is usually carried out by a percutaneous stereotactic technique.

Brainstem tractotomy

The spinothalamic tract can be divided at the medullary level to relieve widespread cervical and facial pain. The risk of operative damage to neighbouring structures is reduced if a stereotactic technique is employed.

Thalamotomy

Stereotactic thalamotomy is useful in patients with long-standing pain or pain which seems to be of central (affective) origin, and in those in whom a more peripheral procedure has failed. Alternatively, stimulating electrodes can be placed in thalamic nuclei and can be activated by the patient using a battery-operated coil placed subcutaneously.

Additional techniques

Cingulotomy

Severe pain is often accompanied by emotional distress, especially in terminal malignancy, so that a technically successful procedure may not provide the expected relief. Addition of a simple tranquillizer may be effective, but in some patients with this 'psychic' pain, stereotactic cingulotomy to interrupt circuits in the limbic system is required.

Sympathectomy

Sympathectomy is also effective in relief of *causalgia*, the burning pain and autonomic dysfunction that results from partial injury to major nerve trunks.

Electroanalgesia

Nerve fibre stimulation rather than destruction has been introduced following the demonstration that stimulation of a peripheral nerve trunk reduces pain sensation over the distribution of the nerve. Activation of A fibres may interfere with the perception of a painful stimulus, possibly at spinal cord level, or there may be a release of enkephalins.

Electrodes are implanted close to the nerve trunk in question, or at higher levels in the nervous system, and can be activated by the patient using a small power pack when he feels the need for more analgesia. Unfortunately these devices are expensive

and give long-term relief in only a small percentage of patients.

Trigeminal neuralgia

The standard treatment of trigeminal neuralgia used to be long-term administration of carbamazepine. However, adverse reactions such as rash, drowsiness and ataxia are frequent, and pain recurrence after months or years is not uncommon. Consequently, radiofrequency trigeminal rhizotomy is now recommended for initial treatment. It produces analgesia without loss of ordinary sensation in the face and the corneal reflex is preserved.

Pain relief in advanced oropharyngeal cancer

Extensive analgesia may be achieved by dividing, through a posterior fossa approach, the 5th nerve, nervus intermedius, 9th and 10th cranial nerves and the upper three cervical nerves on the appropriate side. This is a major procedure in debilitated patients and better results are obtained by stereotactic tractotomy of the trigeminal tract of the upper cervical cord under local anaesthesia.

SPECIAL NEUROSURGICAL TECHNIQUES

Access

Burr holes

Burr holes are simple skull perforations made to remove fluid, pus or blood from the cranium, or to enable instruments to be passed into the brain. The standard burr holes are made in the frontal, parietal and occipitoparietal regions along the pupillary plane (Fig. 37.21). Temporal burr holes may be made immediately above the zygoma to allow access to the middle meningeal artery in extradural haematoma, or directly above the root of the ear to drain a temporal lobe abscess.

After shaving the head, local anaesthetic solution with adrenaline is injected into the skin of the scalp. If the procedure is being done under general anaesthesia, 1:200 000 adrenaline solution is used to assist haemostasis. An incision is made down to bone, any overlying muscle is retracted, and the pericranium scraped away. A small self-retaining retractor is placed in the wound and the skull is perforated using a brace and bit. A burr is then used to enlarge and smooth out the hole. Modern power tools combine

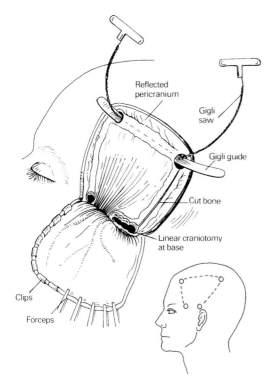

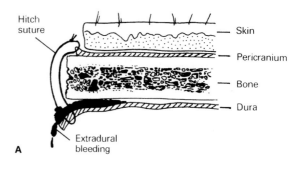

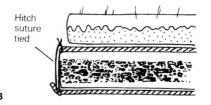

Fig. 37.22 Craniotomy.

Fig. 37.23 Control of dural bleeding with 'hitch' sutures: **A** 'hitch' suture inserted but not yet tied down; **B** 'hitch' suture tied.

these functions. The exposed dura is picked up with a sharp hook and opened using a cruciate incision (see Fig. 37.22).

Craniotomy

A flap of skin and skull is formed which is replaced over the defect at the end of the procedure.

The line of incision is marked out and infiltrated with a solution of local anaesthetic and adrenaline. The scalp incision is made with the assistant compressing the scalp against the skull to reduce bleeding. Artery forceps or clips are then applied to the scalp edges to prevent further bleeding. The scalp flap is elevated, and the lines of incision in the skull are marked by diathermy. The pericranium is incised and scraped away from the lines of incision.

Burr holes are now made. Using a guide, a Gigli saw is used to divide the skull between two burr holes. This process is repeated until the bone flap has been completely separated from the skull. A small muscle attachment is usually left to carry the blood supply to the flap (Fig. 37.22).

This classical technique is being replaced with the quicker and easier method of using a straight incision and self-retaining retraction. Only two

temporal burr holes are needed and the bone flap is cut using a craniotome.

Bleeding from the exposed dura is controlled by diathermy or gelatin packs, or by dural traction. This is achieved by suturing the periphery of the dura to the pericranium around the defect (Fig. 37.23). Raised ICP, as evidenced by a tight dura, may be reduced by mannitol or ventricular puncture.

The dura is opened after elevation on a small hook, and the incision is extended with scissors while the brain is protected by a small swab.

Craniectomy

In urgent situations (e.g. removal of an intracranial haematoma) there may not be time to 'turn a flap'. A single burr hole is then made and extended by piece-meal excision of the skull with bone forceps, making a defect referred to as a craniectomy. The defect may have to be corrected at a later date by insertion of a plastic or metal mould (cranioplasty).

Craniectomy is always used for posterior fossa exploration, as the thick posterior neck muscles cover the area without leaving an unsightly defect.

Laminectomy

The spinal cord and nerves are exposed by partial or complete laminectomy. The skin and underlying

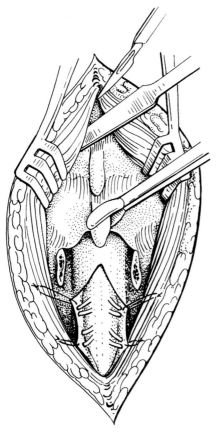

Fig. 37.24 Laminectomy.

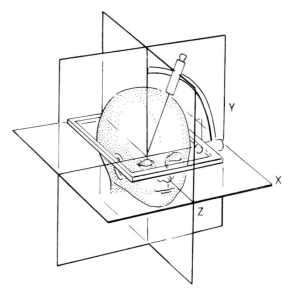

Fig. 37.25 Principles of stereotactic apparatus used to locate (and treat) the target area.

muscles are infiltrated down to the laminae with a solution of local anaesthetic and adrenaline, and an incision is made down to the spinous processes. The wound is held open with a self-retaining retractor. The paraspinal muscles are separated from the processes and lamina, and retracted (Fig. 37.24).

The spinal processes over the desired length of spine are removed at their bases, and the laminae are removed with bone rongeurs, taking care to protect the underlying spinal dura. The dura is incised longitudinally and its cut edges are sutured to the muscles.

In partial laminectomies (or hemilaminectomies) the spinal processes are preserved while the lamina is removed on one side. In *fenestration* procedures for the removal of a prolapsed intervertebral disc, the disc and nerve root are exposed by opening the ligamentum flavum at the appropriate level and, if necessary, removing a small piece of adjoining lamina.

Stereotactic surgery

Most frames for stereotactic surgery employ the Cartesian coordinate system with three fixed intersecting planes at right angles – coronal, sagittal and horizontal (Fig. 37.25). The position of a point in space can be defined in all three planes, and a probe moved precisely to that point.

The instrument is securely fastened to the skull (or spine) and, using specially prepared brain or spinal stereotactic atlases, the coordinates of the target area are determined. Accuracy may be improved by injection of radio-opaque material to outline the ventricles or by obtaining electrical recordings from known areas. Under fluoroscopy, on which a measuring grid also appears, the tip of the probe is advanced to the target area. A lesion is made by cutting (using a leucotome), freezing (using a cryoprobe), heating (by radiofrequency electrode) or irradiation (using isotopes). Alternatively, stimulating electrodes may be left in situ. Recent renewed interest in the technique has centred on its use for accurate tumour biopsy or excision and for interstitial radiation.

Section 10
PRACTICAL PROCEDURES

38
Practical procedures

CONTENTS

and most are helped by a description of sensations they are likely to experience before these occur. Where appropriate, informed written consent should be obtained.

GENERAL PRECAUTIONS

It is important to be aware of the potential danger of inappropriately ascribed results, and of the infective or trauma risk to patient, operator and assistant during any practical procedure. These risks are minimized by following a few simple rules:

- Label all specimens clearly with the patient's full name and some other means of identification such as an identifying number, address or date of birth. The source of the specimen, its nature and the date taken, must also be noted. It is good practice to label specimens immediately after placement in the container.
- Needles should not be 're-sheathed', suture needles should be held in an appropriate instrument, and all disposable sharp instruments discarded by the operator should be placed in an appropriate container. These measures minimize the risk of 'needle-stick injury' to operator and assistant.
- Drapes and other soiled equipment should be placed in appropriate containers.
- Gloves and gown should only be removed after all used instruments and disposable equipment have been placed in appropriate containers.

INTRODUCTION

Every practical procedure performed on a conscious patient should be preceded by an explanation which should include the reasons for the procedure and what it will entail. Appropriate reassurance should always be given. Many patients find comfort in continuing reassurance throughout the procedure

ASEPTIC TECHNIQUE

Transmission of infection is an ever-present problem, and the hands must be washed before and after every practical procedure. As a minimum precaution the skin should be cleaned with an antiseptic solution before all procedures, sterile instruments used and clean gloves worn. For some procedures, such as central venous catheterization, bladder catheterization, insertion of chest drains and lumbar puncture, a full aseptic technique must be used.

Procedure

- An assistant is essential to open non-sterile packs and 'drop' required instruments or solutions onto the sterile field.
- Hand washing for aseptic techniques ('scrubbing-up') should last a full 3 minutes. The hands and forearms are wetted under a running tap and thoroughly washed with an antiseptic solution such as povidone iodine (Betadine) or chlorhexidine (Hibitane scrub).
- A sterile brush is then used to scrub the hands, in particular the ulnar border of the hand, the interdigital clefts and the nails.
- After completing the wash, the hands are rinsed and held hands-up/elbows down, so that water from the hands runs from the elbows into the sink.
- The hands are dried on a sterile towel and the operator puts on a sterile gown and gloves. Thereafter, the operator must not touch anything other than sterile equipment or instruments.
- The operative field is now cleaned with an antiseptic solution such as povidone iodine or chlorhexidine, using sterile instruments and swabs. The area prepared should be much greater than the anticipated operative field and cleansing should start from the centre of the field and work outwards.
- The operative field is now encircled with sterile drapes which are secured so as to leave the operative field at the centre and provide the operator with as wide a sterile surrounding as possible.

LOCAL ANAESTHESIA

Local anaesthetic drugs are potentially toxic. In general, efficacy is related to correct placement, and toxicity to total dose. Where doubt exists about placement or a wide area of infiltration is anticipated, it is safer to calculate the maximum recommended dose and dilute it with 0.9% saline to the desired volume.

Lignocaine is the most widely available local anaesthetic and the maximum recommended dose is 3 mg/kg. For most purposes a 0.5% or 1.0% solution is suitable.

Solutions of local anaesthetic mixed with a 1:200 000 concentration of adrenaline are also available. Local anaesthetic agents with adrenaline should not be used in anatomical areas supplied by an end-artery such as the digits.

WOUND SUTURE

Wounds are sutured under as near-sterile conditions as possible with a strict aseptic technique. A few basic principles underlie good wound care.

- Tissue should be handled gently. The wound should not be rubbed with swabs. Blood in a wound is removed by pressing a swab onto it.
- Haemostasis should be meticulous to prevent wound haematoma.
- All foreign material and devitalized tissues should be removed. Where this is prevented by heavy contamination, delayed primary suture or secondary suture should be considered.
- Potential spaces (dead-space) in the wound should be closed using absorbable suture material such as catgut, 'Vicryl' or 'Dexon'. Where this is not possible, a suction drain is led from the potential space before more superficial layers are closed.
- The tension on knots is critical. If they are tied too tightly, the suture line may become ischaemic, leading to delayed healing or non-healing and an increased risk of wound infection. Equally, insufficient tension on the suture may result in failure to appose the wound edges or inadequate haemostasis.

Suturing the skin

Cutting needles are used to suture skin. Non-absorbable sutures (see below) are generally preferred but require subsequent removal. Interrupted sutures have the advantage over continuous sutures that removal of one or two appropriately sited stitches may allow adequate drainage of the wound if it becomes infected. The sutures should be placed equidistant from one another, taking equal 'bites' on either side of the wound. A sufficient number should be inserted to maintain apposition of the skin edges without gaping. The size of bite is determined by the amount of subcutaneous fat and by whether or not the subcutaneous fat has been separately sutured. In the abdomen, the bite is approximately 5 mm on either side of the wound, whereas on the face a 1–2 mm bite is preferred. The wound edge is picked up

Table 38.1 Times recommended for removal of sutures	
Face and neck	4 days
Scalp	7 days
Abdomen and chest	7–10 days
Limbs	7 days
Feet	10–14 days

with toothed dissecting forceps, and the needle is introduced through the skin at an angle as close to vertical as possible and brought out on the other side at a similar angle.

Similar principles apply when using a continuous suture. A subcuticular stitch, inserted as a continuous suture, is preferred by some surgeons and avoids the small pinpoint scars at the site of entry and exit of the traditional suture, or the ugly cross-hatching that results if sutures are tied too tightly or left in too long. Table 38.1 gives the suggested times for removal of sutures.

Cosmetic results as good as those achieved by subcuticular suturing can be obtained by removing sutures in half the times listed in Table 38.1 and replacing them with adhesive strips (e.g. Steristrip). Skin stapling or clipping is used increasingly for scalp wounds but is appropriate for skin closure at any site. Skin clips are supplied in disposable cartridges for single patient use.

Suture materials

Non-absorbable

Non-absorbable sutures may be classified into three groups:

1. Natural braided sutures (e.g. silk, linen) have good handling qualities and knot easily and securely. Their disadvantage is increased tissue reaction and suture line sepsis caused by capillary action of the braided material drawing microorganisms into the suture track. Such materials also lose tensile strength with time, or when wet.
2. Synthetic braided materials (e.g. Nurolon, Ethibond, Mersilene) cause less tissue reaction than natural materials but have good handling qualities and knot easily and securely.
3. Synthetic monofilament materials (e.g. nylon, polypropylene) have less drag through the tissues and cause little tissue reaction. They are free from the capillary effect of braided sutures and cause less suture track sepsis. They handle less well because of increased 'memory' (i.e. they

retain the configuration in which they were packaged). Knots in monofilament sutures are less secure than knots in braided or natural sutures, requiring multiple throws on each knot.

Absorbable sutures

Absorbable sutures may be classified into two groups:

1. Natural materials (e.g. plain catgut, chromic catgut). Catgut is used to suture skin in a few specific indications (e.g. skin of the penis after circumcision, and suture of scrotal skin). Knots are less secure than with braided material.
2. Synthetic materials such as Dexon (polyglycolic acid), Vicryl (polyglycolic plus polylactic acid) and PDS (polydioxonone) are used to close the skin using a subcuticular technique. In small wounds this may mean interrupted sutures with each knot buried, while in longer wounds a continuous subcuticular suture is used.

Around the eyes, 6/0 gauge sutures are recommended and elsewhere on the face 5/0. In the neck, hands and digits 4/0 sutures are appropriate. In other sites 3/0 or even 2/0 sutures are used. For subcuticular wound closure, 4/0 sutures are appropriate.

ABDOMINAL PROCEDURES

Nasogastric tube insertion

A nasogastric tube is inserted to drain stomach contents in conditions such as intestinal obstruction, or to administrate enteral nutrition. In most situations a 14–16 Fr single lumen, radio-opaque nasogastric tube with multiple distal openings will suffice. Double lumen tubes are occasionally used to allow continuous low-pressure suction without the lumen becoming blocked by gastric mucosa.

Procedure

The nose is inspected for any deformity and the more patent nasal passage is chosen for insertion. The patient is placed in the sitting position and a local anaesthetic spray may be used to anaesthetize the nasal passage. The tube is well lubricated with gel and passed backwards along the floor of the nasal passage (Fig. 38.1). A slight resistance may be felt as the tube passes from the nasopharynx to the oropharynx, and the patient should be warned that a retching feeling may be experienced at this point.

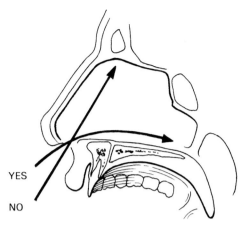

YES

NO

Fig. 38.1 Nasogastric intubation. Note the correct direction for inserting the tube.

nervous system through an open fracture of the base of skull. The oral route is also considered in patients with serious coagulopathy, as passage of the tube through the nose may result in significant haemorrhage. Finally, blind passage of a tube in the early period following oesophagectomy should never be attempted as this may disrupt the anastomosis.

Fine-bore nasogastric tubes

Elemental diets tend to have an unpleasant taste, and are poorly tolerated when swallowed normally. Such diets are best given by infusion through a fine-bore nasogastric tube. These tubes cause less discomfort and are less likely to cause oesophageal erosions than a standard nasogastric tube. They do, however, require great care in insertion as they can easily pass into the respiratory tract.

Procedure

Fine-bore nasogastric tubes have a wire stylet to facilitate passage. The tube is passed in the same way as a standard nasogastric tube. *The position of the tube is confirmed by X-ray*, and only then is the wire stylet removed. Once removed, it must never be re-introduced while the tube remains in the patient as there is a significant risk of the wire perforating both the tube and the oesophagus. The tube tends to collapse if aspirated, and aspiration cannot be used to check its position.

The patient is now asked to swallow and with each swallow the tube is advanced down the oesophagus. Ideally about 10–15 cm of the tube should be placed into the stomach. The oesophago-gastric junction is about 40 cm from the incisor teeth. Most nasogastric tubes have markings which allow measurement of the length inserted. Correct placement of the tube is confirmed by free aspiration of gastric contents, and by auscultation in the epigastrium while 20 ml of air are insufflated.

In patients with head injuries the nasal route is avoided because of the risk of introducing infection, or even the nasogastric tube itself, into the central

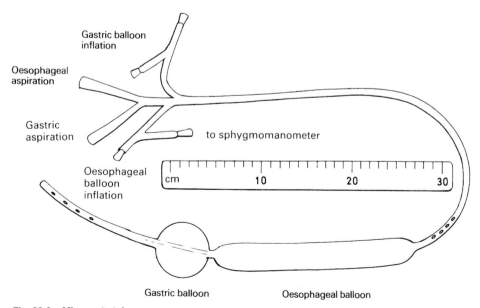

Gastric balloon inflation

Oesophageal aspiration

Gastric aspiration

to sphygmomanometer

Oesophageal balloon inflation

cm   10   20   30

Gastric balloon   Oesophageal balloon

Fig. 38.2 Minnesota tube.

Oesophageal tamponade

The Sengstaken tube is a gastric aspiration tube with inflatable gastric and oesophageal balloons, which compress the distended oesophageal and gastric fundal veins. It is used for emergency treatment of bleeding oesophageal or gastric varices. A modification, the Minnesota tube (Fig. 38.2), has an additional channel to allow the aspiration of saliva from the oesophagus above the level of the oesophageal ballon.

Procedure

The oesophageal and gastric balloons are checked for leaks and then completely deflated prior to insertion. The tube is inserted in the same way as a normal nasogastric tube. However, it is much more uncomfortable and local anaesthesia is recommended for nasal passage. A patient with bleeding varices is unlikely to cooperate fully and the tube may have to be passed with the patient on his side.

About 50 to 60 cm of tube is passed into the patient and the gastric balloon inflated with 30 ml of Gastrografin. An X-ray is taken to confirm position. The gastric balloon is now inflated with 150 ml of water and the tube drawn back until the balloon impacts at the cardia. An assistant holds the tube in this position with slight tension and the oesophageal balloon is inflated with air to a pressure of 30–40 mmHg, checked by attaching a sphygmomanometer. The tube is secured in position with tape to maintain the slight tension. Alternatively continuous traction may be applied.

The stomach is aspirated regularly through the main lumen of the tube. The oesophagus cannot be aspirated through a Sengstaken tube and saliva starts to pool above the oesophageal balloon. The patient is therefore nursed in a semi-prone position so that saliva can be spat out or aspirated from the mouth. With the Minnesota tube these secretions can be aspirated through the fourth lumen.

It is essential to deflate the oesophageal balloon for 5 minutes every 6 hours to avoid the risk of ischaemic necrosis of the oesophageal mucosa. If possible, the pressure in the oesophageal balloon should be reduced to 25 mmHg after 12 hours. The tube is not normally kept in place for more than 24 hours.

Abdominal paracentesis

Abdominal paracentesis is performed to relieve the discomfort caused by distension with ascitic fluid or to obtain fluid for cytological examination. The bladder must be emptied, if necessary by preliminary catheterization. A 'Trocath' peritoneal dialysis catheter (Fig. 38.3) with multiple side perforations

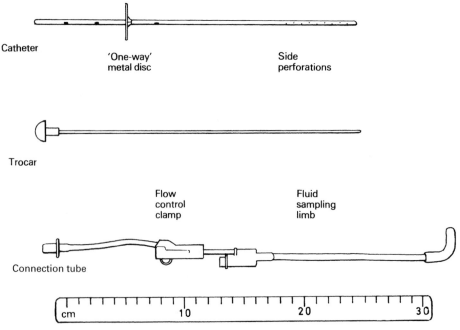

Fig. 38.3 'Trocath' peritoneal dialysis catheter.

over a length of 8 cm is inserted under sterile conditions. The operator scrubs up and wears a gown and gloves. Local anaesthetic is infiltrated at an angle of 70° through all layers of the abdominal wall. This can be done either in the midline (one-third of the way from the umbilicus to the pubic symphysis), or in the right or left iliac fossa (at the junction of the outer and middle thirds of a line drawn from the anterior superior spine to the umbilicus). The depth at which the peritoneum is entered is determined by aspiration with the syringe. The vicinity of scars should be avoided, as adhesions increase the risk of puncture of the bowel.

A 3-mm stab incision is made in the skin with a scalpel. The trocar is introduced into the catheter and the shaft of the catheter is held firmly between left thumb and index finger some 4–5 cm higher than the estimated depth of the peritoneum. This prevents 'overshoot' as the right hand thrusts the trocar and catheter through the abdominal wall into the peritoneum (Fig. 38.4).

The catheter is now advanced further with the left hand while the trocar is withdrawn with the right hand. If any resistance is noted, the catheter is withdrawn 2–3 cm, rotated 180° and then advanced again. The minimum final length of catheter within the peritoneal cavity must be 10 cm. If this position is not obtained, the side perforations of the catheter may lie within the abdominal wall and allow troublesome extravasation of ascitic fluid in the subcutaneous tissues. The one-way metal disc is slid down the catheter to make contact with the skin and secured to it with adhesive tape. The catheter is divided some 4 cm above the metal disc and attached via a connection tube with a flow control clamp to a sterile drainage bag.

Rapid drainage of large volumes of ascitic fluid is avoided as this can result in a marked shift of fluid from the intravascular space into the peritoneal

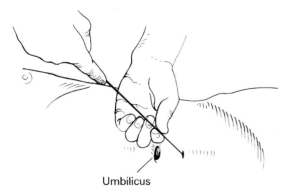

Umbilicus

Fig. 38.4 Insertion of peritoneal dialysis catheter.

cavity, leading to hypotension, cardiovascular instability, and hepatic encephalopathy.

Gastric lavage

The commonest indication for gastric lavage is removal of ingested poisons or drugs. Much less commonly, it is used to lower or raise the body core temperature.

Aspiration of gastric contents is a serious risk. If there is any doubt about the patient's ability to maintain the airway, expert assistance is sought and endotracheal intubation considered prior to the procedure. The patient's level of consciousness, presence of a gag reflex and ability to cough are the most useful guides to the need for endotracheal intubation.

Procedure

After assessing the need for endotracheal intubation, the patient is placed on the left side in the 'recovery position' with a 15° head-down tilt of the trolley. A large-bore gastric tube is introduced into the mouth. A mouth gag is useful to prevent the patient biting the tube. The patient is likely to gag and even vomit, as the tube is passed into the oropharynx and upper oesophagus. The tube is advanced into the stomach and its correct position confirmed by the free flow of gastric contents. If there is doubt, auscultation of the epigastrium during injection of air down the tube will confirm correct placement. About 100–200 ml of warm water (warm to the touch) are passed down the tube into the stomach. The end of the tube is then lowered below the level of the stomach into a collecting bucket and gastric contents will syphon out. The manoeuvre is repeated until the returned water becomes clear. It is important to avoid over-distension of the stomach. Activated charcoal can then be instilled into the stomach to act as an absorbent if this is appropriate. On completion, the tube is removed.

AIRWAY PROCEDURES

Maintaining the airway

The ability to maintain the airway is a basic skill which every doctor, nurse, paramedic and indeed member of the general public should have. Its simplicity belies its importance but it is a life-saving skill which must be learnt through practice.

In the unconscious patient, muscles which normally maintain a clear airway become lax. The tongue and soft tissue fall backwards, particularly in the supine patient, occluding the airway. Maintaining a clear airway allows the patient to breathe or allows the lungs to be ventilated.

Procedure

The simplest manoeuvre is to place the patient on his side with the neck extended in the so-called 'recovery position'. This allows the tongue and soft tissues to fall clear of the larynx and provide a patent airway. The mouth and pharynx should be checked and cleared of debris such as dentures, vomit or food.

Where the patient has to be kept supine, the neck should be extended. The mouth is opened slightly, and the mandible pulled firmly forward by pressure applied behind both angles of the jaw. The mandible is held in this position by closing the mouth and using the teeth as a splint. Forward pressure is maintained behind the angles of the jaw or submentally, avoiding pressure on the soft tissues. In some cases, particularly in edentulous patients, an oropharyngeal airway helps to maintain a patent airway.

Ventilation by mask

The lungs may be ventilated by mask and bag using one of two systems. The first is a rebreathing bag with an adjustable valve and fresh gas supply (which should be present in each anaesthetic room, Intensive Therapy Unit and resuscitation room). The second and more widespread, is the self re-inflating type of bag such as the 'AMBU' or 'Laerdel' bags which do not rely on a gas supply but to which supplemental oxygen can be added. For the inexperienced, this technique is best performed with the help of an assistant.

Procedure

The airway is held patent with the patient supine as described above. A mask is applied to the face and held in position using the thumb and index finger of both hands. The little fingers of each hand are placed behind the angles of the jaw and used to lift the mandible forward. The ring and middle fingers are placed on the mandible to help maintain this position. The assistant squeezes the bag to ventilate the lungs.

With more experience it is possible to maintain a patent airway and hold the mask on with one hand and squeeze the bag with the other.

The laryngeal mask airway

This recently introduced airway is designed to be inserted into the pharynx, and has a cuff which when inflated forms a cup around the larynx. It is not a replacement for endotracheal intubation and does not protect the airway from aspiration. It does however provide a patent airway when positioned correctly and allows effective ventilation of the lungs. As with other procedures, insertion should be learned under supervision.

Procedure

The cuff should be deflated and lubricated with a gel. The patient's head and neck are positioned as for intubation. The mask is held in the right hand and introduced into the mouth, while the left hand is used to maintain the head in the extended position. For women a size 3 is suitable and for men a size 4. Smaller sizes are available for children. The mask is passed backwards over the tongue until resistance is felt. It should then be at the level of the larynx at the upper oesophageal sphincter. The cuff is inflated and the mask should be seen to rise slightly out of the mouth. Position is confirmed by the ability to ventilate the lungs with gentle pressure on a bag system.

Endotracheal intubation

Endotracheal intubation can be life saving. It can maintain a patent airway, facilitate oxygenation, and prevent aspiration. The student is advised to take every opportunity to acquire this skill in the elective situation in the anaesthetic room.

Procedure

The patient's neck is flexed and the head extended at the atlanto-occipital joint. Retaining a pillow under the head but free from beneath the shoulders will usually help to attain this position. Failure to position the patient correctly is one of the commonest causes of difficulty in intubation.

The laryngoscope is held in the left hand and its blade is inserted into the right side of the mouth and passed backwards along the side of the tongue into the oropharynx. The blade is designed to push the tongue over to the left side of the mouth. Care is taken to avoid damage to the lips and teeth. The laryngoscope is *pulled* upwards and forwards, *not* used as a lever, to lift the tongue and jaw and reveal the epiglottis. The blade is advanced to the base of the epiglottis.

Failure to visualize the epiglottis usually reflects the fact that the blade has not been inserted far enough, in which case only the base of the tongue will be seen. Alternatively, it may mean that it has been inserted too far, in which case the upper oesophagus will be seen. The appropriate adjustment in position should be made. The laryngoscope is pulled further upwards and forwards to reveal the vocal cords.

For women an 8.0-mm cuffed tube is usually appropriate and for men a 9.0-mm tube. For children a rough rule of thumb to gauge tube size is age divided by 4 + 4.5 mm. Normally an uncuffed tube is used.

The endotracheal tube is passed through the vocal cords and advanced until its cuff is about 1 cm through the cords. Many endotracheal tubes have a mark to indicate this position. The laryngoscope blade is withdrawn and the cuff inflated to provide an air-tight seal in the trachea.

The most serious complication of endotracheal intubation is failure to recognize misplacement of the tube, particularly in the oesophagus or to a lesser degree, in the right main bronchus. Misplacement is best avoided by direct visualization of passage of the tube between the vocal cords, inspection of the chest wall for equal movement of both sides of the chest, and auscultation for breath sounds bilaterally in the mid-axillary line. Absence of or the presence of only quiet breath sounds in the epigastrium is a further reassuring sign. If there is any doubt about the position of the tube, it should be removed and ventilation instituted by mask.

Tracheostomy

Tracheostomy bypasses the upper airway and has a wide range of indications. These include obstruction of the airway by infection or trauma, or the need to wean critically ill patients from long-term ventilation. In emergency situations, tracheostomy is performed only when other methods of securing the airway and oxygenation are inappropriate or have failed.

Tracheostomy is a procedure for an experienced surgeon. The methods used include formal open surgery, cricothyroidotomy, and percutaneous dilatation.

Changing a tracheostomy tube

It is common practice to change a tracheostomy tube every seven days. Suction must be available.

Procedure

If a cuffed tube is to be inserted, the integrity of the cuff is checked and it is then fully deflated. Lubricant gel is inserted on the cuff and tube. The patient is placed semi-recumbent with the neck extended. If replacement is likely to be difficult, a suction catheter inserted into the old tracheostomy tube can be used as an introducer for the new tube.

The cuff of the old tube is deflated. Secretions often collect above the cuff and enter the trachea when it is deflated causing the patient to cough. Patient and operator should be alert to this. Because the tube is curved, it should be removed with an 'arc-like' movement. The site is then cleaned and any secretions removed. In the spontaneously breathing, stable patient there is no need for undue haste. The new tube is inserted with a similar movement to that employed for removal, and its cuff inflated.

Any signs of respiratory distress should alert one to the possibility of misplacement or occlusion of the tube. The tube and trachea are immediately checked for patency by passing a suction catheter through the tube. If the catheter passes easily into the respiratory tract, usually signified by the patient coughing as the catheter touches the carina, other causes for respiratory distress should be sought.

When the tracheostomy is no longer needed, an airtight dressing is applied over the site after removing the tube. There is no need for formal surgical closure at this stage, as in most instances the wound will close and heal spontaneously. For the first few days, the patient should be encouraged to press firmly on the dressing when he or she wishes to cough, so as to avoid air leakage through the tracheostomy site.

THORACIC PROCEDURES

Intercostal tube drainage

Intercostal intubation is used to drain a large pneumothorax, haemothorax or pleural effusion. To drain a pneumothorax, a size 14–16 Fr catheter is inserted near the apex of the lung in the mid-clavicular line of the second intercostal space.

A lateral approach in the mid-axillary line of the

sixth intercostal space can also be used. This may be easier in muscular patients and has fewer cosmetic problems. Drainage of an effusion or haemothorax requires a larger drain (20–26 Fr) which should be inserted in the 7th to 9th intercostal space in the posterior axillary line. A slightly higher insertion in the mid-axillary line may be technically easier in supine, acutely ill patients.

Procedure

If a low lateral approach is to be used, reference should be made to the chest X-ray to ensure that the drain will not be inserted subdiaphragmatically. A strict aseptic technique must be used. The skin, intercostal muscle and pleura are infiltrated with local anaesthetic. If a rib is encountered by the needle tip, the tip is 'walked' up the rib to enter the pleura above the rib edge. The depth at which the pleural space is entered is determined by aspiration with the syringe. A 1-cm incision is now made in the skin. The shaft of the catheter is held firmly between the left thumb and index finger some 3 cm higher than the estimated depth of the pleura. This prevents 'overshoot' as the right hand thrusts the trocar and catheter through the chest wall in the chosen interspace into the pleural cavity (Fig. 38.5). The point of the trocar is directed towards the apex of the pleural cavity. The catheter is then advanced with the left hand while the trocar is withdrawn with the right hand. The catheter is clamped with a heavy artery forceps and then sutured to the skin with a heavy suture to prevent accidental dislodgement. A

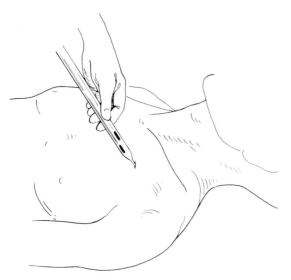

Fig. 38.5   Intercostal intubation with 'Trocath' catheter.

'Z' suture is placed around the incision, wrapped tightly around the drainage tube and tied, thus securing the tube against accidental displacement. A sterile dressing and an adhesive bandage are applied to form an airtight seal and prevent aspiration of air around the tube. The drainage tube is attached to an underwater drainage system. Low-pressure suction may be applied to the drainage bottle to assist drainage or re-expansion of the lung.

Removal of an intercostal drainage tube

The drainage tube may be removed 12 to 24 hours after cessation of drainage. As a precaution in the case of a pneumothorax, the tube is first clamped for several hours and a chest X-ray taken to ensure that there has been no recurrence of the pneumothorax.

Procedure

The 'Z' suture is freed from the tube and can be used to close the wound. Where this is not possible, the suture should be removed totally and a new suture inserted around the wound. The patient is asked to hold his/her breath, and an assistant withdraws the tube after which the skin is firmly closed with the previously inserted suture.

A sterile dressing is firmly applied over the wound and the chest X-ray repeated to confirm that there is no pneumothorax.

Pleural aspiration

Aspiration of fluid from the pleural cavity is performed for diagnostic or therapeutic purposes. Protein or amylase content, and cytological or bacteriological examination may be diagnostic. Complete aspiration of large effusions allows fuller expansion of the lungs and may improve ventilation.

Procedure

Where aspiration is to be undertaken for diagnostic purposes only, a 21-gauge needle and syringe are adequate. In therapeutic aspiration, a larger bore needle, 50 ml syringe and three-way tap system should be used. The procedure is carried out with a strict aseptic technique.

The patient is positioned sitting up, resting his arms and elbows on a table in front. The position and size of the effusion should be outlined by percussion and chest X-ray. The lower border of the effusion is determined, particularly on the right to avoid puncturing the liver. In the case of small effusions, ultrasound guidance is helpful.

The skin, intercostal muscle and pleura are infiltrated with local anaesthetic in the 7th or 8th space in line with the inferior angle of the scapula. A 2-mm stab incision is made in the skin and the needle advanced over the upper border of the rib to avoid damage to the neurovascular bundle. The needle and syringe should be advanced in a downward direction, at an angle of about 70° with continuous aspiration. It should be advanced no further than is required to aspirate fluid freely, thus avoiding damage to the underlying lung.

If the volume of fluid to be removed is greater than the volume of the syringe being used, a three-way tap greatly reduces the risk of air entry and allows emptying of the syringe into a collection vessel (Fig. 38.6); this avoids having to disconnect the syringe each time it is filled. It is normally recommended that no more than 1.0–1.5 litres of fluid be removed at any one time. This reduces the risk of sudden mediastinal shift or the development of pulmonary oedema associated with rapid re-expansion of a collapsed lung. Coughing or pain on aspiration is an indication that visceral pleura is in close contact with the end of the cannula, which should be repositioned or withdrawn.

At the end of the procedure, the needle is withdrawn and a sterile dressing applied. A chest X-ray is taken to assess the amount of residual fluid present and to check for the absence of a pneumothorax.

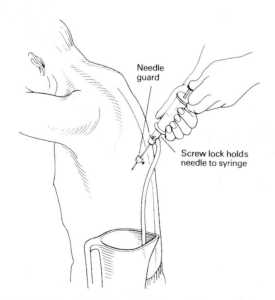

Fig. 38.6 Pleural aspiration. Note screw-lock on needle to maintain position.

VASCULAR PROCEDURES

Venepuncture

The antecubital fossa is the most convenient site as the median cubital vein, median vein of the forearm and the cephalic vein are all easily accessible. Care must be taken to avoid the brachial artery. Sampling from smaller veins on the forearm or the back of the hand may at first sight appear more attractive, but these veins collapse easily on aspiration and adequate samples are difficult to obtain. In cases of extreme difficulty the femoral vein should be considered. This vessel lies medial to the femoral artery which is used as a landmark. In adults a 21-gauge needle is used and in children a 23-gauge or 25-gauge will suffice.

Procedure

A venous tourniquet is applied to the upper arm and the patient encouraged to clench the fist several times to increase venous filling. The position of the vein is identified and the skin cleaned. The needle is advanced through the skin and into the vein with the needle bevel facing upwards. This manoeuvre is carried out in a 'two-step' fashion; first through the skin and then through the vein wall. Entry through the skin with a decisive action causes much less discomfort than a slow hesitant movement. The needle is advanced 2–3 mm into the vein and the position of the needle and syringe stabilized with one hand. The plunger of the syringe is slowly withdrawn with the other hand until the required amount of blood is obtained. The tourniquet is then released, the needle withdrawn and pressure immediately applied over the site of entry into the vein with the arm raised for one minute to prevent haematoma formation, which is painful for the patient and makes subsequent sampling more difficult.

The blood is placed into the appropriate sample tubes after removal of the needle from the syringe. With pre-vacuumed sample tubes, the needle should be left on the syringe in order to fill the tubes. Haemolysis of blood invalidates some results, for example, potassium and phosphate levels. This can be minimized by slow withdrawal of blood into the syringe. It is more likely to occur when smaller needles are used.

Safety measures

Used needles and syringes should be placed in specially reinforced carriers — 'Cin-Bins' — to avoid the risk of needle-stick injury or blood contamination to portering or other staff. To reduce further the risk of blood spillage or contamination to medical and laboratory staff, systems have now been introduced in which the sample tubes themselves are modified so that they may be used as syringes, and sent to the laboratory without the need to transfer blood from syringe to sample tube (e.g. Sarstedt Monovette®).

Venepuncture for blood culture

This procedure is carried out for microbiological culture and identification of organisms which may be present in the blood. The procedure is similar to venepuncture but particular care must be taken to avoid contamination. The skin must be thoroughly cleaned and a strict 'no-touch' technique used.

Procedure

A venous tourniquet is applied as before. The patient's skin is thoroughly cleaned using an appropriate solution and a sterile swab or cotton wool ball. Venepuncture is performed without the operator touching the skin around the site of entry of the needle. After withdrawal of the needle, it is removed from the syringe and a second sterile needle substituted. This is then used to introduce the appropriate aliquot of blood into the blood culture bottles (both aerobic and anaerobic culture bottles should be used). Exact volumes of blood required and the number of bottles filled will depend on local laboratory policies. All blood culture bottles should be sent immediately to the laboratory or, if this is not possible, placed in an incubator at 37° until transport is available.

Peripheral venous cannulation

Most intravenous infusions are given into the forearm. The veins of the leg are generally avoided because of the greater risk of thrombosis. Intravenous cannulae should not be sited over joints, if possible, as this necessitates splinting of the joint reducing the free use of the arm by the patient. Even with splinting, cannulae are subject to more movement in these positions and are prone to more complications.

A wide range of cannulae are commercially available but all consist essentially of an outer flexible sheath and an inner metal needle. A 16-gauge or 18-gauge cannula will suffice for most purposes in adults. Where rapid infusions of large quantities of fluid are required, a larger cannula should be used.

Procedure

A venous tourniquet is applied and the site of insertion chosen. The skin is cleaned and local anaesthetic infiltrated intradermally at the site of the insertion. Venepuncture is made in the 'two-step' fashion described above and confirmed by a 'flashback' of blood into the cannula. The cannula is advanced 2–3 mm into the vein. The cannula sheath is then advanced into the vein with one hand while the metal needle is partially withdrawn with the other.

Once the cannula is fully inserted into the vein, the tourniquet is released and gentle pressure applied over the vein at the tip of the cannula. The metal needle is then fully withdrawn from the cannula and the giving set, previously primed with normal saline, is connected. The cannula and distal 10–15 cm of the giving set are securely fixed to the skin with adhesive tape.

It is wise to insert the cannula as far distal as is practical as this allows a further attempt to be made more proximally on the same vein in the case of failure. This avoids fluid leaking out of the vein through a more proximal recent puncture site. In the case of repeated failure, help from a more experienced colleague should be sought sooner rather than later. This not only reduces discomfort, but leaves more potential cannulation sites available.

Cannulation sites should be inspected regularly for signs of swelling, erythema or tenderness which may indicate extravasation, thrombophlebitis or infection. If any are present or the patient complains of pain at the site, the infusion must be stopped and the cannula re-sited.

Extravasation may cause tissue necrosis. Thrombophlebitis occurs more readily when small veins are used, or when the pH of the infusate differs significantly from blood pH. The chances of infection increase the longer a cannula is left in situ and infusion sites must be changed regularly.

Bolus injections through an intravenous cannula should not be made without first ensuring that the cannula is patent and that there is no extravasation.

Venous cutdown

This may be carried out for access for fluid replacement or for access to the central veins for long-term parenteral nutrition or drug administration.

Venous cutdown for fluid replacement is rarely

required except in seriously hypovolaemic patients, usually following trauma. The most common site is the long saphenous vein at the ankle. Other sites include the basilic vein in the antecubital fossa and the cephalic vein in the delto-pectoral groove. It should only be regarded as a temporary measure for resuscitation.

Venous cutdown to the cephalic or external jugular veins for long-term central venous access is standard practice in many centres.

Procedure

Venous cutdown is performed with an aseptic technique. Local anaesthetic is infiltrated over the site, and a transverse incision is made in the skin over the vein which is then identified by blunt dissection. The vein should be cleared for a distance of 1–2 cm. The distal end of the vein is ligated with an absorbable ligature. The proximal end of the exposed vein is elevated to prevent backflow of blood, using a second absorbable ligature.

A transverse incision is then made in the vein. A large-bore cannula is passed through the skin 2 cm below the skin incision and guided into the vein. The cannula is advanced beyond the proximal ligature, which is then tied securely. The intravenous infusion is commenced.

The wound is closed with non-absorbable sutures and the cannula sutured to the skin to prevent accidental displacement. A sterile dressing is applied.

Central venous catheter insertion

Placement of a central venous catheter is indicated for monitoring of the central venous pressure (CVP) and for prolonged drug administration or parenteral nutrition.

Insertion is carried out with a strict aseptic technique as infection is one of the commonest complications of this procedure. If the catheter is to be used for drug therapy or parenteral nutrition, the procedure should be carried out in the operating theatre using a 'cut-down' technique. The common sites of insertion of catheters into the superior vena cava are from the internal jugular vein in the neck (Fig. 38.7), from the subclavian vein (Fig. 38.8), or occasionally from a peripheral vein in the antecubital fossa. A variety of cannulae and catheters are available but in general they are one of three types: (1) an extra long intravenous cannula; (2) a catheter inserted through a large cannula; (3) a catheter inserted over a wire (Seldinger technique). Each has advantages and disadvantages.

Internal jugular vein cannulation

Several approaches are described, but the high approach at the level of the thyroid cartilage carries the least risk. The right internal jugular vein is preferred as this provides a straighter route into the superior vena cava and avoids the risk of damaging the thoracic duct on the left. In general the 'Seldinger technique' is used and several commercial kits are available with the necessary equipment.

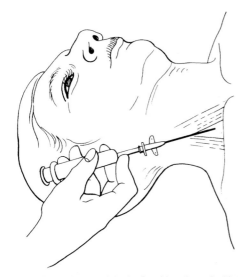

Fig. 38.7 Cannulation of the internal jugular vein. Note the triangle between the sternal and clavicular heads of the sternocleidomastoid muscle.

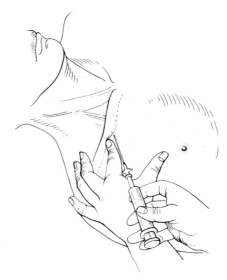

Fig. 38.8 Cannulation of the subclavian vein.

Procedure

Remove any pillows and position the patient slightly head-down with the patient's head turned to the left. Using an aseptic technique, clean and drape a wide area around the right side of the neck.

Identify the carotid artery at the level of the thyroid cartilage with the index and middle finger of the left hand. The internal jugular vein lies just lateral and parallel to it. A bleb of 1% lignocaine is injected into the skin at the proposed puncture site.

Using an 18-gauge needle on a 10-ml syringe held in the right hand, advance the needle through the skin just lateral to the carotid pulsation, at an angle of 60° to the skin and in the line of the vein. Free aspiration of blood confirms the position of the vein. This manoeuvre is repeated to place a larger (16 gauge) needle in the vein. The flexible 'J' end of the guide wire is now passed through this needle into the vein and the needle removed over it. This leaves the guide wire in the internal jugular vein. The dilator is now passed over the wire into the vein and then withdrawn. The manoeuvre is repeated with the catheter, but this time the wire is removed leaving the catheter in situ. In most adults, no more than 15 cm of catheter need be advanced into the vein to ensure correct placement. The catheter is fixed in position and a chest X-ray taken to check the position.

Subclavian vein cannulation

Several approaches to the subclavian vein are described but usually a subclavicular one is used. Any approach to the subclavian vein carries a significant risk of causing a pneumothorax or puncturing the subclavian artery. As with all procedures, but particularly with this one, it should be learnt under close supervision by an experienced operator. The 'Seldinger technique' is generally used to insert a subclavian catheter.

Peripheral venous catheterization

In theory this is the safest approach as it avoids the risk of pneumothorax. Haemorrhage from accidental arterial puncture or as a result of a coagulopathy can be controlled by pressure. Thrombosis and thrombophlebitis are however more frequent than when either the subclavian or internal jugular routes are used. Normally the long catheter is placed through a large cannula.

Procedure

Apply a venous tourniquet to the arm and select a suitable vein in the antecubital fossa through which the catheter can be passed up the basilic vein. Prepare the site using an aseptic technique and infiltrate over the vein with local anaesthetic. Insert the cannula into the vein as for normal intravenous cannulation and withdraw the needle. Pass the long catheter through the cannula into the vein. The venous tourniquet is now released.

Advance the catheter up the basilic vein and into the superior vena cava. A guide is often provided to gauge the length of catheter inserted. Difficulty is often experienced in advancing the catheter past the axilla. Extension of the arm may help overcome this problem.

The insertion cannula is now withdrawn from the vein leaving the long catheter in place, and the whole secured to the arm with adhesive tape. A chest X-ray is taken to confirm placement.

General points on central venous cannulation

- Air embolism is always a risk, even in the head-down position.
- When using a guide-wire, always hold it at some point along its length whilst it remains in the patient.
- Blood should be easily aspirated from the catheter if correctly positioned.
- A chest X-ray should always be taken to confirm the absence of a pneumothorax and correct position. A rough guide to position is that the tip of the catheter should lie at the level of the carina on X-ray.
- Cannulas inserted for intravenous nutrition are tunnelled in the subcutaneous tissue to emerge on the chest wall at a distance from the site of entry into the vein (Fig. 38.9). This minimizes the risk of sepsis spreading down the tract direct into the vein.

Measurement of central venous pressure (CVP)

The CVP is the pressure in the superior vena cava as it enters the right atrium. The zero point is taken as the level of the right atrium. With the patient lying supine, the midaxillary line is the surface marking to use as the reference point and assumed to represent zero or the level of the right atrium (Fig. 38.10). It is often convenient to mark the skin position to provide consistency in the recordings. An alternative surface

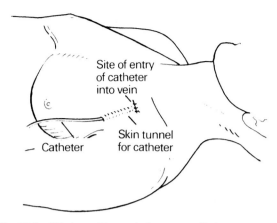

Fig. 38.9 Skin tunnel for central venous catheter.

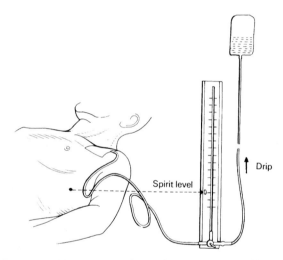

Fig. 38.10 Measurement of central venous pressure. Note the midthoracic point (marked by a black dot) which is used as the zero reference point.

reference point is the junction of the second rib and the sternum. In the supine patient this is considered to lie 5 cm above the right atrium. Whichever reference point is being used, confusion is avoided by remembering that the pressure being measured is in relation to the level of the right atrium. Consistency of the recordings is achieved by always using the same reference point with the patient in the supine position. A water manometer is normally used to measure this pressure.

Procedure

The water manometer system is primed with 5% dextrose prior to connection to the central venous catheter. The zero point on the manometer scale is levelled with the chosen reference point. The column is then filled to a higher level than the expected pressure and opened to the central venous catheter. The water column is allowed to fall and equilibrate. Fluctuations of the column with respiration are a reassuring sign of patency and correct positioning. The CVP is the level of the column at end-expiration.

Arterial blood sampling

Arterial blood sampling is undertaken to measure arterial P_{O_2}, P_{CO_2}, $[H^+]$ and standard $[HCO_3^-]$. The radial artery at the wrist is the site of choice. The brachial artery at the elbow and the femoral artery may also be used.

A heparinized sample is required to prevent blockage in the blood gas analyser due to coagulation of the sample. There are several commercially available pre-heparinized syringes but an ordinary 2-ml syringe which has been pre-heparinized as described below will suffice.

Procedure

If the syringe is not pre-heparinized, draw up to 0.5 ml of 1000 units/ml heparin into the syringe. The plunger is then fully withdrawn following which the air and excess heparin are expelled from the syringe. The residual heparin will be sufficient to anticoagulate the sample. A 23-gauge needle is suitable for arterial puncture.

Define the course of the artery by palpating the pulse between the index and middle fingers held 2 cm apart. The skin is cleaned and the needle with its bevel upwards introduced through the skin at an angle of about 60°. The needle is then advanced into the artery. Correct positioning is confirmed by blood pulsating into the syringe under pressure; 1–1.5 ml of blood is normally sufficient.

The needle is withdrawn and an assistant applies firm pressure over the puncture site for 3 minutes to avoid haematoma formation. The needle is removed from the syringe and any air bubbles expelled before capping the syringe. The syringe is gently inverted several times to ensure mixing of the heparin. The sample is sent immediately for analysis. Where delay is anticipated it should be transported in ice.

URINARY PROCEDURES

Urethral catheterization

This procedure may be carried out to relieve urinary retention or to determine urine output when it needs to be closely monitored. Occasionally, catheterization is necessary to facilitate nursing the incontinent patient. Anatomical obstruction may often be the cause of urinary retention in the male. It is particularly important to avoid forcing the passage of the catheter in this procedure and if difficulty is experienced, assistance should be sought. A full aseptic technique is required for both male and female catheterization.

Procedure in the male

The shaft of the penis is held with a sterile swab and the urethral orifice cleansed with a non-alcoholic, non-iodine containing solution. The foreskin, if present, is retracted. A 14 or 16 Fr catheter is used and lubricated with lubricant gel (Fig. 38.11). The shaft of the penis is held with a sterile swab in the left hand and traction applied to elongate the urethra.

The urinary catheter is introduced into the urethra with a 'no-touch' technique and advanced to its full length (Fig. 38.12). Correct placement is confirmed by the passage of urine down the catheter. If this does not occur, suprapubic pressure may assist. With the passage of urine through the catheter, the balloon on the catheter is inflated with the recommended volume of sterile water (generally 10–30 ml of water).

The catheter is gently withdrawn until the balloon engages the bladder neck, and connected to the drainage tubing. The foreskin, where present, should be replaced over the glans to prevent paraphimosis.

Procedure in the female

A 16–18 Fr catheter is suitable for this procedure. The labia minora are separated with the thumb and

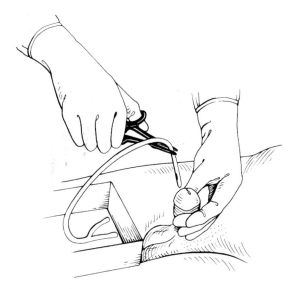

Fig. 38.12   Catheterization.

fingers of the left hand to expose the urethral meatus on the anterior vaginal wall. The pudenda are now swabbed with antiseptic solution. Two swabs are used, each being swept once across the pudenda from anterior to posterior and then discarded.

In general, the catheter need only be inserted for half its length before the passage of urine confirms correct placement. The balloon is inflated and withdrawn until the balloon impacts in the bladder neck.

Suprapubic catheterization

This procedure is only appropriate when the bladder is distended and urethral catheterization has failed or is contraindicated. It is carried out with a full aseptic technique.

Procedure

The position of the bladder is determined by percussion. Where available, ultrasound guidance is of assistance. Generally the point of insertion lies two finger-breadths above the pubic symphysis in the midline.

The area is cleaned and draped. Local anaesthetic is then infiltrated through all layers of the anterior abdominal wall using an 18-gauge needle. The depth and position of the bladder can be gauged by the free aspiration of urine through this needle. The needle is withdrawn and a stab incision made in the skin. The trocar and catheter are advanced through the incision, into the bladder (Fig. 38.13). Entry into

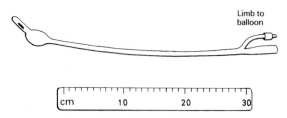

Fig. 38.11   Foley balloon catheter.

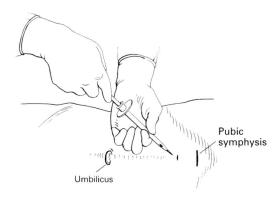

Fig. 38.13 **Suprapubic catheterization.**

the bladder is confirmed by the loss of resistance, at which point the catheter is advanced as the trocar is withdrawn. Free passage of urine confirms correct placement.

The catheter is now secured in place and a sterile dressing applied.

CENTRAL NERVOUS SYSTEM PROCEDURES

Lumbar puncture

Lumbar puncture is carried out to obtain a sample of cerebrospinal fluid (CSF) for diagnostic purposes, to measure the CSF pressure or to introduce materials into the CSF. It is important to examine the patient beforehand for evidence of raised intracranial pressure, examining in particular the fundi for evidence of papilloedema. Lumbar puncture in such patients may result in 'coning'. The advent of computerized tomography (CT) scanning has provided a non-invasive aid to the detection of raised intracranial pressure and in some conditions, such as subarachnoid haemorrhage, has removed the need for lumbar puncture.

Procedure

Lumbar puncture is carried out using a strict aseptic technique. The patient is placed on one side (usually left) with the back at the edge of the bed or trolley. The patient is then asked to curl up as much as possible to flex the lumbar spine and thus open up the interspinous spaces.

The skin is thoroughly cleaned and drapes applied. Then the space between the spinous pro-

cesses of the third and fourth lumbar vertebrae is identified by the point at which a vertical line dropped from the highest point of the iliac crest crosses the spine. Local anaesthetic is infiltrated into the skin and subcutaneous tissues to a depth of about 2 cm. A small stab incision is made in the midline, midway between the two spinous processes.

For most purposes a 22-gauge spinal needle is adequate. The needle is inserted through the stab incision and advanced in the midline in a slightly headward direction (see Ch. 9, Fig. 9.4). Entry into the subarachnoid space is felt with a distinct loss of resistance, and will occur in most adults at a depth of 4–6 cm from the skin.

The stylet is withdrawn from the needle and the position confirmed by the free flow of CSF. If the subarachnoid space is not entered, or bone is encountered, check that the needle has been advanced in the midline. This is best done by observing (from the side) the angle of the needle in relation to the patient's back. If the needle is in the midline, withdraw it and re-insert it in a slightly more headward direction. If the patient experiences pain, a nerve has been touched. The needle should be immediately withdrawn and repositioned.

Once the procedure is complete the needle is withdrawn and a sterile dressing applied. The patient is usually advised to remain supine for at least 12 hours to minimize the risk of developing a 'spinal' headache. Persistent headache may be a result of continued CSF leakage through the puncture in the dura. In these circumstances an anaesthetist should be asked to advise on an epidural 'blood patch'. With modern needles, the risk of CSF leakage is lessened, and the advice to remain supine for 24 hours may be unnecessary.

DRUG ADMINISTRATION

The importance of correct prescription and administration of drugs cannot be overemphasized. Drugs once administered can rarely be retrieved, particularly when they are administered intravenously or intramuscularly. Very few drugs have specific antagonists, with the important exceptions of opiates and benzodiazepines. It is good clinical practice to check drugs with an assistant, particularly where dilutions are involved. Important and useful sources of information include the manufacturer's data sheet, national formulae, hospital formulae and hospital pharmacy drug information services.

Practice points

- Use generic names wherever possible.
- Print generic and, if indicated, proprietary names clearly on the prescription card.
- Check that the correct drug is to be administered.
- Check the patient's identity, particularly if you do not know them.
- Label syringes clearly with the drug, concentration and the time and date drawn up.
- Check the compatibility of the diluent.

- Check calculations when diluting drugs or administering on a body weight basis.
- Check that the correct route of administration in the correct concentration is being used and that the time over which the drug should be given is correct.
- Carry out checks with an assistant.
- It is good practice to administer only drugs you have drawn up yourself and checked with an assistant, or drugs which have been prepared under conditions which you are satisfied will result in the patient receiving the correct therapy.

Section 11
MEDICO-LEGAL ISSUES

39

Medico-legal problems

CONTENTS

Consent to treatment

A doctor may not force recommendations on a patient. Treatment performed without consent may amount to assault and result in litigation. In every instance, the patient should be given as much information about proposed treatment as the doctor considers to be in his or her best interest. For minor procedures such as venepuncture verbal consent is adequate, but for operative procedures written consent must be obtained. The nature and purpose of the operation are explained to the patient by a doctor. The patient is then asked to sign a consent form which the doctor countersigns. For patients under the age of 16 years, informed written consent of the parent or guardian is obtained.

If immediate treatment is necessary to save the patient's life, verbal consent is acceptable. When the patient's condition does not allow even this, the proposed treatment should be discussed with a near relative. If none is readily available, the patient should be given such treatment as the doctor considers necessary to preserve life and health.

In the UK, if a patient is compulsorily detained under the Mental Health Act, treatment immediately necessary to preserve life and health may be given without consent. For all other procedures, the informed written consent of the patient should be obtained before an operation is performed. If the patient is unable or unwilling to give his consent to a non-urgent operation, it should not be performed. If this prohibition jeopardizes the patient's health, the surgeon and psychiatrist should act in good faith and in the best interests of the patient.

Patients with mental illness who are not compulsorily detained under the Mental Health Act have exactly the same rights as other patients.

Jehovah's Witnesses who consent to operation but refuse to consent to transfusion of blood or blood products place the surgeon in a dilemma. If the surgeon agrees to the limitations set by the patient, a conditional consent form prepared by one of the medical defence societies should be signed by the patient and countersigned by the surgeon and a witness.

The operation

Pre-operative examination

Every patient about to have an operation under general anaesthesia must be examined pre-operatively. The responsibility for this may rest with either the surgical staff or the anaesthetic staff. The declared policy of the individual surgical unit should be known to all staff working in it. The history should include a list of previous operations and previous anaesthetics (noting any untoward reactions to either), past history and a systematic enquiry including current drugs and known allergies. In addition to a full physical examination, urinalysis must always be performed. A full blood count and electrolyte estimation, chest X-ray and electrocardiogram (ECG) are prudent for all but the shortest examinations under anaesthetic. The decision as to whether a patient is fit for anaesthesia and the proposed operation rests with the anaesthetist and the surgeon in consultation.

Premedication

Ideally, the premedication should be ordered directly by the anaesthetist. In many instances, however, local policy dictates that the surgical staff prescribe the premedication. The anaesthetist should be consulted if there is any doubt about the drug or the dose to be given.

Safeguards against wrong operations

Performing a wrong operation or operating on the wrong patient is both avoidable and indefensible. A series of safeguards to prevent these disasters has been recommended by the medical defence societies.

- All patients should wear identity bracelets including forenames, surname and hospital number. This is checked when the patient is sent to theatre. In paediatric wards the identity bracelet is of the type which cannot be removed by the child.
- The operation list shows the patient's full name and hospital number. The nature of the operation is written in full, never abbreviated.
- Patients are sent for by name and number by the senior nurse in the operating theatre.
- The anaesthetist checks that the correct patient has been brought to the anaesthetic room.
- The surgeon sees the patient and reviews the case notes before anaesthesia is commenced.

The following safeguards are recommended to prevent an operation on the wrong side, limb or digit.

- The side to be operated on is marked by the surgeon with indelible ink before the patient comes to theatre.
- The words 'right' and 'left' are written in full in the patient's notes and on the operation list.
- To avoid ambiguity in describing digits, the fingers are described as thumb, index, middle, ring and little finger and the toes are described as great, second, third, fourth and little toe.

Discharge against medical advice

When a patient decides to discharge himself from hospital and the doctor feels that discharge is not in the best interest of the patient, the reasons for this advice are clearly explained. The patient is asked to sign a form which indicates that he is voluntarily taking his own discharge from hospital against the advice of his doctor. His signature on this form is witnessed by two persons. The general practitioner is informed about the patient's discharge from hospital, his condition and any further treatment which is considered advisable.

When the patient has a mental illness, the doctor may feel that there are grounds for compulsory detention under the Mental Health Act. The mental welfare officer is then contacted. If he agrees that detention under the Act is in the best interest of the patient or society, he will make application to the Court for formal admission to a mental hospital and compulsory detention.

Confirmation of death

It is the statutory duty of the doctor who has attended the deceased during his last illness to supply a death certificate to the Registrar of Deaths. Although a certificate may be issued if the body has not been seen after death, it is desirable that identification and examination are performed. The pupils are tested for reaction to light. The precordium is auscultated for heart sounds and the optic fundus is inspected with an ophthalmoscope for fragmentation of blood in the retinal vessels.

There are circumstances in which a death certificate should not be issued until the death has been reported to the coroner in England and Wales or the procurator-fiscal in Scotland. These include sudden death when the doctor has not seen the patient before or (in England and Wales) when a doctor has not attended the deceased within 14 days of death; death after trauma or neglect or in suspicious, unnatural or violent circumstances; death during an operation or before recovery from an anaesthetic; death within 24 hours of admission to hospital; and deaths about which complaints or litigation may be expected.

If the doctor is in any doubt about issuing a death certificate, he should discuss the matter first with the coroner or procurator-fiscal.

Cremation

Before a cremation may take place, two medical certificates are required: Forms B and C. Form B is completed by the usual medical attendant of the deceased or the doctor signing the death certificate. Form C is completed by a medical practitioner of at least five years' standing who is neither a relative of the deceased nor a partner of the doctor completing Form B. A fee is payable for each certificate.

Removal of tissues for transplantation

Under the Human Tissues Act of 1961, a registered doctor who is satisfied that life is extinct may remove the required organ for transplantation provided either the deceased has requested in writing or orally in front of two witnesses that his body be used for therapeutic purposes, medical education or research, or the person in possession of the body is satisfied that the deceased expressed no objection and the next of kin have no objection to removal of tissues for transplantation.

The increasing use of life-support systems to maintain respiratory function in patients with severe head injury or spontaneous intracerebral catastrophe has resulted in the definition of stringent criteria of 'brain death'. When these criteria have been confirmed independently by two senior doctors, withdrawal of the life-support system may be considered after discussion with the patient's next of kin. Members of transplant teams should not be involved in these decisions. If the relatives are favourably disposed towards tissue transplantation, organs may be removed before the life-support system is disconnected.

Clinical research

Clinical research presents moral and ethical problems rather than legal ones. Proposed research projects should be presented in detail to the Hospital Ethical Committee. Approval may be expected when the research project has a direct bearing on the illness for which the patient is being treated and does not involve additional invasive or painful investigations. Ethical criteria are stricter when the research project may contribute to the advancement of knowledge but is of no immediate benefit to the patient. Nevertheless, approval is usually given provided there is no unnecessary pain and no risk to the patient's health or well-being. If ethical doubt persists, the matter is referred to a medical defence society.

Informed verbal consent is always obtained from the patient and obtaining written consent is prudent in all but the simplest projects.

Laboratory requests and reports

Great care must be taken in labelling and completing all laboratory request forms and in labelling specimen containers. Inappropriate advice may result from incorrect information on the request forms, incorrect or insufficient samples, or by sending the request form for one patient with the specimen from another. The greatest potential hazard is in blood transfusion, where labelling errors may result in a fatal incompatible blood transfusion. Before blood transfusion is commenced, the patient's name, hospital number, date of birth, blood group and serial number on each unit of blood are checked, at the patient's bedside, on both the laboratory form and the blood bag label to ensure that they correspond. This is confirmed by a second observer.

Laboratory reports must be scrutinized and acted upon without undue delay, and individual surgical units must define policies to ensure that important information is not overlooked. Important outstanding reports may be available by telephone from laboratories at certain times and so permit earlier treatment of critically ill patients than would be possible by awaiting the 'routine' arrival of the written report. Such communications should be made directly to the ward doctor or written in a book specially kept for this purpose.

Confidentiality

The professional relationship between a doctor and his patient is based on the understanding that information which is given to the doctor in his professional capacity is confidential. There are, however, instances in which a breach of professional secrecy is justified. In Court, a doctor may be directed to divulge information. He may request that this information is disclosed in writing but, if this is overruled, failure to comply risks prosecution for contempt of court. Professional secrecy may also be breached when a doctor feels he has a duty to protect the patient or an innocent third party from avoidable harm. There are three common situations in which this problem arises.

1. *Fitness to drive a motor vehicle.* If, for example, a patient is subject to fainting or fits or to a lack of motor coordination which will impair his ability to drive safely, efforts should be made to persuade him to notify the licensing authority. The introduction of the driving licence valid until the 70th birthday has placed a great burden of responsibility on the driver to report any disability and an equal burden of responsibility on the doctor to persuade him to do so. If the patient does not agree to divulge the information himself, it is considered ethical for the doctor to disclose it to the licensing authority.

2. *Non-accidental injury to children.* When a doctor suspects he is dealing with non-accidental injury to a child, it is considered ethical to disclose confidential

information. Health authorities should be able to investigate actual or possible cases of non-accidental injury to children. If this service is not available, the children's officer of the local authority, or the officers of the National Society for the Prevention of Cruelty to Children, are appropriate persons to inform. The doctor should advise the parents that it is in the interests of the child to disclose clinical information to the appropriate authority and that it is preferable to do so with their agreement.

3. *Police investigation of a crime.* A doctor may be asked to divulge information given in confidence. Only if it clearly appears to be in the interests of public safety to do so, should the information be given. In doubtful cases, the prudent doctor will consult his Defence Society or hospital legal advisor.

In all other circumstances, requests for confidential information should be denied unless the patient has given informed written consent.

Notifiable diseases

All doctors must remember that certain diseases are by statute notifiable to health authorities. Those which may be encountered in surgical wards include dysentery, erysipilas, tuberculosis and infective enteritis.

All cases of diarrhoea of undetermined cause, of gas gangrene and clostridial wound infections, and of suspected serum hepatitis should be reported to the hospital infection officer without delay, as should any unusual 'runs' of wound or other infections in the ward.

At present, testing for human immunodeficiency virus (HIV) antibody can only be performed if the patient gives his informed consent.

The police

There are frequent occasions in surgical practice when the doctor comes into contact with the police. Even when the police are acting in the interests of the patient, information should only be disclosed with the consent of the patient. As has been stated previously, the doctor may be faced with difficult decisions when the police are investigating a crime allegedly committed by the patient. The duty of the doctor in possession of information which might assist the police in their pursuit of a criminal is not clear in law and must be left to individual conscience and judgement. In most circumstances the doctor will seek guidance from his Defence Society or hospital legal advisor before divulging to the police

any information received in professional confidence. However, when the nature of the crime is extreme or the potential dangers to society are great, the doctor may feel that these factors take precedence over the rules of professional secrecy.

When an inpatient is in police custody, it is usual for a police officer to remain with him during his stay in hospital. When there is no accompanying police officer, the police may request information about the time of discharge of the patient from hospital and this should be given. When a patient is brought to hospital after a road traffic accident, the question of driving under the influence of alcohol frequently arises. The police may request a blood sample for blood alcohol analysis. The doctor in charge should be satisfied that neither the request for the sample nor the actual taking of it will be prejudicial to the patient's condition. The sample should not be taken by the hospital staff but by a police surgeon. Blood taken by a hospital doctor from an unconscious patient as part of the routine admission investigations should not be made available to the police. If requested, it may be preserved in the hospital and released later if the patient or the legal representative consent.

Court appearance

Most doctors will at some time be required to appear in court. For the junior doctor this will usually be as a witness to fact if he/she has been involved in the care of the patient in the case. For the senior doctor it will usually be as an expert witness whose specialized knowledge is such that he/she is called solely to express an opinion.

Legible and comprehensive notes (see below) must be made when treating any patient, not just those whose case is likely to result in legal proceedings. They must be referred to before appearance so that a clear knowledge of the facts is available.

Divulgence of professional confidence in Court is discussed below.

Clinical records

The importance of accurate and legible clinical records in hospital practice cannot be overemphasized. Complaints against hospital doctors frequently allege that clinical examinations have been omitted or have been cursory. Claims that inappropriate treatment has been given are less common. Oral evidence to refute this is more likely to impress the court if it is backed up by a contemporary entry in the clinical notes. It should be remembered that in the event of a complaint against a doctor, a court may require the case records to be examined by the medical advisors of the complainant. Facetious or derogatory entries should never be made in case notes.

The Data Protection Act (1984) allows any patient access to data about him- or herself. If requested, a copy of the data and an interpretation must be provided. Exemptions to this access exist but have yet to be tested in Court.

Case notes remain the property of the Secretary of State but, as indicated above, there are occasions when a court may order compulsory disclosure of clinical notes. In such instances the applicant issues a summons to the doctor or hospital accompanied by written evidence to justify the application. The doctor or hospital may then request a hearing at which the arguments for and against the production of case notes are heard. If the court orders the production of the case notes, they are disclosed to the applicant's medical advisors only and not to his legal advisors or to the applicant himself. Whenever such applications are made, the doctor should seek advice from his Defence Society or hospital legal advisor immediately.

Professional negligence

Negligence may be defined as a failure to display the competence and to exercise the care which might reasonably be expected of the doctor and which results in damage to the patient. Two common examples which affect junior hospital doctors are prescribing an antibiotic for a patient who is known to be hypersensitive to it and failing to X-ray a patient in whom there is clinical doubt about bone injury. More obvious examples of negligence are operation on the wrong patient, limb or digit.

When a letter of complaint is received from a patient or his lawyer, the case notes should be carefully perused and a factual report about the case made. Copies are sent first to the doctor's defence society and to the hospital legal advisor. A further copy is retained by the doctor. All correspondence including the letters of complaint, threats of proceedings or claims for compensation are forwarded to the Defence Society or hospital legal advisor. If the incident involved an instrument, needle, swab or foreign body, this should be retained where possible.

Index